THE BIOLOGY OF
DISEASE VECTORS

THE BIOLOGY OF DISEASE VECTORS

Edited by

Barry J. Beaty and
William C. Marquardt

UNIVERSITY PRESS OF COLORADO

Published by the University Press of Colorado
P. O. Box 849
Niwot, Colorado 80544
(303) 530-5337

The University Press of Colorado is a cooperative publishing enterprise supported, in part, by Adams State College, Colorado State University, Fort Lewis College, Mesa State College, Metropolitan State College of Denver, University of Colorado, University of Northern Colorado, University of Southern Colorado, and Western State College of Colorado.

Library of Congress Cataloging-in-Publication Data
The biology of disease vectors / edited by Barry J. Beaty and William
    C. Marquardt.
        p.   cm.
    Includes bibliographical references and index.
    ISBN 0-87081-411-7 (alk. paper)
    1. Insects as carriers of disease.   2. Insects—Molecular aspects.
  I. Beaty, Barry J.   II. Marquardt, William C.
  RA639.5.B56 1996
  614.4'32—dc20   95-32509
                                              CIP

This book was set in Adobe Caslon and Adobe Gill Sans.

Cover photo: A female *Aedes triseriatus* mosquito. Photograph by Dr. Stephen Higgs.

The paper used in this publication meets the minimum requirements of the American National Standard for Information Sciences—Permanence of Paper for Printed Library Materials. ANSI Z39.48–1948
∞

10   9   8   7   6   5   4   3   2   1

CONTENTS

CONTRIBUTORS

Barry J. Beaty, Ph.D.
Department of Microbiology and Arthropod-Borne
and Infectious Diseases Laboratory
Colorado State University
Fort Collins, Colorado 80523 USA

Norbert Becker, Ph.D.
Director, KABS
Europlatz 5
6700 Ludwigshofer am Rhein, Germany

William C. Black IV, Ph.D.
Department of Microbiology and Arthropod-Borne
and Infectious Diseases Laboratory
Colorado State University
Fort Collins, Colorado 80523 USA

Susan E. Brown, Ph.D.
Department of Entomology
Colorado State University
Fort Collins, Colorado 80523 USA

Jonathan O. Carlson, Ph.D.
Department of Microbiology and Arthropod-Borne
and Infectious Diseases Laboratory
Colorado State University
Fort Collins, Colorado 80523 USA

Bruce M. Christensen, Ph.D.
Department of Animal Health and
Biomedical Sciences
University of Wisconsin
Madison, Wisconsin 53706-1581 USA

Frank H. Collins, Ph.D.
Division of Parasitic Diseases
Centers for Disease Control, DHHS
4770 Buford Hwy.
Chamblee, Georgia 30341 USA

E.W. Cupp, Ph.D.
Department of Veterinary Science
University of Arizona
Tucson, Arizona 85721 USA

Elizabeth W. Davidson, Ph.D.
Department of Zoology
Arizona State University
Tempe, Arizona 85787-1501 USA

Anne Marie Fallon, Ph.D.
Department of Entomology
219 Hodson Hall
University of Minnesota
St. Paul, Minnesota 55108-6125 USA

James A. Ferrari, Ph.D.
Department of Biology
California State University
San Bernardino, California 92407 USA

Kenneth L. Gage, Ph.D.
Division of Vector-Borne Infectious Diseases
Centers for Disease Control, DHHS
Fort Collins, Colorado 80523 USA

Scott W. Gordon, Ph.D.
Department of Microbiology
Colorado State University
Fort Collins, Colorado 80523 USA

Hilda Guzman, M.S.
Center for Tropical Diseases
Department of Pathology
University of Texas Medical Branch
Galveston, TX 77555-0605 USA

Robert W. Gwadz, Ph.D.
Laboratory of Malaria Research
National Institutes of Health, DHHS
Bethesda, Maryland 20892 USA

Henry H. Hagedorn, Ph.D.
Department of Entomology
University of Arizona
Tucson, Arizona 85721 USA

Miranda C. van Heusden, Ph.D.
Department of Biochemistry
University of Arizona
Tucson, Arizona 85721 USA

Stephen Higgs, Ph.D.
Department of Microbiology and Arthropod-Borne
and Infectious Diseases Laboratory
Colorado State University
Fort Collins, Colorado 80523 USA

Frederick R. Holbrook, Ph.D.
Arthropod-Borne Animal Diseases Research Laboratory
Agricultural Research Service, USDA
Laramie, Wyoming 82071 USA

Anthony A. James, Ph.D.
Department of Molecular Biology and Biochemistry
University of California
Irvine, California 92717 USA

Marc J. Klowden, Ph.D.
Division of Entomology
University of Idaho
Moscow, Idaho 83843 USA

Marcelo Jacobs-Lorena, Ph.D.
Department of Genetics
Case Western Reserve University
Cleveland, Ohio 44106 USA

Fotic C. Kafatos, Ph.D.
European Molecular Biology Laboratory
Meyerhofstrasse 1, D-69117
Heidelberg, Germany

Dennis L. Knudson, Ph.D.
Department of Entomology and Arthropod-Borne
and Infectious Diseases Laboratory
Colorado State University
Fort Collins, Colorado 80523 USA

William C. Marquardt, Ph.D.
Department of Biology and Arthropod-Borne and
Infectious Diseases Laboratory
Colorado State University
Fort Collins, Colorado 80523 USA

Barry R. Miller, Ph.D.
Division of Vector-Borne Infectious Diseases
Centers for Disease Control, DHHS
Fort Collins, Colorado 80523 USA

Carl J. Mitchell, Ph.D.
Division of Vector-Borne Infectious Diseases
Centers for Disease Control, DHHS
Fort Collins, Colorado 80523 USA

Chester (Chet) G. Moore, Ph.D.
Division of Vector-Borne Infectious Diseases
Centers for Disease Control, DHHS
Fort Collins, Colorado 80523 USA

Leonard E. Munstermann, Ph.D.
Yale University School of Medicine
New Haven, Connecticut 06510 USA

Roger S. Nasci, Ph.D.
Division of Vector-Borne Infectious Diseases
Centers for Disease Control, DHHS
Fort Collins, Colorado 80523 USA

Maung Maung Oo, Ph.D.
Department of Genetics
Case Western Reserve University
Cleveland, Ohio 44106 USA

Susan Palchick, Ph.D.
Metropolitan Mosquito Control District
2099 University West
St. Paul, Minnesota 55104-3431 USA

Susan M. Paskewitz, Ph.D.
Department of Entomology
University of Wisconsin
Madison, Wisconsin 53706 USA

Joseph Piesman, Ph.D.
Division of Vector-Borne Infectious Diseases
Centers for Disease Control, DHHS
Fort Collins, Colorado 80523 USA

Karamjit S. Rai, Ph.D.
Department of Biology
University of Notre Dame
Notre Dame, Indiana 46556 USA

José M.C. Ribeiro, Ph.D.
Department of Entomology
University of Arizona
Tucson, Arizona 85721 USA

William S. Romoser, Ph.D.
Department of Zoological and Biomedical Sciences
Ohio University
Athens, Ohio 45701 USA

Kenneth R. Stark, B.S.
Department of Molecular Biology and Biochemistry
University of California
Irvine, California 92717 USA

Walter J. Tabachnick, Ph.D.
Arthropod-Borne Animal Diseases Research
Laboratory
Agricultural Research Service, USDA
Laramie, Wyoming 82071 USA

Robert B. Tesh, M.D.
Center for Tropical Diseases
Department of Pathology
University of Texas Medical Branch
Galveston, TX 77555-0605 USA

Rex E. Thomas, Ph.D.
Paravax, Inc.
1825 Sharp Point Dr.
Fort Collins, Colorado 80526 USA

Stephen K. Wikel, Ph.D.
Department of Entomology
Okahoma State University
Stillwater, Oklahoma 74708 USA

Jennifer L. Woodring, Ph.D.
Arthropod-Borne and Infectious Diseases
Laboratory
Colorado State University
Fort Collins, Colorado 80523

Liangbiao Zheng, Ph.D.
European Molecular Biology Laboratory
Meyerhofstrasse 1, D-69117
Heidelberg, Germany

Rolf Ziegler, Ph.D.
Department of Biochemistry
University of Arizona
Tucson, Arizona 85721

PREFACE

The 19th and early 20th centuries were exciting times in investigations on transmissible diseases. Pasteur, Koch, Bruce, Grassi, Schaudinn, Ross, and scores of other individuals found and described many microbial and eukaryotic disease agents. Organisms were cultivated from diseased humans and animals, vaccines were developed, and immunity was studied for use in diagnosis and prevention of disease. Koch's postulates were promulgated and used to prove that various microorganisms were the causes of diseases.

As it became clear what kinds of agents decimated both human and animal health, effective control techniques were instituted by newly established public health entities. Water treatment and sewage treatment improved. Quarantine was practiced to prevent the spread of diseases that were transmitted directly from one person to another. Vaccination for smallpox, typhoid fever, and diphtheria reduced both morbidity and mortality. Antibiotics and other chemotherapeutic agents improved so that many serious diseases seemed to be a thing of the past. By the mid-1950s effective vaccines all but eliminated such childhood scourges as poliomyelitis. Smallpox was globally eradicated in 1977. Many predicted that infectious diseases had been conquered.

Despite these successes, failures lurked in the background. The dark shadow was cast by many vector-borne diseases, which had complex epidemiologies and reservoirs in various animals other than humans, and flared up unpredictably. The vector-borne agents included the whole spectrum of infectious agents: viruses, rickettsia, bacteria, protists, and helminths. Except for the blood flukes (*Schistosoma* spp.), most of the disease agents were found to be transmitted by arthropods: lice, bugs, mosquitoes, black flies, midges, sand flies, ticks, and mites.

The disease agents were studied and their life cycles were described. The vectors were classified, raised in the laboratory, and their intimate habits probed. Nevertheless, malaria, dengue, trypanosomiasis, filariasis, and the viral encephalitides simmered and surged periodically. Vaccines were developed for some, such as yellow fever. Drugs were developed for malaria and trypanosomiasis, among others. Source reduction for control of insect vectors was effective when continual effort could be given to maintaining the system, but outbreaks persisted.

A turning point came in the late 1930s with the development of DDT. An effective, broad spectrum, persistent insecticide, it had all of the qualities that a good insecticide was thought to have. DDT aborted a typhus outbreak in North Africa and Italy in WWII. It controlled mosquitoes and thus could control mosquito-borne diseases. In the 1950s investigators thought that malaria could be eradicated by killing mosquitoes with DDT and by administering chloroquine to humans to prevent and treat cases. Good insecticides, good drugs, and a concerted campaign meant that success was at hand. But it was not to be, and we are now resigned to containing malaria and keeping its depredations at an acceptable level.

Wherein lay the problem in eradicating malaria? Part of it was economics and politics; as soon as eradication was imminent, other diseases gained priority and money was shifted elsewhere. Evolution also intervened as the mosquitoes developed resistance to insecticides and the malaria organisms became resistant to chloroquine.

In other vector-borne diseases, reservoirs maintained disease agents in the wild, and the agents essentially disappeared between outbreaks in the human population. Plague would break out in rodents and then disappear, perhaps after causing some human infections and deaths. Typhus would become epidemic in difficult times, disappear, and then reappear to visit another disaster on humanity. Dengue waxed and waned and then spread from the Pacific Rim throughout the tropical world. New diseases, such as the tick-borne Lyme disease, emerged.

By the 1980s it became clear that the campaigns against various vector-borne diseases were at a stalemate at best. The long-term support of vector-borne disease research by institutions such as the Rockefeller Foundation, the Walter Reed Army Institute of Research, the U.S. Army Medical Research Institute of Infectious Diseases, and the National Institutes of Health in the United States and other institutions in many parts of the world laid the groundwork for a shift in emphasis in research involving vector-borne diseases. New molecular techniques, genetic cloning, genomic mapping, and the ability to transform organisms permitted identifying and expressing genes in ways that would not have been believed a few years earlier. A molecular biological revolution was under way in laboratories across the globe.

In the early 1980s the John D. and Catherine T. MacArthur Foundation initiated and supported a program to increase knowledge at the molecular level of the main parasitic diseases of humans: malaria, trypanosomiasis, leishmaniasis, and filariasis. The result was an influx of investigators with expertise in immunology, biochemistry, and molecular biology who focused on these disease agents. A new cadre of individuals was recruited into parasitology.

In 1989 a similar program was initiated by the MacArthur Foundation; the Network on the Biology of Parasite Vectors was formed. Eight academic and research institutions were joined in the network. One component of the program involved training a new generation of vector biologists. To help accomplish this, an annual course called the Biology of Disease Vectors was initiated. The first effort was undertaken at Colorado State University in June 1990. The course

was subsequently offered at Colorado State University through 1993 and at the Institute of Molecular Biology and Biotechnology in Crete in 1994.

The objectives of the course have been to introduce molecular biologists to medical entomology, to give experience to medical entomologists in molecular concepts and methods, and to develop a worldwide network of vector biologists. As the instructors and organizers gained experience, it became clear that the course was unique and that much of the information presented would be valuable to those who could not attend. Thus, in 1992, the decision was made to publish a multiauthor textbook based on the course, *The Biology of Disease Vectors*. The volume follows much the same pattern of exposition as the lecture portion of the course but has been considerably expanded. It includes: basic knowledge of arthropods of medical and veterinary importance; epidemiology, development, physiology, feeding, and metabolism, especially as they pertain to vectors; population biology and genetics; and methods of surveillance and control. In each chapter the emphasis has been on cutting-edge molecular biological approaches that illuminate the difficult problems facing vector biologists. Because of the nature of the material covered, this book complements rather than replaces other medical entomology textbooks, for example, *Medical Insects and Arachnids* by Lane and Grosskey (Chapman and Hall, New York, 1993) and *Medical and Veterinary Entomology* by Kettle (C.A.B. International, Wallingford, U.K., 1990). *Entomology in Human and Animal Health* by Harwood and James (Macmillan Publishing Co., N.Y., 1979) is no longer in print.

The contributors are drawn mostly from the faculty of the course and the MacArthur network, but a number of other investigators agreed to contribute chapters. Because it is so directly connected to the course, the organization of the text and the chapters are different from other medical entomology texts. Contributors were given considerable latitude in selecting and organizing the information presented in their respective chapters. Some contributors presented their information in conventional textbook form with minimal referencing; others chose to present their material more in the form of a review article. We are indebted to them all for providing their expertise and for completing their chapters in a timely fashion. We are also indebted to the MacArthur Foundation and to Dr. Denis Prager for support of this effort.

When we began editing this volume, we hoped to produce a landmark textbook in vector biology. We have tapped the talents of 45 investigators and leaders in vector biology (s.l.), and their chapters provide state-of-the-art introductions into their respective areas of research. The contributors all have active research programs, and it was only through a labor of love that they took their time to produce readable, current summaries of knowledge. As editors, we thank them for their efforts, and we hope that we have achieved our objectives.

Because of the support of the MacArthur Foundation for the Network on the Biology of Parasite Vectors, research and educational opportunities are influencing vector biology. More than 150 students from all over the world have attended the 2-week course. Their total immersion in the subject has introduced them to a number of areas of vector biology. They have also made friends and colleagues that, we hope, will last a lifetime. The network is established, the techniques are at hand, and the individuals have been trained by experts in the field. We expect and anticipate great things from both students and faculty who have participated in the disease vectors course.

Perhaps we are on the edge of what will become known as a new golden age of medical entomology. Let us hope that is true.

Barry J. Beaty
William C. Marquardt

1. INTRODUCTION TO ARTHROPODS AND VECTORS

William C. Marquardt

INTRODUCTION

The history of the control of transmissible diseases is a grand tapestry of successes that have given us longer and more secure lives. Conquests of livestock diseases have improved the quality of our lives through safer and more efficient systems of food and fiber production. Early scientific investigators working with diseases contended not only with superstitions about the causes of diseases but with inadequate methods for determining possible disease agents.

It is remarkable that even before the germ theory of disease was established in the latter half of the 19th century, Edward Jenner (1749–1823) developed an immunizing agent for smallpox. In certain areas of Britain it had been observed that smallpox and cowpox seldom occurred together. In 1796 Jenner inoculated a boy with cowpox from the hands of a milkmaid and two months later exposed him to material from a smallpox patient. The boy was protected. Despite this and further successes, battles raged in Europe and in North America concerning Jenner's method of preventing smallpox. Deaths had occurred following vaccination, and it was therefore considered by some to be too unpredictable.

As knowledge of infectious agents developed, Louis Pasteur in France and Robert Koch in Germany isolated and identified various bacterial agents that cause disease in humans, domestic animals, and silkworms. They, and others, firmly established the germ theory of

disease and laid the groundwork for immunization, quarantine, chemotherapy, and sanitary disposal of human waste, which have greatly reduced the effects of bacterial diseases.

Koch's Postulates were developed to properly associate and identify disease agents with disease entities. The four steps promulgated were (1) the agent must be isolated from a host exhibiting the disease, (2) the organism must be grown in pure culture, (3) the organism must be reintroduced into another uninfected host and cause the disease, and (4) the organism must be isolated anew in pure culture. Such rigor was crucial to advancing knowledge of infectious diseases.

Early studies on bacterial and parasitic diseases focused on diseases transmitted directly from one host to another. However, other means of transmission soon became apparent. As early as 1848, Joseph Nott first proposed that yellow fever and malaria were transmitted by mosquitoes. At about the same time, the life cycles of tapeworms were being studied and shown to have more than a single host. It is generally considered that Sir Patrick Manson's studies on elephantiasis caused by the roundworm *Wuchereria bancrofti* were crucial in opening the minds of disease investigators to arthropod vectors. In 1878 Manson showed that the mosquito *Culex quinquefasciatus* transmitted this roundworm to humans. Again, a crucial observation guided future generations of investigators.

Toward the end of the 19th century, scientists discovered a number of vector-borne diseases were found to be transmitted by arthropods. In 1893 Smith and Kilbourne discovered that the causative agent of Texas cattle fever was transmitted by the cattle tick *Boophilus annulatus*. In 1897 Sir Ronald Ross showed that malaria was transmitted by mosquitoes. In 1881 Carlos Finlay postulated that yellow fever was transmitted by mosquitoes, and Walter Reed and his coworkers proved it in the field in 1901.

One hundred years after these epochal discoveries, we have means of controlling many diseases that are transmitted directly from one person or animal to another. Good water and sewage treatment prevent many fecally transmitted diseases. Immunization prevents transmission of diphtheria, typhoid fever, measles, poliomyelitis, and other bacterial and viral diseases. Smallpox was eradicated in the late 1970s—possibly the only instance in which humans have purposely caused the extinction of an organism.

Despite these enormous strides, controlling disease agents transmitted by arthropod and molluscan vectors has proven to be difficult. Diseases predicted to be eradicated in short order, such as malaria and schistosomiasis, are not only still with us but increase in incidence each year. The viral disease dengue, or breakbone fever, affects millions of individuals annually in the Caribbean and Southeast Asia; dengue hemorrhagic fever and dengue shock syndrome result in thousands of deaths as well.

Scientists once believed it possible to eliminate malaria, but each year it still affects more than 200 million persons and causes at least 2 million deaths. Biological and human factors have caused a resurgence of the disease. The mosquitoes that vector malaria have become resistant to insecticides, the causative agent has become resistant to antimalarial drugs, and efforts at control or eradication have given way to economic and political realities.

Various mosquito-borne encephalitides, such as Saint Louis encephalitis (SLE), western equine encephalitis (WEE), eastern equine encephalitis (EEE), and California encephalitis (CE), circulate in wild birds and small wild mammals. On occasion, a virus can enter human and domestic animal populations

and result in a serious outbreak of disease. Such a disease complex is referred to as a zoonosis, or a disease transmitted between humans and other animals. We have considerable information about the epidemiologies of these encephalitides; however, we are often incapable of predicting when outbreaks may occur in humans and have only rudimentary tools available to stop transmission once an outbreak has begun.

Transmission of yellow fever virus by mosquitoes was demonstrated in the early 20th century and is one of the truly historic and heroic events in the development of our knowledge of vector-borne diseases of humans. In 1881 Carlos Finlay in Cuba postulated that the virus was transmitted by mosquitoes. When the Panama Canal was begun in 1879, yellow fever and malaria essentially shut down the French and subsequent U.S. attempts to complete the project.

The Yellow Fever Commission was established in 1900 under the direction of Major Walter Reed. Army volunteers and members of the commission carried out a number of experiments to determine the mode of transmission for yellow fever. Transmission was shown to take place only through the bite of a mosquito, *Aedes aegypti*, not by contact with infected individuals, their clothing, or contaminated water. *Ae. aegypti* was found to be a container breeder common in and around houses. This knowledge allowed the mosquito population to be controlled by source reduction (see Chap. 28). The discovery not only enabled completion of the Panama Canal in 1914 but also improved the quality of life for many tropical areas. The periodic outbreaks of yellow fever that occurred in temperate seaports could then be controlled, because it was known that outbreaks occurred when mosquitoes were taken north in sailing ships. Effective vaccines were later developed that further reduced the risk of infection.

But yellow fever has not gone away. It periodically breaks out in West African countries such as Nigeria, and thousands of deaths often occur. In another epidemiological pattern in South America, the virus circulates among small primates high in the rain forest canopy, and humans become infected when trees are cut to build roads and petroleum pipelines. The mosquitoes end up on the forest floor and can transmit the virus to humans. This epidemiological pattern is referred to as jungle yellow fever.

Attempts to eradicate *Ae. aegypti* in North America have been unsuccessful. In the early 1960s a campaign was undertaken to eradicate *Ae. aegypti* from the United States. It was almost successful, but *almost* is not enough. The campaign was abandoned, and the yellow fever mosquito has resurged in the southern United States and throughout all of the American tropics.

Lest it be thought that attempting control is fruitless, levels of control have been achieved that allow us to live in relative security from some vector-borne diseases and for livestock to be raised in areas that were formerly extremely hazardous. An example of control of a vector-borne disease of livestock is the conquest of Texas cattle fever (red water fever, splenic fever, babesiosis), which was a scourge of cattle in areas of the southern and southwestern United States during the 19th century. Smith and Kilbourne determined that the causative agent was transmitted by the tick *Boophilus annulatus*. Studies showed that the tick had a limited host range; that it usually spent its life cycle on one animal; that it could not survive a winter with significant frost; and that the agent, *Babesia bigemina*, a protistan, was transmitted from one generation of ticks to the next through the egg, transovarial transmission.

At first, control and eradication programs were based on tick control, quarantine of cattle, and leaving pastures vacant until the ticks died. No cattle were shipped out of an infected area until they had been inspected and declared to be free of ticks; cattle entering the United States from Mexico were also inspected and treated for ticks. Eradication efforts were begun in the first decade of the 20th century and were completed about 25 years later in the early 1930s. This is another success story that is a tribute to investigators who laid the groundwork in the field and the veterinarians in disease control who kept their objective firmly in mind for three decades.

Other successes include vaccines that protect livestock from some mosquito-borne viral diseases such as WEE and, as previously mentioned, the control of malaria, which has been all but eradicated in the United States.

Most of the techniques used for controlling and eradicating vector-borne diseases were developed during the early 20th century. Source reduction, insecticides, biological control, vaccination, chemotherapy, and personal protection were all laid out, in principal, nearly a century ago. Many are still effective; others succeeded initially but failed later for a variety of reasons. Investigators must now incorporate new approaches that will allow them to move to the next level of control to alleviate the effects of vector-borne diseases on human and animal health.

ARTHROPODS

This section provides fundamental information about arthropods in general and insects and acarines in particular. It serves as a basis for much of the information in the following chapters on the physiology and molecular biology of specific groups of vectors. Appendix 1 describes zoological classification and provides some details on binomial nomenclature.

Members of the phylum Arthropoda are defined as being bilaterally symmetrical, with an exoskeleton of chitin and jointed legs. They are metameric, i.e., the body exhibits true segmentation in which there is replication of body parts such as muscles and nerve ganglia. Arthropods show tagmatosis, a phenomenon in which segments of the body are modified and grouped together to form mouthparts and body regions such as the thorax of insects. Growth is achieved through a series of molts; the exoskeleton is shed, and the new skeleton underneath expands and hardens. The digestive tract is complete, i.e., the organisms have a mouth, a tubular digestive tract, and an anus. The nervous system is ventral and typically has a series of ganglia that are related to the body segments. The body cavity is a hemocoel: blood is pumped from the heart through a series of blood vessels that eventually empty into the body cavity. The circulatory system is termed "open." because the blood is not contained within vessels. Reproduction is sexual but takes a number of forms.

Familiar members of the phylum are lobsters, crabs, shrimp, centipedes, millipedes, daddy longlegs, insects, ticks and mites, and spiders. (Fig. 1.1). This heterogeneous grouping consists of more than 1 million species and is the largest phylum of the animal kingdom. The

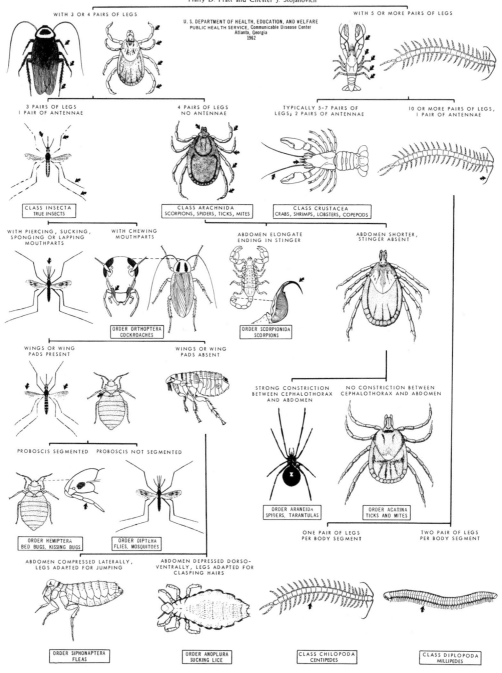

PICTORIAL KEY TO MAJOR CLASSES AND ORDERS OF ADULT ARTHROPODS OF PUBLIC HEALTH IMPORTANCE

Harry D. Pratt and Chester J. Stojanovich

1.1 Representatives of the major groups of arthropods

phylum is so large that this book is limited to the relatively few arthropods that serve as vectors of parasitic agents.

The heterogeneity of the phylum Arthropoda is significant for two reasons. First, four probably phylogenetically distinct groups have been placed in the phylum. Members of a phylum typically descend from a single, primitive ancestor at some earlier geologic time. Because there are four ancestors in the phylum Arthropoda, it is a somewhat artificial grouping. Second, because the taxon is polyphyletic, generalizations about members of the phylum must be stated with care. For example, all arthropods grow by passing through a series of molts in which the exoskeleton is shed, a new skeleton is formed, and significant growth takes place while the new exoskeleton is still soft. While this pattern is common in the phylum, the control of growth and molting as well as the body forms are entirely different between, say, the crustacea and the insects.

Insects

These interesting and lovely creatures form the most successful group among all animals when the number of species and the niches they have occupied in the biotic world are considered. If any group of animals deserves the title of being ubiquitous, the insects do. There can be as many as a million species, and they are found everywhere.

We tend to think of the insects as being noxious or harmful animals, but that is hardly the case. The greatest proportion of them do not adversely affect human welfare; in fact, most insects are probably beneficial. They pollinate economically important plants, control certain harmful insects, and provide food for both fish and birds.

Of course, many harmful insects do exist. They can harm crops, serve as vectors of disease agents, or simply be pests. We should view them dispassionately, however. First, a moral judgment on their activities is not fair; they simply have moved into available ecological niches, and they do what comes naturally—feed and reproduce. If they harm crops when feeding, it is often because human cropping methods have promoted monoculture and have allowed the explosion of

populations of insects that feed on that plant. If they transmit infectious agents while feeding on blood, that is merely incidental to the insect's having discovered blood as a rich source of protein and other nutritious elements.

This book is concerned with insects that serve as vectors of disease agents, but we must also view them as parasites in their own right. Parasitism can be defined as a relationship between two different species in which the smaller (parasite) is physiologically dependent upon the larger (host), the prevalence of the parasites and the intensity of infection in the host population are overdispersed or nonrandom, and the parasite species has a higher reproductive potential than the host species.

Parasitism among insects has taken many forms and occurs in adults and preadults. Some investigators refer to bloodsucking insects such as mosquitoes or black flies as micropredators. However, according to the usual definition of parasitism, mosquitoes and other bloodsucking dipterans are well-defined parasites. Likewise, many insects, particularly Diptera, are parasitic as larvae. Various families of flies have larval forms that are parasitic in vertebrate hosts. Cattle grubs, for example, have larvae that make 9-month-long migrations in the bodies of cattle and each spring drop out of the skin to pupate in the ground. The adults emerge when the weather warms up, and they live only to copulate and lay eggs for the next generation. The adults have vestigial mouthparts and survive on the reserve food provided by the larvae.

In addition to their arthropod characteristics, insects have 3 distinct body regions: head, thorax, and abdomen (see tagmatosis in the previous section) (Fig. 1.2). They have a single pair of antennae located on the head, eyes are both simple and compound, and both may be present in any one species. Each of the 3 pairs of legs on the thorax emerges from a different section of the thorax (pro-, meso-, and metathorax). The parts of the legs, starting proximally, are the coxa, trochanter, femur, tibia (-iae), and tarsus (-i). Wings are found in adult insects, but they can be lost secondarily, as in fleas. Wings, which are primitive extensions of the exoskeleton, are located on meso- and metathorax segments. Mouthparts are fundamentally the same in all insects

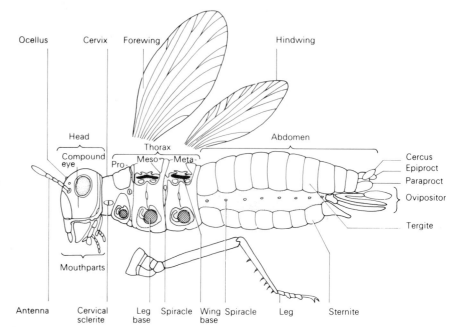

1.2 The external anatomy of a generalized insect. From William S. Romoser and John G. Stoffolano, Jr. *The Science of Entomology.* Copyright © 1994 Wm. C. Brown Communications, Inc., Dubuque Iowa. All rights reserved. Reprinted by permission.

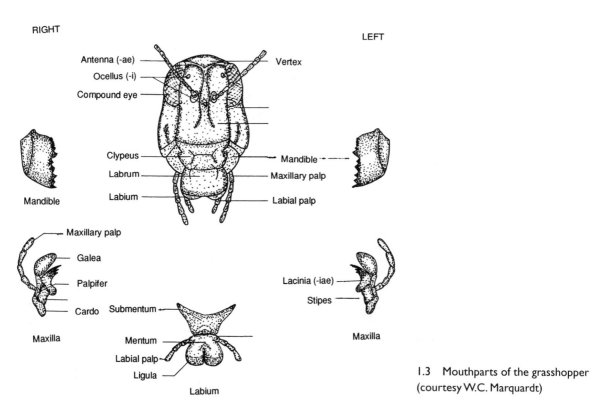

1.3 Mouthparts of the grasshopper (courtesy W.C. Marquardt)

(Fig. 1.3), but they are highly modified for various types of food, including blood and tissue (see the following section). The respiratory system consists of a tracheal system that ramifies and extends throughout the body of the insect (Fig. 1.4). Most often there are separate sexes (Fig. 1.5). Growth and molting are controlled by hormones (see Chap. 17).

Classification

Classification of the members of the class Insecta is based on (1) the type of metamorphosis exhibited by the insect; (2) wings (number, type, and venation); (3) mouthparts; (4) proportions of the major body parts, e.g., large head or constriction between the thorax and abdomen; and (5) setation, or hairs, on various parts of the body.

Metamorphosis. The importance of the pattern of development or type of metamorphosis is difficult to overstate (Fig. 1.8). It underlies food habits, relation to the host, and means of control. Just below the level of Class is the level Series. Three patterns of development exist for insects.

1. Ametabola. Early instars are indistinguishable from the later ones except that the organism grows slightly larger with each molt. Examples are the orders Thysanoptera and Protura. These organisms are of no importance in medical entomology.

2. Hemimetabola. A gradual change occurs from early instars until the final one in which sexual maturity is reached and the wings (when present) become functional. Body proportions change with each molt, and the wing buds appear some time before the final molt. This series is also referred to as the Exopterygotoa because the wings develop externally.

The best-known example of a hemimetabolic insect is the grasshopper (Fig. 1.8). The 1st instar nymph emerges from the egg in early spring. It feeds and molts through the summer, and by the 4th instar nymph, small wingpads extending from the thorax are evident. The final molt produces a winged, sexually mature adult.

Included in Hemimetabola are the orders Ephemeroptera (mayflies), Hemiptera (bugs and kissing bugs), Mallophaga (biting or bird lice), Anoplura (sucking lice), Blattaria (cockroaches), and Dermaptera (earwigs).

3. Holometabola. A striking change occurs in the final larval instar before the adult stage when reorganization of the body takes place in the pupa. The egg hatches to release a larva that feeds and grows through a series of molts until the final larval stage. The organism then forms a pupa in which complete reorganization of the body takes place. After a period of time, the winged, sexually mature adult emerges.

The best-known example of a holometabolic insect is a butterfly (Fig. 1.8). The egg hatches to release a tiny caterpillar that feeds and molts several times. In some species, larval development can require only a week or 2; in others, such as the *Manduca sexta* (tobacco hornworm), larval growth can take place through most of the summer. At the end of larval development, the organism spins a cocoon and undergoes reorganization within it. At least 2 weeks are typically required for development in the pupa to take place. Then the adult winged butterfly or moth emerges.

Included in this series are many insects of medical and veterinary importance such as Diptera (mosquitoes, biting midges, sand flies, horse flies), Siphonaptera (fleas), Hymenoptera (bees, wasps, ants), and Coleoptera (beetles).

Wings. Most ordinal names of insects refer in some way to the wings. Orthoptera (grasshopper, cricket, praying mantis) have two pairs of straight wings, and Neuroptera (lacewings) have wings with an extensive network of tiny veins. The Diptera (flies, mosquitoes) have only two wings; the second set is reduced to a pair of knoblike structures, halteres, that are used for balance. The Siphonaptera (fleas) have sucking mouthparts (*siphon-*) and lack wings (*-aptera*). The numbers of pairs of wings (0, 1, 2) and their structure are important in classification. The primitive insect wing has many veins whereas reduced wing venation occurs in more advanced insects such as Diptera and Lepidoptera. Terminology for wing venation varies somewhat with order of insect, and the ability to identify an insect by its wings is important.

Mouthparts. Feeding structures in insects take many forms. Tagmatosis has occurred in the formation

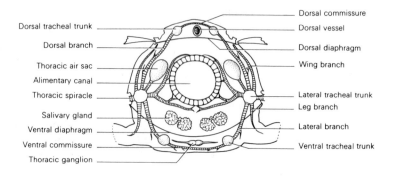

A

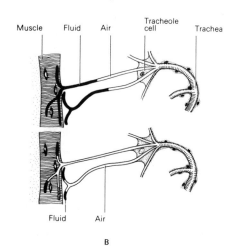

B

1.4 Tracheal system of an insect. From William S. Romoser and John G. Stoffolano, Jr. *The Science of Entomology.* Copyright © 1994 Wm. C. Brown Communications, Inc., Dubuque Iowa. All rights reserved. Reprinted by permission.

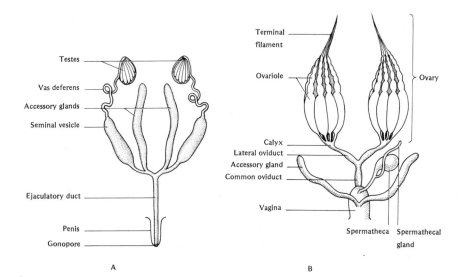

1.5 Female (A) and male (B) reproductive systems of an insect. From William S. Romoser and John G. Stoffolano, Jr. *The Science of Entomology.* Copyright © 1994 Wm. C. Brown Communications, Inc., Dubuque Iowa. All rights reserved. Reprinted by permission.

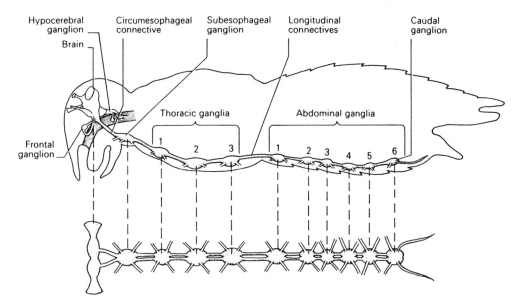

Figure labels (top):
Hypocerebral ganglion · Circumesophageal connective · Subesophageal ganglion · Longitudinal connectives · Caudal ganglion · Brain · Frontal ganglion · Thoracic ganglia (1, 2, 3) · Abdominal ganglia (1, 2, 3, 4, 5, 6)

1.6   Nervous sytem of a generalized insect. From William S. Romoser and John G. Stoffolano, Jr. *The Science of Entomology.* Copyright © 1994 Wm. C. Brown Communications, Inc., Dubuque Iowa. All rights reserved. Reprinted by permission.

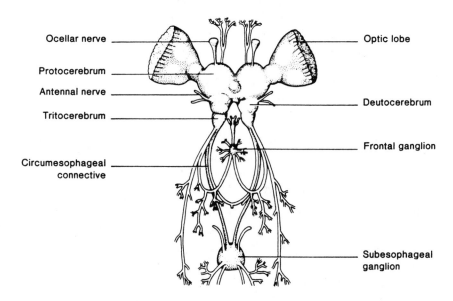

Figure labels (bottom):
Ocellar nerve · Protocerebrum · Antennal nerve · Tritocerebrum · Circumesophageal connective · Optic lobe · Deutocerebrum · Frontal ganglion · Subesophageal ganglion

1.7   Brain and stomatogastric nervous system of an insect. Clyde F. Herried. *Biology.* Copyright © 1977 Macmillan Publishing Company, Inc. Reprinted with permission of Simon & Schuster.

of the heads of insects, and the mouthparts represent primitive legs that have been altered through evolution into feeding structures. The grasshopper's (Fig. 1.3) mouthparts resemble mouthparts of blood- and tissue-feeding insects, except that they are specialized for cutting tough plant material. Two bloodsucking insects (Fig. 1.9), the *Rhodnius* (kissing bug) and the *Anopheles* (mosquito), have evolved to become capillary feeders. Both have developed feeding tubes that deeply penetrate skin; however, different elements of the mouthparts of each of these insects have evolved to serve similar functions. The mandibles in *Rhodnius* are short and serve as an anchor in the skin, whereas the mandibles of the mosquito are long and serve to cut tissue as the mouthparts are inserted into the skin. The kissing bug's salivary canal is located in the maxilla; in the mosquito it is a part of the hypopharynx. Other differences can also be seen in the figures.

Intestinal Tract

Figure 18.2 is a generalized diagram of an insect digestive tract that shows a regionally differentiated organ system. As the food moves from the foregut to the midgut to the hindgut, the food is stored, further triturated, digested, and absorbed; the residue is then dehydrated and deposited as feces. The long, slender Malpighian tubules function in the excretion of the end products of nitrogen metabolism and in water and inorganic ion balance. See Chapters 18 and 19 for additional detail on the intestinal tract, especially of vectors.

Tracheal System

The respiratory system originates in pores along the lateral marginal of the thorax and abdomen. These pores lead to chitinized tubules that ramify and extend throughout the body of the insect (Fig. 1.4).

Reproductive System

Insects reproduce by some form of sexual reproduction. Generalized diagrams of male and female insects show similarities between the sexes (Fig. 1.5 A and B). In a few instances, portions of the reproductive system are used in species identification and in aging certain species. The spermatheca is used in identifying fleas at the species level. Identification of sand flies is partly based on an examination of the

male copulatory structures. In mosquitoes, ovarial dilations are used to determine how many egg batches a female has laid, and the ramifications of the tracheal system indicate whether a female mosquito has laid a batch of eggs.

Nervous System

The nervous system of insects is derived from and reflects their metamerism, or segmentation (Fig 1.6). In the thoracic and abdominal regions, ganglia are associated with each of the segments. Because the main sense organs and feeding structures are in the head, the greatest complexity of the nervous system is also in the head, and many parts have evolved from segmental ganglia. For example, the brain has 3 portions, the protocerebrum, the deutocerebrum, and the tritocerebrum (Fig. 1.7). The brain apparently evolved from the ganglia of 3 legs of a primitive ancestor of the insects and therefore consists of 3 lobes.

It is important to note that the nervous system serves not only for short-term coordination but for long-term coordination as well. The corpora cardiaca and the corpora allata are associated with the hypocerebral ganglia; both serve essential roles in molting as well as other physiological activities (see Chap. 13).

ACARINES

The subphylum Chelicerata is a major group of the arthropods. The group is important from an evolutionary standpoint; many fossils of this group, which demonstrate arthropod evolution, have been found. They are also important for economic and medical reasons because they transmit agents of disease. The characteristic on which the group is based is the presence of the chelicera. Chelicerae are mouthparts that are typically slender, pointed structures that pierce the integument of the prey or host; chelicerates most often feed on liquefied food.

Included in the subphylum are fossils such as the eurypterids, "living fossils" such as the horseshoe crab, and evolutionary backwaters such as the pyncogonids, an obscure group of marine spiderlike animals. We are concerned here with the class Arachnida, which includes spiders, harvestmen, scorpions, sun spiders,

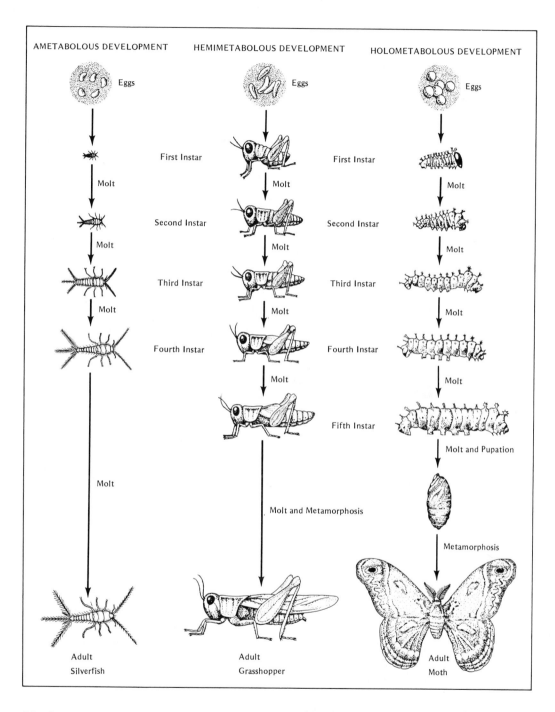

AMETABOLOUS DEVELOPMENT   HEMIMETABOLOUS DEVELOPMENT   HOLOMETABOLOUS DEVELOPMENT

Eggs

Eggs

Eggs

Molt

First Instar

First Instar

Molt

Molt

Molt

Second Instar

Second Instar

Molt

Molt

Molt

Third Instar

Third Instar

Molt

Molt

Molt

Fourth Instar

Fourth Instar

Molt

Molt

Fifth Instar

Molt and Pupation

Molt

Molt and Metamorphosis

Metamorphosis

Adult
Silverfish

Adult
Grasshopper

Adult
Moth

1.8   Patterns of development in insects. From Clyde F. Herried, *Biology.* Copyright © 1977 Macmillan Publishing Company, Inc. Reprinted with permission of Simon & Schuster.

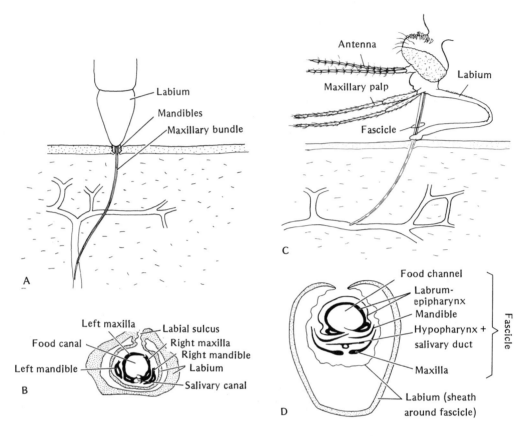

1.9   Mouthparts of a kissing bug and a mosquito. R.F. Harwood and M.T. James, *Entomology in Human and Animal Health 7/E*. Copyright © 1979 Macmillan Publishing Company, Inc. Reprinted with permission of Simon & Schuster.

and mites. The term "mite" includes both ticks and mites even though they are usually classified separately.

In addition to the chelicerae, arachnids have another set of mouthparts called pedipalps that either manipulate food or have sensory functions, depending upon the taxonomic group. There is no head as such major body regions are fused and are only vaguely differentiated. They lack antennae, and the eyes are simple. Members of the group have four pairs of legs at some stage of the life cycle. Developmentally, the young forms appear to be much like the adults; as they grow to larger stages, the body proportions remain much the same. Members of some groups continue to molt and grow after reaching sexual maturity.

Ticks and Mites

The acarines (subclass Acari) are called mites, and the group includes those organisms that we refer to as ticks. Ticks are giant mites, and although they have some distinguishing characteristics, they are referred to separately only because they are so large.

Mites are ubiquitous and have invaded a huge number of free-living and parasitic niches. Most mites are free-living and feed on detritus such as decaying organic matter or are predaceous. Parasitic mites feed on both plants and animals. The chelicerae are important because they allow the mites to puncture the integument of the plant or animal and feed upon the liquids inside. The parasitic forms transmit disease agents of both plants and animals.

About 35,000 species of mites have been described, and new species of both free-living and parasitic mites are described each month in journals devoted to acarines, insects, plant pathology, parasitology, and medical entomology.

The following works provide an introduction to the literature on mites and the diseases they transmit. Woolley (1988) and Evans (1992) are both general textbooks on acarines that contain a great deal of fundamental information. The chapter references provide a good starting point to the literature. McDaniel (1979) is a good handbook for identification of mites; it is useful for those with only moderate knowledge of mites. Hoogstraal's (1970–1982) 7-volume bibliography provides an excellent source of literature on all aspects of ticks.

Structure

All mites have much the same basic structure, although evolution within the acarines has produced some species that seem to be quite different. The body regions are not clearly defined except for the gnathosoma, or capitulum (Fig. 1.10). The gnathosoma is made up of the mouthparts chelicerae, pedipalps, and hypostome (Fig. 1.11). The rest of the body is called the idiosoma, but further subdivisions are often used. The podosoma bears the legs, and the opisthosoma is the region posterior to the legs. The opisthosoma is roughly equivalent to the hysterosoma, where the reproductive system is located. The anus is subterminal, and the genital opening lies at the level of the coxae of the 4th pair of legs. Leg terminology is similar to that of insects, except that mites have an additional segment. The leg parts from proximal to distal are coxa, trochanter, femur, patella, tibia, tarsus, and caruncle and claw.

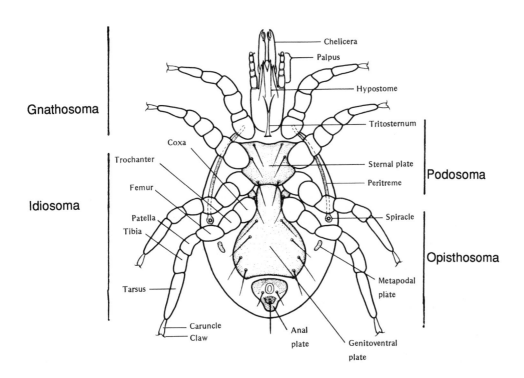

1.10   A generalized mite, ventral surface

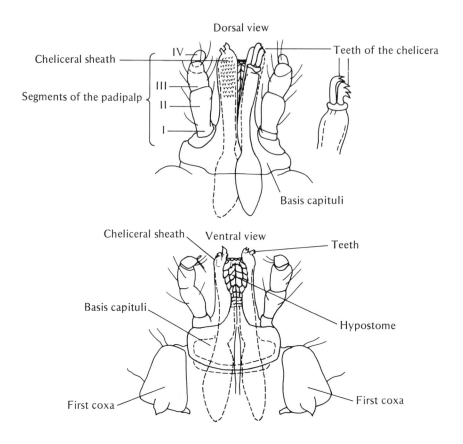

1.11   Mouthparts of a tick, dorsal (A) and ventral (B)

Classification

Not surprisingly, enormous diversity exists within the mites group. Classification has evolved over the past two centuries, but there is still lack of agreement among acarologists on a number of taxonomic groupings within the subclass. Woolley (1988) provides a useful and conservative approach to classification.

The following principal characteristics are used in classification of the mites, especially at the higher taxa: cheliceral type, pedipalp structure, stigmatal structure and tracheae, gnathosoma structure, hypostome, structure of the idiosoma, and the life-cycle pattern.

The subclass is divided into two cohorts, Parasitiformes and Acariformes (Table 1.1). The orders of interest to medical and veterinary entomology-acarology are Gamasida, Ixodida, Actinetida, Astigmata, and Oribatida. These orders contain mites that are either parasites themselves or serve as vectors of disease agents. The oribatids, for example, are free-living mites, but some of them serve as intermediate hosts of tapeworms of grazing animals.

Life Cycle

The life cycle of the mites has the following stages:

$$Egg \rightarrow Larva \rightarrow Nymph \rightarrow Adult$$

The stages are similar to one another in morphology except that the larva has 3 pairs of legs and both the

TABLE 1.1   The Cohorts and Orders of the Subclass Acari

COHORT PARASITIFORMES

Order Opilioacarida

Primitive mites that are purplish, violet-blue, or greenish-blue; they have the greatest number of primitive characters of members of the cohort; the podocephalic canal is absent; coxal glands are present and empty into sternal taenidia associated with the subcapitular groove; sometimes called "synthetic acarines" because of the combinations of characters that bridge the major groups, actinotrichid and anactinotrichid mites. Found mainly in warm, arid climates. *Opilioacarus, Panchaetes, Paracarus.*

Order Holothyrida

Large (2–7 mm), strongly sclerotized mites; oval in outline and tortoise-like in shape; body has 2 regions: the gnathosoma and an unsegmented idiosoma. Slight dorsal epistome is present near the anterior end; hairy in some families but hairless and glabrous in others; color ranges from bright red to dark brown; lack ocelli and tritosternum; 2 pairs of stigmata present; irritating to the mucous membranes of mammals and birds. Generally found in forests of tropical regions; predatory and detritovores. *Holothyrus, Allothyrus, Hammenius.*

Order Gamasida

Often referred to as Mesostigmata; lateral stigmata are located opposite coxae II and IV or between coxae III and IV; stigmata usually accompanied by an elogated peritreme, a groove or tube that extends anteriorly from the stigmata; no tracheal connections are associated with the peritreme; tracheae originate at the stigmata; the peritreme is reduced in some parasitic species; an epistome, or tectum capituli, covers the chelicerae; the gnathosoma is usually distinctly separated from the idiosoma so that the palps and chelicerae, the hypostome and gnathosomal base are easily seen; chelicerae are usually chelate-dentate; palps are leg-like with an apotele of 2 or 3 tines on the tarsus; usually heavily sclerotized with colors that are brown or reddish-brown; adults have an entire dorsal plate; the gonopore in the female is transverse and lies between the coxae. Free-living and parasitic forms. Parasitic forms are often hematophagous on the skin, in the nasal passages or lungs; members of the family Varroaidae are found in honeybees, in which they may cause economic losses. *Dermanyssus, Pneumonyssus, Ornithonyssus, Rhinonyssus, Varroa.*

Order Ixodida

Typically referred to as "ticks"; often classified as Metastigmata; stigmata are located posterior to coxae IV (Ixodidae or hard ticks) or anterodorsal to coxae IV (Argasidae or soft ticks); generally large, 2 mm to 2 cm in length; hypostome has recurved teeth; stigmata present but without sinuous peritreme; palps have 3 or 4 segments but withut claws, leglike in Argasidae, and with knifelike edges and a fused tibiotarsus in Ixodidae; Haller's organ present and on leg 1; genital aperture intercoxal in both males and females usually between coxae I and II; anal valves are subterminal. Parasitic, hematophagous. *Dermacentor, Boophilus, Haemaphysalis, Amblyomma, Argas, Ornithodoros, Otobius.*

TABLE 1.1 (Continued)   The Cohorts and Orders of the Subclass Acari

COHORT ACARIFORMES

Order Actinetidida

Body divided by a dorsosejugal suture with the gnathosoma distinct, but the rest of the body regions variable; genital and anal apertures dorsal in some groups; ocelli, when present, are propodosomal and lateral; 1 or 2 pairs of stigmata are usually located in the region of the gnathosoma at or near its base or with the chelicerae; peritremes present or absent; chelicerae exposed or hidden; palps vary from simple free or adpressed forms to fang-like raptorial types; leg segments may be reduced or missing, and some forms may lack some legs; pronounced sexual dimorphism. Detritovores, predators, parasites. *Cheyletiella, Demodex, Tetranychus, Eriophyus, Pyemotes.*

Order Astigmata

Soft-skinned mites, usually colorless or light coloration; movable gnathosoma usually visible from above and sometimes covered by the propodosoma; infracapitulum bears 2 pairs of setae; chelicerae usually exposed and work in a vertical plane; palps are simple and have 1 segment; idiosoma oval without evidence of external segmentation and lacking overlapping sclerites; sparse setation; integument finely striated in many species; genital apertures ventral. Detritovores, predators, phoretic, parasites. *Psoroptes, Sarcoptes, Chorioptes, Pneumocoptes, Dermatophagoides.*

Order Oribatida

Distinguished by the presence of the trichobothrium (pseudostigmata) and its sensillium (pseudostigmatic organ) located at the posterolateral corners of the prodorsum, function not thoroughly known; body usually divided by dorsosejugal suture into the propodosoma and the hysterosoma; gnathosoma may be found in a camerostome because of the projection of a prodorsal sclerite over the chelicerae; sexual dimorphism is rare; openings to the tracheae are on the coxae of the legs, and no external stigmata are visible. Free-living, some species serve as vectors of anoplocephalid tapeworms. *Liacarus, Camisia, Veloppia.*

---

nymph and adult have 4. Sexes are separate and often dimorphic.

Within the pattern described, a number of variations in the life cycles are possible. More than a single nymphal stage can occur, or the nymph can be lacking in a few species. There can be quiescent stages such as the nymphochrysalis of the chiggers (Trombiculidae). Adult females usually die after laying eggs, but in the soft ticks (Argasidae), females can continue to lay eggs for many months. The life cycles described in the following section are useful for obtaining a grasp of the fundamentals of acarines.

Life cycle of *Sarcoptes scabiei*. (Fig. 1.12). This organism comes in a number of varieties according to the host on which it is found; the varieties are host-specific to a great extent. These organisms cause scabies in humans and other animals, but it should be noted that there are at least two other genera of mites that also cause scabies. Scab mites are not vectors of disease agents, but nonspecific bacterial infections can be seen in the skin of infected hosts.

Transmission of scab mites takes place through close contact between hosts, and it is probably the adult female that is transferred. She burrows into the skin and lays eggs in the sinuous tunnel that she forms. The egg develops and releases the larval stage, which feeds and molts to the nymph. The nymph then molts and forms the adult. In females, there are two nymphal stages; in males there is only one. The life cycle of the female requires 14 to 17 days, and the male requires 9 to 11 days.

Life cycle of a chigger. Members of this family of mites (order Actinetida, family Trombiculidae) serve as vectors of a few disease agents, notably scrub typhus, or tsutsugamushi fever, for which the causative agent is *Rickettsia akamushi*. Chiggers are cosmopolitan, but scrub typhus occurs only in the western edge of the Pacific rim.

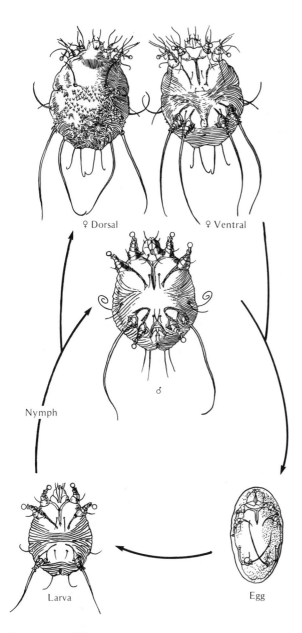

♀ Dorsal   ♀ Ventral

Nymph

♂

Larva   Egg

1.12 Structure and life cycle of *Sarcoptes scabiei*. Reprinted with permission from Macmillan Publishing Company.

The developmental cycle has more stages than the stereotypical acarine life cycle (see Fig. 1.13). Curiously enough, the larval stage is parasitic, but all others are free-living. The rate of development, of course, is determined by temperature, but in tropical climates, development takes place year-round. In warm weather, chiggers complete the life cycle in about 40 days. Some common chiggers include *Leptotrombidium*, *Euschoengastia*, *Trombicula*, and *Eutrombicula*.

Argasid ticks. Soft ticks (order Ixodida, family Argasidae) are leathery in appearance and often quite wrinkled (Fig. 1.14). The pattern of development in the soft ticks (Fig. 1.15) relates to their feeding pattern. Most soft ticks feed intermittently and only for a few minutes. There are typically 3 nymphal stages, but there can be more or fewer depending upon the species.

Soft ticks transmit a few infectious agents, among them the causative agent of African swine fever *(Borellia recurrentis)* and its relatives. These ticks most often associate with birds and rodents that reside in nests and burrows. Soft ticks generally do not associate with the host except to feed for short periods.

Ixodid ticks. Hard ticks form a relatively cohesive group with strong similarities in both structure and their life cycles (see Fig. 1.16). All have egg, larva, nymph, and adult stages. The variation in the life cycles relates to the number of individual hosts in the life cycle of any one species. There are 1-host, 2-host, and 3-host life cycles.

In a 1-host cycle, the tick remains on the same animal during the larval, nymphal, and adult stages (Fig. 1.17). It drops off only when the female has been fertilized and has engorged with blood. *Boophilus annulatus* is the vector of *Babesia bigemina*, Texas cattle fever.

In a 2-host cycle, both the larva and nymph remain on the same host (Fig. 1.18). In some cycles, the tick remains on the same host during the nymphal and adult stages. The engorged nymph drops off, molts to the adult stage, and then seeks a new

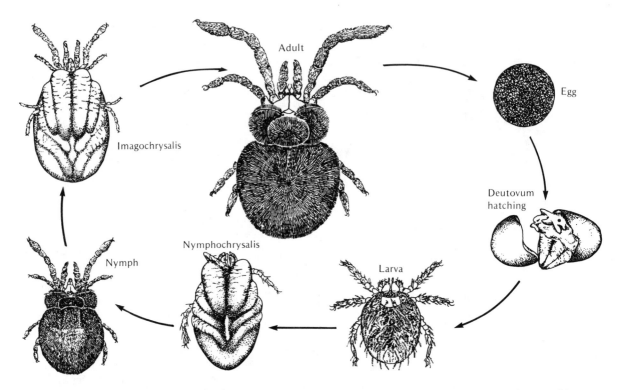

1.13   Structure and life cycle of a chigger. Reprinted with permission from the Annals of the Entomological Society of America.

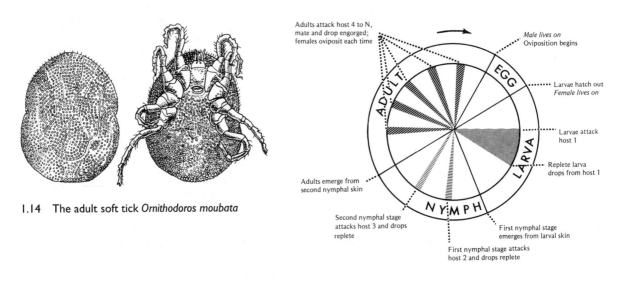

1.14   The adult soft tick *Ornithodoros moubata*

1.15   Life cycle and feeding pattern of a soft tick

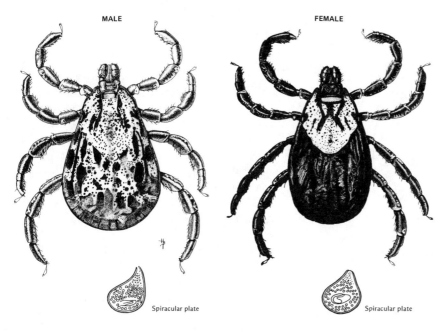

MALE   FEMALE

Spiracular plate   Spiracular plate

1.16   A hard tick, *Dermacentor andersoni,* male (A) and female (B)

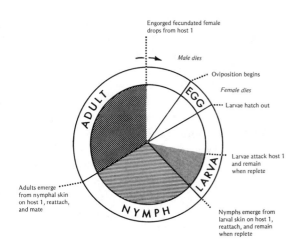

Engorged fecundated female
drops from host 1

Male dies

Oviposition begins

Female dies

Larvae hatch out

ADULT

EGG

LARVA

NYMPH

Larvae attack host 1
and remain
when replete

Adults emerge
from nymphal skin
on host 1, reattach,
and mate

Nymphs emerge from
larval skin on host 1,
reattach, and remain
when replete

1.17   A 1-host tick life cycle

host on which to feed. *Rhipicephalus evertsi* in Africa and *Dermacentor variabilis* in North America are examples of 2-host ticks.

In the 3-host life cycle, each stage feeds, drops off, molts, and then seeks a new host (Fig. 1.19). Examples of 3-host ticks are *Dermacentor andersoni, Ixodes ricinus,* and *Rhipicephalus sanguineus.*

Dermacentor andersoni (wood tick, or Rocky Mountain spotted fever tick) is a good example of a 3-host tick. In temperate climates, it requires a full year to complete its life cycle; in a cold climate such as in Canada, it requires at least 2 years—and sometimes 3—to complete the life cycle from egg to egg.

The adult seeks a host late in winter or early spring and attaches to a large animal such as a porcupine, canid, felid, or rabbit. Humans are incidental hosts and usually not part of the life cycle. The adult feeds for about a week, the males and females copulate, and the female drops off to lay her eggs. An average of 6400 eggs are laid by a female over a 3-week period.

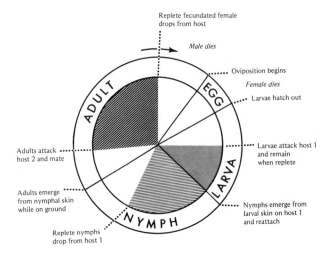

1.18   A 2-host tick life cycle

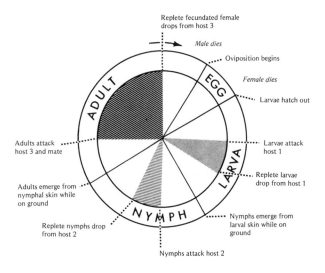

1.19   A 3-host tick life cycle

The egg develops a fully formed larva and hatches in about 35 days and then feeds on a small rodent such as a deer mouse for 3–5 days. The larva molts and remains unfed until the next year. The nymph becomes active in late winter and seeks a rodent such as the golden-mantled ground squirrel on which to feed. The nymph feeds for about a week, drops off, and molts to the adult stage. The adult then seeks a host on which to feed.

INFECTIOUS AGENTS

Symbiosis is defined as an association between two different species of living organisms. Lichen, which is an association of an alga and a fungus, is a good example of symbiosis. Other examples include fish that associate with sea anemones, barnacles on whales, *Remora* fish and sharks, and so forth.

Parasitism is a form of symbiosis and implies potential damage to the host by the parasite. Commensalism is a variation on parasitism in which there is no discernible damage to the host. Mutualism is a symbiotic relationship in which both partners benefit.

Parasitism is found among all groups of living organisms. Depending upon the taxonomic group, the terminology varies. Viruses, rickettsiae, bacteria, fungi, and yeasts are generally referred to as being infectious or microbial agents. Parasites in the limited sense are protozoa or protists and helminths. Arthropods that are parasites are said to infest a host. An infestation has been defined as being caused by a parasite that does not multiply in its host, but this definition has a number of inconsistencies and is only used occasionally.

Among living organisms, prokaryote or eukaryote, protistan or metazoan, parasitism is common. All of the major animal phyla except the echinoderms and chordates have parasites. Parasitism is also common among the mollusks, platyhelminths, annelids, and arthropods.

Parasitism often is spoken of disparagingly as if parasites are defective or are otherwise degenerate. Nothing could be farther from the truth. Parasites are highly specialized organisms that have moved into vacant ecological niches. Damaging the host is not intentional; pathogenesis is not generally advantageous to the parasite. However, this book is concerned with the various parasitic agents that either directly or indirectly have detrimental effects on human welfare. We hope these chapters will aid in mitigating the effects of parasites on their hosts and thereby improve the quality of human life.

CONTROL OF TRANSMISSIBLE DISEASES

One purpose of this book is to describe new means of controlling vector-borne diseases. Traditional methods that can be used in the control of all infectious diseases, vector-borne or not, will also be examined. The following list represents all of the general methods now available:

1. Administer or apply toxicants.

2. Reduce populations of reservoir hosts.

3. Reduce populations of vectors.

4. Induce immunity either naturally or artificially to a pathogen or vector.

5. Modify the environment through a physical change.

6. Avoid areas or activities of high risk, i.e., change behaviors.

7. Protect the individual or group by a barrier-quarantine or other physical barrier.

8. Alter the genome of the vector or vertebrate host.

9. Separate age classes of potential hosts.

10. Test for the presence of the disease agent and remove the infected hosts.

Toxicants

This broad category includes drugs that prevent and cure diseases, insecticides used to reduce populations of vectors, and inorganic substances that are toxic to either reservoir hosts or parasites. Basically, these chemicals interfere with the normal physiology of the target organism. The ultimate effect is at the cellular level and can interfere with nucleic acid synthesis, membrane structure, mitochondrial functions, and so on.

In Western medicine, when quinine was used to treat malaria it was probably the first instance of a chemical being used to treat a specific transmissible disease. During the past 60 years, a new armamentarium has been developed to treat and prevent transmissible diseases: sulfonamide drugs, antibiotics, antimalarials, and anthelmintics, among others. Since the development of DDT in the late 1930s, the chemical-pharmaceutical industry has made enormous strides, not only in developing new drugs and insecticides (s.l.) but also in designing molecules to have specific physiological effects (see Chap. 29).

Population Reduction of Reservoir Hosts or Vectors

With few exceptions, all vector-borne diseases of humans are zoonotic. The disease agent in question often cycles silently in populations of wild animals (see Chap. 4) and infects human populations under special circumstances. The system can often be manipulated so that the risk to human or animal health is reduced by lowering the probability of contact with the reservoir host(s) or the vector(s).

Immunity

Immunity is a specific response to an infectious agent or antigen. Immunity and resistance are not the same; resistance is an inherent character and is nonspecific. Immunity develops upon contact with a parasitic agent, or it can be induced artificially through vaccination or purposeful exposure to an agent.

Immunity nearly always develops when a host is exposed naturally to a parasite. In most instances the host becomes ill; if it survives it will usually be immune for a period of time—often for life. Artificial immunity is induced through vaccination. A living agent or part of an agent is injected into a host, causing immunity so that the host does not become ill upon challenge.

Immunity can be used to protect the individual and the population against an infectious agent. Populations are protected when a certain percentage of the potential hosts have been immunized; however, with some diseases, such as malaria, more than 99% of the population must have protective immunity to prevent transmission.

Environmental Modification or Management

Another method of controlling vector-borne diseases is physically changing the environment to make survival of the parasite or its vector unlikely. Regarding vectors, source reduction is a method of management. Source reduction is a physical change in the environment that makes survival or reproduction for the vector difficult.

Eliminating domestic garbage reduces populations of house flies. In the case of mosquitoes, various environmental modifications, such as draining fields, can reduce the habitat of the larvae (see Chap. 28).

Avoidance of High Risk Areas or Activities

This method involves changing behavior so that the probability of contacting a vector is reduced. River blindness (see Chap. 7) is a disease caused by a roundworm that is transmitted by black flies. The black fly larvae live in well-oxygenated streams and adults migrate out from them to spread the infection. When the risk becomes too great, people living near streams must leave the area for high ground.

Quarantine and Barriers

The term "quarantine" is derived from the Italian word "forty." Quarantine was practiced as early as 1374 in Venice in an effort to prevent the introduction of plague. Persons disembarking from ships were held in designated areas for 40 days before they could mix with the citizens of Venice. Now, modified quarantine is used for individuals with especially virulent infections that are readily transmitted to others. Britain has strict quarantine laws to prevent the introduction of rabies by dogs and cats; the animals must be kept isolated for 6 months before being allowed to mingle with the general populace.

To control African trypanosomiasis in cattle, barriers are established to prevent the migration of the vectors (tsetse). Because tsetse do not migrate far, brush and trees are cleared from a 2 km-wide area, which prevents flies from crossing the barrier (Chap. 10).

Another barrier used is a bednet, which prevents bloodsucking flies such as mosquitoes from reaching people while they sleep. If bednets are properly and diligently used, they are an effective means of preventing mosquito-borne diseases such as malaria.

A novel barrier is the use of zooprophylaxis. In instances where mosquitoes prefer to feed on livestock rather than people, keeping cattle near a house reduces the probability of the mosquitoes feeding on people. There are instances on record in which the introduction of tractors caused an increase in vector-borne diseases of humans.

Biological Control

Biological control is defined as the use of parasites and predators to control vectors of disease agents (see Chap. 31). Control of mosquitoes can be accomplished by introducing predators such as predaceous mosquito larva *(Toxorhynchites)* or fish that feed on mosquito larvae *(Gambusia)*.

Genetic Alteration of a Host

Genetic change can be induced in either the vertebrate host or vector. In many vector-borne diseases genetic changes have been induced in vertebrates and invertebrates by both natural and artificial means. Humans who test negative for the Duffy blood group are resistant to vivax malaria. Mosquitoes have become resistant to insecticides. The malaria parasite has become resistant to antimalarial drugs such as chloroquine.

Only modest success has been achieved in inducing changes in vectors to control vector-borne diseases (see Chap. 33). One significant success in genetic control is the sterile male technique as it applies to screw worms *(Cochliomyia hominovorax)* in the Western Hemisphere.

Separation of Age Classes

Although we use this method implicitly in some cases of human infectious diseases, it applies most often in diseases of livestock. Because all animals, including humans, live in a cloud of infectious agents, one means of lessening these agents' detrimental effects is to reduce the onslaught on young animals. Young animals are usually susceptible to nearly all parasites, and can succumb if they are exposed to many agents at one time. However, if their exposure can be limited both in the numbers and species of infectious organisms they have the opportunity of developing immunity. Thus, newborn animals are kept separate from those that are more than 3 months old.

Test and Remove

This method is used solely with livestock. An individual animal is first determined to be infected or ill with a specific disease. If the animal tests positive, it is removed from the herd and disposed of. Tuberculosis in dairy cattle was controlled in North America and Western Europe by a test-and-slaughter program. On occasion, hoof-and-mouth disease has been introduced into North America, and the control method used was to destroy all exposed animals, whether sick or not. Prior to the development of second generation insecticides such as DDT, scabies was controlled solely by a test-and-slaughter program.

SUMMARY

The field of vector biology stands on the threshold of rapid advances. There is a solid base of information in systematics, life cycles, morphology, and physiology from which to step into the future. Molecular techniques developed within the last two decades have opened up areas that previously were not possible to investigate. Biology has ridden on the coat tails of chemistry, physics, and mathematics during the 20th century, and it continues to do so. However, the discoveries in genetics, especially the Taq enzyme, which has allowed the polymerase chain reaction to be developed, and restriction nuclease enzymes, which have allowed the sequencing of DNA, have led the way for extraordinary discoveries—with more to come.

As these and other molecular and mathematical techniques are applied to vectors of disease agents, new approaches will be developed and novel control methods will be forthcoming. The remainder of this book describes better methods of control and points out the gaps in our knowledge that impede progress toward ameliorating vector-borne human and animal diseases.

APPENDIX 1.1   Zoological Classification

Kingdom (currently five)
  Phylum
    Class
      Cohort
        Order
          Superfamily (-oidea)
            Family (-idae)
              Subfamily (-inae)
                Tribe (-ini)
                  Genus
                    Subgenus
                      species
                        subspecies

Classification of plants and animals is a hierarchical classification that places related organisms in closely related groups at the lower levels of classification. Thus, two mosquitoes with similar characteristics in the genus *Culex* that are slightly different morphologically are placed in different species; examples are *Cx. tarsalis* and *Cx. pipiens*. The farther removed animals are from one another evolutionarily, the higher they are placed in the classification. Insects and flatworms are placed in different phyla. The protozoan that causes malaria and the virus that causes LaCrosse encephalitis are placed in different kingdoms.

All organisms must be placed in a phylum, class, order, family, genus, and species. The other levels of classification, such as cohort and subfamily, are optional. Not included here are such levels as subphylum, superclass, suborder, and infraorder, which are optional. In instances where there are many organisms in the taxonomic group, the super- and sublevels are used by those specializing in the organisms in question. These distinctions allow finer gradations to be included in the classification, thereby showing evolutionary relationships not otherwise possible.

From the level of superfamily down to tribe, the endings of the taxa are standard. Thus, all ticks are in the superfamily Ixodoidea; the hard and soft ticks are in the families Ixodidae and Argasidae, respectively. One can then refer to the ixodids and argasids as common names, but the group is nevertheless identified with precision.

Levine (1973) proposed standardized endings for all of the taxa down through subfamily. His objective was to allow ready communication about the level of classification. The standardized endings have not been widely accepted, but the suggestion has much to recommend it.

In literature, certain inflexible rules apply to animals at the levels of genus and species. For example, "*Passer domesticus* (Linnaeus, 1758) Johnson, 1896" is the full, scientific name of the English sparrow, slightly altered to allow us to use it as an example. The generic and specific names are in italics, and the name is always written this way. The generic name is always capitalized; the specific name, never. The specific name is not used alone; it has no content unless the generic name is included. There are a number of animals with the specific name *domesticus*. Without the generic designation, the reader does not know what is being referred to.

In the literature, the full generic name is given when it is first used, and then only the beginning letter of the generic name is cited when referring to it. *Passer domesticus* should be used for the first citation; thereafter *P. domesticus* is permissible. When referring to the genus only, "*P.*" alone is not used.

Linnaeus provided the first published description of the organism in 1758. Actually, the bird was included in the 10th edition of Linnaeus's *Systema Naturae*, the standard reference in classification. When an "L." appears after the name of an animal, it means that Linnaeus included it in *Systema Naturae*, his life's work.

In this example, the second name, "Johnson, 1896," is a fiction but demonstrates another principle. The first author described the organism adequately, but it was later placed in another genus; thus, the second author's name and date of the reclassification are included in the full name. The parentheses around the first name indicate an adequate description but erroneous placement at the generic level.

A description of a new species is published only once, and it must be published in a printed document that is widely distributed. Normally this means publication in a scientific journal; however, many new species are described in specialized taxonomic monographs. A new species cannot be described in an abstract given at a meeting because the description is inadequate or the details are given only verbally. Therefore, if an investigator finds a new species and wishes to discuss it at a scientific meeting, the new species may be alluded to, but the name is not used in the title of the abstract. If the name is given in the abstract, it will be declared void, and another name must be assigned when real publication is undertaken.

Above the generic level, the rules of zoological nomenclature are less demanding. An investigator who has worked on, say, black flies (Simuliidae) can make a major revision in the classification of the family and erect a dozen new subfamilies. General acceptance by the scientific community is the only criterion for inclusion. Each year a number of these major revisions are proposed, and it is only the merit of the proposal and the scientific reputation of the investigator that determine acceptance.

REFERENCES AND FURTHER READING

Borror, D.J., D.M. DeLong, and C.A. Triplehorn. 1976. *An introduction to the study of insects.* 4th ed. New York: Holt, Rinehart, and Winston.

Borror, D.J., and R.E. White. 1970. *Field guide to the insects of North America north of Mexico.* Boston: Houghton Mifflin.

Evans, G.O. 1992. *Principles of acarology.* Wallingford, U.K.: CAB International.

Hoogstraal, H. 1970–1982. *Bibliography of ticks and tick-borne diseases.* 7 vols. Cairo, Egypt. Spec. Publ. USNAMRU No. 3. Washington, D.C.: Smithsonian Institution.

Levine, N.D. 1973. Standardized endings for the higher taxa. *Syst. Zool.* 7:134–135.

Marquardt, W.C., and R.S. Demaree Jr. 1985. *Parasitology.* New York: Macmillan.

McDaniel, B. 1979. *How to know the mites.* Wm. C. Brown. Dubuque, Iowa.

Romoser, W.S., and J.G. Stoffolano Jr. 1993. *The science of entomology.* 3rd ed. Dubuque, Iowa: Wm. C. Brown.

Storer, T.I., I. Usinger, J.W. Nybakken, and R.C. Stebbins. 1979. *General Zoology.* 5th ed. New York: McGraw-Hill.

Woolley, T.A. 1988. *Acarology: Mites and human welfare.* New York: John Wiley & Sons.

2. COMMON PROBLEMS OF ARTHROPOD VECTORS OF DISEASE

José M.C. Ribeiro

INTRODUCTION

Hematophagy, the habit of feeding on blood, has evolved independently in several disparate animal taxa (e.g, leeches, ticks, insects, and bats). Even within a single insect order, it probably evolved independently in several families, as in the Diptera. This peculiar feeding habit was quickly exploited by parasites to find new hosts. Finding a host; locating blood within the vascular system; digesting this unique meal; fighting the microorganisms and parasites associated with the meal; and in the adult female arthropod, converting blood nutrients into yolk protein are all common problems of arthropod vectors. Thus, the solution to each problem defines the scenario that leads to parasite development and transmission. This independent evolution toward a common set of problems has led to some quite independent solutions or strategies, and different pathogen transmission scenarios. This chapter reviews the physiology of bloodsucking arthropods from a problem-solving perspective; it is aimed at the reader lacking an extensive background in entomology.

The independent evolution of hematophagy was shaped by other more general strategies, such as life-cycle development and method of feeding of the vectors. Three life-cycle patterns exist, i.e., ametabolous, holometabolous, and hemimetabolous (see Chap. 1). Hemimetabolous insects exhibit incomplete metamorphosis. Thus the insect that hatches from the egg (a nymph) looks quite similar to the adult but lacks wings or developed reproductive organs. As is true for all arthropods, immature insects grow by molting, having from 2 to 5 or more juvenile instars, with the last molt resulting in an adult. Holometabolous insects undergo a complete metamorphosis, with 4 distinct developmental stages. These life-cycle strategies affect the way we look at the immature insect stages in the disease transmission cycle and in vector control strategies.

FINDING A HOST

Two different strategies are used by bloodsucking arthropods to find their hosts. They either actively search for prey, attempting to maximize their chances (e.g., tsetse or tabanid—the mugger strategy), or they live close to their hosts—in their dwellings, nests, or even their fur (e.g., triatomine bugs, lice, and ticks—the stealth approach). These host-finding strategies define the type of association between the arthropod and its host. An adult tabanid or tsetse actively searches for a suitable host much like a tiger or lion does. These insects associate with their prey only during feeding time and can be considered micropredators. Lice, however, spend little or no time finding a host because they are associated with their host's body most or all of their lives, being true ectoparasites. Other insects that use the stealth approach, such as fleas, some ticks, and triatomine bugs, associate with their hosts' nests or dwellings. If a nest is an extension of an organism (an extended phenotype), these organisms are also true parasites (nest parasites). Combinations of strategies also exist. For instance, *Anopheles gambiae* adults rest in human dwellings most of the time, thus maximizing the chances of being close to a blood source.

Independent of the strategy, hungry arthropods use different cues for locating meals (Hocking 1971). Visual cues are important for micropredators that feed during the day (tabanids, tsetse, black flies, and some mosquitoes). Black flies and mosquitoes appear to prefer certain colors to land on, and large moving objects elicit the attention of tsetse, which normally feed on large ungulates. Tabanids that normally live in flat habitats such as pasture land are attracted to large contours that block the sky. These cues are used to design traps for these insects. One type of trap designed for tabanids has a large, black sphere to which the insects are attracted.

Other visual cues, such as light traps, are also exploited to trap flying insects. These traps are used at night and use a source of light and a fan to collect the insects. The light source is important to attract insects that disperse at night and that use a punctiform light source for navigational purposes. Normally these sources are distant, as with stars, and they generate a linear path for the dispersing insect. When the light appears to be close, the insect approaches it in a spiral path and is eventually sucked into the trap.

Odor also attracts an insect to its host. Carbon dioxide and water vapor (from breath) and lactic acid (or lactic acid oxidation products)—a common molecule in human sweat—elicit the attention and movement of hematophagous insects toward a host. The lactic acid receptor in the antenna of *Aedes aegypti* has been the object of elegant work in this regard. Butanol, a product of bacterial fermentation in ruminants that is excreted in their urine, is a potent attractive agent to tsetse and can be used to further increase the efficiency of tsetse traps. Carbon dioxide (CO_2), breathed out by hosts, is also a powerful cue for most bloodsucking arthropods. A source of CO_2 (such as dry ice) and sticky paper can be used to collect questing ticks. CO_2 can also be used as a bait for mosquito traps, such as the widely used CDC light traps (see Chap 27).

For insects feeding at night, when the environmental temperature is low and light is not available, orientation toward heat becomes an important cue. Triatomine bugs possibly "see" irradiated heat as well as convection currents. Night-feeding mosquitoes and some species of black flies also move toward a heat source that has a temperature compatible with that of a host.

Like other animals, bloodsucking insects also have a circadian cycle, and different vectors feed at different times of the day. This behavior thus influences vector control. For instance, many *Aedes* and *Psorophora* mosquitoes as well as black flies have crepuscular feeding habits, meaning that they have 2 activity cycles during the day, one early in the morning, and another late in the afternoon. They usually will not bother a sleeping individual, but they can spoil a late afternoon barbecue. As mentioned earlier, most tabanids and tsetse are day feeders. *Anopheles gambiae* and *An. funestus*, important malaria vectors in Africa (Chap. 5), and *Culex pipiens*, the main vector of urban filariasis (Chap. 6), are all night biters, their activity peaking between 10:00 P.M. and 2:00 A.M. The different cues mentioned previously are more or less important according to the feeding schedule. For instance, *Aedes aegypti*, a crepuscular mosquito (that also bites in the middle of the day but with less intensity), quests for its prey between 50 cm (centimeters) and 1 m (meter) from the ground. It senses CO_2, water vapor, and lactic acid, which are all heavier than air and thus close to the ground. The mosquito does not seek objects with temperatures higher than 37° (or time would be wasted investigating rocks heated by the sun), but it does pay attention to moving objects. However, *Culex* mosquitoes will quest high in a room for ascending warm air currents given off by a warm body and then dive in on those currents.

Where the arthropod feeds is also important. In malaria control, exophagic vectors (those that bite humans outside their houses) and endophagic vectors (those that bite inside the house) require different control strategies. Endophilic vectors (those that rest indoors) are usually controlled by indoor residual insecticide spray programs; their exophilic counterparts, which rest outdoors, are not as well controlled.

FINDING BLOOD

Once the bloodthirsty arthropod has landed or crawled on a host's skin, a close-range search begins. Chemoreceptors, located either at the tip of the mouthparts or in the antenna, inspect the surface for appropriate flavors. Mosquitoes touch, without attempting penetration, a possible host's skin several times, moving a few millimeters to either side until deciding to penetrate the skin. Some arthropods are extremely finicky and refuse most hosts. Indeed, some bird-associated soft ticks feed exclusively on particular host species, starving when unable to find their preferred host species.

Mechanoreceptors are also present in the tips of mouthparts and signal appropriate positioning of the feeding stylets for penetration. Again, 2 strategies for finding blood are utilized. In the ice-pick approach, a thin tubing (the feeding fascicle) pierces the victim and cannulates a blood vessel (solenophagy, or vessel feeding). In the ax approach, the insect's stylets slash through the skin, and the insect sips blood that oozes out from the hemorrhage (telmophagy, or pool feeding). Tsetse, mosquitoes, and triatomine bugs, for example, have independently evolved tubular mouthparts and use the ice-pick approach, whereas tabanids and black flies use the ax approach, employing a scissorlike cutting tool that effectively reaches the blood vessels of thick-skinned animals. The first approach often goes unnoticed by the host because the mechanical damage is less and does not elicit defensive behavior. The second approach is very noticeable, and it can only be performed in hosts without much defensive behavior or by arthropods sturdy enough to withstand such adverse host reactions as being beaten by a cow's tail or even being rolled over on (a feat survived by ticks and tabanids). Alternatively, arthropods feed on a site that cannot be groomed, for example, along the midline of the belly, around the anus, or in the ears.

After penetrating the host's skin, a pharmacological battle takes place between the vector and host. When feeding on blood, insects must somehow counteract host's defenses against blood loss, or the hemostatic process. Hemostasis is a redundant phenomenon in which platelet aggregation, blood coagulation, and vasoconstriction prevent blood loss from injured tissue. Consequently, insects that feed on blood have evolved a sophisticated array of salivary antihemostatic components used to locate blood during probing or for maintaining flow during feeding (Ribeiro 1987). Antiplatelet, anticoagulant, and vasodilation agents are found in the saliva or salivary glands of many blood-sucking arthropods, allowing them to efficiently steal blood (Chap. 20).

Although most blood-feeding takes no longer than an hour and is commonly completed in only a few minutes, hard ticks remain attached to their hosts for days or weeks, allowing time for inflammatory cells to invade the site of feeding (Chap. 34). Natural host–tick associations are devoid of significant host disruption caused by tick feeding, but nonnatural associations are often disrupted by such reactions (see Chap. 34). Indeed, guinea pigs serve as hosts for most ticks when exposed the first time, but after 2 weeks they usually reject more than 95% of the ticks. Antitick salivary antibodies and the accumulation of basophils occur simultaneously at the feeding site as well as considerable accumulation of edema. However, the pharmacological mediators of edema are many, and different vertebrate species have different mediators to accomplish the same goal. For instance, guinea pigs produce enormous amounts of histamine at tick feeding sites; many guinea pigs have exceedingly high numbers of basophils, which are histamine-rich. Mice, on the other hand, have few or no basophils and produce edema mainly via bradykinin and anaphylatoxin production. It has been proposed that natural tick–host associations are made possible by the tick producing salivary substances that antagonize their host's inflammatory and edema-promoting mediators. For example, the tick *Ixodes scapularis* has a salivary enzyme that destroys bradykinin and anaphylatoxin, the main edema-promoters in mice and rats, but it has no antihistamine activity. This same tick can feed repeatedly on its natural host, *Peromyscus leucopus* mouse, but it is rejected by guinea pigs previously exposed to it (Ribeiro 1988).

Salivary gland homogenates have been used as antitick vaccines. Although they work well in nonnatural associations, they do not work in natural associations, perhaps because ticks counteract their natural hosts' immunity so effectively. Recently, tick gut antigens employed as vaccines against *Boophilus microplus* have been used successfully (Chap. 34). Immunized cattle can lyse the gut of their ectoparasites in less than 24 hours. This new approach uses concealed antigens, or antigens to which the hosts have not been exposed. Several research groups are presently engaged in developing similar antimosquito vaccines and in investigating their effect on malaria development within the vector.

Because saliva is always injected into the host while the arthropod is searching for food, many viral, bacterial, and protozoan parasites have developed means of invading the salivary glands of their vectors and are delivered to their vertebrate hosts in such a vehicle. Most arboviral diseases (some of which can be transmitted mechanically), Lyme disease, malaria, babesiosis, theileriosis, and some African trypanosomiasis, are transmitted this way. Thus, the parasite must first recognize and then accumulate in significant numbers in the salivary gland of their vectors. Specific recognition of the salivary glands of *Anopheles dirus*, but not that of *An. freeborni*, has been demonstrated for sporozoites of *Plasmodium knowlesi*, and the molecular mechanisms for the recognition of the vector salivary glands by sporozoites of malaria is currently being researched.

As insects penetrate or lacerate their host skin, they are also salivating and tasting whatever is available (ticks salivate and suck through the same canal, whereas insects have independent tubes for each function). It appears that purine nucleotides provide the flavor that most bloodsucking arthropods are looking for. Depending on the tick or insect, adenosine, AMP, ADP, ATP, or 2,3 diphosphoglycerate have been shown to stimulate the uptake of a warm saline meal through a membrane in most bloodsucking arthropods. Anopheline mosquitoes are the least discriminating and drink almost anything isotonic that is offered under a warm membrane. The taste receptors are usually located high in the food channel, near the cibarial pump (much like a peristaltic pump), which is used to bring the blood into the gut. In some species an additional pharyngial pump aids in this process. Because most purine nucleotides are inside red blood cells (and thus not available in the plasma), it is presumed that the shearing forces acting at the pump release the nucleotides from the erythrocytes.

In fleas infected with the plague bacillus, the bacilli accumulate in the insect foregut, the chitinized region containing the feeding pump system. The massive accumulation of bacilli forms a plug (occurring only in a narrow temperature range) that disrupts the feeding process of the flea vector, causing it to regurgitate the bacteria into the victim. Thus, because the flea cannot feed, it becomes permanently hungry and contacts many more hosts than it would normally otherwise. Thus increased disease transmission results (Chap. 11). The sand fly *Leishmania* has recently been shown to produce a chitinase that not only helps to disrupt the peritrophic matrix (Chaps. 9 and 19) but also destroys the valves associated with the feeding pump, presumably reversing the normal flow of pumping and injecting the parasites into the vertebrate host. Like the blocked flea, the infected sand flies have difficulty feeding, which similarly increases transmission of the pathogens.

Bloodsucking arthropods usually take large meals from their hosts. Some, such as mosquitoes and triatomine bugs, average 3–10 times their own weight in blood (Chap. 18). Others, such as hard ticks, often take on more than 100 times their initial weight. This strategy reduces the number of times the arthropod must locate and contact a host. The triatomine bug *Rhodnius prolixus* feeds only once for each molting period, for example. It changes from egg to adult in about 6 months, spending less than 1 hour feeding. Selective pressure must have also acted to allow the development of antihemostatic compounds that speed the act of feeding, thus decreasing vector-host contact time. Because the arthropods have taken on an enormous amount of blood, locomotion or flying becomes difficult; they usually cannot move very far after feeding, and thus a suitable resting place must be at hand (or at wing). Some insects rapidly eliminate water from the meal to reduce their weight.

Some blood-feeding insects, though, feed a little at a time and often feed several times a day (e.g., tabanids and tsetse), which probably indicates that contact with the host poses little danger. Additionally, because they feed a little at a time, they are in better shape to follow a pack of migrating or moving animals, such as ungulates. This feeding behavior also facilitates mechanical transmission of pathogens, e.g., *Trypanosoma evansi*.

The control of ingestion is performed by stretch receptors located in the gut or crop of the arthropods. When the abdominal nerves in mosquitoes and *Rhodnius* are severed in surgery, the insects feed until the abdomen bursts. Normally, as the blood meal stretches the abdomen, signals are sent to the brain that then arrest the feeding reflex. Then another reflex, which warns the insect to flee the host begins, and the insect seeks a suitable resting place, so that digestion and water loss can take place.

WATER BALANCE: SOMETIMES TOO LITTLE, SOMETIMES TOO MUCH

Insects have a much more difficult time conserving water than most vertebrates because they have a large relative surface-to-volume ratio (surface area decreases with the square root of the side of a cube; volume decreases even more as the cubic root of the side). Insect cuticle is impermeable, containing waxes that seal moisture within. However, because of their relative impermeability, a problem arises in gaseous exchanges with the atmosphere. For this purpose, the spiracles that guard the entrance of the tracheal system are closed most of the time. For brief moments, they open and smooth muscles associated with the trachea contract, helping to expel the air within them—an efficient system for saving water.

Some hematophagous insects (e.g., bugs, lice, stable flies, and tsetse) feed exclusively on blood, whereas others (mosquitoes, black flies, and sand flies) drink water and sugar solutions and thus are more flexible in their ability to maintain water balance. Ticks, however, have developed an intriguing system to capture water vapor from ambient air. They secrete a hygroscopic saliva (produced in their type I acini of the salivary glands; see Chap. 20), which is spread over their palps. This saliva captures moisture from the atmosphere and is then ingested. Some soft ticks (e.g., *Ornithodorus* spp.) have been found to remain alive for more than 10 years without a blood meal—and without desiccating—thanks to this mechanism. Tick species differ in their ability to capture and retain moisture. Some obtain sufficient moisture from 60% relative humidity, but some need 70% or more to achieve water uptake (as measured by the relative humidity in which ticks lose or gain weight). This physiological capability defines their habitat. *Ixodes scapularis* ticks (vector of *Borrelia burgdorferi*, the etiological agent of Lyme disease), for example, have been shown to be inefficient in capturing and retaining moisture. This inefficiency probably explains the prevalence of these ticks in humid areas with extensive ground cover, i.e., in areas with dense leaf litter.

The problem of maintaining the proper water balance can also be affected by the insect taking in too much water during a blood meal. Indeed, ingesting several times their own weight in blood in a few minutes makes moving or flying difficult for arthropod vectors and increases their susceptibility to predation or unhappy accidents. One obvious solution is to lose the maximum amount of water as quickly as possible. Indeed, a 5th instar *Rhodnius* nymph, weighing 30 mg, can ingest 300 mg of blood in less than 15 minutes and urinate 150 mg within 6 hours, or 5 times its body weight in 6 hours—almost a whole body weight in urine per hour!

Elegant studies with isolated Malpighian tubules of *Rhodnius* have been conducted, and diuretic hormones have been isolated (Maddrell 1992). These hormones must be present in the bug's hemolymph a few seconds after ingestion of the meal, and the insect can start urinating on the host while still feeding. Indeed, this flow of urine washes out the insect rectum, carrying with it the protozoan *Trypanosoma cruzi*, which is thereby delivered to the vertebrate host's skin. Hormonal regulation of water transport from the midgut to the hemolymph and from the hemolymph to the Malpighian tubules has been the subject of study in many laboratories. A number of neuropeptides and the role of serotonin in this process have been recently characterized (Spring 1990; Wheeler 1990).

Ticks, again, have solved the problem of excess water in a different way; indeed, soft ticks (Argasidae) have solved it differently from hard ticks (Ixodidae).

Soft ticks, which in general feed for periods of minutes to one hour (although some can become attached to their hosts like hard ticks), have developed a unique filtration apparatus, the coxal glands. These glands look much like a vertebrate nephron, opening at the base of the legs (thus the name). The tick integument is lined with smooth muscle that contracts and creates the necessary filtration pressure for the system to work. A dilute saline solution and some protein is eliminated in this process, which starts while the tick is still feeding. Spirochetes causing relapsing fever are also found in the coxal fluid, which is one way they are transmitted by the vector to the vertebrate host. Hard ticks, which feed for several days while attached to their hosts, absorb the meal's water from the gut to the hemolymph, from where most of it is pumped back into the host as saliva (the process of plasmapheresis). Ticks secrete water mostly through the anterior end, whereas the excretory region produces a powdery, uric acid–rich material, although a more diarrheic consistency has also been reported in some species, such as *Amblyomma*.

DIGESTING THE BLOOD MEAL

Blood is a unique meal rich in proteins and essential amino acids but deficient in carbohydrate, fat, and adequate amounts of many B vitamins. Accordingly, all insects that feed exclusively on blood, such as the triatomines, lice, bed bugs, and adult tsetse (which are ovoviviparous) have bacterial symbionts that either supplement the blood with B vitamins or balance the diet by converting proteins to carbohydrates (glyconeogenesis). Without these endosymbionts the insects do not mature sexually, or the adults are infertile. These endosymbionts live in the insect gut, either free (as in triatomines), or in mycetoma, special structures of the gut (as in tsetse or lice).

Some insects store the blood in an inert digestive organ before delivering the meal, in small amounts, for digestion to the intestine (Chap. 18). Tsetse have a crop, a diverticulum of the gut, to which the ingested blood goes; the anterior midgut of *Rhodnius* serves the same function. Endosymbionts are located in the anterior midgut of triatomines. Other insects (such as mosquitoes, sand flies, black flies, and fleas)

deliver the meal directly to the gut, in which it is completely digested.

Within the Diptera, an inert membrane, the peritrophic matrix, is secreted around the blood meal within a few hours of ingestion (Chap. 19). The peritrophic matrix is common to all insects and consists mostly of chitin. Recently it has been demonstrated that malaria ookinetes and *Leishmania* secrete a chitinase to escape this structure and thereby survive and multiply.

Digestion of the blood meal by vectors also presents different approaches in cell biology strategy. Ticks, instead of secreting the digestive enzymes into the gut lumen, secrete a hemolysin, and then slowly pinocytose the gut contents by intestinal cells, resulting in the intracellular digestion of the meal by lysosomal enzymes.

Insects secrete digestive enzymes to the lumen of the gut, where digestion takes place. Most insects digest the blood proteins using serine proteases (e.g., trypsin) secreted into the lumen. Further digestion of the smaller peptides is accomplished by amino- and carboxypeptidases either free in the lumen or associated with the gut microvilli. These enzymes, as expected, have neutral-to-alkaline pH optima for activity, as in the case of their mammalian counterparts. In triatomines, however, the proteolytic enzymes have properties of the sulfhydryl proteases similar to the lysosomal cathepsins and, accordingly, pH optima of around 5.0 (Gooding 1972; Billingsley 1990; Terra 1990).

In an unfed insect, the level of the proteases in the gut is small, but within a few hours or days after taking blood, protease levels can rise 20-fold. The enzymes are induced by the presence of a proteic meal. In *Aedes* spp., a small amount of one type of early trypsin is produced following stretching of the gut, but the main trypsin is not produced if the meal does not contain protein. It appears that if this early "scout" trypsin is produced and peptides are generated, the main trypsin is then synthesized. This process is still poorly understood, and is the subject of current research.

Because most of the lipids and carbohydrates in bloodsucking insects must be made from amino acids, excess nitrogen has to be conveniently excreted. This process is accomplished by the synthesis of uric acid. Indeed, most of the white component of the feces of bloodsucking insects is uric acid, which is secreted by the Malpighian tubules into the insect rectum. The rectum also contains the remains of the blood meal, which includes black hematin from hemoglobin. Analysis of the shape and composition of insect feces found in resting boxes (Nuñez boxes) has been a component of triatomine bug surveillance in areas that were treated with insecticide for Chagas' disease control. Analysis of fecal uric acid also allows metabolic studies on the efficiency of energy conversion from blood to egg production in mosquitoes, in combination with other metabolic measurements.

In some holometabolous insects, such as mosquitoes and sand flies, although only the adult female takes blood, both adult males and females take sugar meals (which can be obtained in nature from honeydew, flower nectar, rotten fruits, etc.). The sugar meal supplies important energy so that the female can find a host and the male can find a female. Salivary glands of these insects often have glycosidases, and more glycosidases are also found in the gut microvilli. The requirement for a sugar meal by the infected sand fly was demonstrated more than 50 years ago as being essential for *Leishmania* to become infective to vertebrates, but the underlying reason is obscure.

Vector-borne parasites have to cope with the digestive system of their host. They must either escape from the gut before enzymes appear (viruses can be digested if they do not invade the gut cells quickly) or adjust to their presence, as do *Typanosoma* or *Leishmania* spp. These protozoa inhabit the gut of the host and have dense surface glycolipidic coats that cannot be digested by their vector's enzymes. Note that the adaptations of these parasites to survive in a proteolytic environment probably preadapted them to feel at home within a macrophage phagolysosome.

FIGHTING PARASITES

Insects have mechanical barriers that prevent easy penetration of microorganisms. A hard integument and the peritrophic matrix isolate the insect cells reasonably well from the outside world (Chap. 19). However, once these barriers are trespassed, a number of physiological processes take place to defend against the invaders. These processes are not peculiar to bloodsucking arthropods but are common to most arthropods. Invertebrates do not have the capability of producing antibodies, but they are capable of both cellular and humoral reactions that fight infections (Chap. 23).

GROWTH AND EGG DEVELOPMENT

Arthropods have difficulty growing up because of their rigid exoskeleton. Thus, all arthropods digest as much as possible of the old exoskeleton (through hydrolytic enzymes released by the epidermal cells that lie under the integument), and by ingesting air (or water) expand the gut until the old skeleton/integument bursts. After the arthropod walks out of the old skin, the new flexible integument expands further and then is hardened by melanization and sclerotization of the cuticle. The insect continues to grow internally into the space that was previously filled with air. In some insects, actual increase in size during a developmental instar can also occur, which is accomplished by an exoskeleton that is not entirely rigid but consists of hard plates joined by less sclerotized membranes (accordion style).

Arthropods that feed on large quantities of blood have to accommodate this large volume within a hard exoskeleton. This can be accomplished by the accordion strategy mentioned or by cuticular plasticization, a phenomenon found in triatomine nymphs and hard ticks. The cuticle of a hungry tick or triatomine does not extend and breaks easily if pulled. However, in *Rhodnius*, a few minutes after starting the meal the cuticle becomes plasticized, i.e., it can be pulled to a thin membrane similar to Parafilm. This can be accomplished in vitro by addition of serotonin to the cuticle, and it involves a water flow from the medium to the cuticle made by the epidermal cells underlying the tissue. The hydration of the cuticle allows the cuticular proteins to roll over one another. Little chitin is found in this plasticizable cuticle.

After hatching from the egg, the insect undergoes a number of molts to reach the larger immature forms before a final molt to the adult stage (Chaps. 1 and 17). Two hormones play a key role in this growing process. Ecdysone (actually 20-OH ecdysone, the active hormone) is produced in the prothoracic glands and is the molting hormone. It has anabolic activity, increasing protein synthesis and mitotic activity in most tissues. In each molting cycle there are usually 2 bursts of ecdysone production, the last one just before molt. Juvenile hormone (JH), a terpenoid lipid, is the other key hormone. It is produced by the corpora allata, an endocrine organ behind the brain. When molts occur in the presence of sufficient amounts of juvenile hormone, the insect molts to an immature stage, thus its name. In the last molt, it is the absence of juvenile hormone that triggers the differentiation process of metamorphosis to the adult stage.

Plants have developed insecticides that exploit the hormonal system of insects. Among them, a class of plant compounds (precocenes) destroy the cells that produce juvenile hormone because they are suicide substrates for the hydroxylation reactions that are part of the synthetic process. Young insects that have been treated with precocene molt in the absence of juvenile hormone to become precocious (but sterile) adults. Another source of plant compounds with insecticidal activity are analogs of juvenile hormone. When insects are exposed to these compounds in their last molting cycle, metamorphosis is disrupted, leading either to the death of the insect (the most common outcome in holometabolous insects), or the production of an organism with both immature and adult characteristics (e.g., hemimetabolous insects) that is sterile. Synthetic juvenoids have been developed and are widely used for mosquito control in the United States.

After the last molt, the prothoracic gland disappears; previously scientists thought that ecdysone was not produced in adult insects. However, both ecdysone and juvenile hormone are produced in adults and play a role in egg development. In *Rhodnius*, juvenile hormone has a positive role in egg development; ecdysone, produced by the ovary, has a negative feedback to JH production via the corpora allata. In mosquitoes both hormones are needed sequentially for egg development. A number of additional hormones are currently under study and many others have been identified and their structures elucidated.

POPULATION STRATEGY

Arthropods develop eggs and their young using 2 different strategies (Chap. 24). At one extreme are the *r* strategists, which produce small offspring in large numbers. Typically, female Ixodid ticks lay over 1000 eggs after feeding. They efficiently convert virtually all their body tissues into eggs before dying. Most other blood-feeding insects also produce a relatively large egg batch from a single meal (e.g., 100–200 for mosquitoes; 30–40 for triatomine bugs), and many batches are produced by an adult, following a blood meal. Tsetse, on the other hand, is a *K* strategist and produces only a few offspring that are larviposited in nature in a fairly advanced state of development. Indeed, tsetse are ovoviviparous and produce only 1 larva that hatches in the fly's ovary, where it is nurtured by a milk gland until the final larval instar. This larva is then deposited by the parent fly in the soil, where it immediately burrows in and then pupates. It does not feed until molting to an adult fly. In the laboratory, a tsetse can produce at most 6–8 pupae and probably fewer in the field.

These 2 contrasting egg allocation strategies are important to consider in vector control strategies. For example, control techniques that kill 75% of the adult tsetse can actually lead to local eradication of flies by reducing the basic reproductive rate of these insects to below one; thus the population continuously decreases at each generation until it reaches zero. However, in control strategies for mosquitoes, nearly 100% of the larvae must be destroyed for local eradication purposes. Indeed, traps have been developed for tsetse control that significantly reduce local populations, but this strategy cannot be expected to work as easily with an *r* strategist.

ACKNOWLEDGMENTS

I am grateful to Rosane Charlab, Eddie Cupp, Henry Hagedorn, Mark Novak, and Roberto Nussensweig for helpful comments on the manuscript.

REFERENCES

Billingsley, P.F. 1990. The midgut ultrastructure of hematophagous insects. *Ann. Rev. Entomol.* 35:219–248.

Gooding, R.H. 1972. Digestive process of haematophagous insects I—A literature review. *Quaest. Ent.* 8:5–60.

Maddrell, H.P., and M.J. O'Donnell. 1992. Insect Malpighian tubules: V-ATPase action in ion and fluid transport. *J. Exp. Biol.* 172:417–429.

Ribeiro, J.M.C. 1987. Role of arthropod saliva in blood feeding. *Ann. Rev. Entomol.* 32:463–478.

Ribeiro, J.M.C. 1988. Role of saliva in tick-host interactions. *Exp. Appl. Acarol.* 7:15–20.

Spring, J.H. 1990. Endocrine regulation of diuresis in insects. *J. Insect Physiol.* 36:13–22.

Terra, W.R. 1990. Evolution of digestive systems of insects. *Ann. Rev. Entomol.* 35:181–200.

Wheeler, C.H., and G.M. Coast. 1990. Assay and characterization of diuretic factors in insects. *J. Insect Physiol.* 36:23–34.

3. VECTOR BEHAVIOR

Marc J. Klowden

INTRODUCTION

The single characteristic that best predicts whether an arthropod will be involved in the transmission of pathogens is probably its behavior. Lacking the behaviors that bring it to a host and allow it to feed on blood, the arthropod is unable to transmit infectious agents. No matter how anatomically and physiologically suited it otherwise may be to harbor pathogens, without the necessary behavior patterns, it cannot be a vector. Thus, understanding whether a particular behavior will be expressed by a vector provides us with a clearer understanding of the dynamics of vector-borne diseases. Also, if our intent is to control vector populations, it certainly helps to know, and possibly predict, where the vectors are and what they are doing. This chapter will outline some of the basic behavior patterns that directly and indirectly contribute to the success of insect vectors, focusing mostly on mosquitoes, for which we have the most information.

FIXED-ACTION PROGRAMS

If, during the course of your education, your mind has ever wandered while you listened to an incredibly boring class lecture, you may have focused your attention on some of the extraneous behaviors of the lecturer. Ear-pulling, nose-scratching, beard-stroking, pocket-stuffing, and wandering behaviors usually abound. Many people characteristically display such unconscious behaviors when under stressful conditions, and these behaviors are fairly universal and cross-cultural.

As much as we prefer to distance our own species from the stereotyped behaviors so characteristic of "less sophisticated" animals, these behaviors are basically similar to the fixed-action patterns that are found throughout the other members of the animal kingdom.

From a physiological perspective, the expression of behavior can be considered as a temporal series of muscle contractions that are usually expressed and coordinated in groups, comprising the stereotyped behavior programs. This is probably best illustrated in the mollusk, *Aplysia californica*. Living in an aquatic environment, the snail is surrounded by fairly uniform conditions of temperature and salinity. The buoyancy of the water simplifies locomotion. The 20,000 or so neurons that make up the central nervous system are adequate to meet the demands of its relatively simple existence, and it is usually occupied with feeding and reproducing. When it lays its eggs, however, *Aplysia* engages in a relatively complex series of behaviors involving the cessation of locomotion and ingestion, increases in heart and respiratory rates, and the execution of specific behaviors that provide the eggs with some degree of protection during their development. These behaviors are controlled by a family of egg-laying hormone genes that are expressed in the bag cells of the central nervous system. Injection of a bag cell extract into snails that normally would not engage in egg-laying behavior elicits the entire repertoire of egg-laying behaviors. Four homologous genes have been identified that encode a family of neuropeptides that

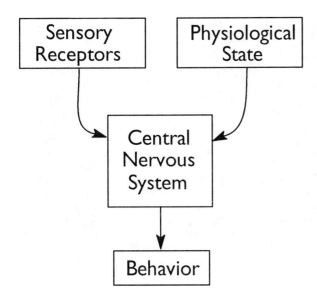

3.1 Interaction between sensory receptors and endogenous physiological state in determining the behaviors an insect will express

act on various target tissues to coordinate the expression of egg-laying behavior. Thus, *Aplysia* must only abide by the chemical signals that cause the biologically appropriate expression of these preprogrammed fixed action programs (Scheller and Axel 1984; Scheller et al. 1984).

Similarly, most insect behaviors appear to be displayed according to the simple scheme in Figure 3.1. In response to signals from the external environment that are perceived by sensory receptors, and signals from the internal environment (e.g., hormones that convey information about physiological state), the stimulus is associated with the proper biological response by the central nervous system. This proper association arose as a result of natural selection fine-tuning the relationship between an organism and its environment over many millions of years, eliminating the behaviors that were not adaptive and ultimately producing an appropriate, sometimes complex, behavior from a given stimulus.

EVOLUTION OF HEMATOPHAGY

Before vectors could acquire the blood-feeding habit, molecular, morphological, and ecological adaptations must have occurred (Chap. 20). Hematophagy is believed to have evolved through 2 major routes in insects (Waage 1979). In the first route predaceous or plant-feeding animals, with mouthparts and digestive tracts already morphologically and physiologically preadapted for piercing tissues, took a short evolutionary hop and shifted their feeding preferences to the rich resource of vertebrate blood. This may have resulted when the predaceous insects that fed upon the numerous other insects that lived in the vicinity of vertebrates ultimately evolved a preference for the vertebrates themselves, or when insects that were preadapted for feeding on nectar from flowers serendipitously punctured the skin of vertebrates. The second possible route was for insects that had no preadaptations for hematophagy to gradually develop a more intimate association with potential vertebrate hosts. This evolutionary route proposes that they fed first on the organic matter in nests, moved to dung and sloughed skin from the host, and finally to skin and blood. Morphological and physiological adaptations then would have evolved along with these changes in feeding substrate.

The ability to tap this store of blood opened up a rich, highly concentrated source of food, but in the more primitive dipteran suborder Nematocera, this resource is only exploited by the females of hematophagous species. Males in these groups lack the mouthparts and the behavior programs necessary to feed on blood; they survive on carbohydrate from plant nectar or the honeydew that often covers vegetation. The females also feed on this carbohydrate to derive energy for flight (Nayar and Van Handel 1971). It is thought that blood-feeding by the female allows her to reproduce by providing her with the exogenous protein for yolk synthesis. In the more phylogenetically advanced dipterans, the trend is for both males and females to feed on blood. Both sexes of the tsetse fly are obligate blood feeders and use the amino acid proline rather than carbohydrate to fuel flight. Another trend has been toward the increasing importance of the larval stage in the accumulation of nutrients needed for adult reproduction. Those species that are autogenous are able to develop an initial batch of eggs without a blood meal because their larvae have acquired the needed protein and carry it over into the adult stage. In anautogenous species, as well as in autogenous ones, adult protein deficits must be met by feeding on blood.

RECEPTOR PHYSIOLOGY

Compared to the skin of vertebrates, the integument of arthropods is relatively insensitive. The impermeable outer cuticle that covers the living epidermal cells of terrestrial arthropods is sprinkled with sensory receptors that are exposed to the environment at strategic places, minimizing water loss yet transducing key bits of environmental information into electrical signals that can be interpreted by the central nervous system (CNS) (Fig. 3.2). However, if all the richness and diversity of environmental information reached the simple CNS, it would undoubtedly overwhelm it. Consequently, many of the sensory receptors, especially those involved in olfaction, are finely tuned so that their sensitivities are greatest toward certain biologically relevant compounds; much of the rest is ignored. These relevant visual, chemical, and sometimes auditory stimuli are perceived by the sensory receptors and then sent to the CNS for integration and association.

There are at least 2 likely ways in which the process of sensory transduction, the translation of environmental energy into electrical signals by the CNS, occurs. When there is a need for highly specific recognition, such as for sex pheromones, specific receptors are present that are sensitive to only a narrow range of substances. These labeled lines send a clear message to the CNS that a specific substance is present in the environment. Thus, a receptor sensitive to a sex pheromone, for example, would synapse with the CNS and initiate upwind flight of the insect to its source when stimulated. The firing of an individual receptor may be sufficient to initiate this behavior. In contrast, across fiber patterns may be generated in the CNS by many nonspecific generalist receptors that are stimulated to

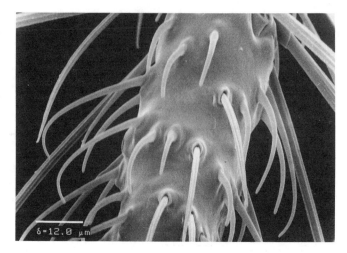

3.2   Sensilla on the antenna of a mosquito

different degrees as a result of their overlapping sensitivities. This pattern from the various receptors, including thermoreceptors and photoreceptors as well as chemoreceptors, is integrated and associated with the proper behavioral response. Behavior only ensues when the CNS receives the correct pattern, or search image, from the field of stimulated receptors. There are examples of information reaching the CNS by both labeled lines and across fiber patterns.

ACTIVITY PATTERNS

Before host-seeking can begin, the nervous system of the vector, and the vector itself, must be in a receptive state. This is reflected in behaviors that make it more likely to receive stimuli, or what may be termed spontaneous activity levels. The behaviors generally show a species-specific circadian rhythmicity, increasing at certain times of the day with 1 or more peaks (Bidlingmayer 1974), and appearing to reflect CNS activity rather than that of peripheral receptors (Bowen 1992a). The older literature defines this as "appetitive behavior," or behavior in search of a stimulus, but this term is rather teleological and imparts motive. "Ranging behavior," used to describe the flight of the tsetse fly in the absence of host stimuli (Vale 1980), is probably a more accurate definition. Although some species of tsetse are more likely to respond to stimuli when resting, others are more responsive when they encounter stimuli during these ranging flights.

In some cases, the activity patterns of vector populations have been synchronized with those of the parasites they transmit. For example, microfilariae of *Brugia malaya* and *Wuchereria bancrofti* exhibit a circadian periodicity in the peripheral blood that coincides with the activity patterns of their mosquito vectors, suggesting that the filariae have adapted a periodicity that facilitates their transmission (Wharton 1963). Parasites infecting the vector may also alter its circadian activity, flight range, and feeding behavior (Husain and Kershaw 1971; Hockmeyer et al. 1975; Rowland and Lindsay 1985; Berry et al. 1986).

During this species-specific circadian window, other factors may modulate the expression of activity. For example, the age of the vector can influence activity levels. Shortly after emergence, there may be a brief period during which it is oblivious to host stimuli, and older individuals may respond much differently than when they were younger (Nayar and Sauerman 1973; Zimmerman and Turner 1984; Packer and Corbet 1989). The age structure of a vector population and effects of age on behavior are particularly relevant, given that an older vector is more epidemiologically important by virtue of its increased opportunity to acquire and transmit pathogens. Nutritional state also affects the intensity of activity peaks; as the period of food deprivation lengthens, activity patterns in insects often become more intense (Brady 1975; Nelson 1977). Insemination, but more specifically male accessory gland substances, also modifies the species-specific circadian activity patterns (Jones 1981; Jones and Gubbins 1977, 1978; Rowland 1989; Chiba et al. 1992), perhaps in order to synchronize mating activities. When all factors contribute to the increase in activity levels, they make the vector more likely to encounter host stimuli, and it may then find itself in the vicinity of a host.

HOST PREFERENCE AND RECEPTOR SPECIFICITY

Although a wide range of animals serve as hosts for hematophagous arthropods, individual arthropod species are often specific for a particular host. The human biting index, the proportion of a mosquito population that feeds on humans, is a measure of both host preference and host availability in an area as well as an indication of the importance of a particular species as a vector of human pathogens. Based on this index and the origin of ingested blood determined by serological tests, a species can be arbitrarily labeled as anthropophilic, more likely to feed on humans, or zoophilic, more likely to feed on other animals. These preferences have been correlated with genetic markers (Coluzzi et al. 1977, 1979). Host preferences undoubtedly developed as a result of host availability and the need to partition hosts to reduce interspecific competition for resources, and it does not necessarily follow that because a vector has selected a host, it has done so optimally. For example, *Aedes aegypti*, which feed readily on humans, produce more eggs when fed on guinea pigs, rats, or birds than on humans because of their higher isoleucine content relative to human blood (Briegel 1985). Based on resting habits, species may be further classified as endophilic, remaining within human habitations for most of the gonotrophic cycle, or exophilic, spending most of their time outside.

The same metabolic by-products that serve as potential kairomones, or chemicals used in host location, are produced by all living things, but what may account for the host specificity is their proportion, and thus the pattern that is presented to the insect CNS to activate behavior. Some hematophagous insects utilize very specific stimuli. The genus *Corethrella* (Diptera: Corethrellidae) contains autogenous species, not known to be vectors, that feed on the blood of frogs. The females are specifically attracted to the sounds of tree frogs and ingest blood from them, behavior that may allow them to undergo subsequent gonotrophic cycles (McKeever and French 1991). The black fly, *Simulium euryadminiculum*, is attracted to loons by secretions of their uropygial glands (Lowther and Wood 1964).

SIGNALS USED IN HOST LOCATION

Locating a host amid all the distractions in the environment poses a special problem for hematophagous arthropods. The simple task of finding food must be translated into a series of simple sequential behavioral subroutines, each involving stimuli from a host that affects the host-seeking arthropod in a different way. The subroutines are not isolated programs but rather appear to form an integrated series of step-wise stimulus-response events (Dethier 1957). Consequently, what we refer to as host-seeking behavior can be explained as the result of a number of behaviors initiated and governed by many different stimuli—sometimes even the same stimuli acting differently on the insect over a range of concentrations. It loosely encompasses all the orientation behaviors an arthropod employs to find a host. Once the vector's host-seeking behavior locates the host, it alights and blood-feeding behavior, another behavioral chain that employs different close-range stimuli, usually follows. The host-seeking steps may be bypassed in the laboratory but are of critical importance, because those individuals that feed when placed directly on a host are not necessarily those that will seek it from a distance (Mitchell 1981). The term "host-seeking" is itself teleological, because the arthropods never really seek a host as such but simply respond to host kairomones by orienting in their direction.

To a hematophagous vector, the host is merely the packaging for the nutritious fluids found within it. However, because blood is undetectable from afar, hematophagous species cue in on the metabolic by-products of living things that are associated with the presence of blood. These kairomones are released as discontinuous filaments or packets of stimuli, broken up by the wind as they move downwind, much like the dispersion pattern of a smoke plume from a chimney (Murlis et al. 1992). The concentration of a component within an area of the plume is determined by both molecular diffusion and turbulent diffusion, the latter being the major determinant of plume development (Murlis et al. 1992). As turbulence tears the plume apart, the host-seeking insect finds the odor molecules not in a uniform gradient but in a series of odor islands that it must hop between.

Insects responding to pheromone plumes have been studied most intensively; they appear to engage in an upwind optomotor anemotaxis, initiated and modulated by olfactory stimuli and steered by endogenous behavioral programs (Bell and Tobin 1982). As they zigzag within and between plumes in a sustained flight, the odor stimuli act as releasers of fixed action programs that eventually lead the insects to their source. Our concepts of the orientation of vector species to odor molecules are thus based largely on the long-distance orientation of lepidopterans to sex pheromones. Note that the relationship between 2 individuals of the same species attempting to find each other to mate is not the same as that of an individual of 1 species hunting another; their flying strategies might therefore be different. However, in support of the concept, wind-tunnel experiments with mosquitoes have suggested that they do engage in similar tactics. When they first encounter host odor stimuli, they continue to fly without making any turns, but upon leaving the odor plume, their turning rate accelerates, increasing the probability they will reenter the plume (Daykin et al. 1965). Similarly, tsetse flies turn upwind when they enter a plume and turn sharply if they fly out of it (Gibson and Brady 1985, 1988). To explain the optomotor anemotaxis in night-flying mosquitoes that are unable to make full use of visual cues, Gillett (1979) suggested that their tendency to fly low (where the wind gradient is the steepest) and their frequent dipping during flight allows them to sample the wind direction by detecting the wind shear as they dip.

Although we are beginning to understand how insects orient within an odor plume, there is virtually nothing known about the mechanisms of long-distance orientation in arthropod vectors. The maximum distance for which mosquitoes have been shown to orient to host stimuli is between 20 and 35 m (Gillies and Wilkes 1968; Edman 1979); tsetse respond to ox odor plumes as far as 90 m downwind (Vale 1977). Migratory flights by some species, such as the saltmarsh mosquito, *Ae. taeniorhynchus*, can range as far as 40 km from breeding sites (Provost 1957), but this does not appear to be initiated in response to host stimuli. Blood-feeding hemipterans, such as *Rhodnius prolixus* and *Triatoma infestans,* which locate their hosts by crawling on the ground, use mainly the short-range stimuli of heat and odor, with secondary cues from vision and vibration (Wigglesworth and Gillett 1934).

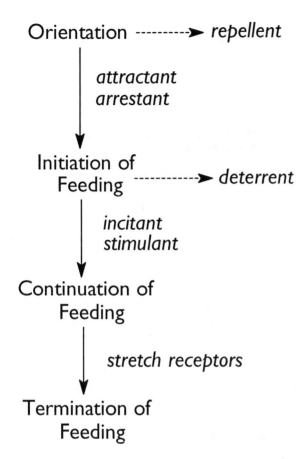

Orientation ‑‑‑‑‑‑‑‑▶ *repellent*

│

attractant
arrestant

▼

Initiation of
Feeding ‑‑‑‑‑‑‑‑▶ *deterrent*

│

incitant
stimulant

▼

Continuation of
Feeding

│

stretch receptors

▼

Termination of
Feeding

3.3   Characterization and behavioral effects of host stimuli

One of the most satisfactory descriptions of the step-wise nature of host-seeking and feeding behaviors is the scheme originally described by Lindstedt (1971) for phytophagous species (Fig. 3.3). In it, a series of behavioral steps are mediated by cues from the host. Attractants are those stimuli to which an arthropod responds by orienting toward its source. The most universal attractant for many species of hematophagous arthropods is carbon dioxide (Gillies 1980; Warnes and Finlayson 1985; Sutcliffe 1986; Takken 1991). CO_2 is normally present in the atmosphere at levels of less than 0.1%, and emanations from hosts can potentially increase these concentrations for as much as 80 m downwind. An active, ranging insect responds not as much to the presence of CO_2 as to the change in the concentration it encounters. Increases in the firing rate of mosquito carbon dioxide receptors have been measured with increases of as little as 0.01% of the gas (Kellogg 1970); changes in behavior have been identified with increases of as little as 0.03% (Eiras and Jepson 1991). Other attractants include octenol, lactic acid, acetone, and unidentified components in animal urine (Acree et al. 1968; Vale 1980; Takken and Kline 1989; Takken 1991), although these are generally synergistic with carbon dioxide and seldom are effective by themselves. Tsetse flies are attracted by both odor and visual cues. The contrast of a host against its background is an important factor in this attraction and enables the tsetse to distinguish distant targets. Indeed, it has been proposed that the pattern of stripes in zebras may have evolved as a defense against biting flies (Waage 1981). By obliterating the animal's sharp visual edge, the stripes make the zebra less likely to be bitten when visual stimuli are the predominant cues in host-seeking. Traps often incorporate illumination in conjunction with other attractants to increase catches at night. The reason insects respond in this way is poorly understood; they may simply be aberrant, as in the case of moths, which are attracted to porch lights. Strong moonlight is often correlated with increased activity in mosquito populations (Bidlingmayer 1974; Charlwood et al. 1986).

It is not enough to be attracted from a distance. Additional behavioral programs must be called into play in order to terminate flight and initiate feeding when the vector approaches the host to alight and feed. Arrestants are stimuli thought to terminate host-seeking behavior when they come into play as closer-range stimuli, such as heat, humidity, and visual cues. Host color, shape, and movement are probably more significant in day-flying insects.

Once on the host, incitants initiate probing. In mosquitoes, this probing is characterized by a series of rhythmic thrusts through the skin of the host, allowing the insect to locate blood from either capillaries or pools (Griffiths and Gordon 1952). Infection with parasites may enhance the ability of mosquitoes to locate blood; when the parasites impair hemostasis, they allow the mosquitoes to find blood more rapidly and thus enhance their own transmission (Ribiero et al. 1985; Rossignol and Rossignol 1988). This probing behavior, associated with the accompanying salivation, is alone sufficient for parasite transmission (Kelly and Edman 1992).

Once blood ingestion commences, phagostimulants in the blood promote the continuation of feeding. Many hematophagous arthropods use adenosine phosphate nucleotides in host blood as phagostimulants (Sutcliffe and McIver 1979; Galun 1987). These nucleotides are also involved in hemostasis; apyrases contained within the injected saliva are able to hydrolyze ATP and ADP, and thus can inhibit normal platelet aggregation and lessen the duration of probing and feeding (Ribiero 1989). Unlike phytophagous species, hematophagous arthropods do not appear to be affected by feeding deterrents once blood ingestion has begun.

If feeding stimulants continue to promote ingestion, the digestive tract will fill with blood and distend the abdomen. Obviously, this feeding behavior must be ultimately terminated lest the vector burst. This termination is accomplished by internal stretch receptors that monitor abdominal distention (Gwadz 1969). Although the specific location of these stretch receptors has yet to be determined, there is considerable evidence for their existence. If a mosquito has just ingested a large sugar meal that causes abdominal distention, it will ingest less blood because its stretch receptors are triggered sooner.

Another behavior (Fig. 3.3) is initiated by repellent compounds. Strictly defined, a repellent is a substance that causes orientation away from its source. By this definition, the chemicals we use to keep hematophagous arthropods from biting are not repellents because they fail to induce this movement. In fact, the most effective and frequently used repellent, "deet" (N,N-diethyl–3-methylbenzamide), has been reported to be an attractant at low concentrations (Mehr et al. 1990). In the model for repellent activity initially presented by Wright (1975) and later modified by McIver (1981), repellents work by creating a pattern in the CNS that the insect does not recognize. By masking the host odors in this way, the "repellent" prevents the insect from matching its sensory across-fiber pattern with the correct behavioral program that will allow it to orient in the direction of the stimuli, and it therefore fails to locate the host. Mosquitoes exposed to host stimuli plus deet in an olfactometer first orient toward the source, but when they get closer, they fly about, apparently unable to precisely identify the origin of the stimuli.

MECHANISMS THAT INHIBIT HOST-SEEKING BEHAVIOR

There are certain hazards inherent to a life of hematophagy. Although ectoparasites that live continuously on a vertebrate host seldom need to worry about their host's behavior, host-seeking insects must often contend with the interference of their feeding by the defensive behavior of their hosts. A tiny animal approaching a host many times its size to feed on blood in order to reproduce is taking a considerable risk. It makes no sense to take these risks and expend energy when the risks would not affect reproductive potential; once blood is ingested and eggs begin to mature, another meal does not normally increase fecundity significantly. The failure of gravid females to engage in host-seeking is reflected in the relatively small numbers normally recovered from attractant traps in the field. Mechanisms have apparently evolved in many species that minimize these risks and allow host-seeking behavior to be expressed only when it is biologically appropriate.

Two mechanisms that inhibit host-seeking behavior have been identified in *Ae. aegypti*. The first is based on abdominal distention. If allowed to feed to repletion, *Ae. aegypti* mosquitoes ingest enough blood to cause the abdomen to swell. This distention triggers stretch receptors in the anterior portion of the abdomen that inhibit host-seeking behavior until the meal has been digested and excreted (Klowden and Lea 1978, 1979b). If the blood volume is below the distention threshold for that individual, host-seeking behavior continues until a blood volume in excess of the threshold is ingested. Thus, a mosquito discouraged by the defensive behavior of its host and prevented from feeding to repletion continues in its attempts to acquire a full meal. However, this persistence depends on nutritional state; sugar-fed mosquitoes are more likely to continue approaching a host when initially discouraged than those that are starved (Walker and Edman 1985).

The second mechanism of host-seeking inhibition is based on a complex cascade of hormonal events that have yet to be precisely identified. This mechanism is initiated if the ingested meal, no matter how large, triggers egg maturation. Mosquitoes fed small blood meals that are below the distention threshold, but that develop eggs, begin to show an inhibition of host-seeking behavior at 30 hr, with a maximal inhibition between 48 and 72 hr. This second mechanism involves the neurosecretory cells of the brain, the ovaries, the fat body, and the male accessory gland substances that have been transferred to the mated female (Klowden and Lea 1979a; Klowden 1981; Klowden et al. 1987; Klowden 1990). Within 8–12 hr following blood ingestion, the ovaries of *Ae. aegypti* produce a factor that initiates the activation of the fat body and the release of a neuropeptide, *Aedes* Head Peptide I, from the neurosecretory cells of the brain and abdominal ganglia (Brown et al. 1994). Both the purified peptide, as well as hemolymph transfused from gravid females into nongravid females, inhibit the host-seeking behavior of the nongravid recipients, apparently by reducing the sensitivity of antennal receptors (Davis 1984). Gravid females are thus less likely to respond to attractants when their sensory receptors fail to recognize them. Following oviposition, host-seeking returns when a nervous system signal from the ovaries signals that they no longer contain eggs (Klowden 1981).

The net result of both these mechanisms reflects the expression of a species' gonotrophic cycle, the concurrence of feeding and egg development (Fig. 3.4). It is commonly assumed that during the gonotrophic cycle, feeding is limited to only once at its beginning. The gonotrophic cycle is therefore a crude but useful tool to estimate the feeding frequency of vector populations;

age-grading of individuals by examining the ovariole dilatations that remain after the eggs have left the ovaries can often determine the number of cycles an individual has undergone (Sokolova 1994). The problem with this concept is that many mathematical models of vector-borne disease erroneously assume that only 1 blood meal occurs during each gonotrophic cycle. In reality, there have been frequent reports of multiple feeding during a single cycle (Boreham et al. 1979; Burkot et al. 1988), and the transmission of pathogens during multiple probing and feeding has also been demonstrated (Klowden and Lea 1981; Kelly and Edman 1992). Multiple feeding can significantly increase the vector potential of a population by increasing the opportunities for acquiring and transmitting parasites.

If, as we discussed, physiological mechanisms are in place that inhibit host-seeking during a gonotrophic

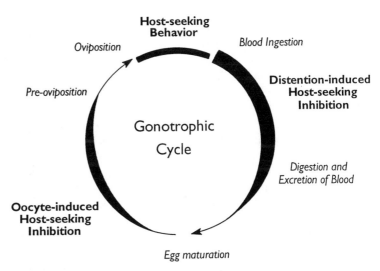

3.4 Physiological events during the mosquito gonotrophic cycle. As a result of host-seeking behavior, the mosquito locates a host and blood is ingested. If the blood meal is large, distention-induced host-seeking inhibition is triggered, tapering off as the blood is assimilated and excreted. Eggs mature from the precursors in the blood, producing oocyte-induced host-seeking inhibition, which gradually develops and then fades. Mature eggs also induce preoviposition behavior, which leads to oviposition. In some mosquitoes that are maintained in the lab under optimal nutritional conditions, host-seeking is confined to the beginning of the cycle.

cycle, then what accounts for this occurrence of multiple feeding in field populations? There are several ways in which vectors might ignore the physiological rules and continue to feed. One factor is undoubtedly the defensive behavior of hosts, which discourages feeding and may limit the size of blood meals (Edman and Kale 1971; Klowden and Lea 1979c; Edman and Scott 1987). Black flies also often fail to acquire replete meals (Barbiero and Trpis 1986). If small meals below or just above the distention threshold are ingested, then it is likely that the insects will return to a host as soon as abdominal distention is reduced. Age is also a factor. Chronologically and gonotrophically older females are more likely to engage in host-seeking when gravid than are younger females (Klowden and Lea 1984). If the insect is undernourished during the larval or adult stages, some of the blood may be utilized by the female for her own reserves, and eggs do not develop at all, with the consequent failure of oocyte-induced inhibition (Feinsod and Spielman 1980). The nutritional state can also affect the intensity of the inhibition when eggs do develop; suboptimally nourished gravid females are more likely to respond to host stimuli than are well-fed gravid females (Klowden 1986). The extent of the behavioral inhibition of host-seeking also is dependent on whether she has mated (Klowden and Lea 1979a), and even on the nutritional state of the male with which she mates (Fernandez and Klowden 1995). Female *Ae. aegypti* that have mated with well-fed males fail to seek a host during oogenesis, but those mated with males maintained on poor adult diets are more likely to continue host-seeking. An unmated mosquito will feed on blood and develop eggs, but the eggs usually can not be oviposited until she has mated.

Then, there are some vector species that routinely do not abide by any of these rules. For example, fully blood-fed and gravid *Anopheles gambiae* continue to seek a host for a blood meal every 24 hr (Klowden and Briegel 1994). Although repletion appears to inhibit host-seeking in this species, egg development does not. Similarly, *Haemogogus janthinomys* mosquitoes show no correlation between host-seeking behavior and the presence of eggs (Chadee et al. 1992). If the mechanisms that inhibit host-seeking indeed evolved

in response to defensive host behavior, it makes sense that day-biting insects such as *Aedes* would be subject to more intense selective pressures than crepuscular feeders such as *Anopheles* and *Haemagogus*, which feed when their hosts are less active and less defensive.

OTHER BEHAVIORS OF VECTORS

To determine what vectors may be doing at any moment, it is necessary to capture them in the act of behaving. This poses little difficulty for the evaluation of blood-feeding behavior, because it is fairly easy for a collector to attract vectors passively using nothing more than his or her inherent scent and a collection aspirator. Consequently, we have relatively more information about hematophagy and all the behaviors that encompass it than about most other behaviors. Common sampling methods generally preclude the direct evaluation of these other behaviors, so for the most part, they have been determined by inference rather than direct observation. Many techniques evaluate insects that are at the end point of their behavioral continuum and are not necessarily observed in the act of behaving. Thus, host-seeking behavior is inferred when insects are recovered from an attractant trap, oviposition behavior when eggs are observed, and mating behavior when females are inseminated. Service (1976) and Muirhead-Thomson (1991) have surveyed recent trap designs and their relative efficacies.

Resting probably occupies most of the adult vector's time, and knowledge of where and when vectors rest is essential in order to expose them maximally to residual insecticides for control. However, searches for resting insects are often unproductive because of inappropriate sampling (Rehn et al. 1950; Bidlingmayer 1971; Bidlingmayer 1985). Attractant traps sample only the host-seeking population, and even relatively nonselective suction traps are biased toward the flying population. Some of the more important vector species may rest in the shelters of humans or other animals before and after they feed on the inhabitants and can be collected within the shelters (Gillies 1955) or trapped in specially designed resting boxes (Edman et al. 1968). Some species may rest in grassy areas exposed to the sun (Bidlingmayer 1971), whereas many others rest in woodlands and "commute" to open areas to feed (Bidlingmayer and Hem 1981).

Surviving the winter presents special problems for poikilothermic animals. Although some vector species overwinter as eggs or larvae, several, particularly mosquitoes in the genera *Culex*, *Culiseta*, and *Anopheles*, overwinter as adults (Mitchell 1988). This overwintering is possible because of special physiological and behavioral adaptations that prepare the female for the winter well in advance of the unfavorable conditions; these adaptations are induced primarily by a juvenile hormone deficiency (Spielman 1974; Case et al. 1977). Among the adaptations associated with the diapause state are a fat body hypertrophy and an uncoupling of the gonotrophic cycle in which blood-feeding no longer is tied to reproduction, or a "gonotrophic dissociation." Although females will often blood-feed if the preliminary host-seeking steps are bypassed in the laboratory (Mitchell 1981), there is some question as to whether this ever occurs in the field, and thus the gonotrophic dissociation may be no more than a laboratory artifact. In *Culex* females, host-seeking and blood ingestion do not naturally occur during diapause because of a reduced sensitivity of lactic acid receptors (Bowen et al. 1988), and the females are unable to utilize the blood even when it is ingested (Mitchell and Breigel 1989). Diapausing females can often be found in artificial shelters that retain an increased humidity (Mail and McHugh 1961), in animal burrows, or on grasses under snow cover (Hopla 1970). Although there must be a behavioral program associated with finding these sites, there have been no attempts to identify this behavior or the mechanism by which these hibernacula are located.

Many hematophagous vectors, with the notable exception of tsetse flies, must also feed on carbohydrate to derive energy for flight and survival (Hocking 1968; Nayar and Sauerman 1975; Foster 1995). As is the case for host-seeking, the expression of sugar-feeding behavior appears to be regulated by a circadian clock (Gillett et al. 1962; Grimstad and DeFoliart 1975; Yee and Foster 1992). Mosquitoes are attracted by floral scents (Thorsteinson and Brust 1962) consisting of cyclic and bicyclic monoterpenes (Healy and Jepson 1988; Jepson and Healy 1988; Bowen 1992b),

although considering the widespread distribution of honeydew on leaf surfaces and the presence of tarsal sugar receptors in many insects (Downes and Dahlem 1987), it is probably not necessary to invoke a sugar-seeking behavioral program at all. Insects may simply be required to land on the upper surface of vegetation to find carbohydrate deposits, and sugar-feeding patterns are often coincident with general activity patterns (Grimstad and DeFoliart 1975).

Mosquitoes often mate in swarms; aggregations of males usually appear at twilight over prominent physical markers, such as fence posts, trees, or bushes. The swarm is not dependent on the interactions of its members; each male engages in swarming and reacts to visual stimuli independently of other males. Simulating the conditions under which swarming will occur has proven difficult and has impeded establishing laboratory colonies of some species. In the field, unmated females can be observed entering these swarms, and after males identify them by their wing beat frequencies, fly off *in copulo* (Bates 1941; Nielsen and Haeger 1960; Charlwood and Jones 1980). Unfortunately, it is difficult to demonstrate that insemination of the female has actually occurred during this ritual, or even that it is only unmated females that enter the swarm. The males bear plumose antennae that are used to identify the wing beat frequency of potential mates (Roth 1948), but some species may also use pheromones for species recognition (Provost and Haeger 1967). In some cases, mating occurs in the vicinity of vertebrate host, with both males and females attracted to host stimuli (Hartberg 1971).

Adult male *Ae. aegypti* become increasingly responsive to female wing beat frequency with postemergence age, corresponding to the maturational extension of their antennal fibrillae (Roth 1948). In male *Anopheles*, the erection of these antennal hairs occurs during a circadian window and is responsible for the daily period of responsiveness of the males to female vibrational stimuli (Nijhout and Sheffield 1979; Beach 1980). As in many other dipterans, male mosquitoes must undergo a rotation of their terminalia before they can mate (Christophers 1915). The muscles in the abdomen that cause this rotation have been identified

(Chevone and Richards 1976), but the releaser that affects them has not.

When a male and female copulate, the male first transfers sperm from the testes and substances produced in his accessory reproductive gland to the bursa copulatrix, a small sac within the female reproductive tract. Female mosquitoes may copulate shortly after emergence, but only mature females are able to retain the semen within their genital tracts (Spielman et al. 1969; Lea and Edman 1972). The length of the post-emergence refractory period is regulated by juvenile hormone (Lea 1968; Gwadz et al. 1971). In the biting stable fly, *Stomoxys calcitrans,* blood ingestion is a prerequisite for production of seminal fluid by the male accessory glands; males cannot inseminate a female without first ingesting a blood meal (Anderson 1978). The male substances then migrate to the sclerotized capsule-like spermathecae (Spielman 1964). Some of the substances also enter the hemolymph and migrate to other locations (Young and Downe 1987), but the sperm remain within the spermathecae and are released for fertilization when a mature egg passes through the oviduct just prior to oviposition.

These male substances can profoundly alter the physiology and behavior of many female arthropods (Lomas and Kaufman 1992; Chen 1984). In mosquitoes, they inhibit subsequent mating activity (Craig 1967), although this inhibition does not last for the life of the female (Young and Downe 1982), and also remove a physiological block that prevents oviposition (Fuchs and Kang 1978; Hiss and Fuchs 1972). Male accessory gland substances also modulate other behaviors; host-seeking behavior during oogenesis is inhibited and preoviposition behavior stimulated in mated mosquitoes. As mentioned previously, mating also affects the levels of spontaneous activity (Jones and Gubbins 1978). Male accessory gland substances can affect reproduction by stimulating autogeny (O'Meara and Evans 1977) and increasing fecundity (Klowden and Chambers 1991).

Polyandry, the insemination of a female by more than 1 male, has been frequently reported for other insects. Although male substances terminate the female mating programs of a number of dipteran species, under some circumstances they mate more than once. This is an important consideration that has implications for any attempts to control vector populations by genetic means (Curtis 1985; Gomulski 1990). If new genes that modify vector competence are to be introduced into a vector population, it would be preferable that after the females mated with the modified males they would become refractory to the advances of native males so that the introduced genes are not diluted. For example, interrupted mating may not prevent the female mosquito from mating again (Gwadz and Craig 1970), and there is also a short postcopulatory period during which a subsequent mating may occur before the effects of the male accessory gland substances are manifested (Craig 1967).

Metamorphosis is thought to reduce the competition between immature and adult insects by dividing the life cycle into stages that occupy vastly different ecological niches. However, in the case of adult insects with aquatic larvae, it means that a behavioral program must exist that allows the adult to change its normal terrestrial routine and return to a habitat conducive to larval survival. For example, the adult female mosquito, although normally attracted to host stimuli, must be programmed to return to water to lay her eggs (Fig. 3.5).

The releaser for this preoviposition behavior in *Ae. aegypti* is a hemolymph-borne factor that is produced during egg development (Klowden and Blackmer 1987). This factor changes the responsiveness of the female to oviposition site stimuli until after the eggs are laid; nongravid females injected with the hemolymph of gravid females are more responsive to oviposition site stimuli. Only mated females respond to oviposition sites when gravid. Unmated females are not only blocked from laying any eggs that develop but also from expending the energy that they would invest in preoviposition behavior when their unfertilized eggs would not be viable (Yeh and Klowden 1990). The female thus needs at least 3 inputs to initiate preoviposition behavior: She must receive a signal from developing eggs that they are mature, a signal from a potential oviposition site, and a signal from male accessory gland substances that tells her she has mated (Klowden 1990).

Once long-distance stimuli bring the female to the oviposition site, other closer-range visual and tactile stimuli invoke the oviposition subroutine that results in the eggs being laid (Bentley and Day 1989). Factors such as color and texture can be distinguished, and females have been shown to preferentially oviposit on certain sites. Theoretically, there are times when host-seeking and preoviposition can both be expressed, but the priorities that gravid females use to decide which behavioral program should be engaged in when they are confronted with both host stimuli and oviposition site stimuli are not yet understood.

As we contemplate novel ways to control vectors, we might well look into how parasites have accomplished the same goals by manipulating their behavior. The parasitic ciliate *Lambornella clarki* infects the ovaries of *Ae. sierrensis,* and induces the females to engage in preoviposition behavior as well as a pseudooviposition, although the insects have been parasitically castrated and contain no mature eggs. The behavior of the mosquito has been manipulated by this parasite in order to distribute itself to breeding sites and to other potential hosts (Egerter et al. 1986). Host-seeking behavior is inhibited at the same time (Egerter and Anderson 1989). Whether the parasite itself has evolved the ability to synthesize and release its own behavior-modifying hormones that mimic those of the mosquito or simply "fools" the infected ovary into inducing the normal array of hormones is an intriguing question waiting to be answered.

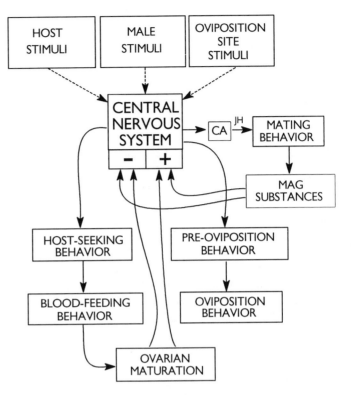

3.5 Control of mosquito behaviors. The central nervous system is alerted that stimuli from potential hosts, mates, and oviposition sites are nearby. With stimuli from a male, the female engages in copulatory behavior once the corpora allata (CA) release juvenile hormone (JH). The male accessory gland (MAG) substances introduced during mating both stimulate and inhibit several behaviors. Host stimuli induce the expression of host-seeking and blood-feeding behaviors, which culminate in the ingestion of blood. Maturing ovaries then initiate a behavioral inhibition of host-seeking, modulated by MAG substances. In the presence of oviposition site stimuli, maturing ovaries, and MAG substances, preoviposition behavior, and ultimately oviposition behavior, are expressed.

REFERENCES

Acree, F.R.B. Tuner, H.K. Gouk, M. Beroza, and C.N. Smith. 1968. L-lactic acid: A mosquito attractant isolated from humans. *Science* 161:1346–1347.

Anderson, J.R. 1978. Mating behavior of *Stomoxys calcitrans*: Effects of a blood meal on the mating drive of males and its necessity as a prerequisite for proper insemination of females. *J. Econ. Entomol.* 71:379–386.

Barbiero, V.K., and M. Trpis. 1986. The engorgement ratio of *Simulium yahense* (Diptera: Simuliidae) at the Firestone Rubber Plantation, Harbel, Liberia. *J. Med. Entomol.* 23:309–312.

Bates, M. 1941. Laboratory observations on the sexual behavior of anopheline mosquitoes. *J. Exp. Zool.* 86:153–173.

Beach, R. 1980. Physiological changes governing the onset of sexual receptivity in male mosquitoes. *J. Insect Physiol.* 26:245–252.

Bell, W.J., and T.R. Tobin. 1982. Chemo-orientation. *Biol. Rev.* 57:219–260.

Bentley, M.D., and J.F. Day. 1989. Chemical ecology and behavioral aspects of mosquito oviposition. *Ann. Rev. Entomol.* 34:401–421.

Berry, W.J., W.A. Rowley, and B.M. Christensen. 1986. Influence of developing *Brugia pahangi* on spontaneous flight activity of *Aedes aegypti* (Diptera: Culicidae). *J. Med. Entomol.* 23:441–445.

Bidlingmayer, W.L. 1971. Mosquito flight paths in relation to the environment. 1. Illumination levels, orientation, and resting areas. *Ann. Entomol. Soc. Am.* 64:1121–1131.

Bidlingmayer, W.L. 1974. The influence of environmental factors and physiological stage on flight patterns of mosquitoes taken in the vehicle aspirator and truck, suction, bait and New Jersey light traps. *J. Med. Entomol.* 11:119–146.

Bidlingmayer, W.L. 1985. The measurement of adult mosquito population changes—some considerations. *J. Am. Mosq. Control Assoc.* 1:328–348.

Bidlingmayer, W.L., and D.G. Hem. 1981. Mosquito flight paths in relation to the environment. Effect of the forest edge upon trap catches in the field. *Mosq. News* 41:55–59.

Boreham, P.F.L., J.K. Lenahan, R. Boulzaquet, J. Storey, T.S. Ashkar, R. Nambiar, and T. Matsushima. 1979. Studies on multiple feeding by *Anopheles gambiae* s.l. in a Sudan savanna area north of Nigeria. *Trans. R. Soc. Trop. Med. Hyg.* 73:418–423.

Bowen, M.F., E.E. Davis, and D.A. Haggart. 1988. A behavioural and sensory analysis of host-seeking behaviour in the diapausing mosquito *Culex pipiens*. *J. Insect Physiol.* 34:805–813.

Bowen, M.F. 1992a. Lack of correlation between peripheral receptor sensitivity and the daily pattern of host-seeking behavior in female *Culex pipiens* mosquitoes. *Bull. Soc. Vector Ecol.* 17:20–24.

Bowen, M.F. 1992b. Terpene-sensitive receptors in female *Culex pipiens* mosquitoes: Electrophysiology and behaviour. *J. Insect Physiol.* 38:759–764.

Brady, J. 1975. 'Hunger' in the tsetse fly: The nutritional correlates of behaviour. *J. Insect Physiol.* 21:807–829.

Briegel, H. 1985. Mosquito reproduction: Incomplete utilization of the blood meal protein for oögenesis. *J. Insect Physiol.* 31:15–21.

Brown, M.R., M.J. Klowden, J.W. Crim, L. Young, L.A. Shrouder, and A.O. Lea. 1994. Endogenous regulation of mosquito host-seeking behavior by a neuropeptide. *J. Insect Physiol.* 40:399–406.

Burkot, T.R., P.M. Graves, R. Paru, and M. Lagog. 1988. Mixed blood feeding by the malaria vectors in the *Anopheles punctulatus* complex (Diptera: Culicidae). *J. Med. Entomol.* 25:205–213.

Case, T.J., R.K. Washino, and R.L. Dunn. 1977. Diapause termination in *Anopheles freeborni* with juvenile hormone mimics. *Entomol. Exp. Appl.* 21:155–162.

Chadee, D.D., E.S. Tikasingh, and R. Ganesh. 1992. Seasonality, biting cycle and parity of the yellow fever vector mosquito *Haemagogus janthinomys* in Trinidad. *Med. Vet. Entomol.* 6:143–148.

Charlwood, J.D., and M.D.R. Jones. 1980. Mating in the mosquito, *Anopheles gambiae* s.l. II. Swarming behavior. *Physiol. Entomol.* 5:315–320.

Charlwood, J.D., R. Paru, H. Dagaro, and M. Lagog. 1986. Influence of moonlight and gonotrophic age on biting activity of *Anopheles farauti* (Diptera: Culicidae). *J. Med. Entomol.* 23:132–135.

Chen P.S. 1984. The functional morphology and biochemistry of insect male accessory glands and their secretions. *Ann. Rev. Entomol.* 29:233–255.

Chevone, B.I., and A.G. Richards. 1976. Ultrastructure of the atypic muscles associated with terminalial inversion in male *Aedes aegypti* (L). *Biol. Bull.* 151:283–296.

Chiba, Y.Y. Shinkawa, M. Yoshii, A. Matsumoto, K. Tomioka, and Y. Susumu. 1992. A comparative study on insemination dependency of circadian activity pattern in mosquitoes. *Physiol. Entomol.* 17:213–218.

Christophers, S.R. 1915. The male genitalia of *Anopheles*. *Ind. J. Med. Res.* 3:371–394.

Coluzzi, M., A. Sabatini, V. Petrarca, and M.A. Di Deco. 1977. Behavioural divergences between mosquitoes with different inversion karyotypes in polymorphic populations of the *Anopheles gambiae* complex. *Nature* 266:832–833.

Coluzzi, M., A. Sabatini, V. Petrarca, and M.A. Di Deco. 1979. Chromosomal differentiation and adaptation to human environments in the *Anopheles gambiae* complex. *Trans. R. Soc. Trop. Med. Hyg.* 73:483–497.

Curtis, C.F. 1985. Genetic control of insect pests: Growth industry or lead balloon? *Biol. J. Linn. Soc.* 26:359–374.

Craig, G.B. Jr. 1967. Mosquitoes: Female monogamy induced by a male accessory gland substance. *Science* 156:1499–1501.

Davis, E.E. 1984. Regulation of sensitivity in the peripheral chemoreceptor systems for host-seeking behaviour by a haemolymph-borne factor in *Aedes aegypti*. *J. Insect Physiol.* 30:179–183.

Daykin, P.N., F.E. Kellogg, and R.H. Wright. 1965. Host-finding and repulsion of *Aedes aegypti*. *Canad. Entomol.* 97:239–263.

Dethier, V.G. 1957. The sensory physiology of blood-sucking arthropods. *Exp. Parasitol.* 6:68–122.

Downes, W.J. Jr., and G.A. Dahlem. 1987. Keys to the evolution of Diptera: Role of Homoptera. *Envir. Entomol.* 16:847–854.

Edman, J.D. 1979. Orientation of some Florida mosquitoes (Diptera: Culicidae) toward small vertebrates and carbon dioxide in the field. *J. Med. Entomol.* 15:292–296.

Edman, J.D., and H.W. Kale II. 1971. Host behavior: Its influence on the feeding success of mosquitoes. *Ann. Entomol. Soc. Amer.* 64:513–516.

Edman, J.D., F.D.S. Evans, and J.A. Williams. 1968. Development of a diurnal resting box to collect *Culiseta melanura* (Coq.). *Am. J. Trop. Med. Hyg.* 17:451–456.

Edman, J.D., and T.W. Scott. 1987. Host defensive behaviour and the feeding success of mosquitoes. *Insect Sci. Appl.* 8:617–622.

Egerter, D.E., and J.R. Anderson. 1989. Blood-feeding drive inhibition of *Aedes sierrensis* (Diptera: Culicidae) induced by the parasite *Lambornella clarki* (Ciliophora: Tetrahymenidae) *J. Med. Entomol.* 26:46–54.

Egerter, D.E., J.R. Anderson, and J.O. Washburn. 1986. Dispersal of the parasitic ciliate *Lambornella clarki*: Implications for ciliates in the biological control of mosquitoes. *Proc. Natl. Acad. Sci. USA* 83:7335–7339.

Eiras, A.E., and P.C. Jepson. 1991. Host location by *Aedes aegypti* (Diptera: Culicidae): A wind tunnel study of chemical cues. *Bull. Entomol. Res.* 81:151–160.

Feinsod, F.M., and A. Spielman. 1980. Nutrient-mediated juvenile hormone secretion in mosquitoes. *J. Insect Physiol.* 26:113–117.

Fernandez, N.M., and M.J. Klowden. 1995. Male accessory gland substances modify the host-seeking behavior of gravid *Aedes aegypti* mosquitoes. *J. Insect Physiol.* (in press).

Foster, W.A. 1995. Mosquito sugar feeding and reproductive energetics. *Ann. Rev. Entomol.* 40:443–474.

Fuchs, M.S., and S.-H. Kang. 1978. Evidence for a naturally occurring inhibitor of oviposition in *Aedes aegypti*. *Ann. Entomol. Soc. Am.* 71:473–475.

Galun, R. 1987. Regulation of blood gorging. *Insect Sci. Appl.* 8:623–625.

Gibson, G., and J. Brady. 1985. 'Anemotactic' flight paths of tsetse flies in relation to host odour: A preliminary video study in nature of the response to loss of odour. *Physiol. Entomol.* 10:395–406.

Gibson, G., and J. Brady. 1988. Flight behavior of tsetse flies in host odour plumes: The initial response to leaving or entering odour. *Physiol. Entomol.* 13:29–42.

Gillett, 1979. Out for blood; flight orientation up-wind in the absence of visual cues. *Mosq. News* 39:221–229.

Gillett, J.D., A.J. Haddow, and P.S. Corbet. 1962. The sugar-feeding-cycle in a cage-population of mosquitoes. *Entomol. Exp. Appl.* 5:223–232.

Gillies, M.T. 1955. The density of adult *Anopheles* in the neighbourhood of an East African village. *Am. J. Trop. Med. Hyg.* 4:1103–1113.

Gillies, M.T. 1980. The role of carbon dioxide in host-finding by mosquitoes (Diptera: Culicidae): A review. *Bull. Entomol. Res.* 70:525–532.

Gillies, M.T., and T.J. Wilkes. 1968. A comparison of the range of attraction of animal baits and of carbon dioxide for some West African mosquitoes. *Bull. Entomol. Res.* 59:441–456.

Gomulski, L. 1990. Polyandry in nulliparous *Anopheles gambiae* mosquitoes (Diptera: Culicidae). *Bull. Entomol. Res.* 80:393–396.

Griffiths, R.B., and R.M. Gordon. 1952. An apparatus which enables the process of feeding by mosquitoes to be observed in tissues of a live rodent, together with an account of the ejection of saliva and its significance in malaria. *Ann. Trop. Med.* 46:311–319.

Grimstad, P.R., and G.R. DeFoliart. 1975. Mosquito nectar feeding in Wisconsin in relation to twilight and microclimate. *J. Med. Entomol.* 11:691–698.

Gwadz, R.W. 1969. Regulation of blood meal size in the mosquito. *J. Insect Physiol.* 15:2039–2044.

Gwadz, R.W., and G.B. Craig Jr. 1970. Female polygamy due to inadequate semen transfer in *Aedes aegypti*. *Mosq. News* 30:354–360.

Gwadz, R.W., L.P. Lounibos, and G.B. Craig Jr. 1971. Precocious sexual receptivity induced by a juvenile hormone analogue in females of the yellow fever mosquito, *Aedes aegypti*. *Gen. Comp. Endocrinol.* 16:47–51.

Hartberg, W.K. 1971. Observations on the mating behaviour of *Aedes aegypti* in nature. *Bull. Wld. Hlth. Org.* 45:847–850.

Healy, T.P., and P.C. Jepson. 1988. The location of floral nectar sources by mosquitoes: The long-range responses of *Anopheles arabiensis* Patton (Diptera: Culicidae) to *Achillea millefolium* flowers and isolated floral nectar. *Bull. Entomol. Res.* 78:651–657.

Hiss, E.A., and M.S. Fuchs. 1972. The effect of matrone on oviposition in the mosquito *Aedes aegypti*. *J. Insect Physiol.* 18:2217–2227.

Hocking, B. 1968. Insect-flower associations in the high Arctic with special reference to nectar. *Oikos* 19:359–388.

Hockmeyer, W.T., B.A. Schiefer, B.C. Redington, and B.F. Eldridge. 1975. *Brugia pahangi*: Effects upon the flight capability of *Aedes aegypti*. *Exp. Parasitol.* 38:1–5.

Hopla, C.E. 1970. The natural history of the genus *Culiseta* in Alaska. Proc. 57th N.J. Mosq. Extermin. Assoc. pp. 56–70.

Husain, A., and W.E. Kershaw. 1971. The effect of filariasis on the ability of a vector mosquito to fly and feed and to transmit the infection. *Trans. R. Soc. Trop. Med. Hyg.* 65:617–619.

Jepson, P.C., and T.P. Healy. 1988. The location of floral nectar sources by mosquitoes: An advanced bioassay for volatile plant odours and initial studies with *Aedes aegypti* (L.) (Diptera: Culicidae). *Bull. Entomol. Res.* 78:641–650.

Jones, M.D.R. 1981. The programming of circadian flight-activity in relation to mating and the gonotrophic cycle in the mosquito, *Aedes aegypti*. *Physiol. Entomol.* 6:307–313.

Jones, M.D.R., and S.J. Gubbins. 1977. Modification of circadian flight activity in the mosquito *Anopheles gambiae* after insemination. *Nature* 268:731–732.

Jones, M.D.R., and S.J. Gubbins. 1978. Changes in the circadian flight activity of the mosquito *Anopheles gambiae* in relation to insemination, feeding and oviposition. *Physiol. Entomol.* 3:213–220.

Kellogg, F.E. 1970. Water vapour and carbon dioxide receptors in *Aedes aegypti*. *J. Insect Physiol.* 16:99–108.

Kelly, R., and J.D. Edman. 1992. Multiple transmission of *Plasmodium gallinaceum* (Eucoccida: Plasmodiidae) during serial probing by *Aedes aegypti* (Diptera: Culicidae) on several hosts. *J. Med. Entomol.* 29:329–331.

Klowden, M.J. 1981. Initiation and termination of host-seeking inhibition in *Aedes aegypti* during oocyte maturation. *J. Insect Physiol.* 27:799–803.

Klowden, M. J. 1986. Effects of sugar deprivation on the host-seeking behaviour of gravid *Aedes aegypti* mosquitoes. *J. Insect Physiol.* 32:479–483.

Klowden, M.J. 1990. The endogenous regulation of mosquito reproductive behaviour. *Experientia* 46:660–670.

Klowden, M.J., and J.L. Blackmer. 1987. Humoral control of pre-oviposition behaviour in the mosquito, *Aedes aegypti*. *J. Insect. Physiol.* 33:689–692.

Klowden, M.J., and H. Briegel. 1994. Mosquito gonotrophic cycle and multiple feeding potential: Contrasts between *Anopheles* and *Aedes* (Diptera: Culicidae). *J. Med. Entomol.* 31:618–622.

Klowden, M.J., and G.M. Chambers. 1991. Male accessory gland substances activate egg development in nutritionally stressed *Aedes aegypti* mosquitoes. *J. Insect Physiol.* 37:721–726.

Klowden, M.J., E.E. Davis, and M.F. Bowen. 1987. Role of the fat body in the control of host-seeking behaviour in the mosquito, *Aedes aegypti*. *J. Insect. Physiol.* 33:643–646.

Klowden, M.J., and A.O. Lea. 1978. Blood meal size as a factor affecting continued host-seeking by *Aedes aegypti* (L.). *Amer. J. Trop. Med. Hyg.* 27:827–831.

Klowden, M.J., and A.O. Lea. 1979a. Humoral inhibition of host-seeking in *Aedes aegypti* (L.) during oocyte maturation. *J. Insect Physiol.* 25:231–235.

Klowden, M.J., and A.O. Lea. 1979b. Effect of defensive host behavior on the blood meal size and feeding success of natural populations of mosquitoes (Diptera: Culicidae). *J. Med. Entomol.* 15:514–517.

Klowden, M.J., and A.O. Lea. 1979c. Abdominal distention terminates subsequent host-seeking behaviour of *Aedes aegypti* following a blood meal. *J. Insect Physiol.* 25:583–585.

Klowden, M.J., and A.O. Lea. 1981. Laboratory transmission of *Brugia pahangi* by nulliparous *Aedes aegypti* (Diptera: Culicidae). *J. Med. Entomol.* 18:383–385.

Klowden, M.J., and A.O. Lea. 1984. Blood-feeding affects age-related changes in mosquito host-seeking behavior during oocyte maturation. *J. Med. Entomol.* 21:274–277.

Lea, A.O. 1968. Mating without insemination in virgin *Aedes aegypti*. *J. Insect Physiol.* 14:305–308.

Lea, A.O., and J.D. Edman. 1972. Sexual behavior of mosquitoes. 3. Age dependence of insemination of *Culex nigripalpus* and *C. pipiens quinquefasciatus* in nature. *Ann. Entomol. Soc. Amer.* 65:290–293.

Lindstedt, K.J. 1971. Chemical control of feeding behavior. *Comp. Biochem. Physiol.* 39A:553–581.

Lomas, L.O., and W.R. Kaufman. 1992. The influence of a factor from the male genital tract on salivary gland degeneration in the female ixodid tick, *Amblyomma hebraeum. J. Insect Physiol.* 38:595–601.

Lowther, J.K., and D.M. Wood. 1964. Specificity of a black fly, *Simulium euryadminiculum* Davies, towards its host, the common loon. *Canad. Entomol.* 96:911–913.

Mail, G.A., and R.A. McHugh. 1961. Relation of temperature and humidity to winter survival of *Culex pipiens* and *Culex tarsalis. Mosq. News* 21:252–254.

McIver, S.B. 1981. A model for the mechanism of action of the repellent DEET on *Aedes aegypti* (Diptera: Culicidae). *J. Med. Entomol.* 18:357–361.

McKeever, S., and F.E. French. 1991. *Corethrella* (Diptera: Corethrellidae) of eastern North America: Laboratory life history and field responses to anuran calls. *Ann. Entomol. Soc. Am.* 84:493–497.

Mehr, Z.A., L.C. Rutledge, M.D. Buescher, R.K. Gupta, and M.M. Zakaria. 1990. Attraction of mosquitoes to diethyl methylbenzamide and ethyl hexanediol. *J. Am. Mosq. Control Assoc.* 6:469–476.

Mitchell, C.J. 1981. Diapause termination, gonoactivity, and differentiation of host-seeking behavior from blood-feeding behavior in hibernating *Culex tarsalis* (Diptera: Culicidae). *J. Med. Entomol.* 5:386–394.

Mitchell, C.J. 1988. Occurrence, biology, and physiology of diapause in overwintering mosquitoes. In: T.P. Monath, ed., *The arboviruses: Epidemiology and ecology*, Vol 1. Boca Raton, FL: CRC Press. pp. 191–217.

Mitchell, C.J., and H. Briegel. 1989. Fate of the blood meal in force-fed, diapausing *Culex pipiens* (Diptera: Culicidae). *J. Med. Entomol.* 26:332–341.

Muirhead-Thomson, R.C. 1991. *Trap responses of flying insects*. NY: Academic Press. 287 p.

Murlis, J., J.S. Elkinton, and R.T. Cardé. 1992. Odor plumes and how insects use them. *Ann. Rev. Entomol.* 37:505–532.

Nayar, J.K., and D.M. Sauerman Jr. 1973. A comparative study of flight performance and fuel utilization as a function of age in females of Florida mosquitoes. *J. Insect Physiol.* 19:1977–1988.

Nayar, J.K., and D.M. Sauerman Jr. 1975. The effects of nutrition on survival and fecundity in Florida mosquitoes. Part 1. Utilization of sugar for survival. *J. Med. Entomol.* 12:92–98.

Nayar, J.K., and E. Van Handel. 1971. The fuel for sustained mosquito flight. *J. Insect Physiol.* 17:471–481.

Nelson, M.C. 1977. The blowfly's dance: Role in the regulation of food intake. *J. Insect Physiol.* 23:603–611.

Nielsen, E.T., and J.S. Haeger. 1960. Swarming and mating in mosquitoes. *Misc. Publ. Entomol. Soc. Am.* 1:71–95.

Nijhout, H.F., and H.G. Sheffield. 1979. Antennal hair erection in male mosquitoes: A new mechanical effector in insects. *Science* 206:595–596.

O'Meara, G.F, and D.G. Evans 1977. Autogeny in saltmarsh mosquitoes induced by a substance from the male accessory gland. *Nature* 267:342–344.

Packer, M.J., and P.S. Corbet. 1989. Seasonal emergence, host-seeking activity, age composition and reproductive biology of the mosquito, *Aedes punctor. Ecol. Entomol.* 14:433–442.

Provost, M.W. 1957. The dispersal of *Aedes taeniorhynchus*. 2. The second experiment. *Mosq. News* 12:233–247.

Provost, M.W., and J.S. Haeger. 1967. Mating and pupal attendance in *Deinocerites cancer* and comparisons with *Opifex fuscus* (Diptera: Culicidae). *Ann. Entomol. Soc. Am.* 60:565–574.

Rehn, J.W.H., J. Maldonado Capriles, and J.M. Henderson. 1950. Field studies on the bionomics of *Anopheles albimanus*. Parts 2 and 3, Diurnal resting places-progress report. *J. Natl. Malar. Soc.* 9:268–279.

Ribeiro, J.M.C. 1989. Vector saliva and its role in parasite transmission. *Exp. Parasitol.* 69:104–106.

Ribeiro, J.M.C., P.A. Rossignol, and A. Spielman. 1985. *Aedes aegypti*: Model for blood finding strategy and prediction of parasite manipulation. *Exp. Parasitol.* 60:118–132.

Rossignol, P.A., and A.M. Rossignol. 1988. Simulations of enhanced malaria transmission and host bias induced by modified vector blood location behaviour. *Parasitol.* 97:363–372.

Roth, L.M. 1948. A study of mosquito behavior. An experimental laboratory study of the sexual behavior of *Aedes aegypti* (Linnaeus). *Am. Midl. Nat.* 40:265–352.

Rowland, M. 1989. Changes in the circadian flight activity of the mosquito *Anopheles stephensi* associated with insemination, blood-feeding, oviposition and nocturnal light intensity, *Physiol. Entomol.* 14:77–84.

Rowland, M., and S.W. Lindsay. 1985. The circadian flight activity of *Aedes aegypti* parasitized with the filarial nematode *Brugia pahangi. Physiol. Entomol.* 11:325–334.

Scheller, R.H., and R. Axel. 1984. How genes control an innate behavior. *Sci. Amer.* 250:54–83.

Scheller, R.H., R.-R. Kaldany, T. Kreiner, A.C. Mahon, J.R. Nambu, M. Schaefer, and R. Taussig. 1984. Neuropeptides: Mediators of behavior in *Aplysia*. *Science* 225:1300–1308.

Service, M.W. 1976. *Mosquito ecology: Field sampling methods.* N.Y.: Halsted Press, 583 p.

Sokolova, M.I. 1994. A redescription of the morphology of mosquito (Diptera: Culicidae) ovarioles during vitellogenesis. *Bull. Soc. Vect. Ecol.* 19:53–68.

Spielman, A. 1964. The mechanics of copulation in *Aedes aegypti. Biol. Bull.* 127:324–344.

Spielman, A. 1974. Effect of synthetic juvenile hormone on ovarian diapause of *Culex pipiens* mosquitoes. *J. Med. Entomol.* 11:223–225.

Spielman, A., M.G. Leahy, and V. Skaff. 1969. Failure of effective insemination of young female *Aedes aegypti* mosquitoes. *J. Insect Physiol.* 15:1471–1479.

Sutcliffe, J.F. 1986. Black fly host location: A review. *Can. J. Zool.* 64:1041–1053.

Sutcliffe, J.F., and S.B. McIver. 1979. Experiments on biting and gorging behaviour in the black fly, *Simulium venustum. Physiol. Entomol.* 4:393–400.

Takken, W. 1991. The role of olfaction in host-seeking of mosquitoes: A review. *Insect Sci. Appl.* 12:287–295.

Takken, W., and D.L. Kline. 1989. Carbon dioxide and 1-octen-3-ol as mosquito attractants. *J. Am. Mosq. Contr. Assoc.* 5:311–316.

Thorsteinson, A.J., and R.A. Brust. 1962. The influence of flower scents on aggregations of caged *Aedes aegypti. Mosq. News* 22:349–351.

Vale, G.A. 1977. The flight of tsetse flies (Diptera: Glossinidae) to and from a stationary ox. *Bull. Entomol. Res.* 67:297–303.

Vale, G.A. 1980. Flight as a factor in the host-finding behaviour of tsetse flies (Diptera: Glossinidae). *Bull. Entomol. Res.* 70:299–307.

Waage, J.K. 1979. The evolution of insect/vertebrate associations. *Biol. J. Linn. Soc.* 12:187–224.

Waage, J.K. 1981. How the zebra got its stripes—biting flies as selective agents in the evolution of zebra coloration. *J. Entomol. Soc. Sth. Afr.* 44:351–358.

Walker, E.D., and J.D. Edman. 1985. The influence of host defensive behavior on mosquito (Diptera: Culicidae) biting persistence. *J. Med. Entomol.* 22:370–372.

Warnes, M.L., and L.H. Finlayson 1985. Responses of the stable fly, *Stomoxys calcitrans* (L.) (Diptera: Muscidae), to carbon dioxide and host odours. 1. Activation. *Bull. Entomol. Res.* 75:519–527.

Wharton, R.H. 1963. Adaptation of *Wuchereria* and *Brugia* to mosquitoes and vertebrate hosts in relation to the distribution of filarial parasites. *Zoonoses Res.* 2:1–12.

Wigglesworth, V.B., and J.D. Gillett. 1934. The function of the antennae in *Rhodnius prolixus* (Hemiptera) and the mechanism of orientation to the host. *J. Exp. Biol.* 11:120–139.

Wright, R.H. 1975. Why mosquito repellents repel. *Sci. Amer.* July 1975:104–111.

Yee, W.L., and W.A. Foster. 1992. Diel sugar-feeding and host-seeking rhythms in mosquitoes (Diptera: Culicidae) under laboratory conditions. *J. Med. Entomol.* 29:784–791.

Yeh, C.-C., and M.J. Klowden. 1990. Effects of male accessory gland substances on the pre-oviposition behaviour of *Aedes aegypti* mosquitoes. *J. Insect Physiol.* 36:799–803.

Young, A.D.M., and A.E.R. Downe. 1982. Renewal of sexual receptivity in mated female mosquitoes, *Aedes aegypti. Physiol. Entomol.* 7:467–471.

Young, A.D.M., and A.E.R. Downe. 1987. Male accessory gland substances and the control of sexual receptivity in female *Culex tarsalis. Physiol. Entomol.* 12:233–239.

Zimmerman, R.H., and E.C. Turner, Jr. 1984. Dispersal and gonotrophic age of *Culicoides variipennis* (Diptera: Ceratopogonidae) at an isolated site in southwestern Virgina, USA. *J. Med. Entomol.* 21:527–535.

4. NATURAL CYCLES OF VECTOR-BORNE PATHOGENS

Jennifer L. Woodring, Stephen Higgs, and Barry J. Beaty

INTRODUCTION

An astonishing variety and number of pathogens are maintained in nature by cycles involving vertebrate hosts and hematophagous (blood-feeding) arthropod vectors. The vector-borne disease cycle consists of a dynamic interaction between pathogen, vertebrate host(s), vector(s), and the environment (Fig. 4.1).

Vector-borne pathogens typically must infect and replicate or develop in both a vector and a vertebrate host. When feeding on blood to support oogenesis or to fulfill other nutritional requirements, the vector can ingest and be infected by pathogens in the vertebrate circulatory system or epidermis. In subsequent blood meals, the vector can transmit these disease agents to new, potentially susceptible vertebrate hosts. The pathogen often exerts little or no deleterious effect upon its arthropod vector, whereas infection of vertebrate hosts can result in serious consequences. Indeed, some vector-borne pathogens cause significant morbidity or mortality in humans and domestic animals. More commonly, the pathogen causes an inapparent or subclinical infection in its natural or usual vertebrate host. In contrast, infection of accidental or tangential hosts can result in serious disease.

Vector-borne cycles appear to be a tenuous mode of transmission and maintenance for pathogens. However, the multitude and diversity of pathogens involved suggests a highly successful strategy. Furthermore, despite enormous effort expended toward controlling them, vector-borne diseases such as malaria, dengue, filariasis, and trypanosomiasis continue to cause morbidity and mortality. The tenacity of these cycles in the face of sometimes drastic human intervention attests to their ability to withstand perturbations. This chapter describes how vector-borne pathogens are transmitted and maintained in natural cycles. Understanding the interactions between pathogens, vectors, and vertebrates allows determination of the weak links at which control efforts should be directed.

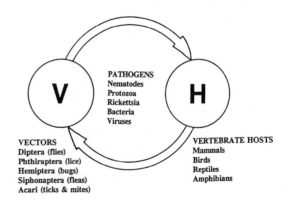

4.1 Principal pathogens, vectors, and vertebrates involved in vector-borne pathogen cycles

ARBOVIRUSES: CYCLES, VIRUSES, VECTORS, AND VERTEBRATE HOSTS

Arboviral Cycles

General Considerations

Arthropod-borne viruses (arboviruses) and arbovirus-vector interactions illustrate the basic mechanisms and generalities of vector-borne pathogen cycles in nature (Fig. 4.2). Arboviruses are naturally maintained in cycles by hematophagous arthropods that

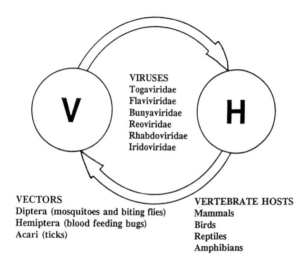

VIRUSES
Togaviridae
Flaviviridae
Bunyaviridae
Reoviridae
Rhabdoviridae
Iridoviridae

VECTORS
Diptera (mosquitoes and biting flies)
Hemiptera (blood feeding bugs)
Acari (ticks)

VERTEBRATE HOSTS
Mammals
Birds
Reptiles
Amphibians

4.2 Principal arboviruses, vectors, and vertebrates involved in arbovirus cycles

biologically transmit virus between vertebrate hosts. The vectors become infected by ingesting viremic blood from a vertebrate host or through transovarial (when a virus crosses the ovaries to enter the eggs) or even venereal transmission. Classically, an arbovirus does not exert a deleterious effect on its vector. In contrast, the same virus can be extremely pathogenic in vertebrate hosts, especially in tangential hosts. Arboviruses do not include the vector-borne plant viruses nor the invertebrate pathogenic viruses such as baculoviruses, iridoviruses, entomopoxviruses, and cytoplasmic polyhedrosis viruses.

Maintenance and Amplification Components

Arboviral cycles can be categorized into maintenance and amplification components. Maintenance is essentially the long-term survival of the virus. Arboviruses can be maintained by ongoing transmission between vertebrate hosts and vectors, by prolonged infections of a host or vector, and by other transeasonal survival mechanisms (see the following section). During periods of little or no transmission, the number of infected hosts and vectors declines. Amplification results in the increased prevalence of infected vertebrate hosts and vectors and ultimately the amount of virus in nature. Amplification can occur with the onset of resumed or increased transmission and compensates for the loss of infected organisms during the maintenance component of the cycle. Thus, amplification is crucial for viral survival in nature. Amplification is also frequently responsible for epidemics of disease in vertebrates. Arboviral cycles are characterized by a dynamic interaction of the virus, the vector, and the vertebrate host (Fig. 4.3). At each step in a cycle, opportunities for and barriers to viral survival exist. The attributes of viruses, vectors, and vertebrate hosts that contribute to the integrity of arboviral cycles are examined in the following sections.

Arboviruses

Arboviral Biology

Viruses differ from other microorganisms in several ways. They are extremely small, ranging in size from 20 nm to 300 nm. The vast majority of arboviruses have small RNA genomes, which code for only a few proteins. Further, arboviruses possess neither an energy generating system nor ribosomes. Thus they are obligate intracellular parasites, completely dependent upon the host cell for their replication and for protein synthesis. Viruses have an infectious stage, the virion, and an intracellular (replication) stage known as the eclipse phase.

Over 500 arboviruses are recognized. Most have RNA genomes and enveloped virions. An arboviral virion is composed of protein and nucleic acid, associated to form the nucleocapsid, with smaller amounts

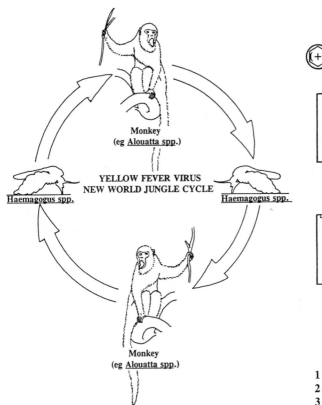

4.3 Simple arbovirus cycle: jungle yellow fever

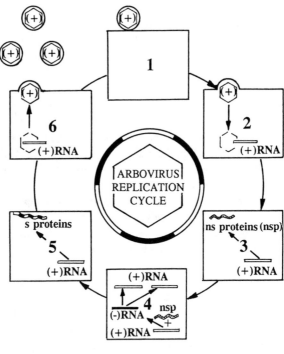

1 = Reception
2 = Penetration and uncoating
3 = Translation
4 = Transcription and replication
5 = Translation
6 = Maturation and budding

4.4 Arbovirus replication in host cells: a positive stranded RNA virus

of lipid and sugars found in the surrounding envelope. When the virion buds through a plasma or other cellular membrane containing virus-derived glycoproteins, it acquires an envelope. Figure 4.4 illustrates the basic steps of viral replication in a cell.

In a productive infection, the virus infects a permissive cell, the sequence of events illustrated in Figure 4.4 occurs, and large numbers of infectious virions result. In an abortive or nonproductive infection, nonpermissive cells permit viral entry but block replication. Infectious virions do not result, although transcription and translation of some viral genes and gene products can occur. Cells that are not susceptible to viral infection or that block infection and replication at a very early stage are termed resistant, or refractory, cells. For example, resistant cells may not have appropriate receptors for viral attachment or entry.

Virus Considerations in Arboviral Cycles

To contribute to the integrity of their own cycles, arboviruses must infect both vectors and vertebrates in such a way as to be transmitted to the next host. Despite relatively small genomes (approximately 10,000 bases), arboviruses must be capable of infection and replication in 2 phylogenetically disparate systems —the invertebrate vector and the vertebrate host. Along with biochemical and physiological differences, significant temperature differences exist between these poikilothermic and homeothermic hosts. In light of these considerations, perhaps it is not surprising that an arbovirus affects the vertebrate and invertebrate quite differently.

For the cycle to remain intact, arboviruses must cause a high-titered viremia (virus in the blood) in the natural vertebrate host. High-titered viremias of long duration increase the opportunity for vector infection and for mechanical transmission of the virus (see below). Viremias of short duration or low titers are less likely to infect vectors. Moreover, the virus should not be unduly virulent, thus killing the vertebrate host before new vectors can be infected. In a "good" host-parasite relationship, the parasite exerts little untoward effect on the usual host because the virus and host have presumably evolved a benign relationship.

Arboviruses must also infect and replicate in the vector to be biologically transmitted to a new vertebrate host or to another vector. Alternatively, viruses that persist on vector body parts can be transmitted mechanically. Arboviruses, by definition, cause little or no detrimental effect on their natural or usual vectors: If the virus deleteriously affected the survival of the vector, the probability of the agent being transmitted to a new vertebrate host would be limited. Recent studies with alphaviruses suggest that some cytopathology can occur in natural vectors, although no effect on transmission could be demonstrated.

Vectors of Arboviruses

Vector Transmission of Arboviruses

For our purposes, a vector is an arthropod, generally hematophagous, that can transmit pathogens from one vertebrate host to another. In some vector species (e.g., mosquitoes), only the females ingest blood and transmit viruses to vertebrate hosts. In other species, such as ticks, both females and males are hematophagous and can transmit the viruses.

Biological versus mechanical transmission of arboviruses. Vectors transmit infectious agents biologically or mechanically. In biological transmission, the pathogens reproduce or develop in the arthropod vector before being transmitted to the next vertebrate host. Arboviruses undergo a propagative mode of development in vectors (Fig. 4.5); other types of vector-borne pathogens may undergo different modes of development.

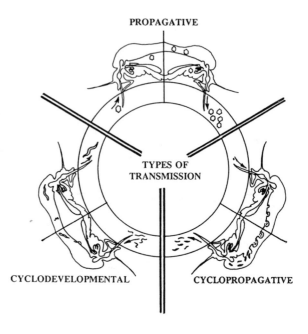

4.5 Three developmental modes of biologically transmitted pathogens

In contrast, for mechanical transmission, the pathogen does not reproduce or develop in the vector; the arthropod merely transmits the pathogen physically from one vertebrate host to another (Fig. 4.6). Most often, the mouthparts of the vector become contaminated with pathogens that are subsequently inoculated into another vertebrate during the vector's next feeding attempt. Transmission is possible only for a short period, until the contaminating virus becomes inactivated. Mechanical transmission has been compared to a "flying pin" method of transmission. In a classic experiment, baby chicks were infected with eastern equine encephalitis (EEE) and subsequently probed either by mosquitoes or by pins. At various time points before biological transmission was possible, noninfected chicks were exposed to the mosquitoes or pins, and mechanical transmission rates were determined (Table 4.1). Pins mechanically transmitted the virus as effectively as the mosquitoes.

TABLE 4.1 Mechanical transmission of eastern equine encephalitis by mosquitoes and pins

Hours	Percent transmission	
Postexposure	Mosquitoes	Pins
0	100	100
1	90	100
4	70	100
20	60	40
70	10	5

Reproduced, with permission, from the *Annual Review of Entomology*, Vol. 6, © 1961 by Annual Reviews, Inc.

Biological and mechanical transmission are neither mutually exclusive nor mutually inclusive. By definition, arboviruses are vectored by propagative biological transmission. However, vectors that biologically transmit viruses can mechanically transmit for several hours after an infectious blood meal. Most hematophagous arthropods could theoretically transmit viruses mechanically, and some nonarboviruses are commonly transmitted in this manner (equine infectious anemia virus by stable flies); others are infrequently transmitted mechanically (Hepatitis B virus by bed bugs). The ability to transmit a pathogen mechanically does not imply a corresponding ability for biological transmission. Usually only a single or a few species are competent for biological transmission because of the multiple barriers the virus must cross (see below). In explosive epidemics, undoubtedly both types of transmission occur. Whether acting alone or in concert, both biological and mechanical transmission can contribute to arboviral cycles. The hypothetical relationship between mechanical and biological transmission is shown in Figure 4.6.

Vertical versus horizontal transmission of arboviruses. Vertical transmission, in which the parent passes the pathogen to its progeny, occurs with some arboviruses (Fig. 4.7). Typically a female arthropod infects her progeny through a transovarial or transovum route. Infected males sometimes vertically infect progeny via seminal fluid; apparently, virus is transferred into the egg through the micropyle during fertilization as the egg passes through the oviduct. Vertical transmission occurs only with biologically transmitted viruses. Horizontal transmission (Fig. 4.7) is classically defined as transmission between vectors via viremia in the vertebrate host. Thus, both biological and mechanical transmission could be considered to be horizontal. In another form of horizontal transmission, arboviruses can be venereally transmitted from male to female mosquitoes. In vector species in which

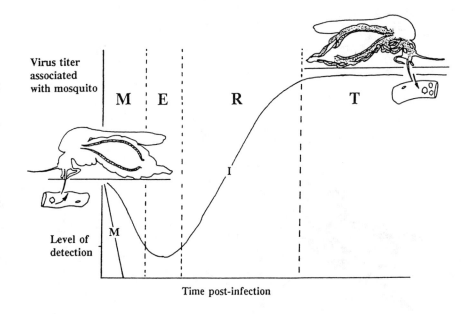

4.6   Viral titer in a vector over time as related to virus transmission. (M) mechanical, (E) eclipse, (R) replication, (T) transmission.

VERTICAL TRANSMISSION (FEMALE TO PROGENY - MALE & FEMALE)

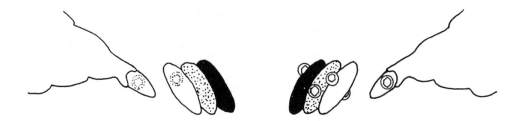

TRANSOVARIAL
(Virus in egg)

TRANSOVUM
(Virus on egg surface)

HORIZONTAL TRANSMISSION (FEMALE TO FEMALE)

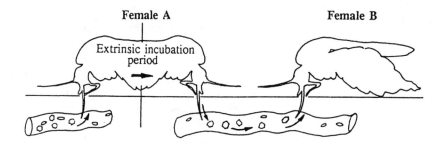

Female A

Female B

Extrinsic incubation
period

HORIZONTAL TRANSMISSION (VENEREAL MALE TO FEMALE)

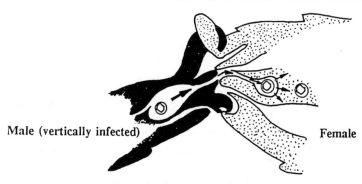

Male (vertically infected)

Female

4.7 Vertical and horizontal transmission of arboviruses

only females are hematophagous, venereal transmission occurs only if vertical transmission to the male has first taken place and the virus has infected and replicated in the male reproductive organs.

Vectorial capacity versus vector competence. Vectorial capacity is the overall ability of a vector species in a given location at a specific time to transmit a pathogen. Quantitatively, vectorial capacity can be defined as the number of infectious bites a person (or other vertebrate of interest) receives daily. Vectorial capacity encompasses the vector interactions with the pathogen and the vertebrate host as well as innate vector characteristics not directly related to either the pathogen or the vertebrate host. Vector population size, longevity, length and number of gonadotrophic cycles, feeding behavior, and diel activity affect the vectorial capacity of a given arthropod population.

In contrast to vectorial capacity, vector competence is the intrinsic ability of a vector (species, strain, individual, etc.) to transmit a disease agent biologically. Vector competence includes susceptibility to infection, permissiveness for pathogen reproduction or development, duration of extrinsic incubation period, and transmission efficiency. Thus, vector competence is restricted to the defined vector-pathogen interaction.

Biological Transmission of Arboviruses

Viral development in the vector. In biological transmission, the period from ingestion of the infectious blood meal to transmission capability is designated the extrinsic incubation (EI) period (Fig. 4.6). During the extrinsic incubation period, the virus infects and replicates in the midgut cuboidal epithelial cells and then disseminates to infect secondary target organs. Virions disperse in circulating hemolymph (vector blood). Once the salivary glands become infected and shed virions into the salivary ducts, the virus can be transmitted to vertebrates during a blood meal. In addition, if the developing follicles of the ovaries become infected, the virus can be transmitted

to the progeny. Arthropod immunity differs from mammalian immunity; once infected with an arbovirus, a vector remains infected throughout its life span. After the EI period, the infective vector can potentially transmit virus to each new vertebrate host during feeding attempts or to new progeny with every period of oviposition.

The duration of extrinsic incubation in a poikilothermic vector depends on the temperature. Within limits, higher temperatures shorten the EI period. The length of the EI also depends on the specific vector and virus involved. A typical EI period would last 10–14 days for a bunyavirus or flavivirus and perhaps 6–7 days for an alphavirus.

Barriers to biological transmission of arboviruses. In any vector-arbovirus system, there are multiple barriers to productive vector infection (Fig. 4.8). The presence or absence of these barriers partially determines the vector competence of the arthropod. Several barriers to productive infection in the vector have been shown or hypothesized at the midgut, salivary gland,

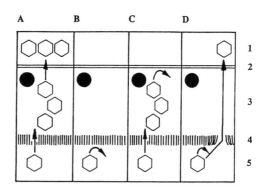

A = PERMISSIVE
B = INFECTION BARRIER
C = DISSEMINATION BARRIER
D = LEAKY

MIDGUT	SALIVARY GLAND	OVARY
1 = Hemocoel	1 = Salivary duct	1 = Follicle
2 = Basement membrane	2 = Secretory surface	2 = Secretory surface
3 = Midgut epithelium	3 = Secretory cell	3 = Follicular epithelium
4 = Brush border	4 = Basement membrane	4 = Ovarian sheath
5 = Gut lumen	5 = Hemocoel	5 = Hemocoel

4.8 Barriers to biological transmission

and ovarian levels and are probably critical to arboviral cycle integrity.

The term "midgut barrier" is loosely used to describe a situation in which the midgut is an impediment to productive viral infection. A midgut barrier has long been recognized as a major determinant of vector competence. A midgut infection barrier, in which the vector is actually refractory to infection, and a midgut escape barrier, in which the midgut cells are infected but the virus does not successfully disseminate to other organs, are also recognized as determinants of vector competence. The midgut barrier can be bypassed experimentally or naturally. Experimentally, interspecific variability in infection rates disappears when mosquitoes are infected by intrathoracic inoculation of virus (see Chap. 35, photo 35.1) or when the midgut is penetrated physically with a needle or by microfilariae. A leaky midgut phenomenon can also occur. In some populations, a certain percentage of the mosquitoes have virus in the hemocoel promptly after ingestion of the blood meal, even before the virus has time to replicate in the midgut. The exact mechanism is unknown; however, the association of leaky midguts with having taken a previous blood meal suggests that damage to midgut integrity is the likely cause.

The midgut barrier is frequently not absolute. A species-specific dose-response phenomenon or infection threshold has been described for a variety of vector-virus systems. Below the threshold, few of the vectors ingesting the blood meal become infected; above the threshold, significant numbers become infected. The infection threshold has been classically defined as the titer in which 5% of the vectors become infected (Fig. 4.9).

Most workers now quantify the threshold using an oral dose infectious for 50% of the individuals tested (OID_{50}). This statistical approach has the advantage of providing a more linear response between dose and infection.

A variety of hypotheses have been proposed to explain midgut infection barriers. Some investigators

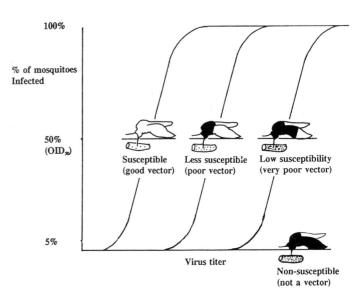

4.9 Infection thresholds for arthropods of differing susceptibilities to viral infection

suggest that the formation of the peritrophic matrix (PM) (see Chap. 19) prevents the virus from contacting and infecting the midgut cells. However, PM formation occurs too late, 24–48 hr after the blood meal, to interfere with infection. It is also possible that refractory arthropods possess specific defensive mechanisms to protect against viral infections. Mucopolysaccharides or other antiviral agents could be secreted into the midgut. Little evidence supporting this hypothesis has been found. Viral inactivation or inappropriate processing of viral surface glycoproteins by midgut enzymes is another potential explanation for the midgut infection barrier. Many now believe that arboviruses are truly enteric viruses of vectors, requiring proteolytic processing for infectivity. Infectivity of bluetongue virus (BTV) and LaCrosse virus (LAC) for their respective vectors is enhanced by proteolytic processing of their virions. Alternatively, nonhomologous vectors might not possess specific receptors for viral attachment. This attractive hypothesis is the subject of a great deal of research, which is discussed later.

Midgut escape barriers have been demonstrated for members of several viral families. In these nonproductive infections, the virus capably infects vector midgut cells and undergoes substantial transcription and translation but does not disseminate from the midgut cells to infect secondary target organs (Fig. 4.8). The virus could be trapped in midgut cells or, less likely, could reach the hemocoel but be unable to infect other organs.

Salivary gland infection and escape barriers have also been described (Fig. 4.8). For infection barriers, the salivary glands are refractory to infection. With escape barriers they become infected, but the virus is not transmitted. For example, *Ae. hendersoni* is not normally a LAC vector despite the replication of infectious virions in the salivary glands. Ovarian infection barriers also exist. When developing follicles do become infected, the virus must replicate and persist through embryogenesis, larval development, and metamorphosis for the adults of the successive generation to be infected. Transovarial infection is relatively rare for most arboviruses and little is known concerning the molecular bases of ovarian barriers.

Genetic determinants of vector competence. Both inter- and intraspecific variation in vector competence have been documented. In a classic study of interspecific variation, different species of mosquitoes were permitted to ingest blood meals from viremic chicks previously infected with EEE. Because all mosquitoes fed at approximately the same time and thus ingested the same dose of virus, the differences in infection and transmission rates reflect interspecific variation in barriers to viral infection and dissemination (Table 4.2).

Intraspecific variability in vector competence also exists. Early studies demonstrated a geographic and genetic basis for vector competence for dengue virus. Subsequent studies revealed a clear geographic distribution in the ability of *Ae. aegypti* to vector yellow fever (YF) virus. The Asian strain of *Ae. aegypti* proved to be a less competent vector for YF than the African and Caribbean strains. This intraspecific variation in vector competence partially explains why the distribution of yellow fever does not mirror that of *Ae. aegypti*, the principal vector in many locations. Both the mosquito and the virus probably originated in Africa. In the Americas, where mosquito strains are competent vectors, yellow fever became established, but in Asia,

TABLE 4.2 Interspecific variation in vector competence

Mosquito	Precent infected	Percent transmitting
Aedes sollicitans	100	75
Aedes triseriatus	100	56
Psorophora ferox	100	15
Anopheles quadrimaculatus	79	0
Culex restuans	45	33
Culex quinquefasciatus	5	0

Modified and reproduced, with permission, from the *American Journal of Hygiene,* Vol. 6, p. 281, © 1954 by the *American Journal of Epidemiology.*

where mosquito strains are less competent, yellow fever failed to establish despite the longer history of trade between Africa and Asia and the seemingly favorable conditions in the Orient.

Many studies have shown a genetic basis for vector competence in mosquitoes. *Ae. aegypti* competence for yellow fever virus has been studied extensively. Lines of *Ae. aegypti* selected for susceptibility and resistance to YF virus react similarly to other flaviviruses. In resistant mosquitoes, viral antigen is restricted to the midgut; disseminated infections are not detected or are delayed. Viral titers are similar in susceptible and resistant lines early in the infection, but titers in susceptible mosquitoes increase later, presumably due to replication in the secondary target organs.

Crosses between resistant and susceptible lines with subsequent backcrosses to the parents were used to elucidate the genetic basis of the 2 phenotypes. Backcrosses of F_1 offspring to the susceptible parent (but not backcrosses to the resistant parent) produced F_2 progeny with infection rates suggestive of a single locus. However, more detailed analyses revealed that the trait is more complex and probably not caused by a single gene. Interspecific and intraspecific variability in vector competence for western equine encephalitis (WEE) virus has been extensively studied. However, actual gene products determining vector competence have not been revealed. Recent work suggests that cell receptors such as laminin may be utilized by viruses to infect midgut cells. The laminin receptor could bind with ligands on the envelope glycoproteins of the arbovirus, thereby permitting entry into the cell. Little evidence indicates that such generic receptors are determinants of vector specificity and thereby function to maintain arboviral cycle integrity. Nonetheless, such receptors could be critical determinants of viral infection of vectors and thus of the midgut barrier. Note that these hypotheses have all dealt with the vector; viral determinants of midgut infection will be discussed later.

Vector Considerations in Arboviral Cycles

Vector incrimination. Although many arthropods are capable of transmitting a given etiological agent, only those invertebrates that are important in maintaining a natural transmission cycle are considered to be primary vectors. Four criteria of vector incrimination are used to identify primary vectors. First, the putative vector must associate with and feed on the vertebrate host under field conditions. Moreover, the seasons and locations of arthropod activity should coincide with the incidence of vertebrate infection. Second, naturally infected vectors must be consistently recovered from the field. Third, the presumed vector must be shown to become infected by feeding upon a viremic host. Fourth, the ability of an infected vector to transmit the pathogen to a new vertebrate host should be confirmed under controlled conditions.

Considerations for biological transmission. In vector-borne disease, the transmission rate is a function of the vector physiology, population dynamics, and behavior. Several attributes of the vector species and populations can aid in maintaining the integrity of arboviral cycles.

As previously defined, vector competence refers to the intrinsic ability of a vector to transmit a disease agent. What interactions make for a competent vector? A good vector species should have a low infection threshold and permit viral multiplication in at least the midgut and salivary glands (and ovaries in the case of transovarial transmission). Further, a high proportion of individuals must transmit virus. In addition, the vector should sustain little or no reduction in fitness or survival despite supporting viral replication. Finally,

the shorter the extrinsic incubation period, generally the better the vector competence because of the potential for the vector to transmit virus to more hosts after becoming infective.

Besides vector competence, many vector attributes potentially increase the vectorial capacity of a population. During host-seeking and feeding activity, the vector must exhibit spatial and temporal patterns that coincide with those of the vertebrate host. Each vector has a characteristic diel activity (active during day, night, or crepuscular period), feeding preference (anthropophilic, zoophilic, etc.), and habitat activity (canopy versus ground feeding, exophilic versus endophilic). Because the vector needs to feed on the vertebrate host, host-feeding preferences can be a major determinant of specificity of arboviral cycles. Some vectors feed on mammals, some on reptiles, some on birds; others are catholic (diverse) in their host choice. In addition, host preference can change during the transmission season. The ability to feed on diverse hosts provides both a survival mechanism when the usual host is unavailable and a mechanism for transmitting virus to new, often tangential hosts. Vector mobility also affects arboviral cycles. A distance traveler is more likely to spread a virus to new susceptibles than a vector that does not travel.

Vector longevity is a major factor in transmission potential and hence vectorial capacity. The longer the vector lives, the more times it will feed after the EI period, resulting in more opportunities for transmission. Long-lived arthropods such as ticks help maintain a pathogen for a long time in the environment. In addition, a shorter gonadotrophic cycle provides more opportunity for transmission as blood is ingested to support production of the next batch of eggs. Arthropods that feed immediately after ovipositing, *Anopheles gambiae* for example, are probably better vectors than those that take more postoviposition rest.

Seasonal and climatic effects on vectors cannot be ignored. Because vectors are small invertebrates, they tend to be sensitive to temperature and humidity. Temperature affects the EI period, vector longevity, gonadotrophic cycle length, and activity. Humidity significantly affects both vector longevity and mobility. Also, water breeders require standing water to reproduce. Thus, cold winters and hot, dry summers substantially reduce mosquito breeding and feeding. Vector inactivity can temporarily disrupt transmission cycles and require that an arbovirus possess a trans-seasonal survival mechanism.

Considerations for mechanical transmission.

Feeding behavior and population density of the vector greatly influence the probability of mechanical transmission. Vectors that exhibit interrupted feeding behavior are likely to transmit viruses mechanically. Interrupted feeding occurs when defensive behavior of the vertebrate host drives the vector away. Typically, the vector will promptly seek another host to complete engorgement. Virus can be transmitted to this second host if the first host supported a viremia capable of contaminating the vector's mouthparts. The likelihood of mechanical transmission increases as vector populations increase for 2 reasons. First, as more vectors feed, the odds that one will successfully transmit the virus increase. Second, vertebrate populations usually become more defensive as vectors become more numerous, thus leading to more interrupted feeding.

Viral factors that facilitate mechanical transmission include viral stability, vertebrate infectivity, and ability to cause a high-titered viremia in the vertebrate host. In general, the more resistant a virus is to environmental degradation, the more likely it is to be mechanically transmitted. Viruses are usually more labile at warm temperatures. Thus, cool temperatures are associated with viral stability and more efficient mechanical transmission. Viruses also differ in their relative infectivity for vertebrate hosts. The more communicable the virus, the longer a sufficient infectious dose can remain on the vector, and thus the greater the probability of mechanical transmission. Finally, the potential for mechanical transmission is directly proportional to the titer of viremia in the vertebrate host. Obviously, when more virus is present in the blood to contaminate the mouthparts of the vector there is more potential that the virus will survive long enough to infect a new vertebrate. Note that all 3 of these factors are interdependent.

Vertebrate Hosts of Arboviruses

Vertebrate Hosts

Any vertebrate that can be infected with virus and develop sufficient viremia to infect subsequently feeding vectors can be considered a vertebrate host. Vertebrates contribute to both maintenance and amplification components of arboviral cycles. Different host names have classically been attached to these different roles, though it should be noted that maintenance and amplification roles are not necessarily mutually exclusive.

The reservoir host usually maintains the virus over long periods of time and experiences no negative effects from infection. The hallmark of a good reservoir host is a high-titered viremia of long duration that can lead to infection of many vectors. Hosts that support recrudescent infections can also be reservoirs. A reservoir host population usually must generate sufficient new susceptible members for ongoing transmission to sustain the viral cycle. Species that breed year round, thus providing a constant supply of new susceptibles, frequently serve in this capacity. In addition to cycle maintenance, migratory or highly vagile reservoir hosts can disperse an arbovirus to new locations.

Vertebrates involved in amplifying the number of infected vectors (and consequently other vertebrates) are called amplification hosts. Amplification hosts reproduce at least annually and provide large numbers of new susceptibles concurrent with vector activity. For example, each spring hatchling birds serve as a pool of new susceptibles. The first birds infected sustain viremias that lead to increasing waves of infection among the vectors and the other susceptibles. Susceptible amplification hosts are usually not present year round (most fledgling and adult birds will have developed immunity), but they provide an important opportunity for the quantity of virus in the environment to increase. For epidemiological purposes, vertebrates serving to bring an arbovirus in contact with vectors that can transmit the viral diseases to humans or livestock can also be amplification hosts.

A tangential host typically is not involved in amplification or maintenance of the virus. In contrast to the usual vertebrate hosts involved in the cycle, tangential hosts support a viremia of relatively low titer. Because transmission to new vectors is reduced or prevented by the low-titered viremia, these hosts are also known as dead-end hosts. Tangential hosts are not important to cycle integrity (unless they distract vectors from the normal vertebrate hosts); however, humans and animals can suffer severe morbidity and mortality when they tangentially enter a disease cycle. Thus, for some serious arboviral diseases, humans and domestic animals are merely tangential hosts. By comparison, reservoir and amplification hosts usually do not develop any major untoward effect resulting from infection. However, some viruses do cause morbidity and mortality in their reservoir hosts (e.g., dengue and BT).

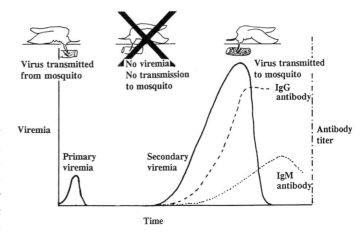

4.10 Viremia and antibody response in a vertebrate host infected by an arbovirus

Pathogenesis in Vertebrate Hosts

The pathogenesis of many arboviruses has been described. Infection probably occurs first in muscle or other cells near the site of the bite and is subsequently transmitted to regional lymph nodes. Viral replication in these tissues leads to a primary viremia (Fig. 4.10), resulting in infection of tissues associated with the vascular system. Viral replication in the vascular system produces a high-titered, long-lasting secondary viremia. Infection of secondary target organs, such as the liver in yellow fever or the central nervous system in encephalitis, ensues. The period required from infection to disease in the vertebrate is termed the "intrinsic incubation period" (as opposed to the extrinsic incubation in vectors).

Several potential syndromes can result from arboviral infection. Inapparent, asymptomatic infections frequently occur, especially in hosts normally involved in a particular cycle. Arboviral infection can also result in clinical manifestations ranging from fever or arthritis to hemorrhagic fever or encephalitis. Obviously, severe morbidity and mortality can result from these serious diseases. As noted previously, tangential hosts are probably more likely to experience severe syndromes, presumably due to lack of coadaptation between host and pathogen. Individuals often respond quite differently to infection with the same virus. Human infection with YF, for example, can elicit

symptoms ranging from an inapparent infection to fatal hemorrhagic fever.

The vertebrate immune response is important during arboviral infections. Unlike arthropods that remain infected for life with arboviruses, most vertebrates respond immunologically to infection (Fig. 4.10). Antibodies limit the duration of the viremia, thus halting further transmission to more vectors. Antibodies also render the individual immune to future infection by the particular virus.

Other arthropod-borne pathogens can develop differently in the vertebrate host, cause their own distinctive syndromes, and elicit incomplete immunity. Details for these other systems are found in the appropriate chapters.

Vertebrate Host Considerations in Arboviral Cycles

Several attributes of a vertebrate host affect its suitability for maintaining an arboviral cycle. Once fed upon by an infective vector, the vertebrate must be susceptible to viral infection and develop a viremia sufficient to infect or contaminate other arthropods, preferably a viremia of high titer and long duration. For biological transmission, a viremia surpassing the infection threshold of the vector species is critical. A high-titered viremia also aids mechanical transmission.

As noted previously, the vertebrate host and vector must share time and space when the vector is actively feeding. Diel activity patterns and accessibility to the vector must be considered. Vertebrates present on the forest floor encounter different vector species than those found primarily in the canopy. Stereotyped behavior of the vertebrate, such as returning to the same vector-infested water hole each evening, can serve to increase vertebrate-vector contact. Interestingly, some medical entomologists attribute air-conditioning and prime-time television viewing to a decrease of arboviral transmission to humans in the United States. Air-conditioning encourages people to limit vector access to their homes (by closing doors and windows), and television keeps people in homes during the twilight hours when many vectors are actively host-seeking. Artifacts also increase vertebrate-vector contact. For example, water jugs and other small containers around village homes provide excellent breeding sites for *Ae. aegypti*, bringing the vector close to humans. Rodent burrows are nonhuman artifacts that are environmentally suitable for both the rodents and their fleas that vector pathogens.

Good vertebrate hosts would ideally fail to exhibit effective defensive behavior that could result in eluding or even killing the vector. Young vertebrates typically are less defensive than adults and can be more susceptible to both vector attack and to arboviral infection than adults. In contrast, defensive behaviors that promote interrupted feeding can increase viral transmission by enhancing mechanical pathogen transmission. An infected vector exhibiting interrupted feeding could potentially transmit virus to more than 1 host per gonotrophic cycle.

Vertebrate behavior influences arboviral maintenance and transmission in yet another manner. Infected vertebrates that roam through vast territories or that migrate to distant locations can bring arboviruses into contact with new vector populations. Hence, disease cycles can begin in new regions or be reintroduced into areas where the cycle had been extinguished. Migratory birds are known to transfer some arboviruses in this manner.

In general, a vertebrate host should not exhibit undue mortality from an arboviral infection, especially

a reservoir host. The exceptions can be fascinating. In its native home of Africa, YF is maintained in monkeys that typically show no clinical symptoms as would be expected. In contrast, in South America, where the virus was probably introduced, YF kills monkeys. YF persists because *Haemagogus* and other canopy mosquitoes transmit it between monkey troops (Fig. 4.3). New susceptibles, born since the previous epizootic, become infected when troops come close and share vectors. Thus, the YF virus reservoir in the Amazon basin moves from region to region with approximately a 25-year periodicity in any given location.

Vertebrates typically develop a long-term immunity to viral pathogens; thus, the absolute size of a vertebrate host population does not indicate its ability to support viral infections. The vertebrates should be adequately fecund to recruit new susceptibles to the population. Epidemic cycles often can be explained in terms of the time required for accumulation of sufficient susceptibles in the population. The Amazon monkeys and YF virus are a good example.

Complexity of Arboviral Cycles

The typical cycle described so far has 1 or more principal vectors maintaining viral transmission between 1 or more species of vertebrate hosts. Many arboviral cycles do not normally involve humans as reservoir or amplifying hosts. Frequently, viruses are transmitted in 2 separate cycles: an urban cycle and a rural, jungle, or sylvatic cycle (frequently called epidemic and endemic cycles), respectively. Humans impinge upon the sylvatic cycle and become infected; they can then transport the virus to urban areas (Fig. 4.11). In rural areas, wild vertebrates are normally the amplification and maintenance hosts; relatively sparse human populations only rarely impinge on the cycles. When humans do become infected, they probably do not contribute to the rural cycle. In contrast, human populations in cities are dense and are likely to include a high percentage of susceptible individuals. Under these conditions, urban vectors, usually well adapted to feeding on humans, can transmit the virus in the susceptible population and cause epidemics.

Commonly, the rural, or sylvatic, cycle maintains the arbovirus. Humans or domestically important species

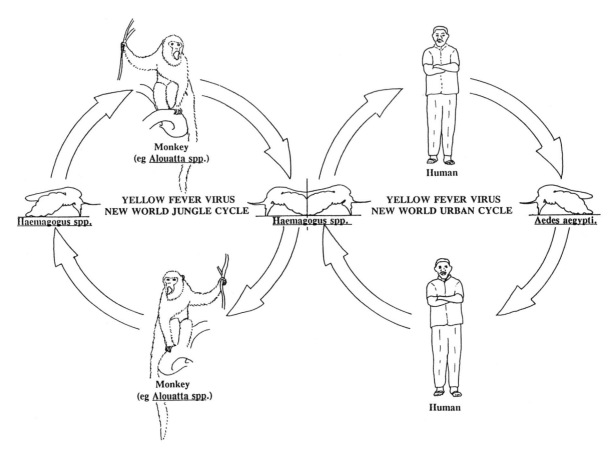

4.11   Jungle and urban yellow fever

become tangentially infected when they intrude on this natural cycle or when conditions bring the cycle in contact with them. In such situations, the vector is frequently catholic in its feeding preferences. The cycle of LAC virus (Fig. 4.12) is a good example. The cycles of WEE and rural Saint Louis encephalitis (SLE) in the American West are also good examples. *Culex tarsalis*, the vector of WEE and rural SLE, prefers passerine hosts and transmits virus between birds. However, the mosquito will feed upon humans and mammals and can thus transmit the virus to tangential hosts. In other instances, the vector can change feeding preferences or lose access to its preferred host, thereby introducing the virus into different vertebrate hosts.

Transseasonality

Whether it be winter in temperate regions or dry seasons in the tropics, vectors are frequently inactive during parts of each year. During these periods, transmission of vector-borne pathogens ceases—a weak link in these disease cycles—and the cycle enters a transeasonal maintenance phase. Several strategies, frequently called overwintering mechanisms (because the research has focused on temperate regions), have been proposed or observed that permit pathogen survival during adverse conditions.

Vectors contribute to viral persistence by 3 principal mechanisms. First, the virus can persist in the adult

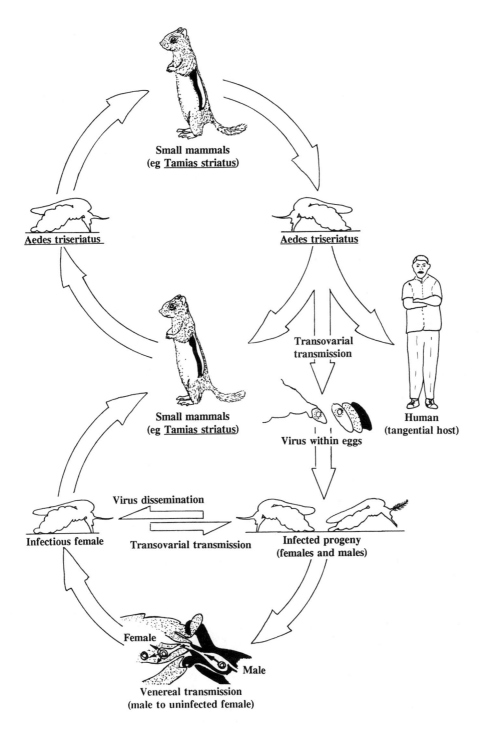

Small mammals
(eg <u>Tamias striatus</u>)

<u>Aedes triseriatus</u>

<u>Aedes triseriatus</u>

Transovarial
transmission

Human
(tangential host)

Virus within eggs

Small mammals
(eg <u>Tamias striatus</u>)

Virus dissemination

Transovarial transmission

Infected progeny
(females and males)

Infectious female

Female

Male

Venereal transmission
(male to uninfected female)

4.12 LaCrosse virus cycle

vector when an infected adult remains dormant during the unfavorable season. For example, SLE virus has been isolated from overwintering adult mosquitoes. Second, the egg (or more rarely juvenile stages), serves as a reservoir for virus when vertical transmission occurs. In the family Bunyaviridae, transovarial transmission is clearly a major mechanism for viral persistence through harsh winters. Third, an undetected arthropod or other metazoan vector can harbor the virus during a season when the known vector is inactive. For example, a cimicid (bed bug) is the overwintering host of Fort Morgan virus, an alphavirus affecting swallows.

Vertebrate hosts also contribute to viral persistence. One or more of the vertebrate hosts can be chronically or persistently infected, thus sustaining long-term viremias. For example, Colorado tick fever virus replicates in developing erythrocytes. When mature erythrocytes enter the bloodstream, they protect the virus from circulating antibodies while causing an effective viremia. Recrudescent viremias can also serve to reintroduce other arboviruses after a period of disrupted transmission. Hibernating reptiles and mammals with delayed viremias have been hypothesized to be involved with the overwintering of alphaviruses and flaviviruses. An arbovirus may actually disappear from an area when the vector(s) become inactive. Migrating species then reintroduce arboviruses to the regions that are seasonally unfavorable to transmission. Some arboviruses, certain Rhabdoviruses for example, have been hypothesized to persist in food chains when the vectors are inactive.

Reservoirs and the Nidus of Infection

Arboviral cycles appear to be extremely tenuous with many opportunities for their disruption. However, as efforts to control vector-borne diseases have shown, these amazingly resilient cycles have proved to be virtually indestructible. The mechanisms that maintain arboviruses constitute the reservoir. In the early days of arbovirology, the vertebrate host was generally called the viral reservoir. When researchers realized that many arboviruses are transovarially transmitted, the definition of a reservoir was expanded to include all of the underlying extrahuman mechanisms by which a specific pathogen population is maintained, including the specialized ecology necessary to support the biological relationships involved. The reservoir is then intimately associated with Pavlovsky's theory of nidality (focus of endemicity). A nidus of infection must contain the components (vectors, vertebrate hosts, habitat) necessary to maintain the virus. The field of landscape epidemiology, which focuses on habitats that are more likely to contain the components needed to sustain arboviral cycles, derives from the nidus concept.

Two principal determinants of the nidus are (1) the presence of competent vectors and (2) the availability of susceptible (nonimmune) vertebrate hosts. The nidus of infection of YF virus in Brazil can be as large as the Amazon basin forest. The nidus could be visualized as a moving wave of YF virus passing from infected to noninfected monkey troops in areas where territories overlap or are contested. In contrast, the nidus could be as small as a homesite or backyard, as for LAC virus, as described in the following section.

TRANSMISSION CYCLE OF LACROSSE VIRUS

Following is a detailed description of the cycle of LAC virus that illustrates the principles of arboviral maintenance and amplification cycles described.

Lacrosse Epidemiology

LAC virus is the leading cause of arboviral pediatric encephalitis in the upper midwestern and eastern United States. Humans are tangential hosts, and infections occur between June and September, with the majority reported in August and early September. Clinical cases are most often observed in children 3–15 years old. Boys are infected more often than girls, presumably because they engage in more outdoor activity and thus experience greater exposure to the vector. Infection of older children or adults typically does not result in encephalitis; a headache and nuchal rigidity (stiff neck) can be the only symptoms of infection.

In the early 1960s, LAC virus was isolated postmortem from the brain of a child who died in LaCrosse, Wisconsin. By the mid-1970s, virtually the entire LAC cycle had been described (Fig. 4.12), with chipmunks and tree squirrels identified as the primary natural vertebrate hosts and *Ae. triseriatus* the principal vector. Most important, the overwintering mechanism of the virus had also been determined; the virus is transovarially transmitted and overwinters in diapausing mosquito eggs. In the spring some adult females emerge immediately ready to transmit to newly born susceptible vertebrate hosts. Males also contribute to the cycle by venereally infecting female mosquitoes during mating.

The natural cycle of LAC virus was identified in a relatively short time. Note that overwintering mechanisms for other arboviral encephalitides, such as EEE and WEE, have yet to be described. Of course, the LAC cycle differs dramatically from the others due to transovarial and venereal transmission of the virus. Flaviviruses are inefficiently transmitted vertically; these viruses apparently infect the eggs during oviposition, not during follicle development as for transovarial transmission. At best, vertical transmission of alphaviruses is poor.

Lacrosse Cycle Components

The Virus

LAC virus belongs to the family Bunyaviridae. It is a member of the California serogroup of the *Bunyavirus* genus. The virion measures approximately 90 nm in diameter and possesses an envelope containing 2 virus-specified glycoproteins. The RNA genome is negative sense and tripartite, and the RNA segments are associated with nucleocapsid proteins. The large RNA segment (L RNA) codes for the viral polymerase, the middle-size RNA (M RNA) codes for the 2 viral surface glycoproteins as well as a nonstructural protein, and the small RNA (S RNA) codes for the nucleocapsid protein and a nonstructural protein.

Aedes triseriatus, the Principal Vector

Ae. triseriatus is the principal vector of the virus. Common throughout the eastern portions of the United States, the distribution of this mosquito extends to the high plains. States bordering the Great Lakes and the Mississippi River historically record the highest incidence of LAC encephalitis. Few cases occur in the southern states, where *Ae. triseriatus* and vertebrate hosts are also relatively abundant. Thus,

considerable intraspecific variability in vector competence exists. The vector, principally a daytime feeder, becomes most active at crepuscular periods.

Those states with high LAC incidence contain oak, hickory, or other climax forest areas that provide exceptional breeding opportunities for *Ae. triseriatus*. This vector oviposits in the tree holes that are especially abundant in oak forests. Other suitable oviposition sites, such as old tires and other water-containing devices, often bring the vector out of the forested areas and into even closer contact with human hosts.

The Vertebrate Hosts

In the upper midwestern states, chipmunks and tree squirrels are the principal vertebrate hosts. Both vertebrate hosts are abundant, coexist with the mosquito vector, and have a relatively high reproductive rate. Active during the day, chipmunks and squirrels are available as hosts for the vectors. Both are permissive to viral infection, develop substantial viremias, and exhibit no apparent negative effect from viral infection. In the forested areas, seroprevalence rates can be exceptionally high, approaching 100% in certain areas. Were it not for transovarial transmission, the arboviral cycles could probably not survive in locations with such high vertebrate host immunity. Each spring, viruses that overwintered in diapaused eggs and replicated in developing mosquitoes are transmitted to newborn, susceptible vertebrates. The arboviral cycle is renewed, and virus prevalence is amplified in nature. Humans are tangential, dead-end hosts.

LaCrosse–Aedes Triseriatus *Interactions*

Productive Infection

In the LAC virus–*Aedes triseriatus* interaction, ingested virus first infects and replicates in cuboidal epithelial cells of the anterior portion of the vector midgut; viral antigen is detected there between 3–6 days postingestion (Fig. 4.13). Viral antigen is subsequently found in the foregut and cardiac portion of the midgut. After approximately 6 days, virus disseminates from the midgut and infects secondary target organs. Viral antigen becomes detectable at 8–9 days in fat body, heart and pericardial cells, and nervous and ovarian tissues. Simultaneous detection of viral antigen in so many organ systems suggests a hemolymph mode of spread of arboviruses in mosquitoes. LAC virus reaches *Ae. triseriatus* salivary gland cells approximately 10–14 days post-infection. The extrinsic incubation period then ends, and the female can transmit the virus to new vertebrate hosts during subsequent blood meals (Fig. 4.13). The virus is virtually pantropic in the vector.

Barriers to Infection

Midgut infection and dissemination barriers, as well as salivary gland and ovarian infection and dissemination barriers to LAC virus, have been described in *Ae. triseriatus*. In addition, intraspecific variation in vector competence for oral susceptibility and transovarial transmission have been demonstrated. For example, *Ae. triseriatus* mosquitoes from Connecticut are much less efficient than those from Wisconsin in transovarial transmission of the virus. The genetic bases of these phenomena remain to be determined.

Because of the complexity of elucidating vector determinants of vector competence, considerable effort has been devoted to investigating viral genetic determinants of virus-vector interactions. Reassortant bunyaviruses were used to determine the molecular basis of virus-vector interactions (Table 4.3). When snowshoe hare (SSH) and LAC reassortant viruses (described according to their large, medium, or small segment composition) infect *Ae. triseriatus* midgut cells, the parental origin of the M RNA segment does not significantly affect infection rates. As quantified by detection of viral antigen, both viruses are equally capable of

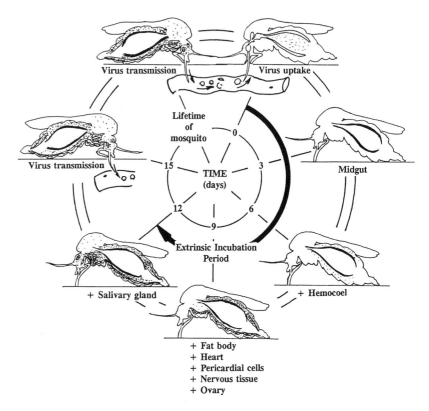

4.13   LaCrosse virus dissemination in *Aedes triseriatus*

infecting midgut cells. Evidently, if efficient infection of midgut cells is principally mediated by specific receptors, then the receptor is not sufficiently discriminatory to distinguish between the LAC and SSH M RNA gene products (glycoproteins).

In contrast to midgut infections, there is a marked difference in the ability of the viruses to escape from the midgut cells or to infect secondary target organs (Table 4.3). Reassortant viruses containing the LAC M RNA segment are significantly more efficient in disseminating than those viruses containing the SSH M RNA segment. The molecular basis of this midgut escape barrier remains to be determined.

The presence of the LAC M RNA segment is also a major determinant of transmission of virus to mice. Viruses containing the LAC M RNA were transmitted

TABLE 4.3 Infection, dissemination, and transmission of LaCrosse, snowshoe hare, and reassortant viruses in *Aedes triseriatus* mosquitoes

Viral genotypes	Percent infected	Percent disseminated	Percent transmitting
LAC/LAC/LAC ⎫ SSH/LAC/SSH ⎬ SSH/LAC/LAC ⎬ LAC/LAC/SSH ⎭	98 (115/117)	98 (113/115)	93 (126/136)
SSH/SSH/LAC ⎫ LAC/SSH/LAC ⎬ LAC/SSH/SSH ⎬ SSH/SSH/SSH ⎭	92 (92/100)	26 (24/92)	35 (36/104)

Modified and reproduced, with permission, from *Virus Research* 10:289–302, © 1988 by Elsevier Science Publishers BV.

by 93% of the mosquitoes; however, those containing the SSH M RNA were transmitted by only 35% of the mosquitoes with disseminated infections (Table 4.3). Thus the M RNA segment seems to be the major determinant of both LAC virus dissemination from the midgut and subsequent transmission by *Ae. triseriatus*. Unfortunately, genetic analysis of bunyaviruses is complicated by the fact that the M RNA segment codes for 2 glycoproteins (G1 and G2) and a nonstructural protein (NsM).

Studies with monoclonal antibody resistant variant viruses (MARVs) revealed that a specific epitope on the G1 glycoprotein was a major determinant of midgut infection of *Ae. triseriatus*. A variant virus (MARV 22) propagated in the presence of a specific monoclonal antibody was deficient in fusion function, was no longer neuroinvasive in mice, and exhibited greatly reduced infectivity for the mosquito midgut (Table 4.4). When the virus reverted at the specific epitope, infectivity for the mosquito was restored.

TABLE 4.4 Phenotypic analysis of parent LaCrosse, MARV 22, and revertant viruses

Virus	Infection rate	Neutralization titer	Fusion index (pH 6.0)
Parent LaCrosse	74% (14/19)	160	>0.8
Variant V22	5% (4/47)	<10	0.2
Revertant Virus	85% (50/59)	320	>0.6

Modified and reproduced, with permission, from *Virus Research* 10:289–302, © 1988 by Elsevier Science Publishers BV.

A mosquito's midgut is replete with proteolytic enzymes after a blood meal, and LAC virus glycoproteins are readily cleaved by such enzymes. Intact virions of LAC virus bind well to vertebrate cells but not to mosquito midguts; however, proteolytic processing of G1 apparently reveals sequences of the G2 glycoprotein, and the processed virions do bind to mosquito midguts. As noted previously, specific mosquito receptors utilized by viruses remain to be elucidated. Interestingly, the 2 glycoproteins of the virus seem to be differentially involved in the various transmission components of the arboviral cycle.

Vertical Transmission

LAC virus vertical transmission to progeny occurs through a transovarial, not a transovum, route. Transmission can be quite efficient; transovarial transmission rates (mothers transmitting virus to progeny) and filial infection rates (percent of progeny becoming infected) can exceed 80 percent. Reproductive tissues become infected concurrently with other tissues. LAC viral antigen has been clearly shown in the follicles in virtually every embryonic cell of the follicle.

Transtadial Transmission and Metamorphosis

LAC virus is efficiently maintained transtadially (between molts) and through metamorphosis, when proteolytic enzymes and nucleases are abundant in the vector. Throughout transtadial passage, virus is detected virtually pantropically. During metamorphosis, virus is apparently preserved in tissues that are not histolyzed. LAC virions can then infect newly developed tissues after metamorphosis.

Horizontal Transmission

Virus is horizontally transmitted (1) to the vertebrate host from the adult female salivary glands or (2) to the adult female from vertically infected males. Females can become infected either horizontally or vertically; males only become infected vertically.

Venereal Transmission

Transovarially infected male mosquitoes can venereally transmit virus to females. Most of the male reproductive tract, including vas, seminal vesicles, and accessory sex glands, permit viral replication. Accessory sex glands accumulate large amounts of virus that can be transmitted to females during mating. If females have not ingested a blood meal, less than 10% become infected venereally; if females have ingested a blood meal, up to 50% become infected. This latter observation suggests a very interesting possible linkage between hormonal status and susceptibility to viral infection.

Lacrosse Nidality

LAC virus is maintained in small forested areas, such as the islands of hardwood forests that are found throughout farming areas of the upper Midwest. Indeed, the nidus of infection can be as small as a backyard if the yard contains at least moderate tree and shrub cover, tree holes, discarded tires or other breeding sites, and vertebrate hosts such as chipmunks and squirrels.

Viruses such as LAC that are efficiently transovarially transmitted can be maintained in rather small geographic regions because virus can be amplified by horizontal and transovarial transmission. LAC can be further amplified by venereal transmission from infected male mosquitoes to noninfected female mosquitoes. Note that infection of new vectors can occur even when the vertebrate host population displays high seroprevalence rates. In fact, the presence of LAC virus antibodies has little effect upon transovarial transmission. Thus, a female could well oviposit 100 infected eggs, even after feeding upon an immune host. In contrast, arboviruses with little or no inefficient transovarial transmission require a constant supply of susceptible vertebrate hosts for horizontal amplification of the virus.

Evolution of LAC Virus in Vectors

General Principles of Arboviral Evolution

The Bunyaviridae, which includes LAC virus, is the largest family of viruses, with over 240 recognized members. Thus, the Bunyaviridae possesses considerable evolutionary prowess. Why is this group so successful? The evolutionary success of the family is probably attributable to their ability to evolve both by intramolecular mutations and by reassortment of the 3 RNA segments (the influenza viruses of arbovirology). Further, the long-term replication of bunyaviruses in their arthropod hosts provides many opportunities for these evolutionary events to occur. Understanding the evolutionary potential of bunyaviruses such as LAC virus in terms of spontaneous mutation rates and in terms of segment reassortment potential is not just an academic exercise. Evolutionary changes in the virus could result in more virulent viruses or viruses capable of being transmitted by different vectors that could introduce the virus to new, susceptible vertebrate species.

Spontaneous Mutations

Spontaneous mutations provide evolutionary potential for all organisms. The spontaneous mutation rate for LAC virus is high; the base substitution error frequency is probably on the order of 10^{-3}. Analyses of isolates of LAC virus from nature substantiate the genomic plasticity of LAC virus; no 2 isolates have identical genomes as evidenced by oligonucleotide fingerprinting (ONF). This is true not only for viruses isolated from different geographic locales at the same or different times but for viruses isolated from the same locale simultaneously. Thus, the major evolutionary mechanism of bunyaviruses is genetic drift via the accumulation of point mutations, sequence deletions, and inversions.

Segment Reassortment

In addition to spontaneous mutations, the evolutionary potential of bunyaviruses is further enhanced by the segmented genome; segment reassortment has been documented to occur in vitro, in vivo, and in nature. For example, the Group C viruses in a small forest in Brazil can represent a gene pool. The 6 viruses are related alternatively by hemagglutination inhibiting antibody (HI), neutralizing antibody (NT), and complement fixation (CF) reactions that assayed M RNA and S RNA gene products, respectively. Reassortment of genomes could result in serious epidemiologic consequences. Either the vertebrate host or the vector could serve as the site for reassortment in such circumstances. Studies attempting to demonstrate bunyavirus genome reassortment in vertebrates have been unsuccessful. Apparently, the acute nature of infection in vertebrate hosts and the development of long-term immunity limits evolutionary opportunities in this host. In contrast, dual infection of *Ae. triseriatus* mosquitoes with 2 bunyaviruses results in high frequency reassortment of the viruses. Resulting reassortant viruses are efficiently horizontally transmitted to vertebrate hosts and vertically transmitted to progeny.

Clearly, the vector can serve as a site for viral segment reassortment, point mutations, sequence deletions, inversions, and so forth. The persistent infection of arthropods, the long life of many vectors (especially ticks), the habit of many vectors of taking multiple blood meals from different vertebrate hosts, and the lack of an effective immune response to viruses in arthropods contribute to arboviral evolution. As these evolutionary events occur, the vector conducts ongoing experimentation by introducing the virus into new vertebrates and potentially initiating an epidemic.

SUMMARY

The vector-borne disease cycle comprises a dynamic interaction between the pathogen, the vectors(s), the vertebrate host(s), and the environment. The pathogen must be capable of reproducing in 2 phylogenetically disparate organisms in such a way as to be biologically or mechanically transmitted to the next vector or vertebrate. Vectors contribute in various ways to cycles. Vector-borne cycles typically undergo maintenance and amplification phases. Several mechanisms can be employed by a pathogen to persist through seasons of reduced or no transmission. Vectors and usual vertebrate hosts frequently suffer little or no adverse effects from infection, though some exceptions cause disease of great medical or veterinary importance. Vertebrates respond immunologically to the pathogen, thereby limiting the duration or intensity of infection. In contrast, vectors are typically infected for life with no untoward effect. Pathogens can be amplified by horizontal and vertical transmission and have evolved mechanisms, which are in most cases poorly understood, for surviving adverse climatic conditions.

Vector-borne disease cycles seem to be a tenuous mode of transmission and maintenance for pathogens. However, the diversity of the pathogens involved and the tenacity of these cycles in the face of sometimes drastic human intervention attests to their ability to maintain and amplify the prevalence of pathogens in nature. Understanding the interactions between pathogens, vectors, and vertebrates will facilitate development of effective and novel control strategies for these important pathogens of humans and animals.

ACKNOWLEDGMENTS

J. Woodring was supported by NIH Training AI grant 07352. This work was supported in part by NIH grant 32543 and the John D. and Catherine T. MacArthur Foundation.

REFERENCES

Beaty, B.J., and D.H.L Bishop. 1988. Bunyavirus-vector interactions. *Virus. Res.* 10:289–302.

Beaty, B.J., and C.H. Calisher. 1991. Bunyaviridae—Natural history. In: D. Kolakofsky, editor, Bunyaviridae. *Curr. Top. Micro. Immunol.* 169:27–78.

Chamberlain, R.W., R.K. Sikes, and W.D. Sudia. 1954. Studies on the North American arthropod-borne encephalitides. Part 6: Quantitative determination of virus-vector relationships. *Am. J. Hyg.* 60:278–285.

Chamberlain, R.W., and W.D. Sudia. 1961. Mechanism of transmission of viruses by mosquitoes. *Ann. Rev. Entomol.* 6:371–390.

Eldridge, B.F. 1990. Evolutionary relationships among California serogroup viruses (Bunyaviridae) and *Aedes* mosquitoes (Diptera: Culicidae). *J. Med. Ent.* 27: 738–749.

Grimstad, P.R. 1983. Mosquitoes and the incidence of encephalitis. In: M.A. Lauffer and K. Maramorosch, editors, *Advances virus research.* Academic Press, New York. pp. 357–438.

Hardy, J.L. 1988. Susceptibility and resistance of vector mosquitoes. In: T.P. Monath, editor, *The arboviruses: Epidemiology and ecology,* Vol. 1. Boca Raton, FL: CRC Press, pp. 87–126.

Karabatsos, N., editor. 1985. *International catalogue of arboviruses: Including certain other viruses of vertebrates.* 3rd ed. San Antonio, TX: American Society of Tropical Medicine and Hygiene. 1147 p.

Ludwig, G.V., B.A. Israel, B.M. Christensen, T.M. Yuill, and K.T. Schultz. 1991. Role of LaCrosse virus glycoproteins in attachment of virus to host cells. *Virol.* 181:564–571.

Miller, B.R., B.J. Beaty, and L. Lorenz. 1982. Variation of LaCrosse virus filial infection rates in geographic strains of *Aedes triseriatus. J. Med. Ent.* 19:213–214.

Miller, B.R., and C.J. Mitchell. 1991. Genetic selection of a flavivirus-refractory strain of the yellow fever mosquito, *Aedes aegypti. Am. J. Trop. Med. Hyg.* 45:399–407.

Monath, T.P., ed. *The arboviruses: Epidemiology and ecology.* Boca Raton: CRC Press, FL.

Paulson, S., and P.R. Grimstad. 1989. Midgut and salivary gland barriers to La Crosse virus dissemination in mosquitoes of the *Aedes triseriatus* group. *Med. Vet. Entomol.* 3:113–123.

Tabachnick, W.J. 1991. Evolutionary genetics and arthropod-borne disease: the yellow fever mosquito. *Amer. Entomol.* 37:14–24.

Weaver, S.C., T.W. Scott, L.H. Lorenz, K. Lerdthusnee, and W.S. Romoser. 1988. Togavirus-associated pathologic changes in the midgut of a natural mosquito vector. *J. Virol.* 62:2083–2090.

5. ANOPHELINE MOSQUITOES AND THE AGENTS THEY TRANSMIT

Robert Gwadz and Frank H. Collins

INTRODUCTION

All mosquitoes are members of the family Culicidae, 1 of the approximately 130 families in the insect order Diptera, the 2-winged flies. Diptera are generally divided into 2 categories, which most taxonomists give subordinal rank: the lower flies, or Nematocera, and the higher flies, Brachycera. The latter group, which includes more than 100 families, is recognized as monophyletic. The approximately 2 dozen families that constitute the Nematocera are a paraphyletic assemblage, but it is not clear which part of the Nematocera is a sister taxon of the Brachycera (Wood and Borkent 1989).

The family Culicidae is typically subdivided into 3 subfamilies: Culicinae, Toxorhynchitinae, and Anophelinae. The Anophelinae includes members of the genus *Anopheles* as well as the small and probably primitive genera *Bironella* (found mostly on or near the island of New Guinea) and *Chagasia* (South America). The *Bironella* species are unique among culicids in that they have 4 pairs of chromosomes: all other mosquitoes have 3. The subfamily Toxorhynchitinae includes less than 70 species, all in the genus *Toxorhynchites*. These are large, non–blood-feeding mosquitoes with carnivorous larvae that prey primarily on the aquatic larvae of other insects, especially mosquitoes. The subfamily Culicinae is by far the largest, with almost 3000 species in over 24 different genera. Most are blood-feeders, although a few have secondarily lost the capacity, and some can facultatively reproduce without access to a blood meal.

The phylogenetic history of the Diptera is not clear. Dipteran-like insects first appear in the fossil record in the late Paleozoic era, and divergence of the higher flies from the lower fly assemblage probably dates from the Triassic (Wood and Borkent 1989). Many of the dipteran families, especially in the lower flies, probably date from a major evolutionary radiation in the early Triassic era that followed the terminal Permian mass extinction. Resolution of phylogenetic relationships among those groups that trace their lineage to this short period of radiation is complicated by the long history of their subsequent divergence (Besansky et al. 1992). Comparison of ribosomal DNA sequences of representatives of the different mosquito subgenera suggests that the Anophelinae diverged first from the ancestral stock, followed by Toxorhynchitinae and then the Culicinae (Boyd 1949). Thus blood-feeding in the Culicidae is ancestral.

Blood-feeding is present in a large number of dipteran families, including the Nematoceran families Culicidae, Corethrellidae, Simuliidae, Ceratopogonidae, and Psychodidae and the Brachyceran families Tabanidae, Rhagionidae, Muscidae, and Glossinidae. Blood-feeding appears to have arisen independently in most if not all of these families, probably in most cases from a carnivorous ancestor but possibly in some cases, such as the Psychodidae, from an ancestor adapted to sucking plant juices.

Of all the blood-feeding groups of insects, the mosquitoes are by far the most important from the point of view of human health. Pathogens causing several of the most important past and present causes of human mortality and morbidity are transmitted by mosquitoes. Toward the end of the 19th century, with the discoveries of Sir Patrick Manson, Sir Ronald Ross, Carlos Finlay, and Sir Walter Reed, mosquitoes were recognized to be vectors of the human filariae, malaria parasites, and arthropod-borne viruses (arboviruses) (Boyd 1949). Today, the 4 species of human malaria parasites, the filarial parasites *Wuchereria bancrofti* and *Brugia malayi*, and a number of arboviruses remain among the principal causes of human mortality and morbidity in the world.

All human malaria parasites are transmitted by mosquitoes in the genus *Anopheles*. In certain parts of the world, *Anopheles* species are also important vectors of human filarial parasites. Although most arboviruses are transmitted by culicine mosquitoes, anophelines were shown to be the sole vectors responsible for several explosive outbreaks of o'nyong-nyong fever in East Africa. Malaria remains the most important parasitic disease of humans in the world today; an estimated 300 million people, of which between 1 and 3 million die each year, are infected with 1 or more species of the parasites. In fact, almost 40% of the world's population lives in parts of the world where malaria is endemic.

In 1977, Knight and Stone described 375 species of *Anopheles* mosquitoes (Knight and Stone 1977). Since then the number has increased to almost 500, primarily because of the discovery that many of the morphologically identified species recognized in earlier publications were actually complexes of cryptic or morphologically indistinguishable species (Collins and Paskewitz 1995). The genus *Anopheles* includes 6 subgenera. Two of the smallest subgenera—*Lophopodomyia* with 6 species and *Stethomyia* with 5—are found in the New World (North and South America) tropics and do not include any species that are known to be malaria vectors. Another small New World subgenus, *Kertezia*, includes 11 forest species, most of

which breed in the leaf axils of bromeliads. Although a few of these species have been marginally involved in malaria transmission in human populations that live or work in close association with the rain forest, today they are of little importance as vectors. The subgenus *Cellia*, composed of 230 or more species, includes many of the most important malaria vectors, especially in the Old World (Asia and Africa) tropics. Mosquitoes of the subgenus *Anopheles*, with over 180 species, were the major vectors of malaria in Europe and North America; today only a few species in this group are involved in malaria transmission. The New World subgenus *Nyssorhynchus*, with more than 40 species, includes most of the important malaria vectors in Central and South America.

MORPHOLOGY AND LIFE CYCLE

All mosquitoes, except members of the genus *Toxorhynchites*, have the same basic developmental cycle. Usually between 50 and 200 eggs are produced by the female 2–3 days after a blood meal. Eggs are typically laid directly on water or a damp substrate likely to be flooded. Many *Aedes* and related species, whose unhatched larvae can diapause for periods of up to a year or more, lay eggs on substrates that will not be flooded for long periods of time. In species that do not diapause, larvae hatch usually within 2–3 days of oviposition and feed by means of mouthparts that in most mosquitoes are adapted to either collecting and filtering microorganisms and detritus from the water—commonly the air/water interface—or for scraping material off surfaces.

All mosquitoes have 4 larval instars, and an aquatic pupal instar that typically takes 2–4 days to complete metamorphosis to the adult. Adults show a marked sexual dimorphism. The females are generally larger and possess mouthparts adapted to piercing; males have mouthparts that are adapted to feeding on liquid sugar sources such as plant nectars and possess long feathery antennae that are used to detect females prior to mating.

Mosquito eggs assume a number of structural forms, but most eggs follow 1 of several basic plans. All anopheline eggs are roughly boat shaped, with protruding bubbles of chorion at the sides that trap air and help the eggs float. Many culicine mosquitoes, especially *Aedes* species, lay eggs that are shaped like elongated U.S.-style footballs; other culicine mosquitoes, especially *Culex* and a number of other genera, lay eggs that stand on the surface of the water in boat-shaped clusters because they are hydrophobic over all but the anterior pole (Chap. 6). The eggs of *Toxorhynchites* species, which are usually laid singly, are spherical. The larvae of different mosquito subfamilies are also relatively distinctive.

All larvae are elongate, with an oval heavily sclerotized head capsula, a thorax, and 9 distinct abdominal appendages. A pair of respiratory spiracles is located on the dorsal surface of the 8th abdominal appendage, and anal papillae, which regulate electrolyte levels by salt and or water uptake (see Chap. 17), are attached to the last appendage. In the larvae of most culicine and toxorhynchitine mosquitoes, the respiratory spiracles are at the end of a long respiratory siphon, and when at rest on the surface, the larvae hang down into the water column. Anopheline larvae, by contrast, do not have an elongate siphon, and when at rest on the surface, where they generally prefer to feed, remain horizontal.

Pupae are also aquatic. The head and thorax are fused into a large cephalothorax from which 2 respiratory siphons emerge. The abdominal segments curl under the cephalothorax and terminate with 2 paddles. Abdominal muscles remain functional throughout the pupal stage, and contraction of these muscles provides effective rapid movement for the pupa. Because air is contained in the region of the cephalothorax in which the adult appendages develop, the pupae are buoyant. When placed in cold water to reduce activity, the pupae float to the surface whereas the larvae sink to the bottom, a difference that is often used in separating larvae and pupae in colonized mosquitoes.

ANOPHELINE MOSQUITOES — GENERAL LIFE CYCLE

Various life-history strategies are found in anopheline mosquitoes. In general, the larval and pupal stages of most species are found in relatively unpolluted water. Common anopheline aquatic habitats include the margins of ponds, lakes, or slow-flowing streams; temporary bodies of water produced by rain, river flooding, or drying rivers and streams; and even water found in such "containers" as rain water cisterns, household water receptacles, and water trapped by the leaf axils of plants such as bromeliads. Many species, particularly some of those important as vectors of malaria, are found in aquatic habitats created by the activities of man, such as flooded agricultural fields, irrigation and seepage ditches, and flooded borrow pits. Most mosquitoes are colonizing species as larvae, preferring to inhabit bodies of water that are, to some extent, temporary and thus relatively free of established populations of predators and competitors.

BIOLOGY OF *ANOPHELES GAMBIAE*, AN IMPORTANT MALARIA VECTOR

An. gambiae, the major vector of malaria in sub-Saharan Africa, is probably the most important vector of a human pathogen in the world. Its life cycle is fairly typical of most anophelines, except that it has an extreme preference for living around human habitations and blood-feeding on people. Typical oviposition sites are small temporary bodies of water exposed to full sunlight, such as small puddles produced by rain. Because the number of available larval habitats increases during rainy seasons, the annual abundance of this mosquito correlates highly with rainfall. The larvae can also be found in agriculturally flooded areas such as rice fields. During the dry seasons, breeding occurs in temporary pools left by drying streams or pools associated with human activities.

Eggs are generally laid directly on the water or on damp soil, often in tiny bodies of water such as those formed by flooded hoofprints or tire ruts. Although eggs typically hatch approximately 48 hours after oviposition, some larvae can remain quiescent in unhatched eggs on damp soil for up to 2 weeks; thus, the population can survive during periods when rainfall is erratic. In addition, the larvae have the capacity to actually crawl some distance across very damp soil, thus enabling them to move to other pools when their habitat dries out.

Larval development is rapid and can be completed in less than a week in very warm conditions with ample food. The larvae are filter feeders and usually feed directly on the surface film of the water by rotating the head 180° so that mouthparts directly face the surface film. Two lateral brushes are used to scoop material on or near the surface film to the mouth. Larvae feed primarily on algae and other microorganisms that concentrate on or near the water's surface. Larvae are also capable of feeding in the water column or on the bottom, but this is not usual.

Pupation typically occurs in full sunlight and can be induced in colonized *An. gambiae* by transferring pans with fully developed 4th instar larvae from the insectary into open and full sunlight. As with larval development, the pupal development period varies, probably from just over 24 hours to as long as 3 or more days, depending on temperature. Adults typically emerge at night.

Both male and female adult *An. gambiae* require at least 24 hours to reach sexual maturity. During this period, the male terminalia, or sexual appendages, undergo a 180° rotation from their upward pointing orientation in the newly emerged male. Many mosquitoes exhibit a swarming behavior that is associated with mating. Typically, such swarms consist primarily of males; the females fly into the swarm to mate. Swarming behavior has not been well documented in wild populations of *An. gambiae*, although it has been seen in laboratory colonies kept in large cages.

In the laboratory, and probably also in the wild, males begin to become active after sundown. The plumes or hairs of their antennae, which are folded against the antennal shaft during the day, open and presumably become receptive to the flight sound of the female. The males detect this sound with a sensory organ, the Johnston's organ, found at the base of the antenna. Males are thus attracted to the nearby females, and mating occurs in flight. Wild female mosquitoes probably mate with only 1 male. Both males and females are generally found inside houses, and although outdoor mating swarms have been described, it is possible that adults mate in houses as well.

Mated female *An. gambiae* seek a blood meal only at night; they usually become active after sundown. Because this species is highly anthropophilic, they usually take more than 90% of their blood meals from human hosts, usually while the hosts are sleeping. Indeed, *An. gambiae* is clearly attracted to human houses, where they not only feed but also rest after the blood meal. Egg development requires about 48 hours during the warm season, but it can take somewhat longer in cooler months. Oviposition, like blood-feeding, occurs at night. As a consequence, the gravid female generally lays her eggs the second night after she has blood fed and after oviposition searches for another blood meal. Thus during the warmer seasons a female *An. gambiae* is capable of ovipositing every other night.

Because of this pattern of oviposition (followed by blood-feeding), most of the females that actively search for a blood meal immediately after dusk are nulliparous, or have not yet laid their first egg batch. Older, parous mosquitoes tend to feed later at night because they must oviposit before they can blood-feed. This repeated feeding and oviposition has major implications for transmission of pathogens such as malaria parasites, which have a required developmental cycle in the mosquito. Indeed, a minimum developmental time for *Plasmodium falciparum* malaria parasites is about 8 to 10 days; thus, a mosquito requires at least 5–6 blood meals to obtain parasites and then live long enough to transmit parasites—assuming that she oviposited and took a blood meal every 2 days. In general, however, environmental factors such as temperature, wind, and rainfall can interfere with the ability of a female to oviposit and blood-feed on this schedule. Most *An. gambiae* with *P. falciparum* sporozoites in their salivary glands have probably taken at least 3–4 blood meals.

HOST–PARASITE INTERACTIONS

Host Finding

The search for a blood meal is a primary activity of the female anopheline mosquito and is one of the first steps in determining its role as a disease vector. Because most anophelines are anautogenous, requiring at least 1 blood meal for each clutch of eggs produced, the search for blood is an ongoing, repetitive process.

Of equal or even greater importance in determining the role of anopheline mosquitoes as vectors of malaria is the question of host choice. Most of the more important vectors are anthropophilic—they prefer to feed on human hosts. Species that are clearly zoophilic, preferring to feed on animals if given a choice, are seldom vectors. Nevertheless, exceptions to this rule are common. In parts of Central America, the primary malaria vector is *An. albimanus*. Although this species is highly zoophilic, and females are seldom found carrying sporozoites, *An. albimanus* maintains transmission, probably because of its very high population densities.

Host preference appears to be genetically determined; however, opportunistic factors can play a major role. Most mosquitoes feed on alternative hosts if the primary choice is unavailable.

Feeding Behavior

Because Culicines are not only similar to Anophelines but have been studied more often, they consequently provide much information about host-seeking and feeding behaviors in Anophelines. A randomly questing female mosquito that encounters an attractant plume from a potential host reorients her flight and begins to fly upwind toward the host. The composition of the plume is complex, composed of CO_2 and host-related odors. As the mosquito nears the host, physical factors including warmth and moisture can be attractants. (Details of host-seeking are provided in Chap. 3.)

Once on the skin of the desired host, the female mosquito exhibits a stereotypical behavior pattern of penetrating, probing, ingesting blood, and withdrawing. This series of steps has been well described for *Aedes aegypti* and appears to be consistent with what has been observed in a number of anopheline species. The details of the process of blood-feeding is outlined in Chapters 2, 3, and 6.

Phagostimulation in anopheline mosquitoes differs significantly from what has been described in culicines. Mosquitoes such as *Ae. aegypti, Culex pipiens,* and *Culiseta inornata* respond to the presence of adenine nucleotides in the blood meal or in a saline solution by feeding to repletion. Tests on 4 diverse anophelines, *An. stephensi, An. freeborni, An. gambiae,* and *An. dirus* showed that these species did not respond to ATP as an engorgement stimulus. Rather, they readily fed on salt solutions isotonic with serum (Galun et al. 1985). It has been suggested that salivary gland apyrase can affect the probing behavior of anophelines and their ability to find blood (Ribeiro et al. 1985; Ribeiro 1987).

The termination of the feeding process is related to the degree of abdominal distension caused by the blood meal and is under control of the central nervous system. If the ventral nerve cord of *An. quadrimaculatus* is cut anterior to the second abdominal ganglion, inhibitory signals are denied the brain, and the female will not only feed beyond repletion to the point of rupture but often for some time thereafter. Without sensory input from abdominal stretch receptors, this species can imbibe at least 4 times the normal blood meal before rupturing. This response appears to be similar in both anopheline and culicine mosquitoes (Gwadz 1969).

Details of the feeding behavior of anophelines and its relationship to the epidemiology of malaria can be found in the excellent review by Gillies (1988).

CONTROL OF ANOPHELINE MOSQUITOES

The control of anopheline mosquitoes is usually associated with the control of malaria. Unlike their culicine relatives, most anophelines are not particularly abundant and are not normally considered to be pest species.

Although the relationship between anophelines and malaria was not validated until the end of the 19th century, inadvertent vector control was regularly practiced by the ancient Romans and others when they drained swamps and marshes to facilitate land use for agriculture. Similar systems of drainage of fields in the United States in the mid-19th century made spring plowing possible and destroyed the larval breeding sites of the anopheline malaria vectors.

When Grassi and his Italian colleagues demonstrated that anopheline mosquitoes were the vectors of malaria to humans, the concept of malaria control became synonymous with mosquito control. As early as 1899, Ross began a malaria control campaign in Sierra Leone by using kerosene on the surface of larval breeding sites. Soon thereafter major control efforts were mounted in Cuba and later in Panama against *Ae. aegypti*, the vector of yellow fever, and the anopheline vectors of malaria. These campaigns were extraordinarily successful and encouraged future control programs.

During the first half of the 20th century, malaria slowly receded from the temperate areas of Europe and North America. Although there were some notable programs aimed at reducing vector populations, such as the Tennessee Valley Authority flood control and land reclamation project in the southeastern United States, most of the decrease could be attributed to general improvement in land use, drainage, animal husbandry, window screening, and education (Boyd 1949, vol. 2). Where control schemes specifically attacked the mosquito, larvicides such as oil and Paris green powder were normally applied to the breeding sites. The only adulticide available at that time was pyrethrum. The advent of DDT during World War II changed the strategy and permitted an all-out assault on the vectors of malaria (see Chap. 29).

In 1957, the World Health Organization (WHO) initiated the global malaria eradication program. The program's primary strategy was the use of a residual insecticide, DDT, for spraying the walls of houses in malaria-endemic areas (Chap. 29). The insecticide was not intended to reduce mosquito populations but rather to interrupt the transmission of malaria. The only mosquitoes affected by this domiciliary treatment were female mosquitoes that had fed on a sleeping human host and subsequently had moved to the walls to rest. Contact with the insecticide resulted in the death of the mosquito before the malaria parasites could become infectious. In general, the program was a remarkable success. The vectors survived, but malaria was eliminated from Europe and greatly diminished throughout most of the world (with the exception of sub-Saharan Africa, where the program was never implemented).

The resurgence of malaria in many areas where control had been successful coincided with a number of events. The root causes and consequences are still matters of controversy. Among these, the administrative transfer of highly structured malaria eradication services to more diffuse public health administration schemes, the elimination of WHO central funding for these programs and the forced reliance on national support, and the appearance of insecticide resistance in the vector populations signalled the end of the global eradication effort. Country by country, control schemes were less well organized and usually poorly funded. The spread of resistance and the requirement for more expensive but less persistent insecticides has made many control programs unworkable.

Today, anopheline control programs remain associated with malaria control efforts. House spraying with residual insecticides is still practiced in some countries, and if properly implemented, malaria control can be maintained. In general, however, the regular use of insecticides for anopheline vector control is proving to be economically unsustainable and environmentally unacceptable.

Integrated control strategies, successful for some culicine species, work on anopheline species that develop in readily defined larval habitats, e.g., rice fields, ponds, and wetlands. However, many of the more important vector species utilize less defined breeding sites. *An. gambiae* is often found in roadside tire ruts, or the water-filled depression of a bovine hoofprint. In Southeast Asia *An. dirus* breeds in isolated pools deep in the forest. Neither is amenable to control.

Methods for reducing contact between the mosquito vector and the human host are receiving increased attention as a means for reducing malaria transmission. The use of insecticide-impregnated bed nets and curtains has been shown to reduce but not eliminate transmission. However, the widespread utility of these techniques remains to be confirmed (Collins and Paskewitz 1995).

A broad range of strategies for the control of anopheline vectors of malaria have been reviewed by Raftajah (1988) (environmental management), Pant (1988) (adult control), Gratz and Pal (1988) (larval control), Rishikesh et al. (1988) (biological control), and Farid (1988) (man-vector contact).

DISEASE AGENTS VECTORED

Mosquitoes of the genus *Anopheles* are justifiably notorious for their role in the transmission of malaria, the most serious vector-borne disease affecting humans; however, this genus contains members that are also important vectors of human filariasis and, in some cases, arboviruses (Gillies and De Meillon 1968; Gillies and Coetzee 1987). The relationship between anopheline mosquitoes and the malaria parasites infecting humans and their primate relatives is both intimate and apparently exclusive. There is a similar requisite relationship between anophelines and the malarias of African rodents. The avian malarias are usually associated with culicine genera but, in some cases, anopheline species can be involved.

Anopheline Mosquitoes and the Malarias Infecting Humans

The role of anophelines in the transmission of malaria to humans was first described by Grassi and his Italian colleagues, who noted that not all species of *Anopheles* could transmit the parasite. "Anophelism without malaria" was the term used to describe situations in which mosquitoes of this genus were common but malaria was absent. Indeed, although almost 500 species of *Anopheles* in 6 different subgenera have been described, probably no more than 20 species are really important vectors. The most important of these vectors are in the subgenus *Cellia*, which is restricted to the Old World Tropics. The 2 most important determinants of a good malaria vector are its propensity to feed on humans and its mean longevity; most malaria parasites must undergo at least a week or more of development and differentiation in the mosquito host before the mosquito can transmit. However, many anophelines are inefficient or incompetent malaria vectors because they are physiologically incapable of efficiently supporting development of the parasite. The various reasons vectors cannot support parasite growth and development are numerous and, in most cases, undefined. This genetic variability is the rationale on which studies of schemes for disease control through modification of vectorial competence are being based.

Anophelines and the Epidemiology of Malaria

The epidemiology of malaria and the biology of its mosquito vectors are inextricably intertwined. Environmental factors are equally important, affecting the behaviors of the vector, the vertebrate host, and the parasite itself. Consequently, a number of anopheline species have evolved as efficient vectors in diverse habitats, each species with its own unique set of biologic and ecologic requirements. Table 5.1 presents a brief listing of some of the most important vectors affecting humans.

Most of these species have been found to be members of species complexes, each complex consisting of several morphologically identical cryptic species (see Chap. 26); not all have the same capacity for malaria transmission. Malaria vectors can be found well adapted to life in desert oases, rice fields, the margins of running streams, transient pools, mangrove swamps, roof cisterns, and the leaf axils of bromeliads high in the forest canopy. The first requirement is always the presence of water to sustain development of the aquatic larval and pupal stages of the mosquito, and with a few notable exceptions, anopheline larvae require water that is relatively clean.

The anopheline vectors of the nonhuman primates are less well characterized, although many species have been shown in laboratory studies to be competent to transmit malaria parasites of both humans and their primate relatives. Several species, often with arboreal feeding habits, are restricted to feeding on tree-dwelling monkeys and serve as vectors for these animals. It is interesting to note that many of the monkey malarias can also infect humans; infections in human hosts can occur after incidental contact and feeding in the forest habitat. The New World primate malaria parasites *Plasmodium brazilianum* and *P. simium* represent forms of the human parasites *P. malariae* and *P. vivax*, introduced into the New World from Europe and Africa, that have adapted to monkeys as hosts.

The natural vectors of the malarias of rodents are even more obscure. *An. dureni millecampsi* has been implicated as a vector of *P. berghei* in central Africa. In the laboratory, *An. stephensi* and some of the more common colonized vectors can be used for transmission studies.

Anopheline Mosquitoes in Laboratory Colonies

Most of what we know of the physiology, biochemistry, and genetics of mosquitoes has been derived from studies on species from a limited number of laboratory colonies. Most of these studies involved culicine

TABLE 5.1 *Anopheles* species associated with the transmission of malaria

Species	Regions of primary importance
Anopheles gambiae	Sub-Saharan Africa
Anopheles arabiensis	
Anopheles funestus	
Anopheles melas	
Anopheles merus	
Anopheles sergentii	Middle East and North Africa
Anopheles pharoensis	
Anopheles sacharovi	
Anopheles superpictus	
Anopheles labranchiae	Mediterranean
Anopheles superpictus	
Anopheles dirus	Far East
Anopheles fluviatilis	
Anopheles minimus	
Anopheles sinensis	
Anopheles sundaicus	
Anopheles aconitus	
Anopheles maculatus	
Anopheles culicifacies	
Anopheles stephensi	
Anopheles annularis	
Anopheles farauti	Australasian Region
Anopheles punctulatus	
Anopheles albimanus	South and Central America
Anopheles darlingi	
Anopheles aquasalis	
Anopheles pseudopunctipennis	
Anopheles nuneztovari	

mosquitoes and, notably, a single species, *Aedes aegypti* (Clements 1992). As a result, *Ae. aegypti* is regarded by many as the archetypical mosquito. However, molecular data suggest not only that anopheline and culicine species are evolutionarily quite divergent, but that different *Anopheles* subgenera probably preceded divergence of the culicinae and toxorhynchitinae, the other 2 subfamilies in the Culicidae. Generalizations of mosquito biology on the basis of studies of *Ae. aegypti*, other culicines, or any single anopheline species should be viewed cautiously.

Two areas of mosquito biology in which anophelines have received significant attention are cytogenetics and molecular approaches to species identification. Most anophelines possess polytene chromosomes much like those in the genetically well defined fruit flies of the genus *Drosophila*. Material derived from larval salivary glands and ovarian nurse cells of half-gravid adult females of many anophelines has been used extensively in the definition of species complexes. Inversion polymorphisms are common in most anopheline species, and different members within these complexes can often be distinguished on the basis of unique combinations of chromosomal inversions. In nature, these inversions can help to fix genes or groups of genes that can confer adaptive advantages permitting survival under specific ecologic conditions. Many complexes of cryptic species include members that cannot be distinguished on the basis of inversion karyotypes; furthermore, polytene chromosomes with distinct banding patterns are not obtainable from all anopheline species. Therefore, a considerable research effort has recently been directed toward the development of DNA-based techniques for identifying individuals in cryptic species complexes (Collins and Paskewitz 1995).

Anopheline Mosquitoes as Laboratory Hosts and Vectors

There is a significant array of model systems for the study of malaria in the laboratory. None is simple to maintain. The rodent models require the least complex husbandry and can utilize normal rodent-rearing facilities. Laboratory models for the various malarias are handled in a relatively similar manner, be they in rodent, chicken, or nonhuman primate hosts.

1. The infection can be initiated in the vertebrate host by the injection of fresh or frozen parasitized blood from an infected donor, by the bite of an infected mosquito, or by injection of sporozoites derived from an infected mosquito.

2. The vertebrate host is monitored regularly by examining thick and thin blood films stained with Giemsa. Patency is usually determined by the presence of infected erythrocytes in the peripheral circulation of the host.

3. In some infections, the sexual-stage gametocytes appear with the first parasites in the circulation. In infections with *P. falciparum*, mature gametocytes usually begin to appear after the peak of asexual parasitemia. The presence of gametocytes on a film is no guarantee of infectivity to mosquitoes; it is not uncommon to acquire a good mosquito infection when no gametocytes are seen. The demonstration of exflagellation in freshly drawn blood is usually a good indication of infectivity to mosquitoes.

4. When it has been determined that the general parasitemia or gametocytemia is consistent with one's experience with infectivity, mosquitoes can be fed directly on an anesthetized or restrained animal. Alternatively, blood can be drawn from the animal and offered to mosquitoes in a membrane feeding device. In both cases, the mosquitoes can feed on the blood source through the netting at the top of the cage.

5. If infection is successful, oocysts can be detected as early as 5 days after feeding with most species of parasites, although in species with longer sporogonic development, such as the rodent malarias and *P. malariae*, oocysts are often difficult to see before at least 8–9 days. Mosquito midguts stained with 2% mercurochrome in a saline solution can be examined under a microscope, and developing oocysts can be readily identified.

6. Sporozoites can be found in the salivary glands as early as 10 days postfeeding in some species of malaria. Glands can be dissected in saline and examined with phase-contrast optics to facilitate detection of the sporozoites.

7. Once sporozoites are present in the salivary glands, the mosquitoes can be considered to be infectious. Direct feeding on an appropriate naive host can reinitiate the cycle of infection. It is important to note that sporozoite-induced infections can be less virulent than infections initiated by the injection of parasitized blood. Sporozoite-induced infections can also be less infectious to feeding mosquitoes and can require a passage of infected blood to a second animal before maximum infectivity to mosquitoes is achieved. Conversely, continuous blood stage passage of some parasite has resulted in the loss of the capacity to produce infective gametocytes.

The Rodent Malarias

For over 30 years, investigators have used one of several rodent malarias to study the biology of these parasites in their rodent hosts and mosquito vectors (Cox 1988). Although *P. berghei* and *P. yoelli* were originally isolated from several species of Central African rodents (among them, the tree rat, *Thamnomys surdaster*), both species will grow in mice, rats, and hamsters. In the laboratory, *An. stephensi* is the vector of choice. It is a relatively easy mosquito to rear, feeds voraciously, and supports development of the parasites to maturation. *P. berghei* is unique in that its sporogonic development in the mosquito vector requires an incubation temperature between 18 and 21°C. All other malarias—including the other species from rodents—grow best at temperatures above 24°C (Cox 1988).

P. berghei and *P. yoelli* are represented by numerous isolates and strains, and their use has been documented in a significant body of scientific literature relating to malaria, immunology, and vaccine development. *P.*

vinckei and *P. chabaudi* are usually limited to studies in laboratory mice; mosquito infections are more difficult to obtain.

The Avian Malarias

Although there is an extensive literature on the use of malarias of birds as model systems, only *P. gallinaceum* is in regular use today. In most laboratories, the usual vector for this parasite of domestic chickens is *Aedes aegypti;* however, several anopheline species, including *An. quadrimaculatus* and *An. freeborni*, have been shown to be capable of transmission in the laboratory. Recently, a strain of *An. gambiae* has been selected that is fully susceptible to *P. gallinaceum*. Some significant advantages of the chicken malaria model are its relatively low cost, the ease with which chickens are reared, and the reproducibility of the system (Collins et al. 1986). Avian parasites such as *P. relictum*, *P. cathemerium*, and *P. elongatum* are presently seldom used and develop almost exclusively in culicine mosquitoes.

The Simian Malarias

The malaria parasites of the nonhuman primates have, over the years, proved to be important models for studies of malaria. Nevertheless, some limitations are obvious. Monkeys are expensive, and the facilities needed for the proper maintenance of these animals are beyond the reach of many laboratories. However, when appropriate animal holding facilities are available, the simian malarias present a superb opportunity for work with a disease system similar in most respects to what is seen in the human host. Coatney and his coworkers have compiled an extensive monograph on the various malaria species, their hosts, and vectors (Coatney et al. 1971). The following is a brief description of 2 of the more common monkey malarias in regular use.

Plasmodium cynomolgi

P. cynomolgi is a relapsing malaria with tertian (48-hr cycle) periodicity, which is similar in many respects to *P. vivax* in humans. *P. cynomolgi* is, in fact, a complex of morphologically and behaviorally similar parasites that can be differentiated at the antigenic and molecular levels. *P. vivax* is probably just one member of the complex that has moved from radiation in a variety of simian hosts and geographic locations into a human host. Most of the members of the *P. cynomolgi* complex can infect humans, albeit often with a generally mild course of disease. At the same time, it is important to note that although *P. vivax* probably arose from an Old World monkey parasite, it has lost the ability to infect monkeys.

P. cynomolgi readily infects a number of anophelines; *An. dirus, An. freeborni, An. stephensi,* and *An. gambiae* are among the more common species used in laboratory studies. When infected with sporozoites of this parasite, a monkey suffers classic parasitologic relapses.

Plasmodium knowlesi

This quotidian parasite of macaques is unique among the primate malarias in that it completes its cycle in the erythrocyte in 24 hr (quotidian = 1 day). In rhesus monkeys, the usual laboratory host, blood-induced infections are often fatal. Sporozoite-induced infections can be less virulent and are seldom fatal. This parasite does not exhibit the relapse phenomenon. *P. knowlesi* is limited in the number of anopheline species it infects. *An. dirus* is the laboratory vector of choice. The parasite produces oocysts and sporozoites in large numbers in both *An. freeborni* and *An. gambiae*, but these sporozoites do not invade the mosquito's salivary glands.

The Human Malarias

Four species of malaria parasites infect humans: *P. falciparum, P. vivax, P. ovale,* and *P. malariae*. All 4 species infect chimpanzees, and these primates have been used from time to time for specific purposes; however, the cost of purchase and maintenance of these animals, coupled with their designation by international conventions as "threatened," severely limits their utility. *P. falciparum, P. vivax,* and *P. malariae*—but not *P. ovale*—have been adapted to growth in New World owl monkeys of the genus *Aotus*, and *P. vivax* and *P. malariae* have been adapted to squirrel monkeys of the genus *Saimiri*. All these human malarias in these monkey species have been used to infect mosquitoes, but with difficulty. In general, the *Aotus* and *Saimiri* human malaria models have proved most useful in studies that do not involve mosquitoes.

P. falciparum is the only human malaria that can be grown readily in vitro. In addition, this species can be induced to produce gametocytes in culture. When fed to appropriate anopheline species through a membrane, this parasite can initiate normal sporogonic development. Oocysts and sporozoites develop normally, and the salivary glands become infected. When such mosquitoes, infected with cultured parasites, are fed on an appropriate vertebrate host, patent infections develop. Both humans and chimpanzees have been infected by the bites of mosquitoes originally infected from cultured *P. falciparum*. The best in vitro laboratory hosts for *P. falciparum* are *An. dirus*, *An. stephensi*, and *An. freeborni*.

Laboratory Models for Filariasis

An. gambiae is a primary vector of *Wuchereria bancrofti* in rural Africa, whereas *An. faranti* transmits the parasite in the southern Pacific. Although this filarioid nematode parasite has been grown in several monkey species, it has not proved to be a usable laboratory model. *W. bancrofti* remains almost exclusively a parasite of humans.

An. quadrimaculatus has been used as a laboratory host and vector of *Brugia pahangi*. *An. dirus* and other members of the *An. balabacensis* complex of Southeast Asian mosquitoes are natural vectors of *B. pahangi* and *B. malayi* but are seldom used as vectors in the laboratory. Most *Anopheles* species will probably support the development of *B. pahangi*, but because of its relatively easier maintainance, the preferred laboratory vector is *Ae. aegypti*.

REFERENCES

Besansky, N.J., V. Finnerty, and F.H. Collins. 1992. A molecular genetic perspective on mosquitoes. *Adv. Genet.* 30:123–184.

Boyd, M.F. 1949. Historical Review. In: M.F. Boyd. *Malariology, Vol. 1.* Philadelphia: W.B. Saunders. pp. 3–28.

———, ed. 1949. Malariology, Vols. 1 and 2. Philadelphia: W.B. Saunders.

Clements, A.N. 1992. The biology of mosquitoes, Vol. 1. London: Chapman and Hall.

Coatney, G.R., W.E. Collins, McW. Warren, and P.G. Contacos. 1971. The primate malarias. Washington, D.C.: U.S. Government Printing Office.

Collins, F.H., and S.M. Paskewitz. 1995. Malaria: Current and future prospects for control. *Ann. Rev. Entom.* 40:195–219.

Collins, F.H., R.K. Sakai, K.D. Vernick, S.M. Paskewitz, D.C. Seeley et al. 1986. Genetic selection of a Plasmodium-refractory strain of the malaria vector *Anopheles gambiae. Science* 234:607–610.

Cox, F.E.G. 1988. Major animal models in malaria research: rodent. In: W.H. Wernsdorfer and Sir Ian McGregor, editors, *Malaria: Principles and practice of malariology.* Edinburgh: Churchill Livingstone.

Farid, M.A. 1988. Simple measures for interrupting man-vector contact. In: W.H. Wernsdorfer and Sir I. McGregor, *Malaria: Principles and practices of malariology,* Vol. 2. London: Churchill Livingston. pp. 1251–1262.

Galun, R., L.C. Koontz, and R.W. Gwadz. 1985. Engorgement response of anopheline mosquitoes to blood fractions and artificial solutions. *Physiol. Entomol.* 10:45–149.

Garret-Jones, C. 1964. The human blood index of malaria vectors in relation to epidemiological assessment. *Bull. WHO* 30:241–261.

Gillies, M.T. 1988. Anopheline mosquitoes: Vector behaviour and bionomics. In: W.H. Wernsdorfer and Sir I. McGregor, *Malaria: Principles and practices of malariology,* Vol. 1. London: Churchill Livingston. pp. 453–485.

Gillies, M.T., and M. Coetzee. 1987. A supplement to the Anophelinae of Africa south of the Sahara. Johannesburg, South Africa: Publications of the South African Institute for Medical Research No. 55.

Gillies, M.T., and B. De Meillon. 1968. The Anophelinae of Africa south of the Sahara. Johannesburg, South Africa: Publications of the South African Institute for Medical Research No. 54.

Gratz, N.G., and R. Pal. 1988. Malaria vector control: Larviciding. In: W.H. Wernsdorfer and Sir I. McGregor, *Malaria: Principles and practices of malariology,* Vol. 2. London: Churchill Livingston. pp. 1213–1226.

Gwadz, R.W. 1969. Regulation of blood meal size in the mosquito. *J. Insect Physiol.* 15:2039–2044.

Knight, K.L., and A. Stone. 1977. A catalog of the mosquitoes of the world (Diptera: Culicidae). 2nd ed. College Park, Maryland: Entomological Society of America.

Labandeira, C.C., and J.J. Sepkiski Jr. 1993. Insect diversity in the fossil record. *Science* 261:310–315.

Pant, C.P. 1988. Malaria vector control: Imagociding. In: W.H. Wernsdorfer and Sir I. McGregor, *Malaria: Principles and practices of malariology,* Vol. 2. London: Churchill Livingston. pp.1173–1212.

Rafatjah, H.A. 1988. Malaria vector control: Environmental management. In: W.H. Wernsdorfer and Sir I. McGregor, *Malaria: Principles and practices of malariology,* Vol. 2. London: Churchill Livingston. pp. 1135–1172.

Ribeiro, J.M.C. 1987. Role of saliva in blood-feeding arthropods. *Ann. Rev. Entomol.* 32:463–478.

Ribeiro, J.M.C., P.A. Rossignol, and A. Spielman. 1985. Salivary gland apyrase determining probing time in anopheline mosquitoes. *J. Insect Physiol.* 9:689–692.

Rishikesh, N., A.M. Dubitiskij, and C.M. Moreau. 1988. Malaria vector control: Biological control. In: W.H. Wernsdorfer and Sir I. McGregor, *Malaria: Principles and practices of malariology,* Vol. 2. London: Churchill Livingston. pp. 1227–1250.

Wood, D.M., and A. Borkent. 1989. Phylogeny and classification of the Nematocera. In: J.F. McAlpine and D.M. Wood, editors, *Manual of Nearctic Diptera.* Vol. 3. Research Branch Agriculture Canada, Monograph 32. pp. 1333–1370.

6. CULICINE MOSQUITOES AND THE AGENTS THEY TRANSMIT

Roger S. Nasci and Barry R. Miller

Mosquitoes are placed in the family Culicidae, suborder Nematocera of the order Diptera, the true flies. The Culicidae contains over 3500 species divided into 3 subfamilies: Anophelinae, Culicinae, and Toxorhynchitinae (Knight and Stone 1977). In this chapter we examine the 29 genera in the Culicinae and the single genus in the subfamily Toxorhynchitinae.

MORPHOLOGY

Culicine eggs are generally elongate and protected by a rigid, proteinaceous shell that minimizes water loss but permits gas exchange (Wigglesworth 1950) (Fig 6.1). Eggs are soft and white immediately after oviposition but sclerotize and darken within 1–2 hours. The eggs are laid either singly in areas that will flood with water, singly on the surface of water, clustered together in rafts that float on the water's surface, or are attached to aquatic vegetation.

Mosquitoes pass through 4 larval stadia. The larvae are legless and vermiform and, although they breathe air, are uniformly aquatic. The larval body is divided into 3 distinct regions (Fig. 6.2). The head is formed by a rigid capsule and bears the antennae, eyes, and mouthparts. The thorax is broader than the head or abdomen. The abdomen is composed of 10 segments; the first 7 segments are roughly identical and form a long cylinder. The posterior 3 segments are modified and bear the siphon, 4 anal papillae, a variety of scales, sclerotized plates, and hair tufts. The siphon ends in a pair of spiracles that are the respiratory openings to the air. Members of the genera *Coquillettidia* and *Mansonia* have siphons modified into spikelike structures for penetrating plant tissue. Larvae of these genera obtain oxygen from plant tissue instead of from the air. The anal papillae are used for ion regulation.

The pupa is aquatic and, unlike the pupae of most insects, is motile and active. The pupal head and thorax are fused into a cephalothorax that bears 2 large respiratory trumpets (Fig. 6.3). The trumpets maintain contact with the air when the pupa is at the water's surface. Trumpets in the *Coquillettidia* and

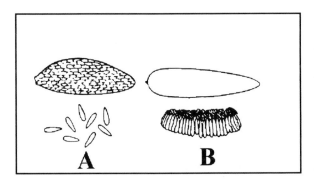

6.1 Eggs of culicine mosquitoes: (A) single eggs of *Aedes* species laid on substrate; (B) egg raft of *Culex* species laid on the water's surface

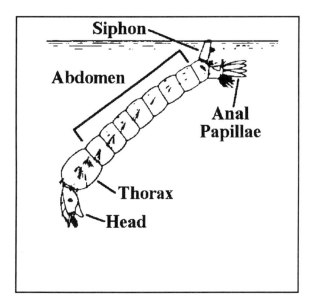

6.2   Culicine mosquito larva

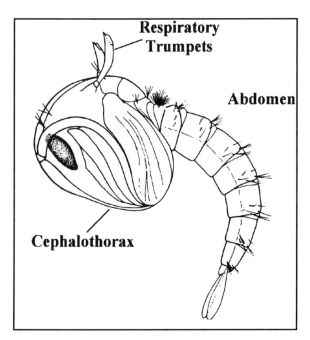

6.3   Culicine mosquito pupa

Mansonia are modified for penetrating plant tissue, as is the larval siphon in these genera. The abdomen is a long, muscular cylinder that is used to propel the pupa in the water.

The adult mosquito has a slender body divided into 3 regions (Fig 6.4). The spherical head bears a large pair of compound eyes, a pair of antennae, a pair of palpi, and the elongate proboscis. The proboscis of the Toxorhynchitinae is long and curves downward. The thorax bears the wings, halters, and 3 pair of slender legs. The wings are long and narrow with characteristic venation patterns. The cylindrical abdomen consists of 10 segments, 8 of which are visible; 2 terminal segments are modified for reproductive functions. The adult mosquito's body, including the legs and wing veins, are covered with hairs and scales in characteristic, species-specific patterns. Sexual dimorphism in culicine and toxorhynchitine adults is readily apparent in the morphology of the maxillary palpi, antennae, and terminal abdominal segments (Table 6.1, Fig. 6.5).

TABLE 6.1   Sexual dimorphism in adult Culicinae and Toxorhynchitinae

Character	Males	Females
palpi	same length as proboscis	⅕ length of proboscis
antennae	dense hairs	sparse hairs
terminalia	claspers	pointed or rounded

LIFE HISTORY

The events that characterize the immature life history of a mosquito are hatching, larval development, pupation, and adult emergence. Embryonic development in the egg is temperature dependent. Generally within a few days to weeks, a fully formed larva develops within the egg and is capable of hatching. Eggs laid on the surface of the water hatch as soon as development is complete. Several species, particularly the floodwater *Aedes*, lay eggs on a substrate that will be flooded and require an exogenous stimulus such as a decrease in oxygen concentration in the water to initiate hatching.

Mosquito larvae use modified mandibles and maxillae to obtain food from the water column or from the substrate. Larval feeding modes are characterized as collecting (filtering-gathering), scraping, shredding, or predation (Merritt et al. 1992). Food consists of microorganisms, detritus, algae, protists, leaves, and living and dead invertebrates. All larvae of the genus *Toxorhynchites* and the larvae of several species in other genera prey on invertebrates, including other mosquito larvae.

During the pupal stage the mosquito does not feed. Larval organs degenerate and are replaced with adult organs from undifferentiated cells in the imaginal discs. When metamorphosis is complete and the adult is fully formed within the pupal cuticle, the pupa swallows air to increase internal pressure, and the cuticle splits along cleavage lines. The adult slowly emerges from pupal cuticle onto the water's surface. The soft adult cuticle then sclerotizes and the adult is able to fly within 10–15 minutes.

Dispersal from the larval habitat varies among species. Several species, such as the saltmarsh mosquito *Aedes sollicitans*, travel several miles aided by the wind in search of blood-meal hosts. Other species may not travel more than a few hundred meters from the larval habitat.

The events that characterize the life of an adult mosquito are mating, feeding, and oviposition. Both male and female mosquitoes become sexually receptive approximately 2 days after adult ecdysis. Male mosquitoes may mate many times, whereas females generally mate only once (Craig 1967). In many species mating occurs when females enter large swarms of flying males that have aggregated in response to environmental cues. In other species, mating is host-associated. Males aggregate near blood-meal hosts and encounter females as they approach the host to feed. Mating also occurs outside swarms in some species. Males locate females using the Johnston's organs of the antennae to orient to the sound produced by the female's wings (McIver 1980). Contact pheromones are involved in the later stages of mating behavior. Sperm transfer requires a complex merging of the

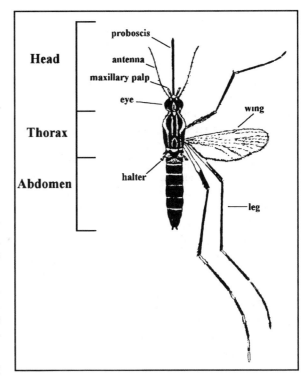

6.4 Culicine mosquito adult female morphology

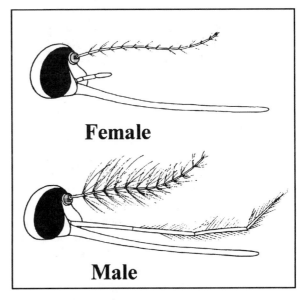

6.5 Sexual dimorphism in the maxillary palps and antennae of culicine mosquitoes

male and female reproductive structures. Inseminated females store sufficient sperm in their spermathecae to fertilize many egg batches.

Both male and female mosquitoes use the long proboscis to obtain nectar and other plant juices as a source of carbohydrates (Magnarelli 1979). The primary sources are floral and extrafloral nectaries. The only exogenous energy source for males is carbohydrates derived from plant juices, and for both sexes plant juices provide energy for survival, routine metabolic maintenance, and flight. In the laboratory, mosquitoes deprived of sugar after adult emergence frequently die within a few days (Nayar and Sauerman 1975). Therefore, feeding on nectar early in adult life is essential for survival.

Large nectar meals are stored in the expansible diverticula associated with the foregut (Friend 1981). When needed, small slugs of the material are shunted from the diverticula to the midgut for rapid absorption. In this way, the midgut is kept relatively empty and free to accommodate large blood meals.

Most mosquito species are anautogenous and require the large amount of protein contained in a vertebrate blood meal for egg maturation. Some species are autogenous and can use protein reserves accumulated during the larval stages to produce the first batch of eggs (Spielman 1973). Few species can produce more than 1 egg batch autogenously. *Toxorhynchites* females subsist wholly on plant nectar and do not take blood meals.

Autogeny is a genetically determined trait; however, expression of autogeny is controlled by environmental factors. Poor larval nutrition resulting from crowded larval habitats or a lack of larval food materials reduces the amount of protein carried over to the adult stage and reduces or eliminates the expression of autogenous egg production in the adult. Anautogenous mosquitoes must engage in complex search and location behaviors before they contact a host and obtain a blood meal (Gillies 1972). When searching for food, mosquitoes use both active and passive strategies. The active search strategy involves flight in search of host cues; mosquitoes using a passive strategy wait for a host to enter the vicinity. Actively searching mosquitoes fly at a right angle to the wind, usually during morning and evening twilight periods. Carbon dioxide and other body odors stimulate the chemoreceptors and indicate the presence of a host. The female responds by turning into the wind and flying toward the host. As the mosquito approaches the host, it uses visual stimuli, heat, and moisture for orientation. Passively searching species use the same cues to identify and locate hosts when they enter the mosquitoes' vicinity.

Once the mosquito has landed on the skin of a host and found a suitable feeding site, the labial sheath of the proboscis slides back to expose a bundle of stylets that is inserted into the skin. The stylets enclose salivary and food canals. While the stylets probe the skin, saliva is injected into the wound. Chemoreceptors detect the presence of blood and direct probing into the lumen of blood vessels below the capillary bed or into the hematoma formed by repeated probing through the vessels. Pumping structures in the head are activated, and blood is shunted into the midgut. Within a few minutes a female can consume up to 4 times her weight in blood. Feeding is terminated by stretch receptors that detect distension of the midgut. The engorged female then flies from the host to a site suitable for digestion of the blood and gonotrophic development. If the mosquito is disturbed during feeding and the volume of blood consumed is below the amount necessary to initiate egg development, the mosquito will attempt to locate another host. If blood meal volume is sufficient to initiate egg development, host-seeking and biting behaviors are inhibited (Klowden 1986).

Mosquitoes are classified as either generalists or specialists with reference to their blood-feeding patterns (Waage 1979). Generalists have the ability to identify and feed on a wide variety of host types. Specialists limit feeding to specific types of hosts, such as *Cs. melanura*, which feeds predominantly on birds, or *Cx. territans*, which feeds predominantly on amphibians. Host use patterns may vary seasonally between geographic regions and as the relative abundance of different hosts changes in an area.

Gonotrophic development may take 2–7 days, after which the female searches for an oviposition site. Visual and chemical cues are used to identify habitats suitable for oviposition and subsequent larval development, and the eggs are placed on or in water or in areas that are destined to be flooded.

The life span of an adult mosquito may be several weeks to months in temperate regions, especially if the species overwinters in the adult stage. In tropical areas adult mosquito life spans are much shorter, ranging from a few days to several weeks.

LIFE HISTORY PATTERNS

Mosquitoes display a great diversity in their life histories. The type of larval habitat, the stage in which the mosquito diapauses, and the number of generations per year (voltinism) are among the traits used to classify life-history patterns. Larval habitats have been described in great detail in the literature. Mosquitoes inhabit salt, brackish, and fresh water and can be found in floodwater as well as in permanent water sites. A standard system of classifying larval habitats proposed by Laird (1988) is listed below.

Aboveground waters	Subterranean waters
flowing streams	natural
ponded streams	artificial
lake edges	
swamps and marshes	
shallow permanent ponds	
intermittent ephemeral puddles	
natural containers	
artificial containers	

Diapause is a period of arrested development in which the mosquito physiologically prepares for survival during long-lasting adverse conditions (Mitchell 1988). In mosquitoes, diapause is usually an adaptation for winter survival. Diapause can occur in either the egg, larva, or adult stage. Diapause is induced by a short photoperiod. Termination of diapause and resumption of metabolic activity usually depend on an increase in photoperiod and/or exposure to cold followed by an increase in temperature. Adult mosquitoes diapause as inseminated, nulliparous females with a reduced blood-feeding drive and suspended ovarian activity. Exposure of larvae and pupae to a short photoperiod induces diapause in the adult stage. Diapausing eggs do not hatch, and both egg and larval diapause are characterized by a suspension of growth and development. Induction of egg or larval diapause may be direct; that is, the egg or larva initiates diapause when exposed to a short photoperiod. However, in several species exposure of the female to a short photoperiod results in diapause induction in the eggs or larvae of her offspring.

Voltinism, the number of generations a mosquito species produces per year, is fixed in some species and variable in others. For example, *Coquillettidia perturbans* and several northern *Aedes* species are univoltine, producing only 1 generation annually. Adults emerge in the spring and lay eggs, which diapause and do not hatch until the following spring. Many other species are multivoltine and produce as many generations as weather conditions permit. Some species that are univoltine in the north are multivoltine at more southern latitudes.

For practical purposes, mosquito species are often grouped on the basis of similarities in life history patterns. A convenient grouping for temperate climate culicine mosquitoes, based on the combination of oviposition pattern, larval habitat, and diapause stage, is shown in Table 6.2. The life history traits not listed in the table (e.g., voltinism, host preference, and mating behavior) are highly variable within most genera and are not useful in this type of classification. However, most mosquito species can be placed in 1 of the life history types.

MOSQUITO CONTROL

Integrated approaches to mosquito control involve using a combination of control activities that is appropriate for the mosquito species and habitat. Mosquito control measures generally include a combination of (1) source reduction (Chap. 28), which eliminates mosquito-producing habitats; (2) larval control; and (3) adult control. Source reduction consists of filling, draining, dredging, or in some way altering the habitat so it is no longer suitable for mosquito larval development. Larval control involves applying a physiological or physical insecticide to the larval habitat (Chaps. 29 and 32) or introducing a parasite or predator into the

TABLE 6.2   Classification of mosquito life history types

Life history type	Eggs and oviposition	Larval habitat	Diapause stage*
Culex	rafts on water	permanent water	adult
Culiseta	rafts on water	permanent water	4th instar larva
Aedes	singly on soil or in container	floodwater, natural or artificial container	egg
Mansonia / Coquillettidia	clusters attached to vegetation	permanent water with emergent vegetation	4th instar larva
Toxorhynchites	singly in containers	natural or artificial containers	4th instar larva

* for diapausing species

habitat to reduce larval populations (Chap. 31). Adult control consists of applying physiological insecticides to the habitat in which mosquito adults are flying or resting. Advances are also being made in genetic control and the reduction of mosquito population densities by the introduction of novel genes or gene combinations.

DISEASE AGENTS VECTORED

Mosquito-Borne Lymphatic Filariasis

The filarioids are tissue-dwelling parasites and are among the most evolved of the parasitic nematodes, the majority of which belong to the large family Onchocercidae. Characteristically, these parasites employ arthropods as intermediate hosts; vertebrate infection occurs when third-stage juvenile worms are deposited on the skin during arthropod blood feeding.

Important human pathogens include *Wucheria bancrofti*, *Brugia malayi*, and *Brugia timori*. Table 6.3 summarizes the World Health Organization estimates of the prevalence of the disease in different endemic areas; little information is available for the African region. The World Health Organization estimates that of some 751 million people at risk, 72.8 million are infected with *W. bancrofti* and 5.8 million with *B. malayi* or *B. timori*.

The development of filariae in mosquito vectors is somewhat similar. The microfilariae are ingested by the mosquito from the host's peripheral blood. The presence of the microfilariae may be more prevalent during defined periods of time in the periodic form. In *W. bancrofti*, for instance, microfilariae are present in

significant numbers in the human peripheral circulation between 2200 hr (hours) and 0200 hr, which overlaps the preferred biting activity of the vector *Culex pipiens quinquefasciatus*. Thus, periodicity may have evolved as a response to the biting activity of mosquito vectors. Mechanisms to explain periodicity are obscure and do not involve the release of a new generation of microfilariae each day. Host-mediated stimuli including reduced arterial oxygen tension and lowered body temperature may be involved. In the areas of the South Pacific, certain *Wucheria* strains exhibit a diurnal presence in the peripheral blood and are referred to as subperiodic forms. Not surprisingly, daytime feeding mosquitoes are the major vectors.

Postingestion, the microfilariae shed their saclike sheaths and migrate through the mesenteron and into the indirect flight muscles of the thorax. In heartworm, *Dirofilaria immitis*, the microfilariae undergo development in the Malpighian tubules. The second juvenile stage (sausage stage) occurs, following a cuticular molt about 48 hr after arrival in the thorax. The infective, filariform 3rd juvenile stage, up to 2 mm long, is produced following a second molt within 2 weeks. The filariform larvae migrate throughout the hemocoel, eventually reaching the labium, in which they escape during vector probing and blood feeding on the vertebrate host. They enter the host's peripheral lymphatics through the wound created by the mosquito's mouthparts and eventually settle in the larger lymph vessels in which they mature into sexually mature adults that produce more microfilariae. Note that the immature forms

TABLE 6.3 Total number of persons living in areas of endemic lymphatic filariasis (in millions)

WHO region	Total population	Population in endemic areas	Filarial infections	
			Wucheria	Brugia
Americas	170	6.5	0.3	0
Eastern Mediterranean	52	3.7	0.2	0
Southeast Asia	1287	493.2	43.8	4.8
Western Pacific	1334	135	2.9	1
Africa	444	113	25.6	0
Total	3287	751.4	72.8	5.8

Modified from 5th report of the WHO Expert Committee on Filariasis, 1992

only develop in the mosquito—they do not increase in numbers (see Chap. 4).

A delicate balance exists between the intermediate mosquito host and the developing immature filarial worms. If too many microfilariae are ingested during blood-feeding, the tissue damage incurred by the vector may lead to a shortened life span and insufficient time for the worms to mature to the infective third stage. The ability of vector mosquitoes to become infected from low-density microfilaraemias (8–11 microfilariae per ml venous blood) has frequently been demonstrated despite the fact that 40–60% of the microfilariae were damaged by the pharyngeal armatures during ingestion.

In humans, the time interval from infection to manifestation of clinical symptoms is variable, but commonly it is 8–16 months; often, signs and symptoms differ from one endemic area to another. In endemic areas a proportion of the population may be microfilaremic, but asymptomatic, for long periods of time. Recent studies have demonstrated that asymptomatic patients have dilated lymphatics and compromised lymphatic function. Acute manifestations of lymphatic filariasis can be characterized by adenolymphangitis accompanied by fever and malaise (in males the bancroftian form may present as acute epididymoorchitis). The primary chronic manifestations of bancroftian filariasis include lymphoedema, hydrocele, chyluria, and elephantiasis.

Over 70 taxa of mosquitoes in the genera *Anopheles, Culex, Aedes,* and *Mansonia* have been implicated as being intermediate hosts for human filarias. A major stumbling block in entomological studies to define vectors involved in transmission of filaria is the lack of species- and stage-specific probes for identifying the major human filarial pathogens. Current DNA probes react with all developmental stages of a given species and therefore cannot differentiate between infected mosquitoes (ingested microfilaria, sausage L2 forms, or encapsulated/aborted infections) and those actually transmitting infective filariform worms. A *B. malayi* filariform (L3) specific monoclonal antibody has been developed and successfully field tested; an equivalent reagent for *W. bancrofti* is needed but unavailable.

Human filariasis, as with many tropical diseases, is almost entirely an affliction of poor communities lacking adequate housing and sanitation. In urban areas vast larval habitats for *Culex pipiens quinquefasciatus* are created by open sewage drains and pit latrines. In recent times rural migration to urban areas and uncontrolled urbanization has favored the spread of *Cx. pipiens quinquefasciatus* and *W. bancrofti* because the urban infrastructure responsible for sanitation and clean water has been overwhelmed or simply collapsed. Clearly, control of human lymphatic filariasis will require not only medical and vector control advancements but a vast improvement in human living conditions where filariae are endemic.

Arthropod-Borne Viral Diseases—Arboviruses

Arboviruses are by definition viral agents that replicate in and are transmitted by members of the phylum Arthropoda. Well over 500 viruses are listed in the International Catalog of Arboviruses and undoubtedly many more exist that are unknown. The majority of arboviruses are not known to infect humans and cause illness presumably because they are unable to replicate in humans or their vectors for various reasons lack contact with humans.

Man's increasing encroachment on remote areas (rain forests to tundra) is dramatically increasing vector-human contact that may lead to the discovery of additional pathogens. Also, the introduction of exotic mosquito vectors into new habitats may alter established arbovirus cycles and significantly increase human exposure to pathogenic arboviruses (Chap. 4). Arboviruses exist in nature from simple to complex cycles; revealing the methods by which these agents endure is crucial in designing prevention and control measures against human and animal disease. A large number of genetic and environmental factors that affect virus transmission have been described. Table 6.4 lists some of the more obvious.

Approximately 100 of the arboviruses can infect humans, and about 40 are known to infect livestock. Vertebrate infection with an arbovirus can be characterized as subclinical when no overt disease is detectable, although the infected animal produces antibodies against the agent. Inapparent infections can be important if the amount of virus in the peripheral circulation is high enough to infect arthropods (reservoir of infection); detection of antibodies (serosurvey) in these vertebrates can serve as a measure of current and past virus activity. Human arboviral diseases are classified clinically by the predominant syndrome caused, namely encephalitis, febrile illness, and hemorrhagic fever. Many arboviral diseases can cause a wide range of symptoms that are not strictly limited to any one of these categories; further, some individuals infected with a particular arbovirus may show only mild symptoms whereas others may have a severe or fatal outcome.

TABLE 6.4   Elements that affect arbovirus transmission and maintenance in nature

Virus	Genetic variants that differ in infectivity
Vectors	Vector competence—susceptibility to oral infection and efficiency of transmission
	Vector population structure—density, longevity, and age structure
	Blood-feeding preference
	Distribution and dispersal
Reservoirs	Ability to develop effective viremia-infectious for vectors
	Vertebrate population structure-density, longevity, and age structure
	Immune status
	Interactions with vectors
	Distribution and dispersal

Modified from Reeves, 1967

It is beyond the scope of this chapter to describe the many viruses that cause human or livestock disease. (See *The Arboviruses: Epidemiology and Ecology*, edited by T.P. Monath, for an excellent review of these interesting and important pathogens.) Table 6.5 presents a synopsis of the more important arboviral pathogens transmitted by Culicine mosquitoes. We will focus on those agents that present a unique or changing ecology and that are currently viewed as important emerging diseases.

Rift Valley Fever

Rift Valley fever virus (RFV), a member of the genus *Phlebovirus* in the virus family, Bunyaviridae, is the agent responsible for Rift Valley fever. Although the disease is primarily a veterinary problem, it appears to be causing increasing human morbidity and mortality during epizootics; thus, much remains to be learned about the various transmission cycles of this agent in Africa. The natural history of the virus is complex and involves both enzootic and epizootic vectors.

TABLE 6.5 Important mosquito-borne arboviruses that cause disease in humans

Arbovirus	Epidemics	Case fatality rate (%)	Disease	Principal human vector
Togaviridae				
Chikungunya	yes	rare	hemorrhagic	*Aedes aegypti*
	yes	0	febrile	
eastern equine encephalitis	yes	50–75	encephalitis	*Coquilletidia perturbans*
Ross River	yes	0	febrile	*Culex annulirostris*
Sindbis	yes	rare	febrile	*Cx. univittatus*
Venezuelan equine encephalitis	yes	0.1–20	encephalitis	*Cx. pipiens* > 30 species
western equine encephalitis	yes	5–10	encephalitis	*Cx. tarsalis*
Flaviviridae				
dengue 1–4	yes	3–12	hemorrhagic	*Ae. aegypti,*
	yes	0	febrile	*Ae. albopictus*
West Nile	no		febrile	*Cx. univittatus*
Japanese encephalitis	yes	30–40	encephalitis	*Cx. tritaeniorhynchus*
Murray Valley encephalitis	yes	20–70	encephalitis	*Cx. annulirostris*
St. Louis encephalitis	yes	4–20	encephalitis	*Cx. pipiens complex,* *Cx. nigripalpus*
yellow fever	yes	5–20	hemorrhagic	*Ae. aegypti, Ae. africanus,* *Ae. simpsoni,* *Haemagogus* spp.
Bunyaviridae				
Rift Valley fever	yes	0	febrile	*floodwater Aedes* spp., *Cx. pipiens*
LaCrosse encephalitis	no	1	encephalitis	*Ae. triseriatus*

Modified from Monath, 1988

The natural history of the virus in sub-Saharan Africa is influenced by the amount and duration of seasonal rainfall. Meegan and Baily in Monath (1988) have proposed that local flooding of "dambos" (standing water in ground pool depressions) stimulates the hatching of floodwater *Aedes* eggs, some of which are transovarially infected with RVF virus. The resulting adult mosquitoes introduce the virus into domestic vertebrate populations in which horizontal transmission occurs. Oviposition by infected mosquitoes replenishes the dambos with infected eggs that hatch during the following rainy season. However, during periods of extremely heavy and prolonged rainfall, not only are large populations of floodwater *Aedes* stimulated to hatch but large populations of secondary vectors also develop, leading to epizootics and epidemics.

Virus persistence mechanisms in North Africa appear to be different. The disease was first recorded in Egypt in 1977 and persisted as an epizootic for 2 years without the benefit of rainfall. Meegan and Baily (1988) postulated that the virus was maintained through horizontal arthropod transmission (biological and mechanical) as well as through aerosol transmission between vertebrates.

Yellow Fever

Yellow fever (YF) virus is the prototype of the genus *Flavivirus* in the family Flaviviridae. It was first recognized as a clinical entity in 17th century Mexico. Until the early 20th century, urban epidemics occurred from tropical areas in the Americas as far north as Boston in the United States. Epidemics of yellow fever also appeared in port cities in France, England, Spain, and Italy. Carlos Finlay was one of the first investigators to propose that the agent causing the disease was transmitted to humans by mosquitoes, specifically *Aedes aegypti*. However, it was not until 1900 that Major Walter Reed demonstrated that an infectious, filterable agent was present in patients' blood and that *Ae. aegypti* mosquitoes were capable of transmission. Later, investigators showed that there existed a "jungle cycle" of yellow fever in both the tropics of South America and Africa. This finding dashed the hopes of those who felt yellow fever eradication was an obtainable goal. Nonetheless, a milestone event in arbovirology occurred in 1937 when M. Theiler and H.H. Smith (1937) reported the attenuation of a wild yellow fever virus (*Asibi* strain) that was useful as a human vaccine. This vaccine (17D) has proved to be one of the most efficacious and safe viral vaccines ever developed; however, its administration requires a "cold-chain" because the virus is of the "live-attenuated" type. This limitation has made routine vaccination of remote populations at risk difficult and expensive.

In the Americas, "jungle," or sylvatic, yellow fever remains a serious problem among rural workers, but urban or *Ae. aegypti*–borne yellow fever epidemics have not been reported for 30 years. The recent introduction of *Ae. albopictus* from Asia into Brazil may have ominous consequences because this mosquito species is a competent vector that is capable of living in both sylvan and urban habitats and therefore could serve as a "bridging" vector, bringing the virus into heavily populated areas from endemic sylvan habitats.

Mosquitoes of the genus *Haemagogus* are the principal vectors of jungle yellow fever in the Americas, blood-feeding in the forest canopy during the midday hours on howler monkeys (*Alouatta* spp.), squirrel monkeys (*Saimiri* spp.), and owl monkeys (*Aotus* spp.) and subsequently ovipositing in tree holes. These monkey species develop effective viremias and commonly develop fatal disease; woolly (*Lagothrix* spp.) and capuchin (*Cebus* spp.) monkeys become viremic but do not develop clinical disease. Sedentary howler monkeys serve as sentinel animals when die-offs at "monkey-trees" happen during the course of an epizootic. Human infection occurs when unvaccinated workers venture into endemic sylvatic habitats for the purposes of forestry, road building, and other agricultural activities.

Endemic and epidemic transmission cycles of yellow fever in Africa are complex and are best evaluated in a biogeographical sense. Primates are also the principal vertebrate reservoirs, developing adequate viremias to infect vectors; dramatic monkey die-offs have not been reported, leading to speculation that the African monkey–virus relationship is more stable and thus precedes the American primate–virus relationship. *Aedes africanus* transmits the virus in humid equatorial zones in the forest canopy to primates; humans inhabiting villages in the forest or on its edge are also fed upon, leading to self-contained "epidemics." The rapid transport of sick individuals from remote areas into large cities has lead to *Ae. aegypti*–borne urban epidemics, most recently in Nigeria. In habitats bordering elevated forests in East Africa, *Aedes simpsoni* serves as a bridging vector linking the sylvan cycle with humans in plantations. The biology of these 2 species with regard to host preferences and habitat utilization is variable between West and East Africa, revealing potential species complexes. Savannah vegetation zones (zones of emergence) border the forested areas and support numerous vector species during the rainy season, including *Aedes furcifer, Aedes taylori, Aedes luteocephalus,*

Aedes opok, *Aedes neoafricanus*, and *Aedes vittatus*. In the still more arid Sahel and Sudan Savannah zones, the primary and epidemic vector is *Ae. aegypti*. Because of its ability to utilize stored water as a larval habitat, large populations form in arid environments, causing large outbreaks when virus is introduced.

The absence of yellow fever in Asia has not been explained despite the abundance of susceptible primates and vectors. Cross-protective flavivirus antibodies (especially dengue antibodies) may subjugate human yellow fever viremias until they are no longer infectious to vectors. A more simplistic explanation is that the virus has never been introduced via a viremic patient under the right set of circumstances to initiate transmission; also, it seems unlikely that a sick West African from a remote village would board a jet flight to Asia.

Because of an effective vaccine, yellow fever is a preventable disease. In 1990 the World Health Organization recommended the vaccine be incorporated into the Expanded Program on Immunization (EPI) and be administered with measles vaccine at 9 months of age in African countries at risk.

Dengue Fever

Dengue fever (DEN) and dengue hemorrhagic fever (DHF), caused by the dengue viruses serotypes 1–4 (genus *Flavivirus*), have become important as human pathogens in recent years. Although the viruses are related, antibodies obtained after infection with 1 serotype are not cross-protective for the other serotypes. In the past, dengue was largely restricted to Asia and the southern Pacific, but following uncontrolled and chaotic urbanization caused by poverty and high fertility rates in tropical areas, dengue has spread to Africa and the Americas, causing significant human morbidity and mortality. As the total number of cases of dengue has increased worldwide, so has the incidence of mortality from dengue hemorrhagic fever. For instance, in the Cuban outbreak of 1981, of about 10,000 people that developed hemorrhagic fever (344,203 dengue cases diagnosed), 158 died.

Why some patients develop hemorrhagic disease following infection with dengue viruses is unknown. One theory suggests that the hemorrhagic manifestations have an immunopathological basis and occur most frequently in those individuals that have been sensitized by a previous infection with a heterologous serotype (see Gubler in Monath 1988). In general, DEN–2 virus has been commonly associated with hemorrhagic fever following a previous infection with DEN–1, DEN–3, or DEN–4.

Although there is evidence for the existence of sylvatic cycles of dengue involving primates and forest *Aedes*, their importance in initiating human epidemics in some settings is debatable because dengue viruses seem to persist in urban areas year after year without a periodic influx from the "jungle." Classic dengue epidemics in urban settings require only dengue antibody naive individuals (children) and large populations of *Ae. aegypti*. Because of its intimate association with humans and their environment, *Ae. aegypti* is the most important mosquito vector of dengue viruses; humans are the principal source of blood, and human utensils (anything that will hold water) are primary sites for oviposition and larval development. In parts of Asia and potentially South America and West Africa, *Ae. albopictus* is an important vector because it utilizes both natural and artificial larval habitats. Adults thrive in rural habitats, sometimes in close association with humans, although they feed on whatever is available (much like *Ae. simpsoni* in the ecology of yellow fever). Vertical transmission of dengue viruses has been demonstrated in the laboratory, and isolations of viruses have been made from mosquitoes reared from field-collected eggs. The importance of vertical transmission in the overall ecology of dengue and yellow fever viruses is difficult to assess.

Vaccines for the dengue viruses are lacking (although several promising candidates are under evaluation); currently, the only demonstrated effective control measure is destruction of *Ae. aegypti* larval habitats. "Sanitation" has proved to be successful over fairly large areas but requires constant and long-term compliance from local communities.

Japanese encephalitis

Japanese encephalitis (JE) virus is distributed widely in Asia with the majority of human cases occurring in China, India, Nepal, and northern Southeast Asia. In

APPENDIX 6.1 Systematics of the Culicinae and Toxorhynchitinae mosquitoes

Family	Subfamily	Tribe	Genus
Culicidae			
	Culicinae		
		Aedeomyiini	*Aedeomyiini*
			Aedes
			Armigeres
			Eretmapodites
			Hemagogus
			Heizmannia
			Opifex
			Psorophora
			Udaya
			Zeugnomyia
		Culicini	*Culex*
			Deinocerites
			Galindomyia
		Culisetiini	*Culiseta*
		Ficalbiini	*Ficalbia*
			Mimomyia
		Hodgesiini	*Hodgesia*

APPENDIX 6.1 (Continued) Systematics of the Culicinae and Toxorhynchitinae mosquitoes

Subfamily	Tribe	Genus
	Mansoniini	*Coquillettidia*
		Mansonia
	Orthopodomyiini	*Orthopodomyia*
	Sabethiini	*Limatus*
		Malaya
		Maorigoeldia
		Phoniomyia
		Sabethes
		Topomyia
		Trichoprosopon
		Tripteroides
		Wyeomyia
	Uranotaeniini	*Uranotaenia*
Toxorhynchitinae		*Toxorhynchites*

Thailand annual attack rates are 10–20 per 100,000. In endemic areas children 3–15 years old are the primary victims. In temperate zones JE outbreaks occur mainly in the months of July, August, and September, reflecting the seasonal buildup of vector populations. Rainfall and temperature are critical in determining the time of emergence and size of mosquito populations. Birds and domestic pigs are important amplifying hosts. The principal vectors are *Culex* species in the *vishnui* subgroup; *Culex tritaeniorhynchus* is the primary vector. Important larval habitats include irrigated rice fields, ditches, and pools. Secondary vectors that have been implicated in virus transmission are *Culex vishnui, Culex gelidus, Culex fuscocephalus, Culex annulus, and Culex annulirostris.* Vertical transmission has been demonstrated; its importance in virus overwintering in temperate regions is unknown. Formalin-inactivated vaccines for human use have been in use since the 1960s. Currently, live-attenuated vaccines are in human trials with promising results.

REFERENCES

Clements, A.N. 1992. *The biology of mosquitoes: Vol. 1. Development, nutrition and reproduction.* London: Chapman and Hall.

Craig, G.B. 1967. Mosquitoes: Female monogamy induced by male accessory gland substance. *Science* 156:1499–1501.

Edman, J.D., and A. Spielman. 1988. Blood-feeding by vectors: Physiology, ecology, behavior and vertebrate defense. In: T.P. Monath, editor, *The arboviruses: Epidemiology and ecology,* Vol. 1. Boca Raton, FL: CRC Press.

Friend, W.G., J.M. Schmidt, J.J.B. Smith, and R.J. Tanner. 1988. The effect of sugars on ingestion and diet destination in *Culiseta inornata. J. Insect Physiol.* 34:955–961.

Gillett. J.D. 1971. *Mosquitoes.* London: Weidenfeld and Nicholson.

Gillies, M.T. 1972. Some aspects of mosquito behavior in relation to the transmission of parasites. In: E. Canning and C. Wright, editors, *Behavioral aspects of parasite transmission.* London: Academic Press.

Gubler, D.J. 1988. Dengue. In: T.P. Monath, editor, *The arboviruses: Epidemiology and Ecology.* Boca Raton, FL: CRC Press. pp. 223–260.

Karabatsos, N., editor. 1985. International catalog of arboviruses, including certain other viruses of vertebrates. *Am. Soc. Trop. Med. Hyg.* 1–1147.

Klowden, M.J. 1986. Coping with inflation: Abdominal distention and mosquito reproduction, In: D. Borovsky and A. Spielman, editors, *Host regulated developmental mechanisms in vector arthropods.* Gainesville: University of Florida Press.

Knight, K.L., and A. Stone. 1977. *A catalog of the mosquitoes of the world (Diptera: Culicidae),* 2nd ed. Thomas Say Foundation. College Park, MD: Entomol. Soc. Am.

Laird, M. 1988. *The natural history of mosquito larval habitats.* London: Academic Press.

Lounibos, L.P., J.R. Rey, and J.H. Frank, editors. 1985. *Ecology of mosquitoes: Proceedings of a workshop.* Gainesville: University of Florida Press.

Magnarelli, L.A. 1979. Diurnal nectar-feeding of *Aedes cantator* and *A. sollicitans* (Diptera: Culicidae). *Environ. Entomol.* 8:949–945.

McIver, S.B. 1980. Sensory aspects of mate-finding behavior in male mosquitoes. *J. Med. Entomol.* 17:54–57.

Meegan, J.M., and C.L. Bailey. 1988. Rift Valley Fever. In: T.P. Monath, editor, *The Arboviruses: Epidemiology and Ecology.* Vol. 1–5. pp. 51–76.

Merritt, R.W., R.H. Dadd, and E.D. Walker. 1992. Feeding behavior, natural food, and nutritional relationships of larval mosquitoes. *Ann. Rev. Entomol.* 37:349–376.

Mitchell, C.J. 1988. Occurrence, biology and physiology of diapause in overwintering mosquitoes. In: T.P. Monath, editor, *The arboviruses: epidemiology and ecology.* Vol. 1. Boca Raton, FL: CRC Press.

Monath, T.P., editor. 1988. *The arboviruses: Epidemiology and ecology.* Vols. 1–5. Boca Raton, FL: CRC Press.

Muirhead-Thompson, E.C. 1982. *Behavior patterns of blood-sucking flies.* Oxford: Pergammon Press.

Nayar, J.K., and D.M. Sauerman. 1975. The effects of nutrition on survival and fecundity in Florida mosquitoes. Part 1: Utilization of sugar for survival. *J. Med. Entomol.* 12:92–98.

Reeves, W.C. 1967. Factors that influence the probability of epidemics of western equine, St. Louis, and California encephalitis in California. *Calif. Vector Views* 14: 13–18.

Spielman, A. 1971. Bionomics of autogenous mosquitoes. *Ann. Rev. Entomol.* 16:231–248.

Theiler, M., and H.H. Smith. 1937. Use of yellow fever virus modified by in vitro cultivation for human immunization. *J. Exp. Med.* 65:787–800.

Waage, J.K. 1979. The evolution of insect/vertebrate associations. *Biol. J. Linn. Soc.* 12:187–224.

Wigglesworth, V.B. 1950. *The principles of insect physiology,* 4th ed. London: Methuen.

WHO Expert Committee on Filariasis. 1992. *Lymphatic filariasis: The disease and its control.* WHO Technical Report, Series No. 821, Fifth Report. Geneva: World Health Organization.

7. BLACK FLIES AND THE AGENTS THEY TRANSMIT

E.W. Cupp

Black flies, also called buffalo gnats, coffee flies, jejens, and Kriebelmücken, are members of the Simuliidae, a small family of nematocerous Diptera composed of approximately 23 genera and 1554 described species (1.3% of the 119,000 species of true flies) (Crosskey 1990). Based on fossil records, it is estimated that this family has been in existence for approximately 160 million years. As is true for many dipterous families, the Simuliidae contains groups of sibling or incipient species-populations that are isomorphic and sympatric but not interbreeding. Thus, accurate identification of taxa often requires not only use of external morphological features described in dichotomous keys but other characters such as banding patterns of polytene chromosomes (usually those in larval salivary glands but occasionally those in the Malpighian tubules of adult females), isoenzymes, and DNA probes (Post and Flook 1992).

Black flies pose significant problems to human and animal health in many parts of the world because of the aggressive, blood-feeding activities of the adult female. The pestiferous nature of certain nearctic univoltine species was first recorded by frontiersmen and missionaries during the early exploration of North America (Crosskey 1990); today within the more temperate parts of North America and Europe, disease syndromes (simuliotoxicosis) associated with salivary secretions during mass feeding by univoltine species

have been described in livestock (Cupp 1986). For example, *Cnephia pecuarum*, the buffalo gnat, has slowly reemerged as a cattle pest in parts of the Lower Mississippi Valley as streams and rivers have been cleaned. Similarly, in South America, several human hemorrhagic syndromes have been described in immigrants and others who enter pristine areas containing large numbers of black flies (Pinheiro et al. 1974; Noble et al. 1974).

Black flies can serve as vectors of viruses and protozoan and helminthic parasites. These pathogens and their vector taxa are listed in Table 7.1. These disease agents include viruses (*Vesiculovirus*-epizootic and enzootic strains of New Jersey serotype of vesicular stomatitis virus; Cupp et al. 1992), protozoans (*Leucocytozoon* and *Trypanosoma* spp.; for an example, see Kiszewski and Cupp 1986), and filarial nematodes. The latter are particularly important because species of *Onchocerca* parasitize both ungulates and humans. Indeed, it seems likely that *O. volvulus*, the causative agent of "river blindness," evolved from an antecedent species that parasitized cattle (Cupp 1986a), suggesting that the domestication of bovids and the attendant change in life-style associated with pastoralism in riverine areas in Africa lead directly to the development of this important human parasite.

TABLE 7.1 Some black fly–associated pathogens and their vectors

Pathogen	Host	Vector
Viruses		
Vesicular stomatitis virus[a]	cattle, horses, swine	*S. bivittatum*[b], *S. vittatum*[c]
Protozoa		
Leucocytozoon spp.		
L. smithi	turkey	*S. slossonae,* *S. aureum,* *S. congareenarum,* *S. meridionale,* *S. jenningsi*
L. simondi	ducks, geese	*S. rugglesi,* *S. innocens,* *S. anatinum,* *S. croxtoni,* *S. euryadminiculum*
L. sakharoffi, *L. berestneffi*	rooks, crows, magpies, jays	*S. ruficorne s.l.,* *S. aureum s.l.*
L. debreuili, *L. fringillinarum,* *L. danilewskyi,* *L. bonasae*	thrushes, passerines, owls, ruffed grouse	*S. vernum s.l.,* *L. S. aureum s.l.*
L. tawaki	penguins	*Austrosimulium* spp.
Trypanosoma spp.	passerines, sparrowhawks, guinea fowl	*S. rugglesi,* *S. latipes*
Filarial nematodes		
Dirofilaria ursi	bears	*S. venustun s.l.*
Onchocerca tarsicola	deer	*S. ornatum,* *P. nigripes*
O. cervipedis	deer	*P. impostor*
O. lienalis	cattle	*S. jenningsi,* *S. ornatum s.l.,* *S. erythrocephalum,* *S. reptans*
O. ochengi	cattle	*S. damnosum complex*

TABLE 7.1 (Continued) Some black fly–associated pathogens and their vectors

Pathogen	Host	Vector
O. volvulus	humans	*S. damnosum* complex, *S. neavei* group, *S. albivirgatum,* *S. exiguum s.l.,* *S. metallicum s.l.,* *S. oyapockense,* *S. ochraceum s.l.*
Mansonella ozzardi	humans	*S. amazonicum s.l.,* *S. oyapockense*
Splendidofilaria fallisensis	ducks	*S. rugglesi,* *S. anatinum*

[a] New Jersey serotype only
[b] Based on field isolation of high-titered virus pool
[c] Based on experimental laboratory results reported in Cupp and Collins (1979)

MORPHOLOGY

Black flies are holometabolous insects with 3 of the 4 life stages occurring in running water (Fig. 7.1). For this reason, some morphological features of the larval and pupal stages are particularly distinctive to the family and serve useful taxonomic purposes.

Egg Stage

The method of oviposition exhibited by gravid females essentially follows 1 of 2 patterns—deposition of ova onto a substrate or ejection of eggs directly onto the water's surface. The females of most species usually oviposit at a fixed time in the 24-hr diel cycle.

Simuliid eggs are ovoid and somewhat triangular in general shape. They lack floats and range in length from 0.1–0.5 mm (Crosskey 1990). The surfaces of black fly eggs are usually smooth and, at the level of light microscopy, free of the types of chorionic markings typical of mosquito eggs. Thus the egg stage of most species lacks obvious characters useful for taxonomic purposes; however, species can be identified on the basis of size and shape of the egg.

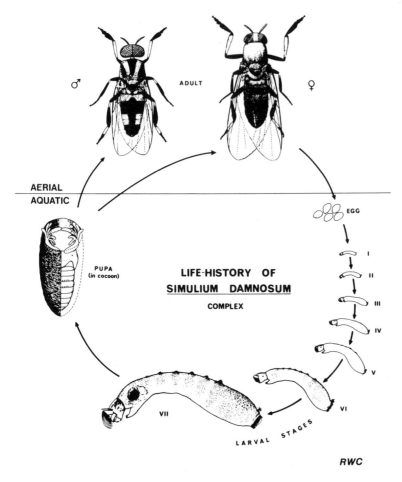

ADULT

♂ ♀

AERIAL
AQUATIC

PUPA
(in cocoon)

**LIFE-HISTORY OF
SIMULIUM DAMNOSUM**

COMPLEX

EGG

I

II

III

IV

V

VI

VII

L A R V A L   S T A G E S

RWC

7.1   Life cycle of the family Simuliidae. The species illustrated is *Simulium damnosum,* an African vector of *Onchocerca volvulus,* the causative agent of river blindness, or human onchocerciasis. The larval stages, or instars, show the general larval growth; their proportions are not exact, and not all species have 7 instars. (From Crosskey, R.W. 1990. John Wiley & Sons. Used with permission.)

years when buried in the moist sandy bottoms of ephemeral streams.

Larval Stage

With rare exception, black fly larvae are filter-feeding organisms found strictly in running water habitats. The larval body is an elongated tubular shape with several distinctive morphological structures that reflect adaptation to an aquatic environment.

The mouthparts are characterized by the prominent anterior "cephalic fans" (Fig. 7.2), which are formed in the embryo by labral outgrowths. These recurved structures, which are really netlike, collect food particles by an internal system of primary and secondary rays, or struts, that are arranged spatially at defined distances. This spacing, in conjunction with the secretion of mucus onto the collecting devices, allows the larva to remove suspended particles from the water column that fall within a certain size range, i.e., 10–150 μm. To do so, the head and upper body must be positioned in such a way that the cephalic fans, which form an arc of 200–250°, point downstream in the current. As particles collect onto and between the parts of the fans, they are periodically cleaned by the action of the mandibles, which lie in the middle of the head capsule between the maxillae. This method of feeding provides the opportunity for a reasonably varied diet for members of the family. Depending on the type of aquatic habitat, nutritional components include bacteria, diatoms, planktonic algae, and organic debris. The latter is the most important constituent in the larval diet. The labrum, which lies anteriorly between the cephalic fans, is a scraping device used to graze and obtain filamentous algae.

As is the case for related nematocerous Diptera, black fly eggs are white when freshly deposited but gradually turn yellow-brown. When laid communally, ova are stacked on top of each other and often form distinctive masses on partially submerged trailing vegetation, sticks, and rocks that can be easily recognized in the field. Eggs are subject to rapid desiccation if placed outside of water. However, some taxa (e.g., *Austrosimulium* spp.) produce ova that can remain viable for several

The labiohypopharynx (Crosskey 1990) is a complicated part of the larval mouth that also helps direct the movement of silk from the larval salivary glands into the aquatic environment. The latter structures are paired, tubelike glands that run the length of the body and secrete a silk that, upon exiting from the appropriate duct within the labiohypopharynx, hardens immediately upon contact with water. The mandibles assist in cutting the silken thread when a sufficient quantity has been produced for rappelling and/or anchoring the larva in the stream.

Black fly larvae anchor themselves within the lotic environment by means of an abdominal proleg (actually the terminal part of the body behind and below the anus), which contains a circle of hooks at its tip. These hooks (which can range in number from several hundred to over 8000 in species that live in cascades [Crosskey 1990]) are placed into the pad of silk that has been secreted onto a suitable substrate. A thoracic proleg, which protrudes antero-ventrally, also has hooks at its tips and serves as an attachment organ. Larvae are thus able to move easily in the running water habitat by using the silken threads and these anchoring devices.

Pupal Stage

The pupal stage is the crucial developmental step in the black fly life cycle that connects the earlier aquatic stages with an aerial-terrestrial existence. This transition requires several subtle physiological and behavioral alterations that precede the more obvious morphological differences evident in the pupa and larva. These differences are associated with the concept of apolysis, in which the cuticle of a developmental

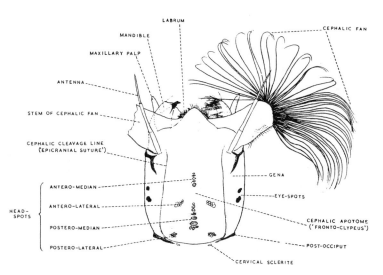

A   Head of larva, dorsal view

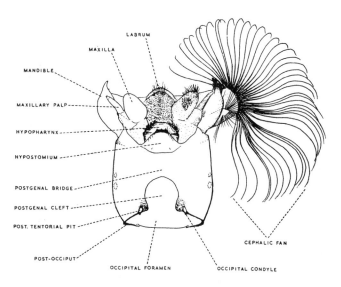

B   Head of larva, ventral view

7.2   The head structures of a larval black fly. A. Dorsal view of the head. B. Ventral view of the head. The cephalic fans are used to trap particulate food from the water. (From Stone, A. 1964. State Geological and Natural History Survey of Connecticut. Used with permission.)

stage in the insect's life cycle separates from the cuticle of the next stage but is not shed or cast off. This process gives rise to a pharate individual that retains the general morphological appearance of its predecessor. Thus, when considering the black fly life cycle, it has been suggested that the pharate pupa (which appears morphologically as a larva) continues to feed and defecate for 4 or more days after the larval-pupal apolysis. Although it also spins its own cocoon, it uses what are essentially the larval silk glands and related structures to do so.

The larval to pupal conversion usually occurs in a silken cocoon that is anchored to the substrate by silken threads. The cocoon of many species is characteristically shaped and can be taxonomically useful. Also, some species pupate without benefit of complete closure inside a cocoon. Regardless, once the molting process is under way, the larval skin is shed so that the pupal gills (located in the thorax) are exposed, thus providing continued access to oxygen. The emergence of these structures (which are covered by a plastron) represent a change in the method of respiration from the larval stage in which O_2 to CO_2 exchange takes place through the cuticle. The pupal gills are branched structures that vary in size and shape within the family.

Ecdysis is completed in a relatively short period of time, and the cast-off larval skin is often entrapped in the pupal case. In this stage, black fly pupae are morphologically similar to other nematocerous Diptera. The head and thorax are fused as a single unit—the cephalothorax—and are rigid whereas the abdomen is flexible. The latter has a series of characteristic hooks that anchor the pupa in the cocoon. The "morphological pupa" is nonfeeding and, in developmental terms, is relatively short-lived because of the rapidity in which pupal–adult apolysis takes place. This major developmental step occurs a few hours after pupation so that the form developing in the cocoon is the pharate adult. This stage respires through an abbreviated structure (the interspiracular trunk) that connects the pupal gills and the adult spiracular network.

Adult Stage

The process of adult development after pupation follows much the same plan as that of related nematocerans, i.e., certain body parts needed for an aerial-terrestrial existence are synthesized de novo from

histolyzed larval tissues whereas other internal structures are carried over from this stage. External body parts such as the adult eyes, antennae, wings, and legs can be seen through the pupal case.

There are also important internal modifications. As reviewed by Crosskey (1990), the larval gut is first partially histolyzed and then reconstructed to form an adult digestive tract that accommodates a liquid diet consisting of blood and/or plant juices. The silk glands also degenerate in the pupal stage and then are reconstituted as salivary glands specifically adapted in the female of many species for blood-feeding.

Once adult morphogenesis is completed, the imago must escape from the aquatic environment. This transition is accomplished by first expelling air from the tracheal system into the pupal case to create a bubble. As the pressure increases, the pupal case is split along a T-shaped line of dehiscence so that the thorax emerges first, followed by the remainder of the body. Because the newly emerged adult remains wrapped in the air bubble, it rises immediately to the water's surface. Unlike many aquatic insects, most black fly species are capable of immediate flight, and adults can quickly move away from the emergence site.

The body of the adult is subdivided into the typical hexapodan tagmata (head, thorax, and abdomen) with some morphological and sensory modifications associated with a parasitic way of life (Jobling 1987) (Fig. 7.3). This is particularly evident in the females of many species, which are dependent upon blood for reproduction and have mouthparts that fit together to form a short, stout proboscis that first cuts the skin and then provides a means for blood transport. Cibarial and pharyngeal pumps located in the head withdraw the blood and transport it into the midgut for digestion. The females of some species are autogenous, i.e., they are capable of maturing at least the 1st clutch of eggs without taking a blood meal.

The skin is first cut by the rasping action of the bladelike mandibles (considerably smaller in the male, which does not blood-feed). The labrum, a hollow structure anterior to the mandibles, is armed with prestomal teeth, which help to anchor the fly during the act of feeding. Because of its morphology and direct connection with the hemocoel, it is likely that this

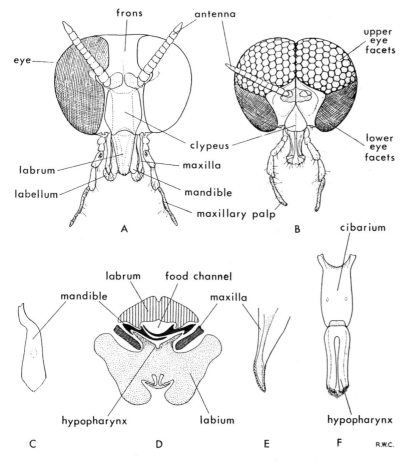

frons antenna

upper eye facets

eye

clypeus

labrum

labellum

maxilla

mandible

maxillary palp

A

B

lower eye facets

cibarium

labrum food channel

mandible

maxilla

hypopharynx labium

hypopharynx

C

D

E

F R.W.C.

7.3 Head structures of adult Simuliidae. A is a female, B is a male, C is the mandible of a female, D is a cross-section of the proboscis of a female, E is the maxilla of a female, and F is the cibarium and hypopharynx of a female. (From Smith, K.V.C. 1973. British Museum of Natural History. Used with permission.)

which directs the flow of saliva into the wound during both probing and feeding, lies posterio-medially to the other mouthparts. Thus, the mandibles, laciniae, and hypopharynx form a functional feeding unit that has been referred to as the syntrophium (see Sutcliffe and McIver 1984). This structure and its general function is similar to the feeding mechanism of hematophagous Ceratopogonidae.

Both sexes have well-developed sensoria on the head that are used for locating sources of nutrition and mating. The adult eyes are sexually dimorphic. However, in the male they are holoptic so that the dorsal hemisphere of each compound eye is covered with enlarged facets for detecting movement of the female within a 180° arc. The female eye is dichoptic, and the individual elements (ommatidia) are of equal size. The females of certain species rely on vision to detect host movement, shape, and color at medium to long ranges. The antennae also contain chemoreceptors that are important to detect host odor. Likewise, Lutz's organ, located on the third segment of the maxillary palps, can be important in detecting CO_2 and other odors.

part of the head is the site of emergence of infective stage larvae of *Onchocerca* spp. (Collins 1979). Together with the mandibles, the labrum forms the portion of the mouth through which the blood meal moves into the foregut of the fly.

The laciniae of the maxillae are also toothed and work in concert with the mandibles to create a subdermal hematoma. These paired structures lie posterio-laterally to the mandibles. The hypopharynx,

Many species within the Simuliidae are strong fliers, as is evident by the structure of the thorax. The vertical flight muscles are extremely well developed and are anchored ventrally to the swollen underside of the mesothorax (the katepisternum; see Crosskey 1990). The wings are short and broad and are strengthened by a series of long veins that run from base to tip; the anal lobe is well developed. As in all winged Diptera, the halteres are located on the metathorax.

LIFE CYCLE

The basic blueprint of the simuliid life cycle is similar to that of other holometabolous insects and consists of egg, larva, pupa, and adult stages. However, unlike most species of Diptera, the black fly development cycle is characterized by a variable number of larval instars that can indicate a physiological adjustment to food quantity and temperature. Thus, the number of instars often range from 6–9, with seven the usual number.

With poikilotherms, ambient temperature controls the rate of development so that the time required for completion of the immature portion of the life cycle is drastically affected. This oddity has been reported for *Simulium sirbanum*, a medically important species (and a member of the *Simulium damnosum* species complex described later) that occurs in the savanna regions of Africa where river temperatures reach 30° C. Larval development of this species can be completed in as few as 4 days, and it has been estimated that as many as 15–20 generations can be completed on an annual basis (Crosskey 1993). This rapidity can be contrasted with many holarctic species that have only 1 generation a year. Here, the rate of development in the overall life cycle is usually regulated by the presence of 1 particular stage (egg or larva) during cold temperatures and can be characterized by diapause in the egg stage or oligopause in the larva (Mansingh et al. 1972). The latter physiological condition is characterized by the ability of the larva to make rapid biochemical-metabolic adjustments to changing water temperatures. For example, at temperatures below 4°C., larvae enter a state of hibernation and show little inclination to feed or undergo growth. Further, high amounts of polyhydric alcohols (e.g., glycerol, sorbitol, and mannitol) are sequestered and used as antifreezes. However, increases in water temperature above 4° significantly elevate O_2 consumption; promote growth; and decrease the levels of the alcohols, with a concomitant rise in trehalose. *Austrosimulium pestilens* and related taxa differ significantly from the life cycle examples described. The immature stages of these species occupy ephemeral streams in semiarid regions of Australia. Because black fly eggs can not withstand desiccation, the ova must remain in contact with moisture trapped by the sandy sediment. Thus, to survive when there is lack of flowing water, the eggs lie dormant in the substrata for several years at a time (Colbo and Moorhouse 1974). As the streams receive water, the eggs are washed from bottom sediments, and the larvae hatch and begin development. Interestingly, to take advantage of temporary streams, the ovaries of females of this species mature within a day or so after engorgement on blood.

BIONOMICS

Simulium (Edwardsellum) damnosum sensu lato is a group of 40 or more sibling species distributed throughout sub-Saharan Africa and the Arabian Peninsula; certain taxa within this complex (termed "cytospecies" based on their designation as species using differences in banding patterns on the larval salivary gland chromosomes) are primarily responsible for transmission of *Onchocerca volvulus*, the causative agent of river blindness. Most members of this group are nonanthropophilic, and little is known about their life cycles. However, based on intensive ecological and behavioral studies conducted on the approximately 12 vector taxa, a general picture of their life cycles and bionomics can be assumed for this diverse group of biting flies.

Depending on the taxon, the immatures of *S. damnosum s.l.* can occur in a variety of aquatic habitats located in savanna (Guinea or Sudan), forest, or transitional geobotanic zones. For example, *S. damnosum sensu stricto* and *S. sirbanum* are found in large rivers of Uganda, southern Sudan, and across the West African savannas in which their population dynamics are regulated to a large extent by seasonal changes in rainfall. Long-distance migration of inseminated gravid females during the rainy season also occurs as a feature of the biology of the savanna forms. Conversely, *Simulium yahense* and related forms are found in small forested streams and are developmentally active throughout the year. However, unlike the savanna cytospecies (and some forest species as well), *S. yahense* is nonmigratory, and adults tend to remain reasonably close to their forested aquatic habitats.

Gravid *Simulium damnosum* females oviposit communally on emergent aquatic vegetation (Muirhead-Thompson 1956). This activity usually takes place at sunset but can also occur at sunrise as well. Prior to egg deposition, groups of females begin to assemble so that when the proper light threshold is reached, aggregation ensues and mass oviposition results. Based on the sequence of events, it has been suggested that communal oviposition can be controlled by 1 or more pheromones, which serve to first attract gravid flies and then to stimulate their oviposition. Consequently, extremely large masses of eggs (numbering in the thousands), held together by a gel-like matrix, accumulate in clumps on the trailing vegetation. The sheer weight of these masses often forces the plant substrate into the water, insuring that a major portion of the freshly deposited ova remain immersed. Embryonation then occurs over a period of 1–2 days (depending on temperature and the level of oxygen within the egg mass), and larvae (sometimes referred to as prolarvae because of the presence of an egg burster on the dorsum of the head) begin hatching.

Once in the aquatic environment, the larva attaches itself to a suitable substrate by spinning a silken pad and then inserting hooks that are on the terminal portion of the abdomen into this pad. From this location, it can then position itself into the current and, by means of its cephalic fans, filter the water passing through them (the head points downstream to place the concave surface of the fans in an upstream direction). The larval diet consists of detritus (finely fragmented organic debris), bacteria, diatoms, filamentous algae, and animal matter (Crosskey 1990). Depending upon availability of food and water temperature, the larval stage can last from 1–4 weeks. In this phase of development, *S. damnosum s.l.* larvae usually pass through 7 instars, although this number varies (a distinctive developmental trait within the Simuliidae).

Adults emerge from the larval habitat encased in a bubble of air and immediately fly to a resting site. Eclosion normally occurs during the day, presumably as a result of the fly's ability to regulate its activity in response to a light-mediated circadian rhythm. Mating usually takes place close to the emergence site.

Males (which emerge first) aggregate into swarms in response to visual markers that stand out against the open sky (for example, the open branches of trees); it is presumed that coupling/mating occurs within the swarm shortly after the females enter it. Detection of the female by the questing males is a visual process, and pheromones probably do not play a role in initial attraction. Instead, the male compound eye is specifically adapted for locating the female. This structure is characterized grossly by a dorso-ventral division with greatly enlarged dorsal ommatidia. The corneal facets in the dorsal portion of the eye are considerably larger than in the ventral eye; the screening pigment also differs, being translucent for light of longer wavelengths and light brown instead of the dark red-brown in the ventral eye. These modifications greatly increase the field of vision and allow the male to detect small, fast-moving objects (females) as well as orient to a swarm marker (Wenk 1965; Kirschfeld and Wenk 1976).

Sperm transfer takes place by means of a spermatophore (Wenk 1965a) that is attached to the genital plate of the female. This ephemeral structure, which is evident in recently inseminated, nulliparous females, consists of a viscous mass that becomes hollowed out to surround the bundle of sperm. The wall of the spermatophore is subdivided into 2 distinct sublayers, presumably assembled from the granular secretory materials seen in the male accessory glands (Raminani and Cupp 1976).

After insemination, the females then ingest nectar and other plant secretions to power their flight in search of a blood meal. This plant diet (composed mainly of carbohydrates) also provides energy to initiate oogenesis and begin the deposition of nonvitellogenic yolk in the ovary. Nulliparous females are often collected at this point of ovarian development (some 24–36 hr after emergence and mating) while seeking the first blood meal. Following engorgement and the initiation of blood digestion, the ovaries undergo further development as vitellogenesis proceeds. Typically, the ovary undergoes a series of characteristic "stages" as yolk accumulates (see Cupp and Collins 1979), ultimately resulting in the production of mature eggs (Christophers' Stage V). During this process, the female feeds daily on a carbohydrate diet to maintain sufficient energy to complete digestion and vitellogenesis. In the *S. damnosum* complex, oviposition then occurs in the late afternoon or early evening as the light intensity begins to decline.

Following egg deposition, a general chronology of postovipositional changes occur that aid in the differentiation of parous (individuals that have fed on blood and that have completed at least 1 gonotrophic cycle) from nulliparous females. Immediately following oviposition, a large sac is formed in the follicular tube. This distension, which represents the space formerly occupied by the mature ovum, is filled with amorphous cellular debris apparently derived from the follicular epithelium and nurse cells. This granular material gradually compacts as the follicular tube begins to contract, resulting in the formation of follicular relicts. The remnants of cellular debris are evident for several days and can be useful in epidemiological studies in which it is necessary to characterize the physiological condition of a vector population and calculate transmission statistics (Cupp et al. 1993). However, these relicts do not readily persist during subsequent gonotrophic cycles as is often the case for many mosquito species, and "physiological age" (number of gonotrophic cycles) cannot be easily estimated.

Depending upon reproductive status (nulliparous versus parous), *S. damnosum s.l.* females can change their search pattern for blood meals. In the savanna region of Cameroon, nulliparous females traveled farther from their riverine habitats than their parous counterparts, often flying several kilometers for a blood meal (appetitive flights). After oviposition, parous flies foraged over a shorter distance and tended to remain closer to the lotic environment. For this reason, transmission of *Onchocerca volvulus* in this setting is particularly intense at the water's edge, and those persons who visit or work in this vicinity (e.g., those fishing, ferrying others, or washing clothes, etc.) are most likely to develop intense parasitic infections. However, in the savannas of West Africa, parous flies were more dispersive, traveling distances of up to several hundred kilometers (Crosskey 1990). Thus human contact with the anthropophilic members of this species group is variable and can occur in agroecosystems (rubber plantations, small farms), river crossings, settlements and villages, and along footpaths and trails.

Blood-engorged and gravid females apparently rest on a variety of substrates, including the undersides of leaves, at the base of clumps of grasses and bushes along rivers and streams, on leaves of trees up to 5–6 meters above ground near the aquatic sites, and on certain food plants (millet and guinea corn). However, more information is needed for this group of species as well as others of medical importance regarding this aspect of their biology.

HOST-PARASITE INTERACTIONS

The general orientation of female black flies searching for a blood meal consists of a series of varied stimuli emanating from the host, including color and silhouette profile, CO_2, and odor. Three hierarchial zones (long, middle, and close range), which correspond to various sensory inputs, have been suggested (Bradbury and Bennett 1974a,b). Long-range orientation is strongly dependent upon host-specific odors; it is probable that these olfactory stimuli initiate host-seeking at distances further than that known for CO_2. For example, several of the forest forms of *S. damnosum s.l.* depend on human sweat as an olfactory stimulus whereas the anthropophilic forms of this species complex in the savanna are not particularly attracted to host odor or exhaled breath.

Middle-range orientation is initiated by a CO_2 stimulus that apparently serves as the principal force in directed orientation (appetitive behavior). CO_2 can also be significant in host finding by nocturnally active, ornithophilic black flies.

Host-seeking at close range is associated with responses to such visual stimuli as shape, color, and size of the host. Movement of the host or its parts can also be significant. These latter factors appear to be important in attracting the savanna forms of *S. damnosum* to human hosts.

Once on the skin of a host, blood-feeding by the female ensues. Peg sensilla located ventrally on the tarsomeres are involved in contact chemoreception and in initiating probing behavior (Sutcliffe and McIver 1979). Heat is also an essential factor in stimulating probing behavior, with adenosine triphosphate serving as a phagostimulant once the skin has been pierced and "tasting" initiated (see Bernardo and Cupp 1986).

During probing and blood-feeding, black flies produce an array of salivary secretions to overcome the vertebrate hemostatic mechanisms. These include anticoagulants (Jacobs et al. 1990; Abebe et al. 1994, 1995), an antiplatelet aggregation factor (apyrase, an enzyme that degrades ATP and ADP, thereby removing the chemical signal necessary to cause aggregation) (Cupp et al. 1993), and a powerful vasodilator that causes a persistent erythema (Cupp et al. 1994). The process of finding blood and engorging is a relatively slow one, with average feeding times of some vector species taking 3–6 minutes. This aspect of feeding is crucial for transmission of *Onchocerca* spp., however, because the parasite is not delivered directly in the saliva but instead must move from its position in the head (or possibly in the thorax) to the labrum-epipharynx from where it erupts subcutaneously into the feeding lesion. Thus the infection process in black fly-associated filariasis (and *Culicoides*-associated filarial infection as well) differs dramatically from that of lymphatic filariasis in which the infective stage larva breaks out of the mosquito's mouthparts onto the surface of the skin and must then enter the puncture wound caused by the stylets.

METHODS OF CONTROL

Black fly control is based primarily on elimination of larvae in their aquatic habitats by means of synthetic insecticides (for example, temephos) and *Bacillus thuringiensis* variety *israelensis* (H–14 serotype), a biological control agent (Luján and Cupp 1991). The elimination of larvae is required for the most part because of the wide range of dispersal by the adult flies following emergence and the cost effectiveness of treating streams and rivers with nonpolluting, nonpersistent control agents. The World Health Organization (WHO) has directed an Onchocerciasis Control Programme in West Africa for the past 2 decades and has successfully eliminated *S. damnosum* vector taxa over a wide part of the savanna region, thereby demonstrating the usefulness of larval control to interrupt transmission of *O. volvulus*.

Ivermectin, a macrocyclic lactone, is also effective in altering transmission of *O. volvulus* when persons infected with the parasite are treated at 6-month intervals (Cupp 1992). Microfilariae are rapidly killed in the skin, and adult females are unable to replenish this stage that is critical for infection of the black fly vector. If used biannually, ivermectin also affects the adult stage by increasing mortality of the female and decreasing male mating success. Because it is so efficacious and favorably tolerated, this drug can be used on a large scale and is currently employed as a major component for onchocerciasis control in both Africa and Latin America.

REFERENCES AND FURTHER READING

Literature Cited

Abebe, M., M.S. Cupp, F.B. Ramberg, and E.W. Cupp. 1994. Anticoagulant activity in salivary gland extracts of black flies. *J. Med. Entomol.* 31:908–911.

Abebe, M., J.M.C. Ribeiro, M.S. Cupp, and E.W. Cupp. 1995. A novel anticoagulant from the salivary glands of *Simulium vittatum* (Diptera: Simuliidae) inhibits activity of coagulation factor V. *J. Med. Entomol.* (in press).

Bernardo, M.J., and E.W. Cupp. 1986. Rearing black flies (Diptera: Simuliidae) in the laboratory: Mass scale *in vitro* membrane feeding and its application to collection of saliva, parasitological, and repellent studies. *J. Med. Entom.* 23:666–679.

Bradbury, W.C., and G.F. Bennett. 1974a. Behavior of adult Simuliidae (Diptera). 1. Response to color and shape. *Can. J. Zool.* 52:251–259.

———. 1974b. Vision and olfaction in near-orientation and landing. *Can. J. Zool.* 52:1355–1364.

Colbo, M.H., and D.E. Moorhouse. 1974. The survival of the eggs of *Austrosimulium pestilens* Mack. and Mack. (Diptera, Simuliidae). *Bull. Ent. Res.* 64:629–632.

Collins, R.C. 1979. Development of *Onchocerca volvulus* in *Simulium ochraceum* and *Simulium metallicum*. *Am. J. Trop. Med. Hyg.* 28:491–495.

Crosskey, R.W. 1990. *The natural history of black flies.* New York: John Wiley and Sons. 711 p.

———. 1993. Black flies (Simuliidae). In: R.P. Lane and R.W. Crosskey, editors, *Medical Insects and Arachnids*, pp. 241–287. New York: Chapman and Hall. 723 p.

Cupp, E.W. 1992. Treatment of onchocerciasis with ivermectin in Central America. *Parisit. Today* 8:212–214.

Cupp, E.W. 1986a. The epizootiology of livestock and poultry diseases associated with black flies. In: K.C. Kim and R.W. Merritt, editors., *Black Flies*, pp. 387–395. University Park, PA: Pennsylvania State University. 528 p.

———. 1986b. Human onchocerciasis: Developmental biology of the parasite. In: G.A. Conder and J.F. Williams, editors, *Proceedings of the Upjohn Symposium on Onchocerciasis/Filariasis*. Kalamazoo, MI: Upjohn. pp. 1–14.

Cupp, E.W., and R.C. Collins. 1979. The gonotrophic cycle in *Simulium ochraceum. Am. J. Trop. Med. Hyg.* 28:422–426.

Cupp, E.W., C.J. Maré, M.S. Cupp, and F.B. Ramberg. 1992. Biological transmission of vesicular stomatitis virus (New Jersey) by *Simulium vittatum* Zetterstedt (Diptera: Simuliidae). *J. Med. Entomol.* 29:137–140.

Cupp, E.W., O. Ochoa, R.C. Collins, M.S. Cupp, C. Gonzales-Peralta, J. Castro, and G. Zea-Flores. 1992. The effects of repetitive community-wide treatment on transmission of *Onchocerca volvulus* in Guatemala. *Am. J. Trop. Med. Hyg.* 47:170–180.

Cupp, M.S., E.W. Cupp, and F.B. Ramberg. 1993. Salivary gland apyrase in black flies (*Simulium vittatum*). *J. Insect Physiol.* 39:817–821.

Cupp, M.S., J.M.C. Ribeiro, and E.W. Cupp. 1994. Vasodilative activity in black fly salivary glands. *Am. J. Trop. Med. Hyg.* 50:214–246.

Jacobs, J., E.W. Cupp, M. Sardana, and P.A. Friedman. 1990. Isolation and characterization of a coagulation factor Xa inhibitor from black fly salivary glands. *Thromb. Haem.* 64:235–238.

Jobling, B. 1987. *Anatomical drawings of biting flies.* London: British Museum (Natural History) and Wellcome Trust. 119 p.

Kim, K.C., and R.W. Merritt, editors. 1986. *Black flies: Ecology, population management, and annotated world list.* University Park and London: Pennsylvania State University Press. 528 p.

Kirschfeld, K., and P. Wenk. 1976. The dorsal compound eye of simuliid flies: An eye specialized for the detection of small, rapidly moving objects. *Z. Nature.* 31(C):764–765.

Kiszewski, A.E., and E.W. Cupp. 1986. Transmission of *Leucocytozoon smithi* in New York. *J. Med. Ent.* 23:256–262.

Laird, M., editor. 1981. *Blackflies: The future for biologic methods in integrated control.* London: Academic Press. 399 p.

Luján, R., and E.W. Cupp. 1991. Human onchocerciasis: New immunodiagnostic assays and control measures. In: K. Maramorosch, editor, *Biotechnology for biological control of pests and vectors.* Boca Raton, FL: CRC Press. pp. 180–192.

Mansingh, A.R., W. Steele, and B.V. Helson. 1972. Hibernation in the black fly *Prosimulium mysticum*: Quiescence or oligopause? *Can. J. Zool.* 50:31–34.

Muirhead-Thompson, R.C. 1956. Communal oviposition in *Simulium damnosum* Theobald. *Nature* 178:1297–1299.

Noble, J. Jr., L. Valverde, O.E. Equia, O. Serrate, and E. Antezana. 1974. Hemorrhagic exanthem of Bolivia. *Am. J. Epidem.* 99:123–130.

Post, R.J., and P. Flook. 1992. DNA probes for the identification of members of the *Simulium damnosum* complex (Diptera: Simuliidae). *Med. Vet. Ent.* 6:379–384.

Pinheiro, F.P., G. Bensabath, D. Costa Jr., O.M. Maroja, Z.C. Lins, and A.H.P. Andrade. 1974. Haemorrhagic syndrome of Altamira. *Lancet* 1:639–642.

Raminani, L.N., and E.W. Cupp. 1978. The male reproductive system of the black fly, *Simulium pictipes* Hagen. *Mosq. News* 38:591–594.

Sutcliffe, J.F., and S.B. McIver. 1979. Experiments on biting and gorging behaviour in the black fly, *Simulium venustum. Physiol. Ent.* 4:393–400.

———. 1984. Mechanics of blood-feeding in black flies (Diptera, Simuliidae). *J. Morph.* 180:125–144.

Wenk, P. 1965. Über die Biologie blutsaugender Simuliiden (Diptera). 2. Schwarmverhalten, Geschlechterfindung und Kopulation. *Z. Morph. Ökol. Tiere* 55:671–713.

———. 1965a. III. Kopulation, Blutsaugen und eiablage von *Boophthora erythrocephala* de Geer im Laboratorium. *Z. Tropenmed. Parasit.* 16:207–226.

Reviews and Important Papers

References by Crosskey (1990, 1993) are the most recent reviews dealing with black flies. Both are excellent, and his 1990 publication is the most comprehensive treatise currently available for the Simuliidae. Another recent source of information is the book edited by Kim and Merritt (1986). Although somewhat dated, the reader is also referred to Laird (1981) for natural history information.

Taxonomic Keys and Aids to Identification

Crosskey (1993) provides geographical keys to the simuliid genera containing human-biting species and to *Simulium* females from Africa that are attracted to and feed on human blood. In addition, this reference contains a substantial faunal and taxonomic literature section. Other details on taxonomy of North American genera can be obtained from chapter 27 (Simuliidae) of the *Manual of Nearctic Diptera* (McAlpine et al. 1981), published by Agriculture Canada. The reader should also consult chapter 10 of *Geographical Distribution of Arthropod-Borne Diseases and Their Principal Vectors*, published by the World Health Organization (WHO/VBC/89.967).

8. BITING MIDGES AND THE AGENTS THEY TRANSMIT

Frederick R. Holbrook

INTRODUCTION

The biting midges (order, Diptera; suborder, Nematocera; superfamily, Chironomoidea; family, Ceratopogonidae) are small, robust flies, generally less than 6 mm long, that are closely related to the Simuliidae (black flies) and Chironomidae (midges). The Nearctic Ceratopogonidae are composed of 4 subfamilies: the Leptoconopinae, Forcipomyiinae, Dasyheleinae, and Ceratopogoninae. The subfamily Ceratopogoninae is further divided into 6 tribes (Culicoidini, Ceratopogonini, Stilobezzini, Stenoxenini, Palpomyiini, and Heteromyiini), 34 genera, and 36 subgenera (Downes and Wirth 1981). They are distinguished by their 15-segmented antennae, which are characterized by sexual dimorphism, and their distinctive wing venation.

Only female ceratopogonids possess biting mouthparts. They take blood from mammals, birds, and reptiles and feed on body fluids from other larger invertebrates such as moths and butterflies and other insects. Certain species, autogenous for the 1st egg batch, require a protein source for subsequent oviposition cycles. Both sexes visit flowers to obtain nectar as an energy source.

These tiny biting flies are second only to mosquitoes as pests of humans and other vertebrates, and in certain areas they are the most frequent biters of humans and livestock. They have been variously called sand flies, punkies, moose flies, no-see-ums, biting gnats, and flying teeth. In areas such as near swamps and salt marshes, their presence can severely curtail outdoor activity, and development near such areas for homes or for recreational purposes can be adversely affected. Their diminutive size allows them to pass through standard mosquito screens. Indeed, a mesh small enough to exclude all ceratopogonids also significantly reduces ventilation. Their bites are accompanied by the introduction of anticoagulants and cause intense pain and itching; the source is often difficult to find. Kettle (1962) stated, "One midge is an entomological curiosity, a thousand can be hell!"

Biting midges cause serious dermatitis and allergic reactions in sensitized individuals. Sensitized livestock, after even 1 bite, often rub against something until large patches of skin become raw and bleed, a condition known as allergic dermatitis, or "Queensland itch." Blood-feeding species are also efficient vectors of such diseases as bird and lizard malaria, equine onchocerciasis, oropouche virus in humans, and bluetongue virus in wild and domestic ruminants. The economic impact of viruses such as bluetongue can be greater than the disease they cause. In North America, the most significant impact of the interrelationship of bluetongue viruses and the vector, *C. variipennis* (Fig. 8.1), is on the international movement of ruminant livestock (including semen and embryos) because bluetongue is a nontariff trade barrier. Currently, the

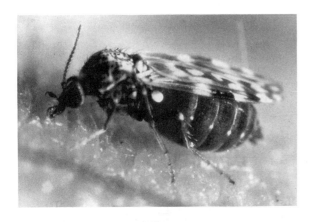

8.1 *Culicoides variipennis,* engorged adult female. Courtesy of E.T. Schmidtmann, Coop. Ext. Serv., University of California.

characteristic serpentine motion when moving through the water.

Pupa

The pupae are comma-shaped and light brown to black, with a pair of dorsal respiratory horns protruding from the prothorax. There are numerous spines, setae, protuberances, and processes that can be used as diagnostic characters.

Adults of the Forcipomyiinae, Dasyheleinae, and Ceratopogoninae are generally similar to each other and differ from the Leptoconopinae. Eyes are approximated, or meeting at the midline, and are usually bare, with uniform facets. Antennae have 13 flagellomeres and exhibit marked sexual dimorphism. Females can

United States is treated as a geographic unit; consequently, all susceptible animals or their living products must be thoroughly tested to receive certification for international shipment, even when lifelong residents of areas in which bluetongue is not present. This testing and resulting lost trade costs the U.S. livestock industry an estimated $120 million yearly.

MORPHOLOGY

Egg Stage

The eggs of biting midges differ between taxa but are usually about 0.25 mm in length, often pale when laid (turning to glossy black), elongate, curved, and pointed at each end. Some species possess characteristic sculpturing or markings.

Larva

The larvae are vermiform, usually pale, and with or without prolegs. They have a characteristically distinctive sclerotized, prognathous head capsule with toothed mandibles and eyespots. There are 3 thoracic and 9 abdominal segments. The larvae of many species exhibit a

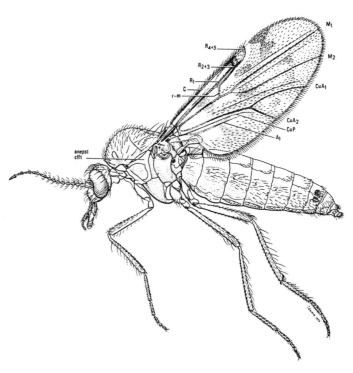

8.2 *Culicoides yukonensis,* female, showing wing venation. J.A. Downes 1981, *Manual of Nearctic Diptera,* Vol. 1, Fig. 28.13 (information from "Agriculture Canada"). Reproduced with the permission of the Minister of Supply and Services, Canada, 1992.

have biting-sucking mouthparts; nonbiting females and males have smaller proboscises and a palpus with 5 segments. For wing venation, see Figure 8.2. The anal lobe is rarely prominent, and the calypter usually does not have fringe. Some genera have a conspicuous pattern of spots. The legs are moderately long, as are the claws. Males with claws are usually bifid at tip (Downes and Wirth 1981).

Culicoides variipennis represents a taxonomic problem that is common in the Ceratopogonidae and related families. This North American disease vector is actually a complex that has been difficult to resolve morphologically. It is composed of 3–5 subspecies, 3 of which (*C. v. occidentalis*, *C. v. sonorensis*, and *C. v. variipennis*) have thus far been confirmed by starch gel electrophoresis. The distribution of bluetongue disease transmission in the United States (Fig. 8.3) is closely correlated to that of *C. v. sonorensis,* (Fig. 8.4), which is the only member of the complex that has been proven a competent vector of the bluetongue viruses.

LIFE CYCLE

In temperate North America, the biting midge *Culicoides variipennis* (Coquillett) is an important vector of bluetongue and epizootic hemorrhagic disease viruses of ruminants and of the parasitic nematode *Onchocerca cervicalis* in horses. This biting midge has been colonized and its life cycle well characterized. At

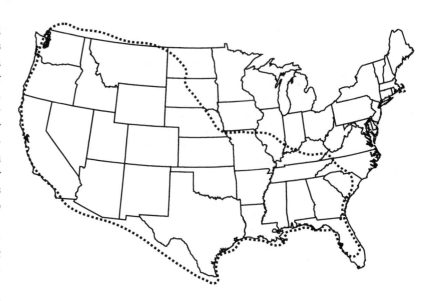

8.3   Seropositive rates of bluetongue (dark portion of each circle) in the United States in a 1977–1978 serosurvey. Metcalf et al., 1981, *Am. J. Vet. Res.* 42:1057–1061, Fig. 1

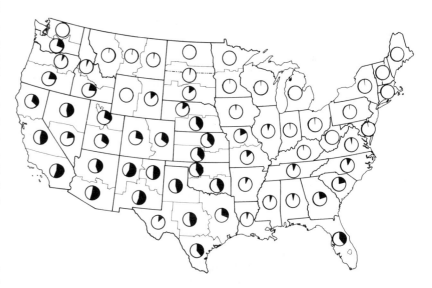

8.4   Geographic distribution of *Culicoides variipennis sonorensis*, the principal vector of bluetongue viruses in the United States

25°C the eggs hatch in 48–72 hr, the 4 larval instars are completed in 10–14 days, and pupal development requires 2–3 days. The adults can mate and blood-feed

2 days after emergence and lay eggs 2–3 days after feeding on blood. Survival is inversely related to temperature; some adults survive a month or more at temperatures below 20°C. Overwintering in temperate climates occurs during the larval stage.

BIONOMICS

The eggs must remain moist. Females lay eggs singly during flight or when crawling near the larval habitat, which is typically damp, with decaying organic matter. Larvae of different species are found at the edges of pools or ponds, in salt marshes, along the banks of creeks, in damp depressions, in tree holes or rock pools, in manure pats, or in collections of rotting plant material. Favorable larval sites are often created by mismanagement of water and waste. The larvae hatch and graze on microorganisms or prey on other small invertebrates; they become cannibalistic when their normal food supply is depleted. The pupae float and often aggregate where drifted by the wind or currents.

The adults emerge, rest, and then disperse for host-seeking, mating, and oviposition. Resting sites are not well described. Mating usually takes place in male swarms, and it is not uncommon to find several species in the same swarm. Some species are autogenous for the first gonotrophic cycle, but multiple cycles do occur. Adults of many species are crepuscular or nocturnal but can be diurnally active on cloudy days or when evening temperatures stay below the activity threshold.

The preferred habitat for the larvae of *C. variipennis* is a permanent pool or pond exposed to direct sunlight, with gently sloping banks free of vegetation, and with a high organic content. Such sites are most often found associated with confined livestock operations, dairy washing water runoffs, waste lagoons, watering holes, or overflowing stock tanks. Larvae have also been found in sewage treatment ponds, septic ditches, and waste ponds at vegetable processing plants. The larvae are tolerant of a wide range of fresh, saline, and alkaline conditions. They are mobile but are usually found concentrated in a band a few cm above and below the water's surface. Under favorable conditions, the larvae can be found in the upper 2 cm of mud. As the temperature drops or the mud dries, they penetrate downward;

larvae have been found several cm deep at the frost margin or aggregated in a compact mass at the bottom of cracks in the mud's surface. Pupation occurs just above the surface of wet mud.

The adults emerge in 2–5 days, and host-seeking, blood-feeding, and mating commence about 2 days after eclosion. Adults are normally crepuscular—their activity usually peaks just after sunset—but they have been observed flying on bright moonlit nights. They have been collected from crevices in the bark of trees and fence posts, and imagoes have been found on vegetation near their place of emergence. The females prefer to feed on large animals and, with some notable exceptions, seldom feed on humans. In the absence of preferred hosts, they are quite opportunistic. Adults have been captured more than 18 km from their point of emergence. Oviposition commences 2 days after feeding; a gonotrophic cycle can be completed in 4–5 days, repeating throughout the life of the adult female. Colonized adult females held at 26°C for more than 15 days experienced a significantly higher cumulative mortality than those held at 20°C (73 % versus 51%) (Hunt et al. 1989).

HOST-PARASITE INTERACTIONS

Culicoides females only fly at wind speeds below 4–7 meters per second (m/s). As with other blood-feeding insects, host-seeking is activated and controlled by a combination of physical, genetic, and chemical stimuli. The size, shape, and color of the host is important. However, because most species feed after sunset, when winds tend to decrease, the chemical factors are probably of greater significance. CO_2 is a powerful attractant for host-seeking females but not males of most species; however, it repels females searching for oviposition sites. In suction and light traps, CO_2 can increase catches by a factor of 10 or more. Another component of animal breath, octenol (1-octen–3-ol), has been shown to attract females of certain species. Ultraviolet (UV) light sources also attract females in varying states of parity, but the role of UV radiation in host-seeking has not been determined. Little is known about the host-seeking behavior of *Culicoides* spp. that prey on other insects. Some catch their prey in flight, whereas others attach to larger insects that are either at rest or in motion and suck their host's juices.

METHODS OF CONTROL

In the 1920s sprays, fumigants, and screens were the recommended methods used to control biting midges. Applications of crude oil, coupled with management practices such as flooding, filling, dredging, and the removal of breeding materials, were used for larval abatement.

In the mid-1940s, aerial applications of chlorinated hydrocarbon pesticides revolutionized pest and vector control; repellents also made their debut. By the 1950s, biting midges were found to be resistant to several of the common chlorinated hydrocarbons, and effective alternative chemicals with less residual effect, particularly the organophosphates, were recommended. The development of insecticidal ear tags for livestock in the 1980s showed great promise, but misuse resulted in the rapid development of resistance.

A number of biological control agents have been proposed, but none have demonstrated sufficient potential to warrant use. The genetic engineering of aquatic agents such as *Bacillus thuringiensis israelensis* and the development of resistant host strains show promise for long-term control.

Current recommendations for *Culicoides* control involve insecticide applications, management practices at developmental sites, repellents, judicious use of ear tags impregnated with insecticides, and preventing access to host animals. The array of available options can be combined into a management strategy that is tailored to the local situation.

DISEASE AGENTS VECTORED

Biting midges (mostly those found in the genus *Culicoides*) have been shown to transmit protozoa, nematodes, and viruses in humans and animals. The organisms for which the vector relationships have been firmly established are shown in Table 8.1. Organisms transmitted to humans are in the Nematoda and viruses. *Mansonella perstans* and *M. streptocerca* in Africa and *M. ozzardi* in the Amazon Basin and the Caribbean Islands of the New World are relatively nonpathogenic filarial parasites. Oropouche virus in South America is the causal agent for the disease of the

TABLE 8.1 Organisms transmitted by Ceratopogonidae

Taxa	Vector species	Vertebrate hosts
Alphavirus eastern equine encephalomyelitis	C. (Selfia) spp., C. spp.	humans, rodents, birds, cattle, marsupials, other primates
Bunyavirus Akabane	C. brevitarsis, C. oxystoma, C. imicola, C. wadai	cattle
Buttonwillow	C. variipennis, C. (Selfia) spp., C. spp.	rabbits, rodentia, chiroptera, cattle, horse, pig, goat, deer
Douglas	C. brevitarsis	cattle, deer, goats, horses, sheep, buffalo
Oropouche	C. paraensis	humans, other primates, birds, rodents
Peaton	C. brevitarsis	cattle, sheep, horses, buffalo, goats, pigs, deer
Jerry Slough	C. variipennis	rodents
Lokern	C. variipennis, C. (Selfia) spp., C. spp.	rabbits, rodents, horses, cattle, pigs, sheep
Main Drain	C. variipennis, C. (Selfia) spp.	horses, rabbits, rodents, cattle, pigs, sheep
Flavivirus Israel turkey meningoencephalitis	C. spp.	turkey
Lyssavirus Kotonkan	C. spp.	humans, cattle, birds, hedgehogs, rodents, sheep, horses

TABLE 8.1 (Continued)   Organisms transmitted by Ceratopogonidae

Taxa	Vector species	Vertebrate hosts
Nairovirus Congo	*C.* spp.	humans, cattle, goats, hedgehogs
Dugbe	*C.* spp.	humans, cattle, rodents
Nairobi sheep disease	*C. tororensis*	humans, sheep, goats
Orbivirus African horse sickness	*C. imicola*	equids, dogs
bluetongue	*C. insignis*, *C. imicola*, *C. nubeculosus*, *C. impunctatus*, *C. debilipalpis*	ruminants
epizootic hemorrhagic disease	*C. schultzei*, *C. kingi*, *C. variipennis*	deer, cattle, sheep
Bunyip Creek	*C. brevitarsis*, *C. schultzei*, *C. oxystoma*	cattle, buffalo, sheep, deer
CSIRO Village	*C. brevitarsis*, *C.* spp.	cattle, buffalo, sheep, deer
D'Aguilar	*C. brevitarsis*	cattle, sheep
Phlebovirus Rift Valley fever	*C. variipennis*, *C.* spp.	humans, sheep, cattle
Protozoa *Haemoproteus*		
canachites	*C. sphagnumensis*	spruce grouse
meleagridis	*C. edeni*, *C. hinmani*, *C. arboricola*	turkey
velans	*C. stillobezzoides*	woodpeckers
Hepatocyctis		
kochi	*C. aderi*	monkeys
simiae	*C.* spp.	monkeys

TABLE 8.1 (Continued)   Organisms transmitted by Ceratopogonidae

Taxa	Vector species	Vertebrate hosts
Leucocytozoon caulleryi	*C. arakawae*, *C. circumscriptus*	chickens
Nematoda *Chandlerella*		
chitwoodae	*C. stillobezzoides*	common crows
quiscali	*C. crepuscularis*, *C. haematopotus*	common grackles
striatospicula	*C. haematopotus*	American magpies
Mansonella (= *Dipetalonema*)		
ozzardi	*C. furens*, *C. phlebotomus*	humans
perstans	*C. grahami*, *C. inornatipennis*	humans
streptocerca	*C. grahami*	humans
Eufilaria longicaudata	*C. crepuscularis*, *C. haematopotus*	American magpies
Icosiella neglecta	*Forcipomyia velox*	green frogs
Onchocerca		
cervicalis	*C. nubeculosus*, *C. variipennis*	horses
gibsoni	*C. shortii*, *C. orientalis*, *C. marksi*	cattle
gutterosa	*C. fulvithorax*, *C. kingi*, *C. krameri*, *C. nubeculosus*, *C. trifasciellus*	bovines
oxystoma	*F. townsvillensis*	cattle
reticulata	*C. nubeculosus*	horses
sweetae	*C.* spp.	water buffalo
Splendiofilaria		
californiensis	*C. multidentatus*	California quail
picacardina	*C. crepuscularis*	American magpies

same name. Oropouche virus is the most important human pathogen transmitted by the biting midges, and numerous outbreaks have been recorded. Although not fatal, it can be severely debilitating for up to 2 weeks. Other viruses causing significant human illness are eastern encephalitis virus in the Americas and Rift Valley fever and Congo viruses in Africa.

REFERENCES AND FURTHER READING

Literature Cited

Holbrook, F.R. 1985. An overview of *Culicoides* control. In: T.L. Barber and M.M. Jochim, editors, *Bluetongue and related orbiviruses*. New York: Alan R. Liss. pp. 607–608.

Hunt, G.J., W.J. Tabachnick, and C.N. McKinnon. 1989. Environmental factors affecting mortality of adult *Culicoides variipennis* (Diptera: Ceratopogonidae) in the laboratory. *J. Am. Mosq. Contr. Assoc.* 5(3):387–391.

Kettle, D.S. 1962. The bionomics and control of *Culicoides* and *Leptoconops* (Diptera: Ceratopogonidae = Heleidae). *Ann. Rev. Entomol.* 7:401–418.

Linley, J.R. 1985. Biting midges (Diptera: Ceratopogonidae) as vectors of nonviral animal pathogens. *J. Med. Entomol.* 22:589–599

Linley, J.R., A.L. Hoch, and F.P Pinheiro. 1983. Biting midges (Diptera: Ceratopogonidae) and human health. *J. Med. Entomol.* 20:347–364.

Wirth, W.W. 1977. Pathogens of Ceratopogonidae (midges). *Bull. WHO* 55 (Suppl)1:197–204

Reviews and Important Papers

Atchley, W.R., W.W. Wirth, C.T. Gaskins, and S.S. Strauss, translators. 1981. *A bibliography and keyword index of the biting midges (Diptera: Ceratopogonidae)*. Washington, D.C.: U.S. Dept. Agric. Biblio. Lit. Agric., no. 13. 544 p.

Keys and Aids to Identification

Blanton, F.S., and W.W. Wirth. 1979. The sand flies (*Culicoides*) of Florida (Diptera: Ceratopogonidae). *Arthropods of Florida and neighboring land areas*. Vol. 10. 204 p.

Downes, J.A., and W.W. Wirth. 1981. Ceratopogonidae. In: J.F. McAlpine, B.V. Peterson, G.E. Shewell, H.J. Teskey, J.R. Vockeroth, and D.M. Wood, coordinators, *Manual of Nearctic Diptera*. Vol.1, Monograph 27. Ottawa, Canada: Agric. Ottawa. pp. 393–421.

Glukova, V.M. 1979. Larvae of the biting midges of the subfamilies Palpomyiinae and Ceratopogoninae of the fauna of the USSR. Nauk, SSSR, Leningrad: *ANSSSR, Opredeleteli po fauna SSSR*, 121, 230 p. (Key to genera, with English translation available through the informal Ceratopogonid Information Exchange).

Murphree, C.S., and G.R. Mullen. 1991. Comparative larval morphology of the genus *Culicoides* Latrielle (Diptera: Ceratopogonidae) in North America with a key to species. *Bull. Soc. Vector Ecol.* 16:269–399.

Wirth, W.W., A.L. Dyce, and D.G. Peterson. 1985. An atlas of wing photographs, with a summary of the numerical characters of the Nearctic species of *Culicoides*. *Contrib. Am. Entomol. Inst.* 22:1–46.

Wirth, W.W., and W.L. Grogan Jr. 1988. *The Predaceous midges of the world: Flora and fauna handbook 4*. New York: E.J. Brill. 160 p.

Wirth, W.W., N.C. Ratanaworabhan, and F.S. Blanton. 1974. Synopsis of the genera of Ceratopogonidae (Diptera). *Ann. Parasitol. Hum. Comp.* 49:595–613.

9. SAND FLIES AND THE AGENTS THEY TRANSMIT

Robert B. Tesh and Hilda Guzman

INTRODUCTION

Sand flies are small bloodsucking Diptera in the family Psychodidae, subfamily Phlebotominae. These tiny flies are of considerable public health importance because they serve as vectors of the etiologic agents of leishmaniasis, bartonellosis, and several arboviral illnesses.

The Phlebotominae are relatively ancient insects that probably appeared during the Lower Cretaceous Period (Lewis 1982). The first description of a phlebotomine (a male of unknown species) was published in Rome by Philippo Bonanni in 1691. The type species, *Phlebotomus papatasi*, was described by J.A. Scopoli in 1786. Historical records suggest that their medical importance was recognized at least as early as 1764; in that year the Spanish physician Cosme Bueno published a book on the folklore about transmission of leishmaniasis and bartonellosis in the Peruvian Andes and noted that local inhabitants of the region believed that both diseases originated from the bite of a small insect called "uta" (sand fly) (Herrer and Christensen 1975).

MORPHOLOGY

Adult sand flies can be recognized by their small size, hairy bodies, erect wings, and relatively long legs and mouthparts (Fig. 9.1). Correct species identification is more difficult; most species are identified by their internal morphology (pharynx, cibarium, spermatheca,

and terminal genitalia), and these structures can be damaged by improper cleaning or mounting (Lewis 1982; Young and Arias 1991). For those inexperienced in sand fly identification, it is recommended that representative specimens be sent to a specialist for confirmation.

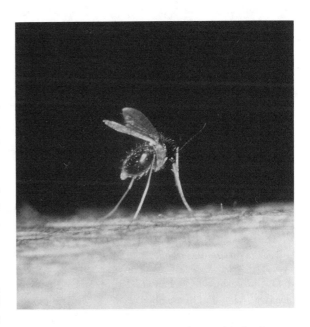

9.1 Adult female sand fly (*Lutzomyia*) immediately after ingesting blood

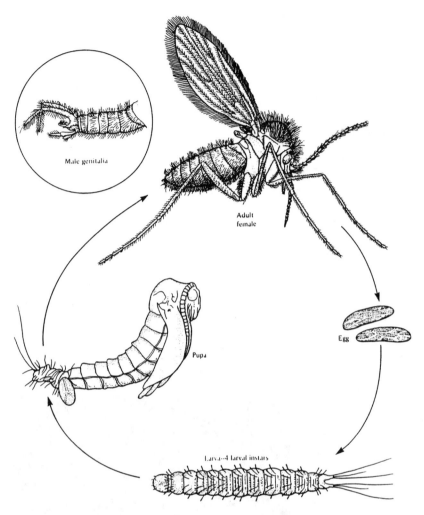

Male genitalia

Adult
female

Pupa

Egg

Larva—4 larval instars

9.2   Sand fly life cycle, showing egg, larva, pupa, and adult. From Marquardt and Demaree 1985. Used with permission.

the medically important species belong to the genera *Lutzomyia* and *Phlebotomus*.

The eggs of about 50 sand fly species have been described. Sand fly eggs are dark and elliptical (Fig. 9.2) and have surface ridges or other protuberances that form patterns typical of the species or species complex (Young and Arias 1991). The larvae are small and caterpillar-like, with a well-developed head capsule, many brushlike setae on the body, and characteristic long caudal setae. Few taxonomic keys are available for the immature stages (Ward 1976).

At present, sand fly species are still differentiated principally by their morphological characteristics; however, this is not entirely satisfactory because females of some closely related species cannot be distinguished (Lewis 1982; Young and Arias 1991; Young and Duncan, 1994). Furthermore, there appears to be considerable intraspecific variation in morphology, host preference, vector competence, mating compatibility, and general ecology among some current taxa, sug-

A number of adult classification schemes have been proposed; the most widely used is that of Lewis et al. (1977), which recognizes 3 genera of Phlebotominae (*Lutzomyia*, *Brumptomyia*, and *Warileya*) in the New World and 2 genera (*Phlebotomus* and *Sergentomyia*) in the Old World. More than 500 different sand fly species have been described; about two-thirds of them are found in the Americas (Lewis 1978, 1982; Young and Duncan 1994; Peril'ev 1968; Abonnec 1972). Most of

gesting that species complexes exist. For example, there is considerable evidence that *Lutzomyia longipalpis*, a widely distributed vector species in tropical areas of South, Central, and North America, is a complex of at least 3 distinct species (Lanzaro et al. 1993; Ward et al. 1988). Modern genetic techniques such as enzyme electrophoresis, cuticular hydrocarbon analysis, DNA sequence polymorphism, and comparative behavioral studies are just beginning to be used. Cytogenetic

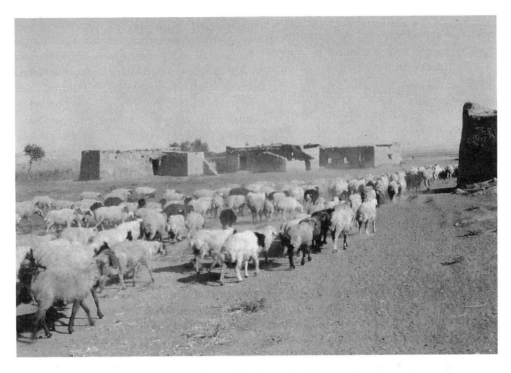

9.3 Desert in central Iran, where sand flies (principally *P. papatasi*) are abundant. In this habitat, the insects were found in rodent burrows and in buildings.

studies of a few sand fly species indicate that the chromosome number in this group of insects ranges from 2N = 6 to 2N = 10 (Kreutzer et al. 1987).

BIONOMICS AND LIFE CYCLE

Although sand flies live in temperate regions, the majority of species are tropical or subtropical in their distribution (Lewis 1978, 1982; Young and Duncan, 1994; Peril'ev 1968; Abonnec 1972). These insects are found in a wide variety of habitats, ranging from desert to rainforest to intradomiciliary (Figs. 9.3 and 9.4). The sand fly life cycle consists of egg, 4 larval instars, pupa, and adult (Fig. 9.2). Sand flies are terrestrial throughout their life cycles, but the precise breeding sites of most species in nature are unknown. Because of their small size and peculiar breeding habits, the immature stages are extremely difficult to locate. On the basis of observations of the behavior of laboratory colonies and of adult resting sites, investigators generally assume that sand fly eggs are laid individually in small batches in protected moist microhabitats such as rock crevices, animal burrows, termite mounds, bases and cavities of large trees, cellars, domestic animal shelters, and among leaves and other organic debris on the forest floor (Young and Arias 1991; Lewis 1978; Peril'ev 1968; Abonnec 1972). Because of the wide diversity of sand fly species and their varied ecological requirements, it is not feasible to describe each in detail. Furthermore, many species are known only from a few isolated collections; apart from their morphology, almost nothing is known about their biology. Consequently, we focus primarily on *Phlebotomus papatasi*, which is one of the better-studied species and is also the sand fly of greatest public health importance.

P. papatasi has a wide distribution in the Old World; it occurs throughout most of the Mediterranean basin,

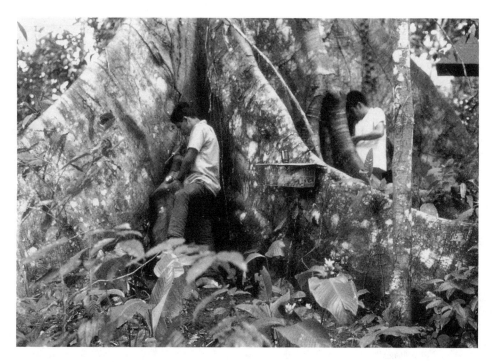

9.4   Collecting sand flies in tropical rain forest in Panama. During the day, the insects were found resting at the bases of large trees and in leaf litter on the forest floor

the Middle East, and the Indian subcontinent (Lewis 1982). In the Indian subcontinent, adult *P. papatasi* are active only during the warmer months of the year (between April or May and September or October, depending upon the latitude). During the colder months, the larvae undergo diapause, allowing the insects to overwinter (Lewis 1978; Peril'ev 1968; Guzman and Tesh, in press). *P. papatasi* is quite anthropophilic and often lives close to humans; it readily enters houses to feed and breeds in adjacent gardens, animal shelters, and cellars (Fig. 9.5)(Peril'ev 1968; Whittingham and Rock 1923; Schmidt and Schmidt 1965; Javadian et al. 1977). However, this sand fly species can also be found in uninhabited desert areas, far from human dwellings, where it rests and presumably breeds in rodent burrows (Fig. 9.6) (Peril'ev 1968). Sand flies are not strong fliers; they usually approach their hosts in short hopping movements along the ground or on vegetation and walls of buildings. In the peridomestic

environment, *P. papatasi* does not travel far from its breeding and resting sites; but in open desert where they can be carried by air currents, they have been reported to travel up to 1500 m (Peril'ev 1968).

P. papatasi is nocturnal in its feeding activity (Schmidt and Schmidt 1965); like other sand fly species, only the female feeds on blood. Although *P. papatasi* readily bites humans, it is basically an opportunistic feeder and feeds on almost any warm-blooded mammal or bird that it encounters (Peril'ev 1968; Javadian et al. 1977). During feeding, sand flies sometimes appear to swarm over their hosts in a frenzy of activity (Ward et al. 1988; Schlein et al. 1984). In some species, courtship and mating take place on the host. During mating, male and female flies take an end-to-end position, connected by their terminalia. Copulation usually lasts 10–15 minutes. An aggregation pheromone released by engorging females has been described in *P. papatasi* (Schlein et al. 1984). At least 2 other mating-aggregation pheromones with farnesene- and diterpenoid-like structures are released by male *Lutzomyia longipalpis* (Ward et al. 1988). Although little research has been done in this area, the available data suggest that some sand fly species communicate via pheromones, using these substances to locate mates and possibly vertebrate hosts.

Theodor (1936) estimated that a fully engorged female *P. papatasi* ingests about 0.5–0.3 μl of blood. The subsequent rate of blood digestion and of ovarian development is largely dependent on the ambient temperature. At 25°C, most laboratory-reared *P. papatasi* develop mature oocytes within 6 days after blood-feeding (Magnarelli et al. 1984). Eggs are laid a day or 2 later if the insects are provided with an appropriate oviposition substrate. The number of eggs produced by an individual female in the 1st gonotrophic cycle ranges from about 10–70 (Magnarelli et al. 1984). However, some *P. papatasi* also develop eggs autogenously in the laboratory if maintained solely on sugar. Although the number of eggs produced by autogenous females is generally less than in blood-fed individuals, the rate of oocyte development is similar. Female *P. papatasi* also take multiple blood meals during a single gonotrophic cycle if an appropriate vertebrate host is available (Schmidt and Schmidt 1965). Because of autogeny and multiple feedings, asynchronous oogenesis is sometimes observed in this species.

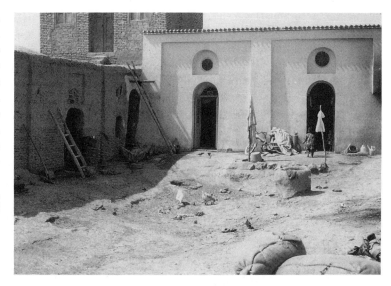

9.5   The interior of a family compound in a village in Iran. This photograph shows the close association of *Phlebotomus papatasi* with humans; large numbers of adult sand flies were present in the animal shelters on the left and in the human living quarters behind.

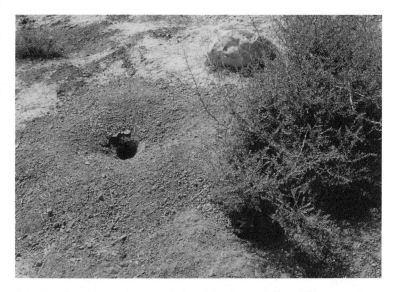

9.6   A rodent burrow in an uninhabited desert area of Israel. Numerous *P. papatasi* adults were recovered from this habitat during the day.

In addition to blood, sand flies also feed on sugars in their natural environment. A variety of sugars have been identified in the guts of sand flies caught in the wild; the most common is fructose (Moore et al. 1987). Sugars provide an energy source for the insects, but there is also evidence that sugars can be important for the development and subsequent transmission of *Leishmania* parasites. Sand flies apparently obtain their sugars in nature from plants and from aphid honeydew (Moore et al. 1987; Schlein and Warburg 1986). *P. papatasi* of both sexes ingest dried sugars on plant leaves and have also been observed to actually pierce the tissues of certain plants, presumably to obtain carbohydrates and/or liquids (Schlein and Warburg 1986).

Most of our knowledge about the biology of *P. papatasi* results from observations of laboratory colonies because the species is one of the easier sand fly species to colonize (Modi and Tesh 1984). The duration of the life cycle of this species largely depends on the ambient temperature and food supply. At 28°C and with adequate food, the period from oviposition until adult emergence ranges from 34–76 days; at 18°C it takes 116–165 days (Guzman and Tesh in press). The wide variation in developmental time among sand flies of the same generation and reared under similar conditions illustrates that *P. papatasi* is not synchronous in its development. This is the case with most sand fly species. Ambient temperature also affects the survival time of adults (Fig. 9.7) (Guzman and Tesh, in press).

HOST-PARASITE INTERACTIONS

Sand flies have small cutting mouthparts; they lacerate the skin and then feed from hemorrhages induced in surface capillaries. The bite usually produces a distinct stinging or burning sensation. While feeding on blood, the insects salivate into the skin of the vertebrate host. Sand fly saliva contains a number of substances whose pharmacologic effects include antihemostatic, vasodilatory, and antiinflammatory or immunosuppressive activity. Most species probably have apyrase in their saliva; this enzyme inhibits platelet agglutination and clotting (Ribeiro et al. 1989). Extracts of salivary glands from *L. longipalpis* contain maxadilan, a potent vasodilatory peptide (Lerner et al. 1991). Salivary glands of *L. longipalpis* and *P. papatasi* also contain

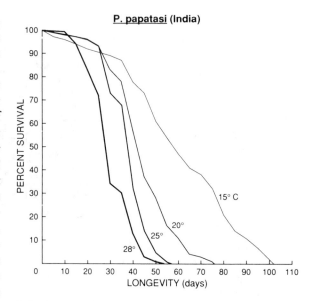

9.7 Survival of *P. papatasi* adults (both sexes) maintained on sucrose solution at four different temperatures (28, 25, 20, and 15°C)

another yet unidentified substance that inhibits macrophages and appears to enhance infection with some leishmanial parasites (Sammuelson et al. 1991; Theodos and Titus 1993). These or similar substances are likely present in other sand fly species as well; however, because *L. longipalpis* and *P. papatasi* are relatively easy to colonize (Modi and Tesh 1984), most pharmacologic studies to date have been done with these 2 species.

The sand fly alimentary tract is divided into 3 broad regions: the foregut, midgut, and hindgut (Fig. 9.8) (Walters et al. 1987)(Chap. 18). The foregut is lined with cuticular intima and consists of the proboscis (mouthparts), cibarium, pharynx, crop (which stores sugar solutions), esophagus, and stomodeal valve. The midgut is lined with epithelial microvilli and is subdivided into anterior (thoracic) and posterior (abdominal) regions. The cardia is considered to be the bulbous region of the anterior midgut, surrounding and just posterior to the stomodeal (or cardiac) valve. The pyloric valve constitutes the terminal end of the midgut and separates this region from the hindgut. The hindgut is also lined with cuticular intima and is subdivided into the anterior intestine (pylorus, ileum, and

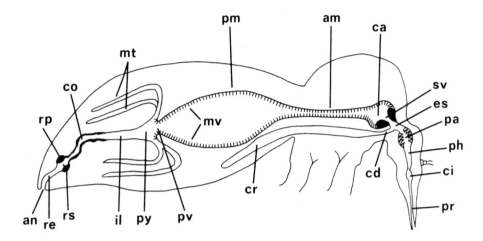

9.8 Schematic drawing of a sand fly in sagittal section, showing the morphology and anatomical divisions of the gut; proboscis (pr), cibarium (ci), anterior pharynx (ph), posterior armature region of pharynx (pa), esophagus (es), crop duct (cd), crop (cr), stomodeal valve (sv), cardia (ca), anterior midgut (am), posterior midgut (pm), microvilli (mv), pyloric valve (pv), Malpighian tubules (mt), pylorus (py), ileum (il), colon (co), rectal sac (rs), rectal papillae (rp), rectum proper (re), and anus (an). From Walters et al. 1987. Courtesy of *Amer. Soc. Trop. Med.*

colon) and posterior intestine (rectal papillae, rectal sac, rectum, and anus). The pyloric region of the hindgut is the expanded area of the anterior intestine just posterior to the pyloric valve; the Malpighian tubules enter into the pylorus. One of the reasons for the special interest in the various subdivisions of the sand fly alimentary tract is that 3 broad classifications of the genus *Leishmania* (Hypopylaria, Peripylaria, and Suprapylaria) have been proposed, based on where the parasites develop in the insect's gut (Lainson and Shaw 1987). The developmental site in the sand fly gut is also used to designate different morphologic forms of these protozoa during their life cycle in the vector (Walters 1993).

After ingestion, blood initially fills the entire midgut, where the peritrophic matrix is formed (Walters et al. 1993). The pattern and formation of the peritrophic matrix varies with sand fly species, but generally it is evident by 12 hr and is fully formed by 36 hr postfeeding. The peritrophic matrix is secreted by the midgut epithelium and appears as an electron-dense, fine-grained secretion containing fibers. It is composed of chitin, glycoprotein, and protein (see Chap.

19). As digestion occurs, the blood meal becomes confined to the posterior midgut. Breakdown of the peritrophic membrane begins at about 60 hr at 25°C, and the digested blood is excreted into the hindgut and eventually passes out the anus.

METHODS OF CONTROL

Because the breeding places of most sand fly species are unknown or not easily accessible, control strategies for these insects have focused mainly on the adult stage. Spraying residual insecticides on houses, animal shelters, and other nearby adult resting sites has been effective in controlling peridomestic sand fly species such as *P. papatasi* and *L. longipalpis* (Young and Arias 1991; Peril'ev 1968; WHO Expert Committee 1990.) Recently, however, insecticide resistance has been reported in *P. papatasi* and *P. argentipes* (Joshi et al. 1979).

Unlike control of periodomestic species, area control of sylvan species is virtually impossible. Attempts to control sand flies in tropical forests by aerial spraying or by ground application of insecticides to tree trunks and other vegetation have had little success (Young and

Arias 1991; WHO Expert Committee 1990; Grimaldi and Tesh 1993). Environmental modification such as clearing forests, eliminating rodent breeding sites, and relocating domestic animals away from human dwellings has been used successfully in some areas to reduce local sand fly populations (Young and Arias 1991; WHO Expert Committee 1990; Grimaldi and Tesh 1993). Personal protective measures such as the use of topical repellents containing diethylmetatoluamide (DEET), screening, and bed nets also effectively reduce sand fly bites.

DISEASE AGENTS VECTORED

Sand flies are vectors of the agents causing bartonellosis, leishmaniasis, and several arboviral illnesses. In addition, their bite also sensitizes some people, producing an urticarial skin reaction referred to by some authors as "harara" (Theodor 1935).

Bartonellosis (Carrion's disease, Oroya fever, verruga peruana) is caused by the bacterium *Bartonella bacilliformis* (Schultz 1968). The disease is currently restricted to the Peruvian Andes and focal areas of Ecuador. A single sand fly species, *L. verrucarum*, has generally been implicated as the vector. Little is known about the life cycle of *B. bacilliformis* outside of its human host.

Phlebotomus (sand fly) fever is an acute nonspecific febrile illness, characterized by severe headache, fever, myalgia, and prostration; it is caused by a number of different viruses belonging to the family Bunyaviridae, genus *Phlebovirus* (Tesh 1988). Most of these agents are transmitted by the sand fly. The disease is most common in the Middle East and Central Asia; *P. papatasi* is the major vector in this region. Many of the phleboviruses are transovarially (vertically) transmitted in their sand fly hosts and overwinter in diapausing larvae (Tesh 1988; Tesh et al. 1992).

Sand flies have also been implicated as vectors of several viruses in the vesicular stomatitis serogroup (family Rhabdoviridae; genus *Vesiculovirus*) (Comer and Tesh 1991). Some of the viruses in this group cause disease in domestic animals as well as in humans.

Sand flies are best known as the vectors of leishmaniasis. After malaria, leishmaniasis is probably the second most important protozoan disease. Leishmaniasis is actually a complex of diseases caused by a number of different parasite species that are capable of producing a wide variety of clinical manifestations (Grimaldi and Tesh 1993). All of the leishmaniases are transmitted by sand flies, and most are zoonoses. Each *Leishmania* species has a unique epidemiologic pattern with different vectors, reservoir hosts, and geographic distribution.

The life cycles of the various *Leishmania* species in their sand fly vectors have the following common features (Walters 1993). Amastigote forms of the parasite are ingested by the insect when it takes a blood meal from an infected vertebrate host. Within 24 hours, the amastigotes transform into promastigotes, which then undergo rapid multiplication within the blood meal. The ingested blood initially enters the anterior midgut of the insect (Fig. 9.8), where it becomes encased within the peritrophic matrix. After about 3 days, the peritrophic matrix disintegrates, and the promastigotes migrate to the hindgut (in the case of peripylarian parasites) or to the foregut and midgut (suprapylarian parasites), where further multiplication and differentiation occur. Some *Leishmania* spp. appear to secrete chitinase, which causes lysis of chitin in the peritrophic matrix and allows the parasites to escape earlier (Schlein et al. 1991). After about 7 days, the parasites move anteriorly to the esophagus-pharynx-stomadeal valve region of the alimentary tract, where they attach to the cuticular lining by flagellar hemidesmosomes (Figs. 9.9, 9.10) (Walters 1993; Walters et al. 1987). Attachment and release of the parasites seem to be controlled by stage-specific sugars on the lipophosphoglycan of the promastigote, which interact with the midgut epithelium of the insect (Pimenta et al. 1992). Transmission of the parasites to the next mammalian host occurs when the infected fly takes another blood meal. The available evidence suggests that transmission occurs by regurgitation of parasites from the midgut during blood-feeding (Schlein et al. 1992).

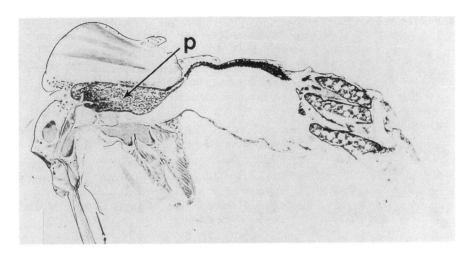

9.9   Parasagittal histological section of a sand fly infected with *Leishmania mexicana*. Note enlargement of the cardia/anterior midgut region, which is full of parasites (P). From Walters et al. 1987. Courtesy of *Amer. Soc. Trop. Med. Hyg.*

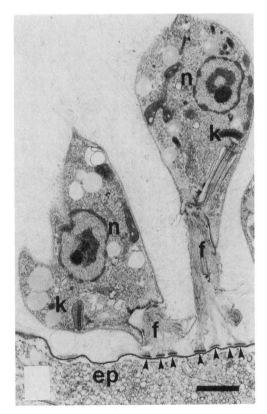

9.10   Promastigotes of *Leishmania panamensis* attached to the interior of the foregut (stomodeal valve) of an infected sand fly via flagellar hemidesmosomes. Symbols are (k) kinetoplast, (n) nucleus, (f) flagellum, and (ep) epithelium of the stomodeal valve. Bar = 1 μm. From Walters et al. 1989. Courtesy of *Amer. Soc. Trop. Med. Hyg.*

REFERENCES AND FURTHER READINGS

Abonnec, E. 1972. *Les Phlebotomes de la Region Ethiopienne (Diptera: Psychodidae). Mem. ORSTOM* No. 55. Paris: ORSTOM.

Comer, J.A., and R.B. Tesh. 1991. Phlebotomine sand flies as vectors of vesiculoviruses: a review. *Parassitologia.* Suppl. 33:143–150

Grimaldi, G. Jr., and R.B. Tesh. 1993. Leishmaniasis in the New World: Current concepts and implications for future research. *Clin. Microbiol. Rev.* 3:230–250.

Guzman, H., and R.B. Tesh. 1995. Effect of temperature and diet on the growth and longevity of phlebotomine sand flies (Diptera: Psychodidae). *J. Med. Entomol.* In press.

Herrer, A., and H.A. Christensen. 1975. Implication of *Phlebotomus* sand flies as vectors of *bartonellosis* and *leishmaniasis* as early as 1764. *Science* 190:154–155.

Javadian, E., R. Tesh, S. Saidi, and A. Nadim. 1977. Studies on the epidemiology of sand fly fever in Iran: part III. Host feeding patterns of *Phlebotomus papatasi* in an endemic area of disease. *Am. J. Trop. Med. Hyg.* 26:293–297.

Joshi, G.C., S.M. Kaul, and B.L. Wattal. 1979. Susceptibility of sand flies to organochlorine insecticides in Bihar (India): Further reports. *J. Commun. Dis.* 11:209–213.

Kreutzer, R.D., G.B. Modi, R.B. Tesh, and D.G. Young. 1987. Brain cell karotypes of six species of New and Old World sand flies (Diptera: Psychodidae). *J. Med. Entomol.* 24:609–612.

Lainson, R., and J.J. Shaw. 1987. Evolution, classification and geographical distribution. In: W. Peters and R. Killick-Kendrick, eds., *The Leishmaniases in Biology and Medicine*, Vol. 1. London: Academic Press. pp. 1–120.

Lanzaro, G.C., K. Ostrovska, M.V. Herrero, P.G. Lawyer, and A. Warburg. 1993. *Lutzomyia longipalpis* as a species complex: Genetic divergence and interspecific hybrid sterility among three populations. *Am. J. Trop. Med. Hyg.* 48:839–847.

Lerner, E.A., J.M.C. Ribeiro, R.J. Nelson, and M.R. Lerner. 1991. Isolation of maxadilan, a potent vasodilatory peptide from the salivary glands of the sand fly *Lutzomyia longipalpis. J. Biol. Chem.* 266:11234–11236.

Lewis, D.J. 1978. The phlebotominae sand flies (Diptera:Psychodidae) of the Oriental Region. *Bull. Br. Mus. Nat. Hist.* (Ent.). 37:217–343.

Lewis, D.J. 1982. A taxonomic review of the genus *Phlebotomus* (Diptera:Psychodidae). *Bull. Br. Mus. Nat. Hist.* (Ent.). 45:121–209.

Lewis, D.J., D.G. Young, G.B. Fairchild, and D.M. Minter. 1977. Proposals for a stable classification of the phlebotominae sand flies (Diptera: Psychodidae). *Syst. Ent.* 2:319–332.

Magnarelli, L.A., G.B. Modi, and R.B. Tesh 1984. Follicular development and parity in phlebotomine sand flies (Diptera: Psychodidae). *J. Med. Entomol.* 21:681–689.

Modi, G.B., and R.B. Tesh 1984. A simple technique for mass rearing *Lutzomyia longipalpis* and *Phlebotomus papatasi* (Diptera: Psychodidae) in the laboratory. *J. Med. Entomol.* 20:568–569.

Moore, J.S., T.B. Kelly, R. Killick-Kendrick, M. Killick-Kendrick, K.R. Wallbanks, and D.H. Molyneux. 1987. Honeydew sugars in wild-caught *Phlebotomus ariasi* detected by high performance liquid chromatography (HPLC) and gas chromatography (GC). *Med. Vet. Entomol.* 1:427–434.

Peril'ev, P.P. 1968. *Fauna of the U.S.S.R.: Diptera.* Vol. 3, No. 2, *Phlebotomidae (Sand flies).* Jerusalem: Israel Program for Scientific Translations.

Pimenta, P.F.P., S.J. Turco, M.J. McConville, P.G. Lawyer, P.V. Perkins, and D.L. Sacks. 1992. Stage specific adhesion of *Leishmania* promastigotes to the sand fly midgut. *Science* 256:1812–1815.

Ribeiro, J.M., G.B. Modi, and R.B. Tesh. 1989. Salivary apyrase activity of some Old World phlebotomine sand flies. *Insect Biochem.* 19:409–412.

Sammuelson, J., E. Lerner, R. Tesh, and R. Titus. 1991. A mouse model of *Leishmania braziliensis braziliensis* infection produced by coinjection with sand fly saliva. *J. Exp. Med.* 173:49–54.

Schlein, Y., R.L. Jacobson, and G. Messer. 1992. *Leishmania* infections damage the feeding mechanism of the sand fly vector and implement parasite transmission by bite. *Proc. Natl. Acad. Sci. USA* 89:9944–9948.

Schlein, Y., R.L. Jacobson, and J. Shlomai. 1991. Chitinase secreted by *Leishmania* functions in the sand fly vector. *Proc. R. Soc. Lond. B* 245:121–126.

Schlein, Y., and A. Warburg. 1986. Phytophagy and the feeding cycle of *Phlebotomus papatasi* under experimental conditions. *J. Med. Ent.* 23:11–15.

Schlein, Y., B. Yuval, and A. Warburg. 1984. Aggregation pheromone released from the palps of feeding female *Phlebotomus papatasi* (Psychodidae). *J. Insect Physiol.* 30:153–156.

Schmidt, J.R., and M.L. Schmidt. 1965. Observations on the feeding habits of *Phlebotomus papatasi* (Scopoli) under simulated natural conditions. *J. Med. Entomol.* 2:225–230.

Schultz, M.G. 1968. A history of bartonellosis (Carrion's disease). *Am. J. Trop. Med. Hyg.* 17:503–515.

Tesh, R.B. 1988. The genus *Phlebovirus* and its vectors. *Ann. Rev. Entomol.* 13:169–181.

Tesh, R.B., J. Lubroth, and H. Guzman. 1992. Simulation of arbovirus overwintering: Survival of Toscana virus (Bunyaviridae: Phlebovirus) in its natural sand fly vector *Phlebotomus perniciosus*. *Am. J. Trop. Med. Hyg.* 47:574–581.

Theodor, O. 1935. A study of the reaction to phlebotomus bites with some remarks on "harara." *Trans. Roy. Soc. Trop. Med. Hyg.* 19:273–284.

Theodor, O. 1936. On the relation of *Phlebotomus papatasi* to the temperature and humidity of the environment. *Bull. Ent. Res.* 27:653–671.

Theodos, C.M., and R.G. Titus. 1993. Salivary gland material from the sand fly *Lutzomyia longipalpis* has an inhibitory effect on macrophage function *in vitro*. *Parasite Immunol.* 15:481–487.

Walters, L.L. 1993. *Leishmania* differentiation in natural and unnatural sand fly hosts. *J. Euk. Microbiol.* 40:196–206.

Walters, L.L., G.L. Chaplin, G.B. Modi, and R.B. Tesh. 1989. Ultrastructural biology of *Leishmania* (*Viannia*) *panamensis* (= *Leishmania braziliensis panamensis*) in *Lutzomyia gomezi* (Diptera: Psychodidae): A natural host-parasite combination. *Am. J. Trop. Med. Hyg.* 40:19–39.

Walters, L.L., K.P. Irons, H. Guzman, and R.B. Tesh. 1993. Formation and composition of the peritrophic membrane in the sand fly, *Phlebotomus perniciosus* (Diptera: Psychodidae). *J. Med. Entomol.* 30:179–198.

Walters, L.L., G.B. Modi, R.B. Tesh, and T. Burrage. 1987. Host-parasite relationship of *Leishmania mexicana mexicana* and *Lutzomyia abonneci* (Diptera:Psychodidae). *Am. J. Trop. Med. Hyg.* 36:294–314.

Ward, R.D. 1976. The immature stages of some Phlebotomine sand flies from Brazil (Diptera: Psychodidae). *Syst. Ent.* 1:227–240.

Ward, R.D., A. Phillips, B. Burnet, and C.B. Marcondes. 1988. The *Lutzomyia longipalpis* complex: Reproduction and distribution. In: M.W. Service, editor, *Biosystematics of haematophagous insects*, Systematics Assoc. Spec. Vol. No. 37. Oxford: Clarendon Press. pp. 257–269.

Whittingham, H.E. and A.F. Rock 1923. The life history and bionomics of *Phlebotomus papatasi*. *Brit. Med. J.* 15 Dec.:1144–1154.

World Health Organization Expert Committee. 1990. *Control of the Leishmaniases.* Tech. Rep. Ser. 73. Geneva: World Health Organization.

Young, D.G., and J.R. Arias. 1991. Phlebotominae sand flies in the Americas. Tech. Paper No. 33. Washington: Pan American Health Organization.

Young, D.G., and M.A. Duncan. 1984. Guide to the identification and geographic distribution of *Lutzomyia* sand flies in Mexico, the West Indies, Central and South America (Diptera: Psychodidae). *Mem. Am. Entomol. Inst.*, No. 54. Gainesville: Associated Publishers.

10. HEMIMETABOLIC VECTORS AND SOME CYCLORRAPHAN FLIES AND THE AGENTS THEY TRANSMIT

William C. Marquardt

INTRODUCTION TO HEMIMETABOLIC VECTORS

Hemimetabolic insects undergo incomplete metamorphosis; thus, the preadult stages are morphologically similar to the adults. This gradual change in body form and the fact that all stages have the same kinds of mouthparts have certain implications for these insects in their roles as vectors of disease agents. All life stages have the same food habits, and they inhabit the same ecological niches. Thus, an immature hemimetabolic insect has the same potential for transmitting a disease agent as does the adult. Holometabolic insects such as mosquitoes, in contrast, occupy distinctly different ecological niches as larvae and adults. Likewise, their foods are different because their mouthparts are different (Chaps. 5 and 6).

Among the orders of insects included in the Hemimetabola are the dragonflies and damselflies (Odonata), grasshoppers and crickets (Orthoptera), mayflies (Ephemeroptera), stone flies (Plecoptera), earwigs (Dermaptera), termites (Isoptera), cockroaches (Blattaria), the 2 orders of lice (Mallophaga and Anoplura), the thrips (Thysanoptera), the so-called true bugs (Hemiptera), and the aphids and leafhoppers (Homoptera). Of these, the Odonata, Orthoptera, Ephemeroptera, Plecoptera, and Blattaria serve as intermediate hosts of a number of helminthic parasites such as digenetic trematodes.

Of the remaining orders, the lice homopterans some hemipterans, and thrips transmit plant and animal disease agents. A number of homopterans and thrips also are biological vectors for viruses of disease agents of plants. They also damage plants directly by feeding on their tissues and juices. In the context of this book, the lice and bugs are of principal interest.

THE BUGS: ORDER HEMIPTERA

The ordinal name Hemiptera means "half wing." These insects have 2 pairs of wings; the forewings have leathery basal portions and membranous distal portions (Fig. 10.1), and the second pair of wings is membranous. Both pairs of wings are held over the abdomen at rest. Hemipterans have piercing-sucking mouthparts well adapted for feeding on plants, small arthropods, and blood. There is usually a distinct pronotum and a pronounced scutellum between the bases of the forewings. The eyes are generally well developed. Antennae are straight with 4 or 5 segments. The sizes of adults range from a few mm to more than 2 cm in length.

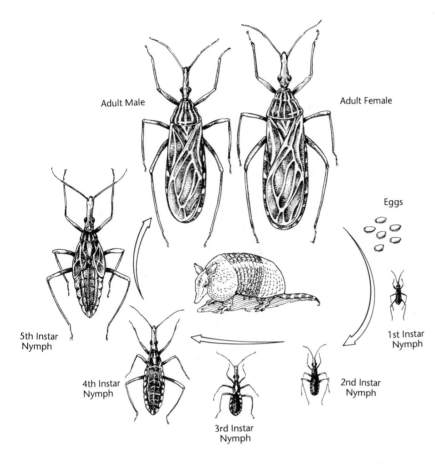

Labels on figure:
Adult Male
Adult Female
Eggs
5th Instar Nymph
4th Instar Nymph
3rd Instar Nymph
2nd Instar Nymph
1st Instar Nymph

10.1   Life cycle of *Rhodnius prolixus* (W.C. Marquardt. Used with permission.)

The members of the Hemiptera comprise 1 of the largest orders of insects, and the group is the largest among the Hemimetabola. More than 23,000 species have been described worldwide, and more than 4500 have been described in the United States. Classification is complex (Henry and Froeschner 1988; Barrett 1991).

Most hemipterans are predaceous or feed on plant juices. Most of them will bite humans if they are handled, and their bites can be painful. Two families are of importance in medical entomology: the Cimicidae (bed bugs) and the Reduviidae (assassin bugs, kissing bugs). Reduviids are both predaceous and hematophagous; members of the subfamily Triatominae feed on blood and serve as vectors of disease agents. A number of species of triatomines serve as vectors of *Trypanosoma cruzi*,

the cause of Chagas' disease (American trypanosomiasis) in the Western Hemisphere. Common names for triatomines are kissing bugs, benchuca, vinchuca, cone-nosed bugs, giant bed bugs, and chinche de monte.

KISSING BUGS
Morphology
Members of the subfamily Triatominae are generally large insects; adults range from about 5–30 mm. Newly hatched first instar nymphs are usually 2–3 mm in length. The head is long and narrow with prominent eyes, and the filiform antennae insert anterior to the eyes. The beak, which contains the mouthparts, has 3 segments and is held back under the head. The thorax typically has a constriction at about its middle, and the abdomen is concave, often with patterning on its margin. The wings fold over one another and fit down into this concavity. The long legs are well adapted for running, and there are 3 tarsi (Fig. 10.1).

Life Cycle
Rhodnius prolixus is an important vector of *Trypanosoma cruzi* in South America and is an example of development in the group. The operculated eggs are 2.5 mm long and, although white when laid, turn bright red within a few hours. Development of the eggs is relatively long, requiring about a month at 22°C and 12 days at 32°C. The first instar nymph is about the size of the egg, or 2.7 mm. Each of the 5 nymphal instars feeds and molts, increasing approximately 1.5 times its original size at each molt. The life cycle in the laboratory requires about 80 days from

egg to adult. Other species vary in the length of the life cycle. For example, *Triatoma infestans* requires about 180 days to develop from the egg to the adult.

Bionomics

Kissing bugs lay their eggs in rodent burrows, or if domiciliated, in cracks and crevices in the house or in areas such as a thatched roof. Those that live in trees oviposit in bird nests, the crowns of palm trees, and epiphytes, for example. The rate of development of the eggs varies with temperature, and they do well over a range of 16–34°C. They are resistant to desiccation; 50% hatch at a humidity as low as 20%.

Triatomines are distributed in the Western Hemisphere. They are found in warm temperate climates in the United States (40° north latitude) as well as throughout much of South America (45° south latitude) (Fig. 10.2). The 5 taxonomic tribes currently recognized are based on both morphology and habitat. Habitat ranges from warm-temperate to tropical climates and from desert habitat to tropical rain forest.

In the wild, bugs associate with burrowing animals such as rodents, or they can be found in epiphytes in rain forest, where they feed on both birds and reptiles. Many species become domiciliated by moving from habitats in the wild to human dwellings because food is plentiful and readily available. Such species usually hide during the day in the walls or roof. The poorer the quality of the housing, the more bugs are likely to be found in it. In studies done in South America, as many as 8500 bugs have been found in a single poorly maintained adobe house.

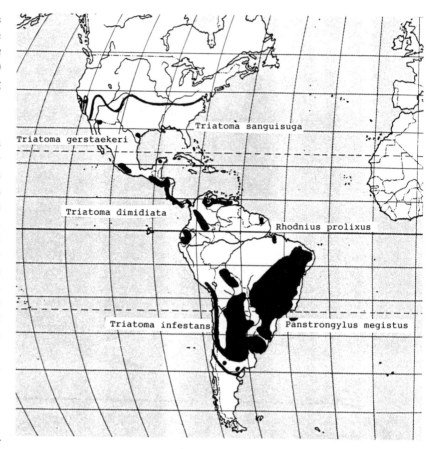

10.2 Distribution of Chagas' disease and some of the major vectors (W.C. Marquardt. Used with permission.)

Adults lay eggs in relatively small batches over a period of several months. *Rhodnius prolixus* lays up to 14 eggs per batch and can lay 30–50 batches. Thus, 1 female can lay 300 eggs in a lifetime. After laying a batch of eggs, the female usually feeds again on blood. At some point the female lays a final batch of eggs and dies. The life span is about 6 months, unusually long for an adult insect.

The term "kissing bug" comes from the predilection of the bugs for feeding on areas of the face where the skin is thin: near the lips and around the eyes. Except for a few species, triatomines feed at night. They congregate in bedrooms in houses and come out of the walls and ceilings while people are sleeping. They are attracted to their hosts by warmth and carbon dioxide; odor also seems to play a role in the attraction. They do not usually cause pain when they feed, and it is assumed that they produce an anesthetic with the saliva that is injected into the wound.

Kissing bugs are capillary feeders. The mandibles are short (Fig. 1.9) and lock into the surface of the skin. The maxillae then are inserted into the skin and probe until a capillary is found. Feeding times range from 3–30 minutes. The volume of blood taken by 1 of the smaller nymphal instars is relatively small, but an adult *R. prolixus* may take nearly 0.25 ml of blood at 1 feeding. Over the life of a kissing bug, it may take from 4–10 ml of vertebrate blood.

Host-Parasite Interactions

Because only adults have wings the nymphs must walk to their source of food. Thus, although many species are good fliers as adults, they seem to prefer to walk to their potential hosts.

Most triatomines that associate with humans are nocturnal, remaining hidden in the house during the day and seeking food at night. The bites, although seldom painful, can cause certain individuals to become hypersensitive and develop red, swollen areas at the sites.

Nearly all kissing bugs have a broad host range. They feed readily on reptiles, birds, and mammals. Thatched roofs are homes to various kinds of animals, and triatomines live there as well, feeding on small lizards and any other vertebrates.

Control

The most effective control for triatomines revolves around source reduction, for example, eliminating places in the house where the bugs can hide during the daytime. Plastering interior walls to cover cracks and using concrete instead of beaten earth for the floor are both effective 1st steps. Replacing thatch with sheet metal is also recommended. Screening doors and windows is effective but prohibitive in tropical climates because it restricts cool air movement at night.

Personal protection, such as a bed net, is advisable. Such nets should have solid, not mesh, tops so that feces from infected bugs do not fall on the sleeper.

Beds or hammocks should also be inaccessible to the bugs to prevent their crawling up to the occupant.

Bugs are peridomestic and feed on domestic animals and companion animals such as dogs and cats. Removing resting sites near these animals is recommended. Habitat near the house that maintains small wild animals should be eliminated. A buffer zone should also be established between the reservoir in the wild and houses.

Residual insecticides have been found to be effective against triatomines. DDT and dieldrin work well, but their use is now prohibited in some countries and discouraged in others. Silicone dusts have been found to effectively control triatomines in the crawl spaces of houses in southern California.

New methods of control are necessary because prevention and control of Chagas' disease requires eliminating contact between humans and triatomines. For example, symbiotic bacteria in the intestinal cells of triatomines provide essential nutrients. Research is under way to develop methods for eliminating the symbiotic bacteria. Blood is rich in protein but is not the perfect food (see Chaps. 2 and 22). Therefore, energy sources from carbohydrates must be obtained from other sources, and certain vitamins must also be synthesized. Intestinal symbionts provide some of these essential nutrients in hematophagous insects. Eliminating the bacteria could kill triatomines.

Disease Agents Vectored

Kissing bugs are the vectors of *Trypanosoma cruzi*, a protozoan that causes Chagas' disease, or American trypanosomiasis. About 24 million people are affected at any one time in Central and South America and perhaps an additional 65 million people are at risk of infection with *T. cruzi* (Fig. 10.2). Although the organisms and occasional cases of Chagas' disease are found in the United States, the disease is not considered to be a major threat to public health. Chagas' disease is a zoonosis with reservoirs of infection in both wild and domestic animals. Reservoirs include rodents such as pack rats, armadillos, dogs, cats, and large domestic animals. Birds and reptiles do not seem to be a part of the epidemiological picture.

Brazilian physician Carlos Chagas discovered the causative agent of the disease in 1909 in the triatomine *Triatoma megista*. He associated the organism with the disease complex that ultimately came to bear his name. However, it was not until the early 1930s that the medical community accepted his findings and agreed that there was indeed a serious problem.

Chagas' disease is a disseminated infection that takes either an acute or chronic course and often results in death. A kissing bug becomes infected when it feeds upon an infected animal or person (Fig. 10.3). Development of the protozoan takes place in the intestine of the bug over a period of 1–2 weeks. When the bug returns to another host for an additional blood meal, it can transmit the agent.

It is important to note that *T. cruzi* is transmitted through the feces of the bug; the bite of the bug does not inoculate the potential host. When a bug feeds, it takes a large amount of blood in a few minutes. Often a drop of feces, teeming with protozoa, is squeezed out of the rectum of the bug. The organisms do not penetrate intact skin but enter the intact mucous membranes of the eye or mouth and small abrasions of the skin.

The so-called good vectors are those that defecate while feeding. Many bugs, such as *Triatoma sanguisuga*, readily feed on humans but are poor vectors because they do not defecate at that time. A good vector's intestine must allow the trypanosomes to multiply so that the rectum becomes full of organisms. The organisms can then be deposited on the skin of the potential host.

The organisms multiply for a few weeks in the region of the skin in which they have penetrated. They cause swelling and inflammation of the tissues at this

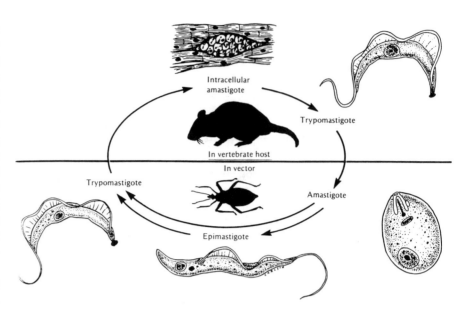

10.3 Life cycle of *Trypanosoma cruzi* (W.C. Marquardt and Demaree, *Parasitology*, Macmillan Co., New York, 1985. Used with permission.)

location (Fig. 10.4), a lesion referred to as Romaña's sign. The organisms then spread to other tissues in the body. Children often do not survive the acute infection, dying within months. If an individual survives the initial, acute infection, the chronic phase then ensues. Damage to the host takes place over many years, and the heart and/or intestinal tract are most often affected.

No effective treatment exists for Chagas' disease. Although 2 drugs are used, unless they are administered early they have little effect. Some individuals develop natural immunity during infection, but it is insufficient to eliminate the infection; it seems only to slow down the course of the disease. Artificial immunity, or vaccination, is not yet available. Control of Chagas' disease therefore depends on controlling vectors and preventing infection through personal protection.

Other protozoa also infect humans; thus, the diagnosis of Chagas' disease is not always straightforward. *Trypanosoma rangeli* and *T. minasense* are also found in humans and are transmitted by kissing bugs. Note that the organisms causing leishmaniasis (Chap. 9) are found in many of the same areas as *T. cruzi*.

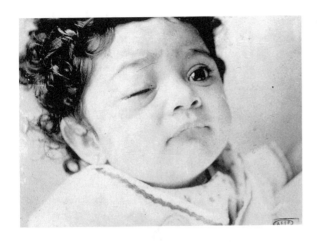

10.4 Romaña's sign in a child. Note the swelling around the eye where a triatomine had fed and *Trypanosoma cruzi* entered the tissue. (Armed Forces Insitute of Pathology Neg. No. 62-3934-6)

THE BED BUGS

Members of this family are associated mainly with birds and remain in their nests transeasonally. Some are associated with mammals, and 2 species live with humans in their dwellings. *Cimex lectularius* is the so-called human bed bug and *C. hemipterus* is the tropical Bed bug; there are 7 species associated with humans in various parts of the world, but these 2 are the most common. Some other genera found on birds are *Leptocimex, Haematosiphon, Oeciacus,* and *Ornithocoris.*

Morphology

Bed Bugs are brownish, dorsoventrally flattened insects that lack functional wings as adults. The adults have wing pads, but the earlier instars do not. The body is covered with many small hairs, or setae. The 3-segmented beak is held back under the head. The human Bed bug, *C. lectularius,* is about 3 mm wide and 5 mm long as an adult and is typical of many members of the group (Fig. 10.5).

Life Cycle

Bed Bugs copulate upon reaching adulthood. It is interesting to note that the male inserts the copulatory apparatus through the exoskeleton of the female and deposits the sperm into her hemocoel. The female

deposits its yellowish eggs, which hatch in about 10 days, in hiding places in a house. There are 3 nymphal instars; each takes up to 3 blood meals between molts. Development is fairly slow and requires from 37–128 days from egg to adult.

Bed Bugs are intermittent feeders and do not reside on the host most of the time. Those that associate with humans find resting sites in beds, behind torn wallpaper, or behind loose baseboards. They remain in these sites until a proper victim appears. Although Bed bugs are not usually seen, they emit a characteristic aroma that can be detected when they are present in large numbers in a house or hotel room. They do not usually cause any pain when feeding, and most people do not know Bed bugs are present until morning. A line of 2–3 reddened wheals on the skin is usually the 1st evidence of Bed bugs in a house.

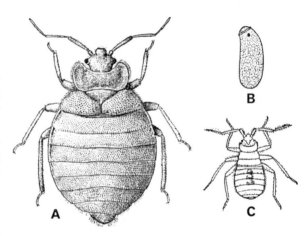

10.5 *Cimex lectularius* adult (K.G.V. Smith 1973. Used with permission.)

Control

When Bed bugs are detected in a home, control involves laundering all clothing and bedding that might have eggs or bugs in it, eliminating hiding places around the room or house, and treating the house and furniture with insecticides. To eliminate the bugs, all 3 steps must be undertaken.

Disease Agents Transmitted

Bed Bugs have all of the characteristics of a good vector. They suck blood, have host preferences but feed on a variety of species, live a long time, and are patient. Oddly enough, they do not serve as vectors of any infectious agents of humans. Laboratory studies have generally shown that a variety of agents survive for a short period in the gut of a Bed bug, but the agents do not replicate and are not transmitted. In hosts other than humans, swallow bugs have been found to harbor Fort Morgan virus and probably transmit it among birds.

THE LICE

There are 2 orders of lice that are closely related, the Mallophaga, the biting or bird lice (Fig. 10.6A), and the Anoplura (Fig. 10.6B), the sucking lice. The life cycles of both are much the same, and their morphologies, except for mouthparts, are also much the same. Both are relatively small insects that lack wings, are dorsoventrally flattened, and have many hairs, or setae, on the body. The life cycles in both consist of egg, 3 nymphal stages, and adults with separate sexes. The mandibles of the Mallophaga are stout, heavily sclerotized structures that are laterally opposed (Fig. 10.7). The mandibles scrape the skin or feathers of the host,

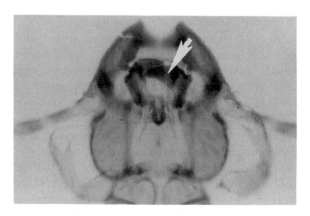

10.7   Mandibles of a mallophagan from a cat. Note the heavily sclerotized mandibles that overlap to facilitate cutting the skin of the host. (W.C. Marquardt. Used with permission.)

or they actually cut the skin and allow blood to come to the surface. The mandibles of the sucking lice are slender structures that are adapted for piercing the skin of the host and taking blood.

Lice are of considerable economic importance as parasites of domestic animals. Five species of biting lice cause weight loss and a fall in egg production in chickens. Large domestic animals such as sheep, cattle, and swine all have lice, which cause reductions in weight gains and reduced production of milk and fiber. Each species of host has its own lice; indeed, each louse has a preferred site on the body of the host.

The Anoplura of humans and the Mallophaga are known to transmit only a few infectious agents, and neither are economically or medically important. Three lice are found on humans: *Pediculus humanus*, the body louse; *P. capitis*, the head louse (Fig. 10.8A); and *Pthirus pubis*, the crab louse (Fig. 10.8B). Of these, the body louse is most important because it is the vector of louse-borne typhus, a scourge of human health all through history (Zinsser 1935). The head louse is not a vector of any disease agents of humans. The crab louse, sometimes called "papillion d'amour," is generally thought of as being transmitted from one person to another during sexual intercourse. That is true, in a sense, but it is really only close bodily contact that allows this louse to transfer between people.

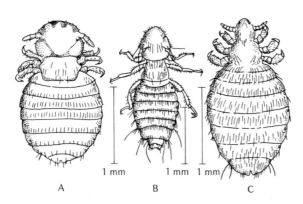

10.6   Representatives of the 2 orders of lice, from a dog. Mallophagans, *Trichodectes canis* (A), *Heterodoxus longitarsus* (B), and an anopluran, *Linognathus setosus* (C). (W.C. Marquardt and Demaree, *Parasitology,* Macmillan Co., New York, 1985. Used with permission.)

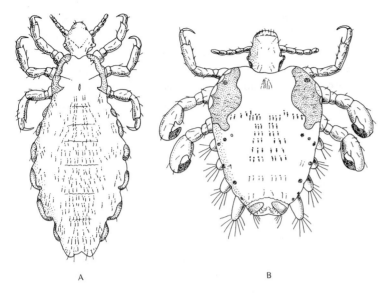

10.8 Lice from humans. A is both *Pediculus humanus*, the body louse, and *Pediculus capitis*, the head louse. B is the crab louse, *Pthirus pubis*.

Morphology and Life Cycle

The body louse and the head louse are identical morphologically, but they are separate breeding populations and therefore should be considered as separate species (Busvine 1978). However, many investigators consider them to be a subspecies (Chap. 26). Adult female lice are 3–4 mm long; the adult male is slightly smaller. They are dorsoventrally flattened and have large numbers of hairs, or setae, directed toward the rear of the body. The head is narrow, and the mandibles exit at the anterior tip of the head.

Eggs of body lice are typically laid in seams of the clothing. A female body louse lays from 275–300 eggs in a lifetime; the eggs hatch in 1–3 weeks. The 3 nymphal instars increase in size at each molt. It has been estimated that populations of body lice can increase 4000–5000 times their weight in 3 months.

Bionomics

Lice do not live long off the host. Unfed lice can live about 10 days, but the nits, or eggs, are quite resistant. Body lice oviposit in the clothing whereas head lice generally attach their eggs to the hairs of the head. Body lice also tend to move into the clothing for a period of time and then return to the skin to feed.

Control

Insecticides are used to control lice. For both biting and sucking lice on domestic and companion animals and on humans, control has been achieved with 2nd generation insecticides applied to the body of the host. Hosts may be dusted, as in the case of chickens; dipped in a liquid insecticide, as in the case of sheep and cattle; or hand-dressed, as in the case of horses. The basic aim is the same in all cases: to get the insecticide in contact with the lice. Humans that have been infested with body lice are dusted with an organochlorine insecticide; when head lice are present, a shampoo with an insecticide is used.

Body lice on humans are rare when personal cleanliness is practiced. Frequent washing of clothing and frequent bathing keep populations low. When personal hygiene is not maintained, populations of lice increase.

Head lice represent a somewhat different situation because they can be found in circumstances in which cleanliness is evident. Outbreaks of head lice are often seen in schoolchildren, and the lice can spread quite rapidly. Public health measures to ensure the whole population is examined and when necessary treated usually eradicates the infestations.

Host-Parasite Interactions

Lice remain on the host at all times. They are transferred from one host to another by close body contact or by sharing clothing. Populations of lice increase under crowded, unsanitary conditions. This happens when artificial or natural disasters disrupt personal hygiene.

Both head, body, and crab lice feed frequently and cause irritation and blood loss. Because they take so much blood, they continually pump partially digested blood out of the anus that soils the clothing of the host. Changes in the skin of persons who harbor large populations of lice have been reported, but they do not have a sound foundation (Scholdt et al. 1979).

Disease Agents Vectored

The principal disease agents transmitted by body lice are *Rickettsia prowazeki,* the cause of louse-borne or epidemic typhus; *Rochalimaea quintana,* the cause of trench fever; and *Borrelia recurrentis,* the cause of relapsing fever. Of these, louse-borne typhus is the most important.

Typhus follows natural and artificial disasters. Typhus is a risk to the human population whenever there is war, flood, famine, or poverty. The organism lies in wait somewhere in the population and breaks out when people are crowded, displaced from their homes, and suffering poor nutrition.

Much of the mystery about typhus focuses on where the organism goes between outbreaks. So far as is known, humans are the only hosts for the *Rickettsia.* This fact alone is unusual because nearly all important human diseases are zoonotic, at least in part. But this disease agent lives only in humans and essentially disappears between epidemics.

Outbreaks occur when crowding and the inability of people to maintain normal cleanliness allow the populations of lice to increase rapidly. Stress and poor nutrition probably contribute to lower levels of immunity as well. The disease affects a few individuals and then spreads rapidly through the community.

Body lice become infected by feeding on a rickettsemic individual, and the organisms then multiply rapidly in the cells of the louse intestines. The infected cells rupture, releasing large numbers of organisms into the lumen of the gut—the gut contents and the feces are especially infectious. The organisms enter the body through a break in the skin or through the unbroken mucous membranes of the eye, nose, or mouth. Organisms remain alive for as long as 60 days in the feces of lice, so an area can remain contaminated for an extended period.

When a person is infected, a generalized or systemic infection results, and the organisms multiply in the endothelial cells of the smaller blood vessels. The incubation period ranges from 5–15 days, and the onset is characterized by fever, chills, general pain, and prostration. At about 5 days after the onset of the disease, a skin rash appears as a result of the breakdown of smaller blood vessels. Recovery begins about 2 weeks after the onset, but mortality ranges from 5–25%. Broad spectrum antibiotics and supportive, nonspecific measures effectively control typhus.

Prevention of typhus is based on louse control and vaccination. A good vaccine is available that prevents the development of disease in most instances. In those individuals in which the vaccine is less effective, the disease that results is generally mild and of short duration.

Typhus has been documented in nearly every war in history. In World War I typhus caused 3 million deaths in Europe; in World War II, there were 100,000 deaths in North Africa. When Allied forces reached Italy in 1944, an outbreak was just beginning that was aborted by the massive use of DDT powder, particularly in the civilian population. Clothing was dusted with guns that were inserted into sleeves and neck openings of clothing. This was an early triumph in the saga of using DDT as a means of controlling insect vectors of disease.

A number of diseases caused by Rickettsiae that have about the same clinical course are transmitted by various arthropods. Among them are scrub typhus, transmitted by chiggers in the Pacific rim area; murine typhus, transmitted by rodent fleas; and Rocky Mountain spotted fever, transmitted by ticks in both the Rocky Mountain region and the eastern states of the United States.

INTRODUCTION TO CYCLORRAPHAN FLIES

General Morphology

The cyclorraphan flies (order Diptera, suborder Cyclorrapha) are those dipterans that are usually considered to be flies. They are heavy bodied, fly well, have large eyes, and several species of them are domiciliated or associated with livestock.

One of the distinguishing characters of the adults is the short, inconspicuous antennae. These antennae consist of 2 segments: the 1st is smaller than the 2nd, which is usually oval and held close to the head. An arista, a plumose fiber that arises on the 2nd antennal segment, is also characteristic of the group.

Life Cycle

Members of the suborder have life cycles that are quite similar to one another. The blue bottle fly, *Calliphora vicina,* is a good general example (Fig. 10.9). Females oviposit in areas in which the larvae are likely to have the proper food. The 1st instar larva hatches from the egg usually after a period of development outside the body of the mother. The larva grows and molts twice to give rise to the 3rd instar larva. At the end of its development, it forms a pupa using the skin of the larva as its protective covering. When pupal development is complete, the larva forces off the operculum, a circular lid (thus the term *Cyclorrapha*), of the pupal case by inflating a structure located between the eyes called the ptilinum. The adult emerges from the pupal case, inflates the wings, dries off, and is ready to fly in a matter of minutes.

Cyclorraphan larvae are maggots; they are stout, often with short, stiff bristles on the body. The head is reduced to a cephalopharyngeal skeleton of which only a pair of small mouthhooks protrude from the anterior end of the organism. These mouthhooks move vertically, in contrast to those of the other suborders in which the mouthparts move laterally. The cephalopharyngeal skeleton is often used in identification of larvae to the species level. The pair of spiracles located at the posterior end of the maggot are also important to identification.

When feeding, larvae use mouthhooks to abrade the surface of whatever they feed on and then consume the liquid or particulate food by mouth. The larvae grow rapidly. For example, the house fly, *Musca domestica,* has an egg that is barely visible to the naked eye, perhaps 0.5 mm long; however, by the 3rd instar it is about 5 mm long. The 3rd instar larvae of cattle grubs, *Hypoderma* spp., measure 20 mm or more. Although larvae may live in a milieu replete with bacteria, they require air, and the posterior spiracles often are visible at the surface, where they obtain oxygen. This is often the case in the parasitic larvae such as cattle grubs or *Dermatobia hominis* of humans in which the posterior spiracles can be seen at a hole in the skin made by the larva.

Most adult cyclorraphans are strong fliers and often buzz quite loudly. Even the relatively small house fly can be heard flying at a distance of a meter. Most adult flies (e.g., the house fly, *Musca domestica,* and the face fly of cattle, *Musca autumnalis*) feed on liquids and have mouthparts adapted for mopping or sponging. Flies that feed on blood (e.g., horn flies) have piercing mouthparts. Others, such as the stable fly, *Stomoxys calcitrans,* and tsetse, have both piercing and mopping mouthparts.

Flies are important to humans from a number of standpoints. Many flies, such as the house fly, are nuisances; *M. vetustissima* of Australia is legendary because of its persistence and its long migration from the northern states. Others, such as the eye gnats, family Chloropidae, are serious pests simply because large numbers often cluster around the heads or open sores of humans or livestock. Because they feed in areas that are rich in bacteria and other potential pathogens, flies can also transfer infectious agents mechanically on their mouthparts, bodies, legs, or in the feces.

A number of families of flies (e.g., Calliphoridae, Sarcophagidae, and Cuterebridae, among others) are composed of flies that have either facultative or obligate parasitic larval forms. The condition in which larvae of flies exist as parasites in the body of a vertebrate is called myiasis. A number of these flies are important in human health, but most are economically important in livestock. The larvae feed on the carcasses of dead animals or may invade the living tissue (as does the screwworm, *Cochliomyia hominivorax*). Some, such as cattle grubs, *Hypoderma* spp., have an annual life cycle in which the larva migrates in the body of the host for about 8 months before emerging from the skin of the back and dropping to the ground to pupate.

Cyclorraphans that feed on blood and tissue fluids as adults cause both economic losses and medical problems through irritation of the skin, blood loss, and transmission of disease agents. Horn flies, *Haematobia irritans,* for example, are reported to cause more than $160 million annual loss to the cattle industry in the United States.

Relatively few cyclorraphans serve as biological vectors of disease agents. Several members of the family Hippoboscidae, the louse flies, are vectors of the apicomplexan protozoa *Haemoproteus* spp., red blood cell parasites of birds. The family Glossinidae contains

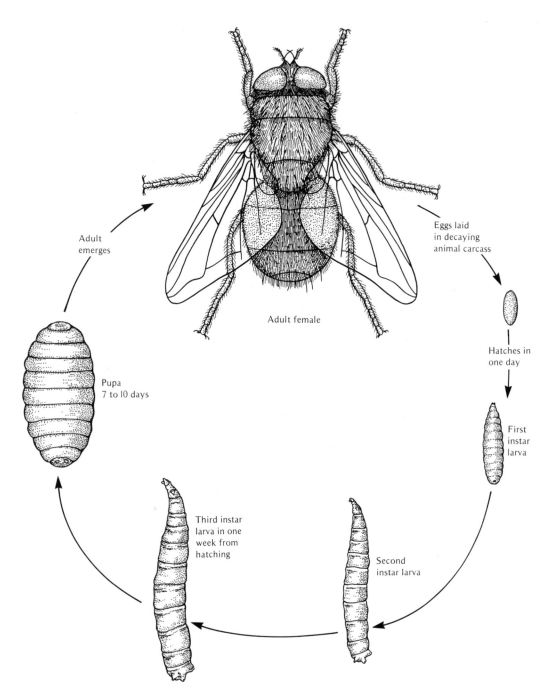

Adult emerges

Adult female

Eggs laid in decaying animal carcass

Hatches in one day

First instar larva

Pupa 7 to 10 days

Second instar larva

Third instar larva in one week from hatching

10.9 Life cycle of *Calliphora vicina*, the blue bottle fly. This fly shows a typical cyclorraphan life cycle with 3 larval stages as well as pupa and adult stages. (W.C. Marquardt and Demaree, *Parasitology*, Macmillan Co., New York, 1985. Used with permission.)

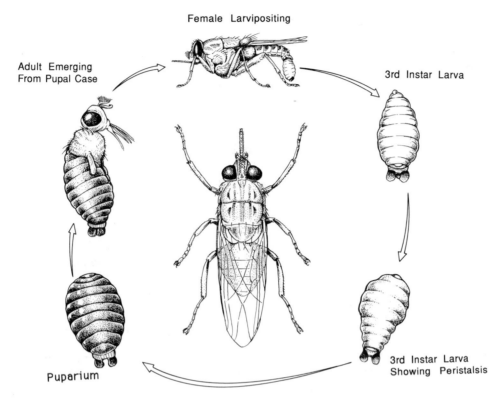

Female Larvipositing

Adult Emerging
From Pupal Case

3rd Instar Larva

Puparium

3rd Instar Larva
Showing Peristalsis

10.10 Life cycle and morphology of a tsetse, *Glossina*. The adult tsetse at rest holds its wings folded over the back, and the mouthparts extended forward. The three larval stages are retained within the body of the female until the 3rd larval instar is fully grown; it is then deposited in a protected area where the larva can burrow into the soil by peristaltic movement. The puparium turns black and remains in the soil until the adult emerges. The fly expands the ptilinum on the head in order to remove the operculum of the pupal case. (W.C. Marquardt. Used with permission.)

a single genus, *Glossina* (tsetse), which are vectors of several species in the kinetoplastid protozoan genus *Trypanosoma*.

GLOSSINIDAE (SUPERFAMILY MUSCOIDEA)

Glossina are distributed only in Africa south of the Sahara Desert to about 25°S latitude. One species, *G. tachinoides,* was found in the Arabian peninsula in the early 1900s, but it is not known whether it is still there. Tsetse once had a wider distribution than the present—fossils have been found in central Colorado, USA.

Morphology
The tsetse (*tsetse fly* is redundant) are all members of the genus *Glossina*. The adults are relatively large flies, 7–14 mm long, with prominent eyes and wings that overlap one another at rest (Fig. 10.10). A diagnostic character of the tsetse is the so-called hatchet cell in the center of the wing (1st M) (Fig 10.11).

Life Cycle
Adult females mate only a single time, and the female averages only about 9 offspring. The tsetse is probably the most highly selected "K" strategist among insects known (Chaps. 2 and 24). Unlike most flies that lay

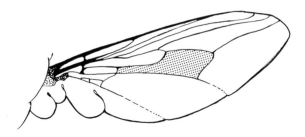

10.11 Wing of a tsetse. The wing is similar to other members of the higher diptera except for the hatchet cell, which is shown shaded and is characteristic of the family. (W.C. Marquardt. Used with permission.)

eggs, or sometimes 1st-stage larvae, the female tsetse retains the larva in the uterus and gives birth to just one 3rd instar larva at a time (Fig. 10.10). During gestation, the larva is fed from so-called milk glands that lie in the hemocoel and empty into the uterus. Three blood meals are required for the maturation of the larva, which are fully grown in 8–25 days.

When the female larviposits, the larva burrows quickly into the soil and transforms within an hour into a pupa. Pupation requires at least 2 weeks or more if soil temperature and moisture conditions are not optimal.

Bionomics

The habitat and the taxonomic groupings of the 23 species of *Glossina* correspond well. The *palpalis* group has members that are mostly forest dwellers, but they are also found near streams and lakeshores. The *palpalis* group is among the most important as vectors of trypanosomes. The group includes *G. palpalis* (2 subspecies), *G. tachinoides,* and *G. fuscipes* (3 subspecies), all of which serve as vectors.

The *morsitans* group are mainly savannah dwellers ranging from forest margins to sahelian- or sudan-type habitats. *G. morisitans* and *G. swynnertoni* are examples of vectors in the group.

The *fusca* group occurs principally in lowland forest, but some species are found at forest edges where the microclimate is somewhat drier than that of the rain forest. This group does not have members that are important vectors of trypanosomiasis.

Tsetse do not ordinarily fly far; they typically remain within an area of a couple hundred m in diameter. Many species pursue moving objects such as animals, humans, or vehicles, most likely seeking both mates and food sources. They cue in on dark, moving objects. Indeed, one method of counting tsetse is to have a team of collectors move through an area wearing dark clothing and vests on which a sticky substance has been applied that traps flies. The flies are later removed and counted.

The riverine species (e.g., *G. palpalis*) remain within about 10 m of the shore. This area usually has a fairly dense growth of trees and shrubs that provide places for the adults to rest. The females oviposit in loose soil in locations that are likely to retain some moisture, such as under fallen logs or where plant growth is heavy.

G. swynnertoni, a savannah species, is more diffuse in its distribution but is found in brushy areas. It tolerates dryness better than the riverine species.

An important method that prevents animals from being infected in the tsetse belt of Africa involves the diurnal feeding habit of tsetse. All species of tsetse feed during the day (a few individuals have been collected at night). Thus, cattle are held in corrals during the day and then let out to graze at night.

Host-Parasite Interactions

Tsetse are generally catholic in their tastes for blood. Both males and females feed on blood. Although they have host preferences, they will feed on any available, warm-blooded host. Most prefer large herbivores as hosts, and a few feed on reptiles such as crocodiles. Relatively few prefer primates; however, because tsetse are opportunistic, they often feed upon humans.

Tsetse, like many other insects, have symbiotic bacteria in the midgut, ovary, milk gland, and fat body. In general, these bacteria are considered to provide essential nutrients to their hosts. This is especially true of those insects that are hematophagous, because blood is an incomplete food (Chap. 2).

Tsetse have 2 species of bacteria in the gut and milk glands, and studies are under way attempting to achieve a genetic transformation in the bacteria. The method currently being used introduces genes into the symbiotic bacteria to interfere with the development and replication of the trypanosomes that they vector. Ideally, the bacteria would produce a trypanostatic or trypanocidal compound that would not be detrimental to the tsetse.

Control

At the turn of the 20th century, when the life cycle of the trypanosomes causing sleeping sickness in Africa was described, tsetse were found to be the vectors. At that time, there was no chemotherapeutic agent to treat the disease in either humans or domesticated animals, and the emphasis on control lay in reducing populations of tsetse. Biological studies showed that the flies did not move much, and for a time it was thought that they had home ranges. It was also observed that the pupae needed moisture and moderate temperatures to survive. Therefore, the 1st control methods were based on source reduction.

For riverine and lacustrine species, the foliage within about 10 m of the water was completely removed, thereby denying the adult flies resting sites and larviposition sites. To prevent the flies from moving from one place to another, trees and brush were completely removed from lanes 2 km wide. Thus the flies were contained, as they do not readily cross broad, grassy areas. Such barriers are effective only temporarily and must be a part of a larger program that includes land use designed to eliminate breeding sites.

As insecticides were developed, they were applied to resting sites. Insecticides actually allowed the concept of selective clearing to be implemented. Low-growing plants were removed, and limbs of trees were removed to a height of about 3 m. This left some desirable vegetation, but eliminated resting sites on the branches of trees and shrubs and allowed hot, dry winds to desiccate the soil where the pupae were deposited.

After World War II, there was a blossoming of 2nd-generation insecticides, the foremost of which was DDT. Moreover, many bombers used in the war lay idle. Thus, whole flotillas of bombers, in formation, roared over the forested areas in which tsetse lurked. They sprayed DDT over huge areas, killing beneficial insects and possibly some tsetse.

Tsetse can be trapped relatively efficiently with the Harris trap, which mimics the silhouette of an ox, or a biconical trap. Such traps are suspended from trees, and the flies, which tend to alight on the underside, crawl through a narrow opening and are retained inside the screen body. Where financial resources and personnel are available, trapping can be effective in reducing the transmission of the trypanosomes discussed later.

The sterile male technique was developed for screwworm control in the early 1950s, and it was thought that it could also be applied to tsetse because they, like the screwworm, mate only once. The development program has gone on for a number of years but has not resulted in effective control in the field.

DISEASE AGENTS VECTORED

The *Trypanosoma* spp. that cause African sleeping sickness in humans and nagana in cattle are vectored by *Glossina* spp. Members of the genus *Trypanosoma* are flagellated protists in the order Kinetoplastida. These organisms have a relatively simple structure (Fig. 10. 12).

The complex of diseases called African trypanosomiasis is contiguous with the distribution of tsetse in sub-Saharan Africa. Sleeping sickness and nagana extend over an area of 11 million km^2, an area roughly equivalent to the 48 contiguous states in the United States. These diseases have been crucial to human ecology in Africa; they influenced the way in which cultures developed and provided a barrier to incursions into sub-Saharan Africa from the north. In the tsetse belt, draft animals such as horses and cattle were difficult, if not impossible, to raise. Thus humans had no additional power to till their fields and no aid to transport on land. Sufficient control of the diseases has now been achieved so that cattle can be raised with only moderate risk in many areas. Even today, though, so-called traction schemes are being developed so that farmers will have some help in tilling their fields. The digging stick is yet to become a thing of the past.

There are various organisms in the genus *Trypanosoma* that cause disease in humans and livestock (Table 10.1). All but 2 of those found in sub-Saharan Africa are vectored by tsetse.

TABLE 10.1   Species of *Trypanosoma* originating in Africa and infecting humans and animals

Trypanosome	Disease	Range	Mammalian Hosts
Transmission by Tsetse			
T. brucei gambiense	Chronic sleeping sickness	Central Africa	Human
T. brucei rhodesiense	Acute sleeping sickness	East Africa	Human, bovids, antelopes
T. brucei brucei	Nagana	Tropical Africa	All domestic mammals, antelopes
T. congolense	Nagana	Tropical Africa	Ruminants, pigs, dogs, equids
T. simiae	Acute or chronic disease	Tropical Africa	Monkeys, pigs, warthogs, possibly bovids, equids, camels
T. vivax	Souma	Central and South America	Ruminants, equids, dogs
T. uniforme	Relapsing fever, occasionally fatal	East and Central Africa; Angola	Ruminants
Mechanical Transmission			
T. evansi	Surra	North and N.W. Africa, Sudan, Somalia—all continents	Ruminants, equids, dogs, monkeys, elephants, etc.
T. equiperdum	Dourine	South America; north, south, and S.W. Africa	Equids[a]

[a] Transmission by coitus

T. brucei and *T. congolense* are important organisms in the broader sense. The 3 subspecies of *T. brucei* as shown in Table 10.1 are morphologically indistinguishable from one another, but they infect different hosts and cause different, but related, diseases. *T. b. gambiense*, once found only in western Africa, is an infection that is obtained by persons living at home in their villages or towns; it is a person-to-person transmission via tsetse. *T. b. rhodesiense* is found in the savannah of eastern Africa and has wild ruminants, the bushbuck, and probably other large ruminants as its normal hosts. Humans become infected when they enter the habitat in which the organism is cycling, an excellent example of a zoonosis.

T. b. gambiense causes a relatively long, chronic disease of 5 years or more before the infected individual dies, whereas *T. b. rhodesiense* causes an acute disease syndrome in which the human host typically dies about 6 months after the onset of signs and symptoms. *T. b. brucei*, by definition, infects large ruminants only, not humans.

The development of these organisms in the tsetse is identical for all subspecies of *T. brucei* (Fig. 10.12). So-called stumpy forms are picked up from the blood of the mammalian host by a tsetse during feeding. They change into promastigotes and multiply in the midgut of the fly. After about 20 days, the promastigotes change to a trypomastigote form, usually referred to as metacyclic trypomastigotes because they follow the replicative phase. It is not until the metacyclic form has been reached that transmission back to a mammalian host can occur.

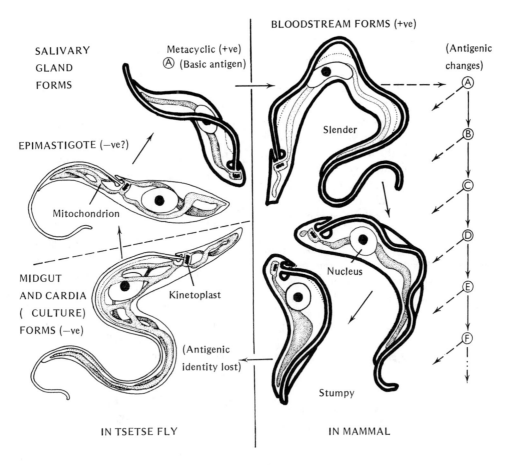

SALIVARY
GLAND
FORMS

Metacyclic (+ve)
Ⓐ (Basic antigen)

BLOODSTREAM FORMS (+ve)

(Antigenic
changes)

EPIMASTIGOTE (−ve?)

Slender

Mitochondrion

MIDGUT
AND CARDIA
(CULTURE)
FORMS (−ve)

Kinetoplast

Nucleus

(Antigenic
identity lost)

Stumpy

Ⓐ
Ⓑ
Ⓒ
Ⓓ
Ⓔ
Ⓕ

IN TSETSE FLY

IN MAMMAL

10.12 Morphology and life cycle of *Trypanosoma brucei*. The trypomastigote form in the bloodstream has a single flagellum attached to the body by an undulating membrane. There is a centrally located nucleus and a kinetoplast which lies close to the basal body of the flagellum. In the bloodstream forms, the mitochondrion is essentially nonfunctional and it lacks internal structure. In the tsetse the promastigote form has a structurally complex mitochondrion and all of the enzymes of the Krebs cycle. The variable surface glycoprotein, shown as the dark line around the body of the bloodstream forms, is antigenic and elicits antibody production in the vertebrate host. The VSG changes periodically so that the antigenic type of the trypomastigote continually changes (see left side of diagram). (W.C. Marquardt and Demaree, *Parasitology*, Macmillan Co., New York, 1985. Used with permission.)

The metacyclic trypomastigotes enter the bloodstream of a new mammalian host when the infected fly takes a blood meal. They develop for a period in the skin and lymph nodes and then multiply in the bloodstream as slender trypomastigotes. Slender forms are not infective for tsetse, but when the stumpy forms begin to appear in the bloodstream, they can successfully infect the fly.

Why all of this changing form and losing and regaining infectivity? The answer is that 2 separate phenomena are happening at the same time. First, bloodstream forms lack functional mitochondria and therefore also lack the complete Krebs cycle and excrete 3-carbon compounds into the bloodstream. The midgut forms regain a functional mitochondrion and have all of the enzymes of the Krebs cycle. The mitochondrion's growth and regression probably influence the body shape of the organisms.

Second, the bloodstream forms have a glycoprotein coat on their surfaces that prevents the immune response from eliminating them (Fig. 10.12). When the stumpy trypomastigotes are picked up by a fly, the glycoprotein coat is lost and replaced by a thinner coat called procyclin. Only when the metacyclic trypomastigote form is regained is the glycoprotein surface coat reformed.

The glycoprotein surface coat on the bloodstream forms is antigenic and leads to immunity in the mammalian host to the trypanosomes. The organisms have been selected, however, to continually change the surface coat, which is referred to as the variable surface glycoprotein (VSG). There seems to be almost no limit to the number of different antigenic coats that any one isolate can produce, and the numbers of trypomastigotes continually rise and fall in the bloodstream as 1 antigenic form is replaced by another every 2–3 weeks.

The continual change in the VSGs has been studied intensively, and many of the mechanisms have been described at the molecular level. From a practical viewpoint, it has been difficult, even impossible, to make a vaccine that is effective against the infection in either humans or livestock. Studies indicate that a vaccine containing several antigenic types may be effective in protecting cattle against trypanosomiasis.

Chemotherapy as a means of controlling African trypanosomiasis has been partially successful. Early in the 20th century organic arsenical compounds were found to be effective against *T. brucei* but were toxic to the mammalian host. With the advent of tryparsamide, moderately successful chemotherapy was at hand. A number of additional drugs have been found and developed, but a highly effective, nontoxic drug that can be given by mouth has not yet been discovered. Drug resistance, such as that which developed against pentamidine, remains a problem. The search for new drugs continues at a modest level, but trypanosomiasis is considered to be one of the orphan diseases because,

though important, it occurs in a part of the world where there is little economic gain to be realized by development and marketing of a drug.

The basis of control of African trypanosomiasis has remained in the domains of source reduction and inadequate chemotherapy and chemoprophylaxis. Trapping adult flies can be successful in reducing transmission in some circumstances.

In recent years, significant advances have been made in the biochemistry and molecular biology of trypanosomes as well as the physiology of the vectors, *Glossina* spp. It is likely that we will see better drugs for both prevention and treatment of the disease. Testing of vaccines has provided encouraging results, and the frustrations of the past may have been overcome. The sterile male technique for reducing populations of tsetse has not yet succeeded, but the development of this means of control is still being pursued. The role of intestinal bacteria in the physiology of the flies has been elucidated rather well, and altering the bacterial flora of the flies may give a means of reducing the populations of trypanosomes.

REFERENCES AND FURTHER READINGS

Barrett, T. 1991. Advances in triatomine bug ecology in relation to Chagas' disease. *Adv. in Dis. Vect. Res.* 8:143–176.

Beard, C.B., S.L. O'Neil, R.B. Tesh, F.F. Richards, and S. Aksoy. 1993. Modification of arthropod vector competence via symbiotic bacteria. *Parasitol. Today* 9:179–183.

Brenner, R.R., and A. de la M. Stoka. 1987. *Chagas' disease vectors*. 3 vols. Boca Raton, FL: CRC Press.

Busvine, J.R. 1978. Evidence from double infestations for the specific status of head and body lice (Anoplura). *Syst. Entomol.* 3:1–8.

Henry, T.J., and R.C. Froeschner. 1988. *Catalog of the Heteroptera, or true bugs, of Canada and the continental United States*. Gainesville, FL: Sandhill Crane Press.

Jordan, A.M. 1993. Tsetse-flies (Glossinidae). In: R.P. Lane and R.W. Crosskey, editors, *Medical insects and arachnids*. London and New York: Chapman and Hall. pp. 333–388.

Lent, H., and P. Wygodzinsky. 1979. Revision of the Triatominae (Hemiptera, Reduviidae) and their significance as vectors of Chagas' disease. *Bull. Am. Mus. Nat. Hist.* 163:123–520.

Sholdt, L.L., M.L. Holloway, and W.D. Fronk. 1979. *The epidemiology of human pediculosis in Ethiopia.* Spec. Publ. Navy Dis. Vect. Ecol. and Control Center. Jacksonville, FL: NAS.

Usinger, R.L. 1944. *The Triatominae of North and Central America and the West Indies and their public health significance.* U.S. Public Health Bull. No. 288.

Usinger, R.L. 1966. *Monograph of the Cimicidae* (Hemiptera-Heteroptera). Vol. 7. College Park, MD: Thomas Say Foundation.

Usinger, R.L., P. Wygodzinsky, and R.E. Ryckman. 1966. The biosystematics of the Triatominae. *Ann. Rev. Entomol.* 11:309–330.

Zinsser, H. 1935. *Rats, lice and history.* Boston: Little, Brown Co.

11 . FLEAS AND THE AGENTS THEY TRANSMIT

Rex E. Thomas

INTRODUCTION

Fleas are members of the order Siphonaptera. They are small, wingless holometabolous insects (Fig. 11.1) that are ectoparasites of warm-blooded animals. Both male and female fleas feed on the blood of a variety of hosts, ranging from pangolins or pandas to bats or birds. Some flea species are ultraspecific in their host preferences. The mountain beaver flea, *Hystrichopsylla schefferi*, is found only on *Aplodontia rufa* in the Pacific Northwest region of the United States. Some flea species parasitize a particular family or genus of vertebrates, such as the flea genus *Anomiopsyllus*, which is associated only with wood rats of the genus *Neotoma* (Barnes 1963). Others, like the cat flea, *Ctenocephalides felis*, are cosmopolitan and feed on many vertebrate hosts. In any case, the life of the flea is closely associated with a host and its environment.

Fleas are thought to be descended from a scorpion-fly-like ancestor (order Mecoptera) (Rothschild 1975). Fossils indicate that members of the order Siphonaptera had evolved to "normal pulicid form and size" as early as the Cretaceous period. A fossil very similar in appearance to a modern sticktight flea (*Echidnophaga* spp.) has been found in lower Cretaceous siltstone in Australia (Riek 1970), and fleas have been found in European baltic amber dating from the Eocene period (Ross et al. 1982). Traub (1980) states that the Siphonaptera must date back to the Jurassic era and arose as a monophyletic order on Pangea prior to continental rifting.

MORPHOLOGY

Adult fleas, like all insects, have 6 legs. The hind pair of legs are especially adapted for jumping. The pleural arch contains a rubberlike substance called resilin (Rothschild and Schlein 1975). The resilin is compressed within the pleural arch and held until a jump is initiated. The flea tumbles through the air toward a potential host with tarsi of the hind legs extended over the back to clasp onto the host's fur. The tarsi of the front 2 pairs of legs extend downward. The effect is to turn the flea into a tumbling grappling hook (Rothschild 1965a).

Adult fleas are ornamented with various densities of spines over the entire body (Fig. 11.2). The number of spines is usually positively correlated to the density of the normal hosts' fur. There are also highly specialized, heavier spines called ctenidial combs that appear in single rows either over the proximal end of the mouthparts, behind the head, over the 1st abdominal segment, or in some combination of these locations. The ctenidial combs and the location of the smaller spines are taxonomically diagnostic for individual flea species. Collectively, they help anchor fleas in the fur of the host. Flea taxonomy is also dependent upon the species-specific structure of the female spermatheca and the male sexual accessory structures.

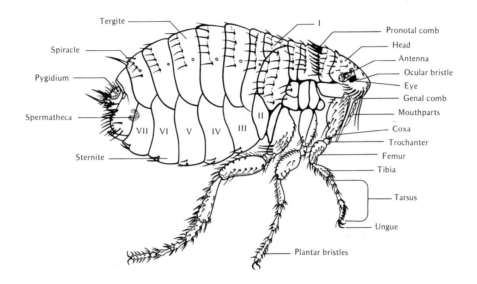

Labels in figure:
Tergite, Spiracle, Pygidium, Spermatheca, Sternite, VII, VI, V, IV, III, II, I, Pronotal comb, Head, Antenna, Ocular bristle, Eye, Genal comb, Mouthparts, Coxa, Trochanter, Femur, Tibia, Tarsus, Ungue, Plantar bristles

11.1   Line drawing of a female cat flea, *Ctenocephalides felis*

LIFE CYCLE

Fleas are holometabolous. The life cycle of the cat flea, *Ctenocephalides felis*, has been described more thoroughly than that of any other flea because of its economic importance (Dryden 1989a) (Fig. 11.3). A blood-fed female *C. felis* lays an average of about 25 eggs per day (Dryden 1989b, personal observation). Development times for the egg, larval, and pupal stages vary depending on temperature and humidity.

The egg-laying behavior of a particular flea species is generally adapted to the behavior of the host. The eggs of *C. felis* are oval, smooth, and dry. They fall from the host's fur and are deposited throughout the host's environment. The predatory or omnivorous hosts, on which *C. felis* apparently evolved, have defined home ranges that they frequently patrol, thus exposing themselves to offspring of their own fleas. The eggs of *Hoplopsyllus g. glacialis* are attached to fur of the arctic hare, and larval development takes place on the host. In this case, the environment off of the host would be extremely hazardous to the egg or larval flea. Other flea species, such as members of the genus *Anomiopsyllus*, lay their eggs singly in the nest of the

host, wood rats of the genus *Neotoma* (Barnes 1963). The activities of these rats center around a nest, and the host returns to the fleas in dependable fashion. Thus, environmental conditions of the nest may be more stable than they might be on the host itself.

Generally, flea eggs hatch within 3–5 days, and 1st instar larvae emerge using "egg-bursters" located on the top of the head capsule. The larval biology and taxonomy of many North American flea genera are reviewed by Elbel (1991). The larval stage has 3 instars with a molt occurring between each instar. During this stage of the life cycle many, if not all, flea species have a dietary requirement for blood. These larvae obtain blood in the form of dried adult flea excreta, which are present either in the fur of the host or in its environs. However, in a case of extreme adaptation, the larvae of 1 flea species, *Nosopsyllus fasciatus*, attach to the abdomen of an adult flea and ingest fecal blood as it passes from the anus (Molyneux 1967). Larvae also may feed on a variety of other organic material in the substrate of the environment.

Third-instar flea larvae enter a prepupal stage in which they spin a silken cocoon. Often the pupal case has detritus, sand, or other debris incorporated into it and is thus well camouflaged. Initially, the pupa inside the cocoon is translucent and immobile; by the end of the pupal stage, the pupa has partially melanized. The pupa remains in the pupal case until host recognition factors such as vibration, temperature increases, carbon dioxide, direct pressure on the cocoon, or some combination of these induce the teneral adult to explode from the cocoon in the direction of the stimulus. In the presence of adverse environmental conditions or the absence of host stimuli, adult fleas may remain in the cocoon for weeks or months. The period of quiescence for the cliff swallow flea, *Ceratophyllus celsus*, can last for many months (Hopla 1993) because cliff swallows do not always return to the same colony every year.

Most adult fleas must take a blood meal to reproduce. Female cat fleas require blood for egg production. Although male cat fleas emerge with fully mature sperm, they require blood for dissolution of an epididymal plug. This may not be true for all flea species.

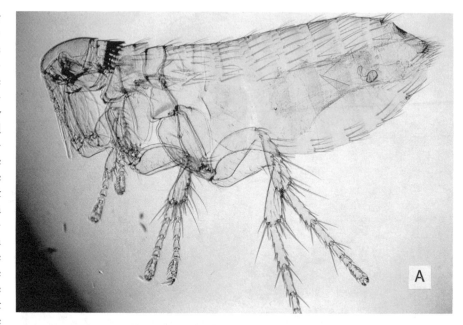

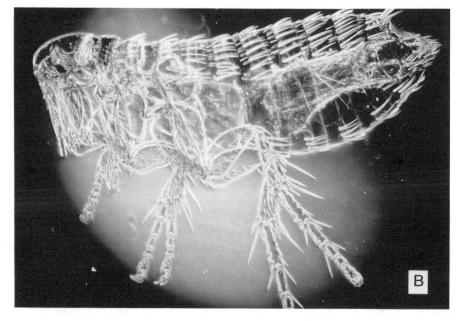

11.2 Female *Pleochaetus exiles* lit from above (A) and Below (B) to show density of the spines.

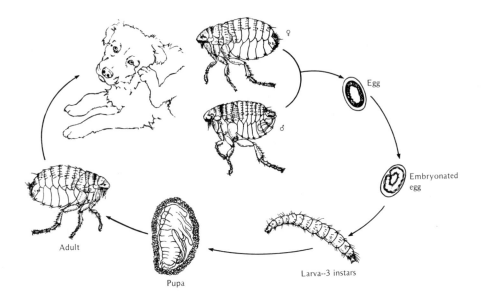

11.3 Life cycle of the cat flea, *Ctenocephalides felis*

HOST-PARASITE INTERACTIONS

Fleas can be obligate parasites of 1 mammal or bird species, genus or family, or they can be nonspecific in host choice. Rothschild (1965b) has described a highly specialized association between the European rabbit (*Oryctolagus cuniculis*) and its flea (*Spilopsyllus cuniculi*). The reproductive behavior of the flea is regulated by the female rabbit hormones that the flea takes in with a blood meal. Once stimulated to reproduce, the flea produces offspring that congregate on the doe rabbit's face at the time her young are born. As she brings her muzzle into contact with the newborn rabbits, the fleas quickly infest the newborns. Many other coevolved associations have been reviewed and described by Traub (1985).

However, some fleas do not require a particular host species as much as the microenvironment of that host. For example, *Peromyscopsylla h. hamifer* occurs throughout the range of its normal host, *Microtus* spp., but only in flood plains in which required soil type or moisture are present (Benton and Miller 1970). The appearance of homogenous populations of the ground squirrel flea, *Hoplopsyllus anomalus*, on giant kangaroo rats (*Dipodomys ingens*, family Heteromyidae) in southern California may be due to these rats filling the niche of the fleas' normal ground squirrel hosts (Tabor et al. 1993). An extreme example of an animal providing the appropriate host environment for a wide variety of fleas is that of *Onychomys leucogaster*, the northern grasshopper mouse. Over 50 species of fleas, including some that are thought to be specific for other rodents, have been collected from *O. leucogaster* in western North America (Thomas 1988).

METHODS OF CONTROL

Flea control consists of 2 different control strategies. The first type of control focuses on cat and dog fleas in and around the home. In this case there is often a pet animal associated with the infestation. The animal must be treated with an external (e.g., flea collar or flea powder) or systemic (e.g., cythiotate or flea juvenile hormone analogue) compound. The animal's resting areas and the range of the animal (e.g., carpets, the yard, and under porches and foundations if accessible) must be treated concurrently. This type of control program is directed at killing all adult and juvenile fleas in the pet's environment at one time. If any of these components is not treated at the same time surviving adult fleas will renew the infestation. Fortunately, now there are compounds (larvicidal compounds and juvenile hormone [JH] analogues) that pass into and through surviving adult fleas to affect egg development and kill larvae that consume adult feces. In the absence of adulticidal compounds, these control infestations over a period of weeks. In combination with adulticides, the compounds affect the offspring of surviving fleas, quickly controlling the infestation. Concepts for flea control on poultry and livestock are similar to those for infestations on pets.

The second type of flea control involves wild animal populations. This is most often undertaken to prevent or reduce the risk of flea-borne disease transmission. In areas where humans are not in contact with disease-carrying wild hosts or their fleas, it is often practical to eliminate the host population. Bait stations that contain a rodenticide such as cholecalciferol (Beard et al. 1988)may be used. This technique eliminates the disease-carrying vertebrate population and starves the infected fleas if no alternative hosts are available. When it is unacceptable to kill the host population, as is the case when an endangered species is involved, it is often preferable to treat host burrows or dens with an insecticide to kill fleas (e.g., permethrin). Of course, when there is a risk of human contact with disease-carrying fleas, it is unacceptable to simply eliminate the vertebrate host population. Flea populations must be controlled concurrently to prevent humans from becoming alternative hosts for starving, infected fleas.

DISEASE AGENTS VECTORED

Plague

Plague bacilli (*Yersinia pestis*) are small, gram-negative, pleiomorphic, nonmotile rods that exhibit bipolar staining with Giemsa or Wayson's stains. The bacilli grow well in various media; the most rapid growth occurs around 28°C. Media for cultivation and isolation of *Y. pestis* are described in Baymanyar and Cavanaugh (1976).

Plague is a flea-borne bacterial zoonosis naturally transmitted among rodent populations. Until recently plague was commonly referred to in the United States as either urban, campestral, or sylvatic. The term "sylvatic" is misleading because it indicates that plague is a forest disease. The name actually comes from the French term "sylvatique," which means "wild." To differentiate this from plague, which occurs in plains habitat, the term "campestral" plague was adopted but only added further to the confusion. Those who currently work with plague use the terms "urban" or "wild" rodent plague.

In areas in which enzootic or epizootic wild rodent plague is found, one or two species of mammals and fleas are invariably responsible for initiating and maintaining the transmission cycle. However, any number of species may be found to carry plague in an area in which the pathogen is present. The transmission cycle is a dynamic ecological interplay between vectors and hosts (Kalabukov 1965). Flea species that vector plague efficiently exhibit a number of characteristics, such as intimate association with hosts susceptible to infection, distribution in geographic areas that support the endemicity of plague environmentally, and enhanced capacity to amplify and subsequently transmit the bacilli.

Early research on vector competence among fleas involved determination of plague transmission potentials at the species level. Kartman (1957) offered a competence estimator that he termed "vector potential." This is the product of values representing the prevalence of the flea in nature, its field infection rate, and an experimentally derived value for its ability to feed on an infected host, become infected and blocked, and transmit to noninfected hosts. In more general terms, we now refer to the latter attributes as vector competence and to the sum of these characteristics as vectorial capacity (Chap. 4).

Fleas that transmit plague most efficiently generally are those that develop a bacterial mass at the proventriculus. Enhanced transmission is assumed to be due to the flea making repeated attempts to feed while the proventriculus is plugged. Blood is drawn up into the proventriculus and washes over the bacterial mass. As the flea's salivary pumps relax, the plague-infected host blood is ejected back into the bite wound, thereby enhancing transmission. The blocking potential of a

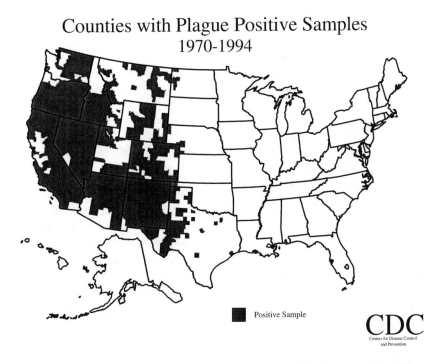

Counties with Plague Positive Samples
1970-1994

Positive Sample

CDC
Centers for Disease Control
and Prevention

11.4   Distribution of plague in the United States (1970–1994). Courtesy of the U.S. Centers for Disease Control and Prevention.

Global Distribution of Plague

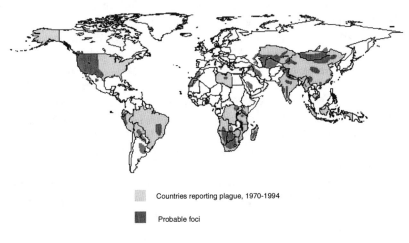

Countries reporting plague, 1970-1994

Probable foci

Compiled from WHO, CDC, and country sources

11.5   Probable present worldwide distribution of plague. Courtesy of the U.S. Centers for Disease Control and Prevention.

flea is possibly the most important factor in defining vector competence.

Appropriate combinations of flea vectorial capacity, distribution, and host association have resulted in many small focal areas of endemic zootic plague within a large geographic region of western North America (Barnes 1982) and throughout the world (Baltazard 1964) (Figs. 11.4 and 11.5). Within these foci, incidence of zootic plague has been noted during epizootic cycles probably triggered by a critical level of susceptible rodents and environmental factors that are favorable to flea populations. However, rodent epizootics are usually rather random in their occurrence both in time and location. This makes the distribution of plague appear to be very fluid over time.

Mammalian Susceptibility to Plague

Mammals vary in their susceptibility to plague. In areas of the world where *Yersinia pestis* is present, plague is primarily reservoired and transmitted via rodent infection (Twigg 1978). Prairie dogs (genus *Cynomys*) are uniformly susceptible to fatal infection with *Y. pestis*, and entire populations, numbering hundreds or thousands of individuals, may be decimated in a single epizootic episode (Lechleitner et al. 1962). Urban rats and mice (*Rattus* spp. and *Mus musculus*) are susceptible to plague, as are felids (e.g., bobcats and house cats), and mortality rates are high. Other rodents, such as the heteromyids (e.g., the genera *Dipodomys*, the kangaroo rats, and *Perognathus*, the pocket mice), are refractory to the disease. Most rodent species, *Onychomys leucogaster*, for example, appear to be represented by populations with various degrees of resistance to plague. Two North American populations of these mice exhibited more than a 10,000-fold variation in their susceptibilities to plague. (Thomas et al. 1988). Carnivores and omnivores exhibit varying degrees of resistance to plague. Mustelids (weasels, badgers, and ferrets), ursids (bears), and canids (domestic dogs, coyotes, and wolves) appear to suffer little from the disease.

Within an enzootic area, the relative susceptibilities of vertebrate hosts often differ from those of the same hosts in other areas (Isaäcson et al. 1981; Thomas et al. 1988). In turn, the relative susceptibility of a flea's host animal plays a large role in defining that flea's potential to vector plague. Thus, the relative importance of flea species as vectors of plague can be unique to a given area (Kartman et al. 1960). Though flea transmission of plague among mammals is most common, transmission from infected animals to predators or omnivores that consume the infected host has also been documented (Thomas et al. 1989; Gasper et al. 1993), and pneumonic transmission among rodents has been suggested by some.

Human Infection

Human plague infections are possible wherever *Y. pestis* is present in nature. Human exposure to plague normally is associated with activities such as working, hunting, or recreating in rural areas where the natural disease cycle is active. Urban exposure may result from epizootic disease among rodents such as tree squirrels (Hudson et al. 1971), or when human sanitation is insufficient to provide a barrier between domestic and wild rodents. This occurs more often in underdeveloped countries or areas experiencing social upheaval. Surveillance and control measures must be maintained in urban areas near natural foci of plague to keep the disease out of urban rodent populations and, thus, away from human populations (Schwan et al. 1985).

The evolutionary and geographic origins of the plague bacillus are much debated. It arose as a flea-borne pathogen either in the steppe region of central Asia or in Africa. It is known that at least 3 pandemics originated in Asia. In the first 2 pandemics, which occurred between A.D. 1300 and 1700, infected fleas were carried by infected rats and humans throughout the Old World. It is estimated that up to 25% of the population of Europe died during plague epidemics of the 14th century. The most recent pandemic is thought to have originated in Hong Kong in the late 1800s. During this time plague was carried aboard ships to North and South America and to South Africa.

Human plague has been called the Black Death and is commonly referred to as bubonic plague. Regardless of its name, plague in its many forms is a disease caused by a single agent, *Y. pestis*. The term "bubonic" refers to the most common initial form of the disease. After an infected flea bites a susceptible host, the plague bacilli commonly take up residence in a regional lymph node and replicate. This replication causes enlargement of the node, forming a "bubo." When the bacilli escape the lymphatic system and enter the bloodstream, the disease has progressed to the "septicemic" stage. During this stage capillary walls begin to leak, and disseminated intravascular coagulation (DIC) occurs, turning the skin black.

If the host survives long enough the bacilli infect the lungs, and the disease becomes "pneumonic" plague. Although flea-bite transmission with the onset of bubonic plague is the most common type of human plague, humans can acquire primary septicemic plague by handling an infected animal. For example, if a hunter receives a cut or is bitten while handling an infected animal, the bacilli directly enter the bloodstream, thus bypassing the bubonic stage. If the disease progresses to the pneumonic stage, it is possible for another human to acquire primary pneumonic plague from the infected individual. Primary pneumonic plague is the most rapidly fatal form of the disease and is of most concern to public health officials. In the United States there have been no documented cases of human-to-human transmission of plague via pneumonic infection in over 75 years. However, there have been 5 cases of primary pneumonic plague transmitted from domestic cats to humans between 1977 and 1993. Domestic cats as a source of human plague infection is an emerging epidemiological problem in the United States (MMWR 1994). It is important to remember that if diagnosed in time, plague is easily treated with a number of antibiotics such as streptomycin or tetracycline.

Plague Transmission and the Genetics of *Yersinia pestis*

Many *Y. pestis* virulence characters are coded for on a 72-kilobase pair (kbp) plasmid (Brubaker 1984; Portnoy et al. 1983). Corresponding 70+ kbp plasmids are found in *Y. pseudotuberculosis* and *Y. enterocolitica* (Portnoy et al. 1984; Portnoy and Falkow 1982); however, *Y. pestis* carries 2 additional plasmids that the congeneric species lack. The largest of these is 90–110 kbp and codes for the capsule that forms around the bacillus when it enters a vertebrate host and for a membrane-bound protein that is toxic to mice. The 3rd and smallest *Y. pestis* plasmid (9.5 kbp) codes for the bacteriocin pesticin and for resistance to this particular bacteriocin (McDonough and Falkow 1989; Sodeinde and Goguen 1988). Pesticin is lethal to the human-pathogenic members of the genus *Yersinia* (Brubaker et al. 1965), including any *Y. pestis* bacilli that lack the plasmid. The specificity of the bacteriocin suggests a mechanism for conservation of the 9.5-kbp plasmid in *Y. pestis* bacilli because strains that lack it will be eliminated from mixed cultures (Ben-Gurion and Hertman 1958). Maintenance of the plasmid results in conservation of other genes on the same plasmid that regulate coagulase and fibrinolysin activities (Beesley et al. 1967; Sodeinde and Goguen 1988; McDonough and Falkow 1989), both of which are important in the flea-borne stage of the transmission cycle. The 9.5-kbp plasmid also has been shown to affect products coded for by the 72-kbp plasmid, indicating plasmid/plasmid interaction (Sample et al. 1987; Mehigh et al. 1989).

The likelihood of proventricular blockage is not equal among flea species (Douglas and Wheeler 1943). As previously mentioned, the block formation potential of a given flea species is considered to be the most important factor in defining its vector potential. As important as block formation may be, the phrase "ability to block" is probably an oxymoron, because this phenomenon appears to be regulated by the plague bacillus. After a flea has taken an infectious blood meal, it is important to the flea-borne transmission cycle that the flea leaves that host to transmit the bacillus to a new host. The fact that fleas are obligate parasites of warm-blooded animals is crucial to the transmission of plague in this sense; when a host dies, the flea usually leaves it to seek a new one (Westrom and Yescott 1975). When the flea is no longer in association with a warm-bodied mammal, an infected blood meal cools to ambient temperature. At temperatures below 27.5℃, the 9.5-kbp plasmid expresses coagulase (Sodeinde and Goguen 1988). Cavanaugh (1971) showed that block formation begins at temperatures below 27.5℃ as infected host blood is coagulated in the flea midgut. The bacilli multiply in the clot and form a partial or complete occlusion that often appears to anchor on proventricular spines. When a blocked flea feeds, many thousands of bacilli per bite can be inoculated into the host.

At temperatures above 27.5°C, which fleas encounter during intimate contact with a new, potentially uninfected host, the plasmid gene that codes for coagulase initiates expression of fibrinolysin (McDonough and Falkow 1989). This enzyme helps dissolve the fibrin network of the block and allows amplified numbers of bacilli to be transmitted in feeding efforts. The fibrinolysin produced by *Y. pestis* also has been implicated as a "spreading factor" (Jawetz and Meyer 1944) because it appears to suppress coagulation at the site of the flea-bite wound.

Upon entry into a vertebrate host, *Y. pestis* is unencapsulated and probably is susceptible to phagocytic activity and complement-mediated lysis. However, at host temperatures (37°C) and in the presence of the low calcium levels present in mammalian tissues, *Y. pestis* expresses products that both protect it from the immune system and are pathogenic for the host (Barve and Straley 1990; Plano et al. 1991; Mehigh and Brubaker 1993). The largest of the *Y. pestis* plasmids (90–110 kbp) codes for the capsule that forms around the bacillus at 37°C (Gaylov et al. 1990). The capsule has several virulence functions: It confers resistance to phagocytic digestion by macrophages (Straley and Harmon 1984), blocks the complement cascade by antagonizing deposition of the C2 and C4 components (Williams et al. 1972), and probably also buffers the bacillus from extremes of pH and temperature because of its reported glycoprotein nature. (It would be interesting to determine whether *Y. pestis* also can modify the pH of phagolysosomes, as has been shown for *Histoplasma capsulatum* [Eissenberg et al. 1993].) Glycoprotein synthesis is rare among the eubacteria. In their analyses of the capsular (Fraction 1) molecule, Bennett and Tornabene (1974) and Glosnicka and Gruszkiewicz (1980) found that the carbohydrate component of this glycosylated protein is primarily galactose. This molecule possibly functions in receptor events. Both human and mouse macrophages have a cell surface receptor with lectin-like properties specific for galactose (Ho and Springer 1982; Cherayil et al. 1990).

Encapsulated plague bacilli reproduce within phagolysosomes of macrophages (Straley and Harmon 1984). Eventually, replicating bacilli kill the macrophages, and encapsulated *Y. pestis* disperse throughout the host body in a septicemic stage. Fraction 1 is the immunodominant antigen in plague infections and antigen-specific titers indicate that antibody against Fraction 1 eventually results in bacteriolysis.

The largest *Y. pestis* plasmid also has been implicated in production of murine toxin (Brubaker 1984). This protein is a bimorphic, membrane-bound exotoxin that reacts specifically with beta-adrenergic receptors of mice (Brown and Montie 1977; Montie 1981). This toxic molecule is released upon bacteriolysis and is lethal to mice in submicrogram quantities. A lipopolysaccharide endotoxin, characteristic of gram-negative bacteria, also is produced by *Y. pestis* and is released upon cell lysis. Its production is probably determined chromosomally.

The 72-kbp plasmid of *Y. pestis* codes for a number of outer membrane proteins (YOPS) that are associated with virulence in the *Yersinia*. The literature pertaining to these proteins, their regulation, and their putative virulence functions has been reviewed by Straley (1988) and Cornelis et al. (1989). The absence of any one of several of the YOPS reduces the virulence of the deficient *Y. pestis* strain.

The plague bacillus apparently can make some flea species better vectors by enhancing block formation when the vector leaves an infecting host. The bacillus actively breaks down the block when the flea finds another warm body with a product that also promotes dissemination of the bacilli from the site of inoculation by antagonizing coagulation of host blood there. Once inside the vertebrate body, *Y. pestis* produces a capsule that appears to both target it for phagocytosis and protect it from phagocytic digestion. This intracellular residence probably affords the bacillus protection from the immune system in early infection resulting, at least in part, from suppression of gamma interferon and tumor necrosis factor by *Y. pestis* (Nakajima and Brubaker 1993). Upon release of bacilli from macrophages that have been overwhelmed by intracellular reproduction, the immune system targets the highly antigenic capsular glycoprotein. Further, Fraction 1 antigen has been shown to cause proliferation of splenic mononuclear cells derived from *Mastomys natalensis* (Arntzen et al. 1991). Release of LPS endotoxin upon cell death is common among gram-negative bacilli; however, *Y. pestis* uses this same principle against the mouse immune system with a 2nd toxin. This mouse-specific protein exotoxin (murine toxin) is also released when plague bacilli are lysed. As noted, this pathogenic bacterium depends upon fleas for transmission; thus, a mouse-specific toxin has significant advantages for the bacillus in expediting the transmission cycle by killing the host and forcing the fleas to seek new, potentially susceptible hosts.

Summary

The interactions between *Y. pestis* and its vectors and vertebrate hosts are truly remarkable. *Y. pestis* virulence characters appear to have coevolved precisely with key components of the natural transmission cycle. For the past 90 years, research on plague in North America has been focused on surveillance and control. Within the past 20 years we have discovered that *Y. pestis* produces products that affect both its vectors and hosts to the benefit of the transmission cycle. We will likely learn that the ability of *Y. pestis* to moderate components of its own transmission cycle varies from area to area subject to differences in biotic and abiotic factors that affect vector-host relationships.

Murine Typhus

Murine typhus is a flea-borne rickettsial zoonosis caused by *Rickettsia typhi* (*R. mooseri*). Except for Antarctica, it can be found worldwide. The primary mammalian reservoirs throughout the world are rats (genus *Rattus*). Domestic cats have been shown to be sources for infected fleas in Texas (Older 1970), and 11% (8 in 75) of opossums (*Didelphis marsupialis*) tested for *R. typhi* antibody in Orange County, California, were seropositive (Adams et al. 1970). Although the number of human cases per year in the United States has dropped from the thousands before 1950 to fewer than 100 in recent years, it is still an important disease worldwide (Azad 1990). In humans the disease has a 5–18 day incubation period followed by violent headache with high fever and chills. A macular eruption occurs about the 4th day after onset. Murine typhus is

much less virulent in the New World (2% mortality) than in the Old World (70% mortality); unfortunately, the reason has not been discovered.

Murine typhus was first reported in the United States in the early 1900s, and by 1939 the fleas *Xynopsylla cheopis*, *Echidnophaga gallinacea*, and *Leptopsyllus sengis* were shown to carry the agent in Georgia (Hubbard 1968). More recently, *Ctenocephalides felis* have been shown to be susceptible to experimental infection with *R. typhi*; this fleas species also may play a significant role in the transmission of murine typhus to humans (Azad et al. 1984). Note that all 4 of these flea species have cosmopolitan distributions.

The murine typhus rickettsiae reproduce within midgut epithelial cells in the flea (Ito et al. 1975). The rickettsiae enter the lumen of the gut upon cellular exfoliation and pass out of the flea in the feces. Human infection occurs when the infected feces are rubbed or scratched into the flea-bite wound.

Azad et al. (1985) demonstrated transovarial transmission of *R. typhi* in laboratory-infected *Xenopsylla cheopis* fleas. This was the first evidence that the rickettsiae infect flea tissue other than the midgut epithelium. Azad and Traub (1989) showed that *Xenopsylla cheopis* fleas infected for at least 21 days could transmit the rickettsiae during feeding in a system that excluded the possibility of transmission via the feces. This was the 1st evidence that murine typhus could be transmitted by other than posterior station transmission.

A typhus-like rickettsia, distinctly different from *R. typhi*, has recently been found in laboratory colonies of *C. felis* (Adams et al. 1990). This rickettsia has since been labeled the ELB agent and has been implicated as the agent of typhus-like disease in humans in the United States. The agent is stably transmitted transovarially in cat fleas (Azad et al. 1992).

Myxomatosis

Myxomatosis is an epizootic disease of rabbits characterized by skin tumors and a high mortality rate in the European rabbit, *Spilopsylus cuniculis*. It is caused by a myxoma virus that is native to South America, but it has spread to the United States and Great Britain (Harwood and James 1979). In Great Britain the primary vector is *Spilopsyllus cuniculi* (Mead-Briggs and

Vaughn 1980). Although it can be transmitted by contact with an infected individual, it has been shown in the laboratory that it can be mechanically transmitted by many bloodsucking arthropods, including fleas. This knowledge was used in a campaign of biological control of European rabbits in Australia in the 1960s. European rabbits were first introduced into Australia in 1859, and by the mid 1900s *O. cuniculis* populations had become intolerably high. After it was determined that native *Echidnophaga myrmecobii* and *E. perilis* fleas were not adequately efficient vectors of myxoma virus to control *O. cuniculis* populations, *S. cuniculi* fleas were imported, infected, and released. In areas in which their populations achieved high enough numbers to represent an infestation of approximately 30 fleas per doe rabbit and 20 fleas per buck, epizootics of fatal myxomatosis were observed to control rabbit populations (Shepherd 1980).

Tularemia

Hopla (1980) pointed out that the Siphonaptera were the first arthropods to be associated with tularemia (*Francisella tularensis*) transmission. However, ticks have since been shown to be the primary arthropod vectors of this zoonotic disease to humans. Hopla stated that the significance of fleas in the ecology of tularemia in the Nearctic region is greatest in the maintenance of *F. tularensis* among cricetid and sciurid rodents. Although *F. tularensis* is rarely identified from fleas in the United States, it has been isolated from at least 6 species of fleas in the former USSR.

It is assumed that the transmission of tularemia by fleas is mechanical, following interrupted feeding on an infected host. However, fleas held for 24 hours after an infectious blood meal still transmitted at a rate of 30%, and *F. tularensis* has been recovered from fleas up to 3 days after an experimentally infected blood meal (Hopla 1980).

Tapeworms

Cat and dog fleas (*C. felis* and *C. canis*) are intermediate hosts of the dog tapeworm *Dipylidium caninum* and the rodent tapeworm *Hymenolepis diminuata*. When fleas are consumed during host grooming, the immature tapeworms are released into the definitive host. After maturation and reproduction of these worms, eggs are passed in the host feces and are consumed by flea larvae to complete the life cycle. Both of these tapeworm species occasionally infect humans.

Cat Scratch Disease

Cat scratch disease is characterized by localized lymphadenitis following a scratch or exposure to cats (Carithers et al. 1969). The etiologic agent was recently isolated from HIV-positive patients suffering from bacillary angiomatosis, which is thought to be an aggressive form of the disease among AIDS patients. The agent was found to be a newly recognized rickettsia and was named *Rochalemaea henselae* (Regnery et al. 1992).

A survey in the San Francisco Bay area of impounded cats found 41% (25 in 61) to be positive for *R. henselae,* with bacteremias as high as 1000 colony-forming units per ml of blood. Additionally, *R. henselae* was cultured from *C. felis* fleas of at least 1 of the 7 cats tested (Koehler et al. 1994). These data leave open the possibility that the true vectors or reservoirs of this disease may be cat fleas.

REFERENCES

Adams, J.R., E.T. Schmitmann, and A.F. Azad. 1990. Infection of colonized cat fleas, *Ctenocephalides felis* (Bouché), with a rickettsia-like microorganism. *Am. J. Trop. Med. Hyg.* 43:400–409.

Adams, W.H., R.W. Emmons, and J.E. Brooks. 1970. The changing ecology of murine (endemic) typhus in California. *Am. J. Trop. Med. Hyg.* 19:311–318.

Arntzen, L., A.A. Wadee, and M. Isaäcson. 1991. Immune responses of two *Mastomys* sibling species to *Yersinia pestis. Infect. Immun.* 59:1966–1971.

Azad, A.F. 1990. The epidemiology of murine typhus. *Ann. Rev. Entomol.* 35:553–569.

Azad, A.F., J.B. Sacci, Jr., W.M. Nelson, G.A. Dasch, E.T. Schmidtmann, and M. Carl. 1992. Genetic characterization and transovarial transmission of a typhus-like rickettsia found in cat fleas. *Proc. Natl. Acad. Sci., USA* 89:43–46.

Azad, A.F., and R. Traub. 1989. Experimental transmission of murine typhus by *Xenopsylla cheopis* flea bites. *Med. Vet. Entomol.* 3:429–433.

Azad, A.F., R. Traub, and S. Baqar. 1985. Transovarial transmission of murine typhus rickettsiae in *Xenopsylla cheopis* fleas. *Science.* 227:543–545.

Azad, A.F., R. Traub, M. Sofi, and C.L. Wisseman Jr. 1984. Experimental murine typhus infection in the cat flea, *Ctenocephalides felis* (Siphonaptera: Pulicidae). *J. Med. Ent.* 21:675–680.

Baltzard, M. 1964. The conservation of plague in inveterate foci. *J. Hyg. Epidemiol. Microbiol. Immunol.* 8:409–421.

Barnes, A.M. 1963. A revision of the genus *Anomiopsyllus* Baker 1904 (Siphonaptera:Hystrichopsyllidae) with studies of the biology of *Anomiopsyllus falsicalifornicus.* Ph.D. dissertation. Berkeley: University of California Berkeley. 218 p.

Barnes, A.M. 1982. Surveillance and control of bubonic plague. *Symp. Zool. Soc. Lond.* 50:237–270.

Barve, S.S., and S.C. Straley. 1990. *lcrR*, a low Ca^{2+}-response locus with dual Ca^{2+} dependent functions in *Yersinia pestis. J. Bacteriol.* 172:4661–4671.

Baymanyar, M., and D.C. Cavanaugh. 1976. *Plague manual.* Geneva: World Health Organization. 65 p.

Beard, M.L., C.E. Montman, G.O. Maupin, A.M. Barnes, R.B. Craven, and E.F. Marshall. 1988. Integrated vector control. Rodenticide may reduce the spread of human plague. *J. Environ. Health.* 51:69–75.

Beesley, E.D., R.R. Brubaker, W.A. Jansen, and M.J. Surgalla. 1967. Pesticins: 3. Expression of coagulase and mechanisms of fibrinolysis. *J. Bacteriol.* 165:19–26.

Ben-Gurion, R., and I. Hertman. 1958. Bacteriocin-like material produced by *Pasturella pestis. J. Gen. Microbiol.* 19:289–297.

Bennett, L.G., and T.G. Tornabene. 1974. Characterization of the antigenic subunits of the envelope protein of *Yersinia pestis. J. Bacteriol.* 117:48–55.

Benton, A.H., and D.H. Miller. 1970. Ecological factors in the distribution of the flea *Peromyscopsylla h. hamifer. Am. Midl. Nat.* 81:301–303.

Brown, S.D., and T.C. Montie. 1977. Beta-adrenergic blocking activity of *Yersinia pestis* murine toxin. *Infect. Immun.* 18:85–93.

Brubaker, R.R. 1984. Molecular biology of the dread Black Death. *ASM News.* 50:240–245.

Brubaker, R.R., M.J. Surgalla, and E. D. Beesley. 1965. Pesticinogeny and bacterial virulence. *Zentralbl. Bacteriol. I. Abt. Orig.* 196:302–315.

Carithers, H.A., C.M. Carithers, and R.O. Edwards. 1969. Cat-scratch disease. *JAMA* 207:312–316.

Cavanaugh, D.C. 1971. Specific effect of temperature upon transmission of the plague bacillus by the oriental rat flea, *Xenopsylla cheopis. Am. J. Trop. Med. Hyg.* 20:264–273.

Cherayil, B.J., S. Chaitovitz, C. Wong, and S. Pillai. 1990. Molecular cloning of a human macrophage lectin specific for galactose. *Proc. Natl. Acad. Sci. USA* 87:7324–7328.

Cornelis, G.R., T. Biot, C.L. deRouvroit, T. Michiels, B. Mulder, C. Sluiters, M.-P. Sory, M. VanBouchaute, and J.-C. Vanooteghem. 1989. The *Yersinia yop* regulon. *Molec. Microbiol.* 3:1455–1459.

Douglas, J.R., and C.M. Wheeler. 1943. Sylvatic plague studies: 3. The fate of *Pasturella pestis* in the flea. *J. Infect. Dis.* 72:18–30.

Dryden, M.W. 1989a. Biology of the cat flea, *Ctenocephalides felis felis. Comp. Anim. Pract.* 19:23–27.

———. 1989b. Host association: On-host longevity and egg production of *Ctenocephalides felis felis. Vet. Parasitol.* 34:117–122.

Eissenberg, L.G., W.E. Goldman, and P.H. Schlesinger. 1993. *Histoplasma capsulatum* modulates the acidification of phagolysosomes. *J. Exp. Med.* 177:1605–1611.

Elbel, R.E. 1991. Order Siphonaptera. In: *Immature insects,* Vol. 2. Dubuque: Kendall Hunt Publishing. pp. 674–689.

Galyov, E.E., O. Yu. Smirnov, A.V. Karlishev, K.I. Volkovoy, A.I. Denesyuk, I.V. Nazimov, K.S. Rubtsov, V.M. Abramov, S.M. Dalvadyanz, and V.P. Zav'yalov. 1990. Nucleotide sequence of the *Yersinia pestis* gene encoding F1 antigen and the primary structure of the protein. *FEBS* 277:230–232.

Gasper, P.W., A.M. Barnes, T.J. Quan, J.P. Benziger, L.G. Carter, M.L. Beard, and G.O. Maupin. 1993. Plague (*Yersinia pestis*) in cats: Description of experimentally induced disease. *J. Med. Entomol.* 30:20–26.

Glosnicka, R., and E. Gruszkiewicz. 1980. Chemical composition and biological activity of the *Yersinia pestis* envelope substance. *Infect. Immun.* 30:506–512.

Harwood, R.F., and M.T. James. 1979. *Entomology in Human and Animal Health.* 7th ed. New York: Macmillan. pp. 228–229.

Ho, M.K., and T.A. Springer. 1982. MAC-2, a novel 32,000 Mr mouse macrophage subpopulation-specific antigen defined by monoclonal antibodies. *J. Immunol.* 128:1221–1228.

Hopla, C.E. 1980. Fleas as vectors of tularemia in Alaska. In: R. Traub and H. Starcke, editors, *Fleas; Proceedings of the International Conference on Fleas; Peterborough, U.K.; June 1977.* Rotterdam: A.A. Balkema. pp. 287–300.

Hopla, C.E. 1993. Cliff swallow ectoparasites: Adaptation and vector relationships. In: D. Borovsky and A. Spielman, editors. Proceedings of the 3rd symposium on host regulated developmental mechanisms in vector arthropods. Vero Beach: Univ. Florida-IFAS. pp. 200–207.

Hubbard, C.A. 1968. *Fleas of western North America.* New York: Hafner Publ. Co.

Hudson, B.W., M.I. Goldenberg, J.D. McCluskie, H.E. Larson, C.D. McGuire, A.M. Barnes, and J.D. Poland. 1971. Serological and bacteriological investigations of an outbreak of plague in an urban tree squirrel population. *Am. J. Trop. Med.Hyg.* 20:255–263.

Isaäcson, M., L. Arntzen, and P. Taylor. 1981. Susceptibility of members of the *Mastomy natalensis* species complex to experimental infection with *Yersinia pestis. J. Infect. Dis.* 144:80.

Ito, S., J.W. Vinson, and T.J. McGuire. 1975. Murine typhus rickettsia in the oriental rat flea. *Ann. N.Y. Acad. Sci.* 266:35–60.

Jawetz, E., and K.F. Meyer. 1944. Studies on plague immunity in experimental animals: 2. Some factors of the immunity mechanism in bubonic plague. *J. Immunol.* 49:331–358.

Kalabukov, N.I. 1965. The structure and dynamics of natural foci of plague. *J. Hyg. Epidemiol. Microbiol. Immunol.* 9:147–159.

Kartman, L. 1957. The concept of vector efficiency in experimental studies of plague. *Exptl. Parasitol.* 6:599–609.

Kartman, L., S.F. Quan, and V.I. Miles. 1960. Ecological studies of wild rodent plague in the San Francisco Bay area of California. *Am. J. Trop. Med. Hyg.* 9:153–157.

Koehler, J.E., C.A. Glaser, and J.W. Tappero. 1994. *Rochalimaea henselae* infection. A new zoonosis with the domestic cat as reservoir. *JAMA* 271:531–535.

Lechleitner, R.R., J.V. Tileson, and L. Kartman. 1962. Die-off of a Gunnison's prairie dog colony in central Colorado: 1. Ecological observations and description of the epizootic. *Zoonoses Research* 1:185–199.

McDonough, K.A., and S. Falkow. 1989. A *Yersinia pestis*-specific DNA fragment encodes temperature-dependent coagulase and fibrinolysin associated phenotypes. *Mol. Microbiol.* 3:767–775.

Mead-Briggs, A.R., and J.A. Vaughn. 1980. The importance of the European rabbit flea *Spilopsyllus cuniculi* (Dale) in the evolution of myxomatosis in Britain. In: R. Traub and H. Starcke, editors, *Fleas; Proceedings of the International Conference on Fleas. Peterborough, U.K.; June 1977.* Rotterdam: A.A. Balkema, pp. 309–314.

Mehigh, R.J,. and R.R. Brubaker. 1993. Major stable peptides of *Yersinia pestis* synthesized during the low calcium response. *Infect. Immun.* 61:13–22.

Mehigh, R.J., A.K. Sample, and R.R. Brubaker. 1989. Expression of the low-calcium response in *Yersinia pestis. Microb. Pathogen.* 6:203–217.

MMWR. 1994. Human Plague–United States, 1993–1994. 43:242–246.

Molyneux, D.H. 1967. Feeding behavior of the larval rat flea, *Nosopsyllus fasciatus* (Bösc). *Nature* 215:779.

Montie, T.C. 1981. Properties and pharmacological action of plague murine toxin. *Pharmac. Ther.* 12:491–499.

Nakajima, R., and R.R. Brubaker. 1993. Association between virulence of *Yersinia pestis* and suppression of gamma interferon and tumor necrosis factor alpha. *Infect. Immun.* 61:23–31.

Older, J.J. 1970. The epidemiology of murine typhus in Texas, 1969. *JAMA* 214:2011–2017.

Plano, G.V., S.S. Barve, and S.C. Straley. 1991. LcrD, a membrane-bound regulator of the *Yersinia pestis* low calcium response. *J. Bacteriol.* 173:7293–7303.

Portnoy, D.A., and S. Falkow. 1982. Virulence-associated plasmids from *Yersinia enterocolitica* and *Yersinia pestis. J. Bacteriol.* 148:877–883.

Portnoy, D.A., H.F. Blank, D.T. Kingsbury, and S. Falkow. 1983. Genetic analysis of essential plasmid determinants of pathogenicity in *Yersinia pestis. J. Infect. Dis.* 148:297–304.

Portnoy, D.A., H. Wolf-Watz, I. Bolin, A.B. Beeder, and S. Falkow. 1984. Characterization of common virulence plasmids of *Yersinia* species and their role in the expression of outer membrane proteins. *Infect. Immun.* 43:108–114.

Regnery, R.L., B.E. Anderson, J.E. Clarridge, M.C. Rodriguez-Barradas, D.C. Jones, and J.H. Carr. 1992. Characterization of a novel *Rochalimaea* species, *R. henselae* sp. nov., isolated from the blood of a febrile, human immunodeficiency virus-positive patient. *J. Clin. Micro.* 30:265–274.

Riek, E.F. 1970. Lower Cretaceous fleas. *Nature.* 227:746–747.

Ross, H.H., C.A. Ross, and J.R. Ross. 1982. *A Textbook of Entomology*. 4th ed. New York: John Wiley and Sons.

Rothschild, M. 1965a. Fleas. *Sci. Amer.* 213:44–53.

———. 1965b. The rabbit flea and hormones. *Endeavour.* 24:162–168.

———. 1975. Recent advances in our knowledge of the order Siphonaptera. *Ann. Rev. Entomol.* 20:241–259.

Rothshchild, M., and J. Schlein. 1975. The jumping mechanism of *Xenopsylla cheopis:* 1. Exoskeletal structures and musculature. *Phil. Trans. Roy. Soc. Lond. B.* 271:457–490.

Sample, A.K., J.M. Fowler, and R.R. Brubaker. 1987. Modulation of the low-calcium response in *Yersinia pestis* via plasmid-plasmid interaction. *Microb. Path.* 2:443–453.

Shepherd, R. 1980. The European rabbit flea *Spilopsyllus cuniculi* (Dale) in Australia—Its use as a vector of myxomatosis. In: R. Traub and H. Starcke, editors, *Fleas;* Proceedings of the International Conference on Fleas; Peterborough, U.K.; June 1977. Rotterdam: A.A. Balkema. pp. 301–307.

Schwan, T.G., D. Thompson, and B.C. Nelson. 1985. Fleas on roof rats in six areas of Los Angeles County, California: Their potential role in the transmission of plague and murine typhus to humans. *Am. J. Trop. Med. Hyg.* 34:372–379.

Sodeinde, O.A., and J.D. Goguen. 1988. Genetic analysis of the 9.5-kilobase virulence plasmid of *Yersinia pestis. Infect. Immun.* 56:2743–2748.

Straley, S.C. 1988. The plasmid encoded outer-membrane proteins of *Yersinia pestis. Rev. Infect. Dis.* 10(suppl. 2):S323-S326.

Straley, S.C., and P.A. Harmon. 1984. *Yersinia pestis* grows within phagolysosomes in mouse peritoneal macrophages. *Infect. Immun.* 45:655–659.

Tabor, S.P., D.F. Williams, D.J. Germano, and R.E. Thomas. 1993. Fleas (Siphonaptera) infesting giant kangaroo rats (*Dipodomys ingens*) on the Elkhorn and Carrizo Plains, San Luis Obispo County, California. *J. Med. Entomol.* 30:291–294.

Thomas, R.E. 1988. A review of flea collection records from *Onychomys leucogaster* with observations on the role of grasshopper mice in the epizoology of wild rodent plague. *Great Basin Nat.* 48:83–95.

Thomas, R.E., A.M. Barnes, T.J. Quan, M.L. Beard, L.G. Carter, and C.E. Hopla. 1988. Susceptibility to *Yersinia pestis* in the northern grasshopper mouse (*Onychomys leucogaster*). *J. Wildlife Dis.* 24:327–333.

Thomas, R.E., M.L. Beard, T.J. Quan, L.G. Carter, A.M. Barnes, and C.E. Hopla. 1989. Experimental plague infection in the northern grasshopper mouse (*Onychomys leucogaster*) acquired by consumption of infected prey. *J. Wildlife Dis.* 25:477–480.

Traub, R. 1980. The zoogeography and evolution of some fleas, lice and mammals. In: R. Traub and H. Starcke, editors, *Fleas;* Proceedings of the International Conference on Fleas. Peterborough, U.K.; June 1977. Rotterdam: A.A. Balkema. pp. 93–172.

Traub, R. 1985. Coevolution of fleas and mammals. In: K.C. Kim, editor, *Coevolution of parasitic arthropods and mammals.* New York: John Wiley and Sons. pp. 295–437.

Twigg, G.I. 1978. The role of rodents in plague dissemination: A worldwide review. *Mammal Rev.* 8:77–110.

Westrom, D., and R. Yescott. 1975. Emigration of ectoparasites from dead California ground squirrels, *Spermophilus beecheyi* (Richardson). *Calif. Vector Views.* 22:97–103.

Williams, R.C. Jr., H. Gerwurz, and P.G. Quie. 1972. Effects of Fraction I from *Yersinia pestis* on phagocytosis in vitro. *J. Infect. Dis.* 126:235–240.

12. TICKS AND MITES AND THE AGENTS THEY TRANSMIT

Joseph Piesman and Kenneth L. Gage

INTRODUCTION

Ticks and mites are biologically distinct from the other arthropods that transmit pathogens to humans and animals. Although the majority of vectors are insects found within the phylum Arthropoda, subphylum Mandibulata, ticks and mites are in the subphylum Chelicerata (Chap.1).

Ticks and mites comprise the subclass Acari within the class Arachnida. The subclass Acari is further divided into the order Parasitiformes and the order Acariformes. The order Parasitiformes contains the ticks (suborder Ixodida) and many parasitic mites (suborder Mesostigmata) of medical and veterinary importance. Parasitic mites are also found in the suborders Astigmata and Prostigmata of the Acariformes. Mites are a remarkably diverse and large taxon. Approximately 35,000 species of mites have been described, but possibly 1 million species remain to be classified (Oliver 1989). The ticks are a relatively small group of about 850 species.

Morphology

The acarine body is divided into 2 sections, unlike the insects, which have 3 (Chap. 1). The business end, or "head," is called the gnathostoma (capitulum in ticks). This contains the mouthparts but no brain. The posterior part of the acarine is called the idiosoma, which contains the podosoma (legs) and the opisthosoma; the opisthosoma is analogous to the distinct abdomen of insects. Internally, the midgut dominates the body, with a fused synganglion acting as the central nervous system.

Life Cycle

The standard life cycle includes 3 life stages: larva, nymph, and adult. The larva has 6 legs; the nymph and adult each have 8 legs. Hard ticks (family Ixodidae) take 1 blood meal per life stage. The Ixodidae larva feeds once and molts to the nymph; the nymph feeds once and molts to the adult; the adult female feeds once, lays eggs, and dies. Soft ticks (family Argasidae) have more diverse life cycles. There can be several nymphal stages in Argasidae: females feed, lay eggs, feed again, and lay eggs several times. Even more diverse are the life cycles of mites, which can have a bewildering variety of nymphal stages.

Soft ticks generally feed quickly, obtaining blood from the host in a matter of minutes. Hard ticks generally stay attached for several days to hosts during a blood meal. Ticks are extremely long-lived with slow life cycles; there are reports of Argasidae going years or even decades between blood meals. The long-lived nature of these creatures and the difficulty of speeding up the life cycle in the laboratory have caused the field of molecular acarology to lag far behind molecular entomology. The importance of ticks and mites in transmitting pathogens demands the investment of more resources in this field.

DIRECT EFFECT OF MITES AND TICKS ON HEALTH

Ticks and mites have a wide-ranging direct effect on the health of humans and animals. Mites in particular are responsible for much misery in both the developing and developed worlds. Human scabies is caused by infestation by the human itch mite, *Sarcoptes scabei*. The egg-laying females of these mites burrow into the host's skin. Discomfort results not only from the burrowing action but also from allergic reactions to antigens produced by these mites. In veterinary practice, mite infestation and the resulting skin disease is called mange. Most domestic animals have their own varieties of skin infesting mites.

A primary cause of asthma is an allergic reaction to the cosmopolitan house dust mite *Dermatophagoides farinae*. Allergy to this mite is common in the United States, Japan, and Europe. Molecular characterization of the allergens produced by house dust mites is an active area of research (Evans 1992).

A direct effect of ticks on human and animal health is a condition known as *tick paralysis*. Certain tick species secrete toxins so powerful that just 1 tick can cause an ascending flaccid paralysis (tetraplegia). Removing the offending tick results in dramatic resolution of the paralysis. The Australian paralysis tick *(Ixodes holocyclus)* is perhaps the best-known tick that causes paralysis. The toxin secreted by *I. holocyclus* is a protein (yet to be characterized). In North America *Dermacentor andersoni* and *Dermacentor variabilis* cause paralysis in young children, and canine paralysis is a common occurrence. The soft ticks *Argas walkerae* and *A. persicus* can induce paralysis in chickens. An extensive literature review of tick paralysis is available (Gothe and Neitz 1991).

Obligate Intracellular Bacteria

Mites and ticks are often infected with obligate intracellular bacteria. A few of these small, nonmotile, gram-negative organisms are important agents of human or animal disease. Others, such as *Wohlbachia* spp., are probably harmless symbionts of their arthropod hosts.

These organisms are currently grouped together within the order Rickettsiales and are referred to collectively, if somewhat incorrectly, as "rickettsiae."

The following is a brief overview of the major groups of obligate intracellular bacteria that are associated with mites or ticks. More detailed reviews can be found in Weiss and Dasch (1981), Walker (1988), and Gage and Walker (1992).

Phylogeny

Classification of the families and genera of Rickettsiales is based on phenotypic characteristics, including the site of growth within the host cells, type of host cells attacked, and mode of reproduction; however, recent phylogenetic studies at the molecular level show that these phenotypic similarities are often due to convergence rather than as a result of shared descent (Weiss 1991).

Within the genus *Rickettsia*, the spotted fever and typhus groups are closely related to each other and more distantly related to the *Ehrlichia* and *Cowdria* (Weiss 1991; van Vliet 1992). The scrub typhus agent (*R. tsutsugamushi*) does not appear to be closely related to any members of the Rickettsiales, and Tamura et al. (1991) have suggested that it be placed in its own genus, *Orientia*. *Coxiella* is probably somewhat related to *Wohlbachia*, but neither of these intracellular bacteria appears to be significantly related to other genera within the order (Weiss 1991). The phylogenetic relationships of the 2 genera (*Anaplasma* and *Aegyptionella*) within the family Anaplasmataceae remain uncertain.

Rickettsiae

Rickettsia are typically coccoid to rod-shaped, grow free within the cytoplasm of host cells, and reproduce by simple binary fission. Lice, fleas, mites, and ticks are the primary vectors for these organisms. The primary reservoirs for acarine-borne *Rickettsia* are the vectors themselves. Vertebrate hosts are probably of minor importance as reservoirs for acarine-borne species, but in some instances they play an essential role as amplifying hosts (Chap. 4) for infecting mites and ticks. At least 7 species of tick- or mite-borne *Rickettsia* cause severe and occasionally fatal illness in humans, but many other species are thought to be relatively nonpathogenic for humans and other mammals. With the apparent exception of *R. bellii*, each of the different species of *Rickettsia* can be placed within one of 3 major serological groups (typhus, spotted fever, and scrub typhus groups).

Humans or animals are exposed to acarine-borne rickettsiae when they enter habitats in which infected mites or ticks are found. Individuals are often exposed while working or during recreational activities such as camping or hiking. Suburbanization of formerly rural areas that are good tick or mite habitats has caused an increasing number of people exposed to rickettsial infections and may be partially responsible for the increased number of Rocky Mountain spotted fever cases observed during the 1970s and 1980s. As discussed later, human alterations of natural environments are also responsible for the existence of many foci of scrub typhus, a mite-borne rickettsiosis of Southeast Asia and nearby islands. Similar environmental disturbances in other regions of the world will likely result in increased amounts of secondary brushy habitats preferred by many tick species. Heavy mouse infestations, often the result of unclean housing, can result in increased human risks of rickettsialpox.

General symptoms of rickettsial infection include rash, high fever, severe headache, chills, malaise, and myalgia. A black crusty lesion, or eschar, can appear at the site where the vector fed. Patients infected with *R. rickettsii* rarely develop eschars, but these lesions are common among individuals affected by other acarine-borne rickettsioses.

The primary site of attack in vertebrate hosts are the endothelial cells lining blood vessels. As rickettsiae multiply within these cells, they eventually destroy them, causing blood vessels to become "leaky"; this disruption of normal circulation leads to the characteristic rash. The precise mechanism of rickettsiae-induced cytopathogenicity has not been described, but there is some experimental evidence that rickettsial phospholipases or proteases play a role (Walker 1988).

Progress in rickettsiology has been linked closely to the development of new and improved techniques for rickettsial isolation and identification. Initially, the only strains of rickettsiae that could be identified were those that were pathogenic for guinea pigs. However,

after techniques were developed for cultivating rickettsiae in the yolk sacs of embryonated eggs, it became apparent that ticks were infected with previously unrecognized rickettsial strains that had very little or no pathogenicity for laboratory animals (McDade and Newhouse 1986).

Vaccine protection, complement fixation, and toxin-neutralization analyses demonstrated that most of these low virulence tick-borne strains were antigenically related to but distinct from the handful of pathogenic tick-borne rickettsiae known from around the world. These assays have been replaced almost completely by the microimmunofluorescence test of Philip et al. (1978). This test is the currently accepted method for distinguishing between rickettsial serotypes and identifying new serotypes (which have often been designated as separate species). Although microimmunofluorescence gives reliable results, the time, expense, and biosafety considerations involved in producing the reagents necessary to perform the assays can limit its performance to some research laboratories specializing in rickettsiology. One drawback to the test is that rickettsiae must first be isolated in tissue culture or embryonated eggs to provide sufficient material for serotype identification. Recently, a polymerase chain reaction/restriction fragment length polymorphism assay has been described that produces results similar to those obtained by the microimmunofluorescence test (Regnery et al. 1991; Beati et al. 1992). This assay has been used to identify rickettsial serotypes in tick tissues without preliminary isolation (Gage et al. 1994) and should be adaptable to specimens preserved in alcohol (Gage et al. 1992). Monoclonal antibodies have also been described that are group- and species-specific and can, therefore, be used to identify rickettsial serotypes in ticks (Walker 1988).

Tick-borne *Rickettsia*. With the exception of *R. canada* and *R. bellii*, all tick-borne species of *Rickettsia* belong to the spotted fever group (SFG). *R. canada* is a typhus group rickettsia that has been identified only in the rabbit tick, *Haemaphysalis leporispalustris* (Philip et al. 1982). This rickettsia does not appear to cause disease in humans, and a report of possible human infection with *R. canada* is suspect because of the lack of specificity of the serological test (Bozeman et al. 1970).

R. bellii was first isolated from *Dermacentor variabilis* collected in Arkansas (Philip et al. 1983). Little is known about this rickettsia, but it does not appear to belong to the typhus, spotted fever, or scrub typhus groups of rickettsiae. *R. bellii* is relatively common in *Dermacentor andersoni* and *D. variabilis* tick populations in different geographic regions of the United States. There is no evidence that it causes disease in humans.

The remaining tick-borne rickettsiae belong to the spotted fever group. This group has an almost worldwide distribution and contains 5 of the 6 acarine-borne species of *Rickettsia* that are pathogenic for humans (Burgdorfer 1980; Walker and Fishbein 1991). *R. rickettsii*, the etiologic agent of Rocky Mountain spotted fever, exists in North, Central, and South America. The primary vectors of the highly pathogenic R-like serotype of *R. rickettsii* in the United States and Canada are *Dermacentor andersoni* and *D. variabilis*. *Haemaphysalis leporispalustris* is the primary vector of the less virulent Hlp-like serotype in these same areas. *R. rickettsii* has been identified in *Amblyomma cajennense* and *H. leporispalustris* ticks in Central America and in *A. cajennense* and *A. striatum* in South America. *A. americanum* is often cited as a vector in North America, but there is little evidence that this tick is naturally infected with *R. rickettsii*. *R. conorii* or closely related serotypes are the etiologic agents of Boutonneuse fever and similar illnesses referred to by various regional names in southern Europe, Africa, the Middle East, and India. The primary vector of classical Boutonneuse fever is *Rhipicephalus sanguineus*. Potential vectors in other areas include other *Rhipicephalus* spp., *Amblyomma*, *Haemaphysalis*, *Hyalomma*, *Boophilus*, *Ixodes*, and *Dermacentor*. The wide range of vectors may actually result from the existence of previously unrecognized serotypes that have been confused with *R. conorii* (Kelly and Mason 1990). *R. sibirica* is found in northern Asia, where it causes North Asian tick typhus. The primary vectors of *R. sibirica* are various species of *Dermacentor* and *Haemaphysalis*. *R. australis* is the etiologic agent of Queensland tick typhus, which occurs in Queensland, Australia. The primary vector is *Ixodes holocyclus*, which feeds not only on small marsupials but on a variety of other species, including man. *R. japonica* is a recently discovered SFG rickettsia that causes human disease in some regions of Japan (Gage and Walker 1992).

Each of the pathogenic SFG rickettsiae has its own characteristic geographic range, tick vectors, and associated small mammal host species; however, the ecological cycles are basically similar for all of these species (Burgdorfer 1980). Our basic understanding of the natural history of tick-borne rickettsioses can be traced back to Ricketts's classic studies of Rocky Mountain spotted fever in western Montana during the early 1900s. Although Ricketts did not isolate the spotted fever agent, he demonstrated that ticks could transmit rickettsial disease. His experiments demonstrated that infected ticks passed rickettsiae from one life cycle stage to the next by either transstadial or transovarial transmission. These results led him to conclude correctly that ticks were the primary reservoirs of *R. rickettsii*. Ricketts also hypothesized that wild rodents could become infected with the spotted fever agent and serve as sources of infection for ticks. Experimental support for this hypothesis was reported more than 50 years later by Burgdorfer et al. (1966).

Transstadial and transovarial transmission are highly efficient mechanisms for maintaining rickettsiae in nature. Transstadial transmission is possibly close to 100% efficient. Transovarial transmission is also highly efficient, with infected female *D. andersoni* transmitting *R. rickettsii* to 30–100% of their progeny. Such high rates of transmission suggest that tick-borne rickettsiae can be maintained indefinitely via transstadial and transovarial transmission, but this assumption has been questioned by McDade and Newhouse (1986). These authors hypothesize that lines of rickettsiae-infected ticks are likely to die out over time because *D. andersoni* ticks infected with *R. rickettsii* have much lower survival and fecundity rates than uninfected ticks. These observations suggest that some mechanism of horizontal transmission must exist if the percentage of infected ticks in an area is to remain relatively constant.

There is evidence that horizontal infection can occur when uninfected ticks feed on rickettsemic hosts (McDade and Newhouse 1986). After being ingested by a feeding tick, rickettsiae invade and multiply within cells of the midgut epithelium. They then escape from the midgut and invade hemocytes within the hemocoel (Chap. 23). Infected hemocytes transport rickettsiae to other tick tissues, including those in the salivary glands and reproductive organs. To transmit rickettsiae to a susceptible host during a blood meal, the tick's salivary glands must be infected. Likewise, transovarial transmission is possible only after the rickettsiae becomes established in the ovaries of adult female ticks. Venereal transmission of rickettsiae from infected male ticks to female ticks during mating apparently does not occur.

Horizontal transmission of rickettsiae via feeding of ticks on infectious host animals is less efficient than transstadial and transovarial transmission. Some hosts may circulate insufficient quantities of rickettsiae to infect ticks because they are naturally resistant or because they have survived a previous infection and are immune (McDade and Newhouse 1986). Infected mammals are rickettsemic for only a few days and, therefore, provide limited opportunities for ticks to become infected. Feeding must take place during periods of peak rickettsemia to ensure that sufficient numbers of rickettsiae are ingested to breach the "gut barrier" and establish a generalized infection (Burgdorfer et al. 1966).

Evidence suggests that tick species are usually hosts for more than 1 serotype of rickettsiae. These organisms cannot be readily distinguished by light microscopy using standard staining techniques such as the Gimenez method; they must be differentiated using the more involved techniques described earlier. The diversity of rickettsiae within a small geographic area is well illustrated by the observation that *D. andersoni* ticks in western Montana were infected with *R. bellii* and 4 different species of SFG rickettsiae (*R. rickettsii* R-like, *R. rickettsii* Hlp-like, *R. montana*, and *R. rhipicephali*). Less than 10% of the more than 3700 ticks examined by hemolymph test were infected with rickettsiae. These results suggest that there is only a slight chance that any tick within a population will be infected with a pathogenic rickettsia capable of causing disease in humans.

Although a given tick species within a geographic area may harbor more than 1 serotype of *Rickettsia*, there is virtually no evidence that individual ticks are infected with more than 1 serotype at a time. Burgdorfer et al. (1981) presented experimental evidence that infection of ticks with 1 serotype may interfere with the establishment of another serotype in the same host tick. Ticks on the east side of the Bitterroot Valley were infected transovarially with a spotted fever group rickettsia that was distinct from the serotypes identified previously on the west side of the valley by Philip and Casper (1981) and others. This rickettsia, which has been designated East Side Agent, is apparently rare on the west side of the Bitterroot Valley but infects more than 80% of the ticks on the east side. Ticks infected transovarially with the East Side Agent could be superinfected with *R. rickettsii* by feeding them on an infected animal, but the latter rickettsia did not invade the ovaries of adult female ticks that were infected with the East Side Agent. Because *R. rickettsii* fails to establish itself in the ovaries of ticks infected with East Side Agent, transovarial transmission does not occur. *R. rickettsii* also failed to become established in lines of ticks infected with *R. rhipicephali* or *R. montana*. This suggests that the phenomenon might be more general and that rickettsial interference could be an important mechanism determining the focality of *R. rickettsii* and other rickettsial serotypes.

Mite-borne *Rickettsiae*. The only mite-borne member of the spotted fever group of rickettsiae is *R. akari*. This rickettsia was first recognized in New York City in 1946 when many residents of a housing complex became ill following infection with a previously unrecognized spotted fever group rickettsia (Lackman 1963; Brettman et al. 1984). The vectors for this agent are nymphal and adult *Liponyssoides sanguineus*, a common ectoparasitic mite of house mice. Transovarial transmission of *R. akari* occurs in these mites. Larval *L. sanguineus* can be infected by transovarial transmission but do not feed on blood, and therefore cannot transmit the infection to vertebrates. Horizontal transmission occurs when uninfected mites feed on rickettsemic house mice. Wild house mice recover from infection and presumably acquire long-term immunity to further infection. Thus, vertebrates appear to be amplifying hosts, but not reservoirs, for *R. akari*.

Relatively little is known about the distribution and possible extramurine cycles of *R. akari*. This rickettsiae probably exists in most areas in which house mice are infested with *L. sanguineus*. Isolates have been reported from the United States and former Soviet Union, and the existence of rickettsialpox in Africa and Central America is suggested on the basis of clinical evidence. A single isolate from a field vole (*Microtus fortis pelliceus*) in South Korea suggests that this rickettsia may be maintained in nature by vectors and rodent hosts other than *L. sanguineus* and house mice (Burgdorfer 1980).

R. tsutsugamushi is the etiologic agent of scrub typhus and has been assigned its own serological group (the scrub typhus group) consisting of 3 major serotypes: Karp, Kato, and Gilliam (Traub and Wisseman 1974). Scrub typhus is transmitted to vertebrates by the larval stages of various species of trombiculid mites (chiggers) within the genus *Leptotrombidium*. Only larval *Leptotrombidium* are parasitic on vertebrates; nymphal and adult stages feed on eggs, quiescent stages, or recently dead carcasses of other small arthropods. The principal hosts of *Leptotrombidium* larvae in most scrub typhus foci are various species of field rats (*Rattus* spp.), but smaller rodents (voles and mice), insectivores, and birds can be important in some areas.

The primary reservoirs of *R. tsutsugamushi* are the mite vectors, which maintain the rickettsiae by transstadial and transovarial transmission. The efficiency of transovarial transmission varies greatly among the different species of *Leptotrombidium*. Uninfected mites can acquire rickettsiae after feeding on infected host animals. These ingested rickettsiae survive for at least 5–15 days but do not spread to the ovaries of adult female mites. Because the ovaries remain uninfected, transovarial transmission does not occur, and new lines of infected mites do not arise from the progeny of these females. Horizontal transmission through infectious feeding does not appear to be important. The possibility of venereal transmission has received little attention and should be investigated.

Scrub typhus is a highly focal disease that persists only in areas that have the 4 basic requirements of the zoonotic tetrad: *R. tsugamushi*, *Leptotrombidium deliense*–group mites, small mammal hosts, and secondary or transitional vegetation (scrub) growing on recently disturbed sites or the banks of waterways.

These restrictions on the distribution of scrub typhus largely result from the habitat requirements of the various species of *Leptotrombidium* vectors. These mites prefer areas that have high humidity, moderate to high air temperatures, abundant hosts for the parasitic larval stages, and moist soil conditions that provide adequate prey for the free-living nymphal and adult stages. These conditions are best fulfilled in areas in which vegetation has been removed and replaced by secondary vegetation or scrub that consists of various mixtures of grasses, herbs, and smaller woody species. Clearing land for agriculture, logging of primary forests, abandonment of fields, and war are likely to lead to the formation of suitable conditions for establishments of scrub typhus foci.

Ehrlichia

Ehrlichia are coccoid, ellipsoidal, or pleomorphic organisms that, unlike *Rickettsia*, grow within membrane-bound vacuoles. As they multiply within these vacuoles, they form characteristic grapelike clusters, or morulae. Ehrlichia infect primarily circulating lymphocytes, but some species (*E. canis*, *E. chafeensis*, *E. sennetsu*, and *E. risticii*) infect primarily monocytes; others (*E. equi*, *E. phagocytophila*, and *E. ewingii*) are usually found in granulocytes. Platelets are the primary target cell for *E. platys*, a pathogen of dogs. Many of the recent advances in knowledge of ehrlichiae have been made possible by improved culture techniques that have allowed sufficient quantities of organisms to be grown for serological and molecular analyses (Fishbein and Dawson 1991; Ristic et al. 1991).

Interest in *Ehrlichia* has increased greatly during the last decade because of the discovery that 2 previously unknown ehrlichiae, *E. chafeensis* and *E. risticii*, were the etiologic agents, respectively, of recently recognized diseases in humans (human ehrlichiosis) and horses (monocytic equine ehrlichiosis). At least 3 species of ehrlichiae have been shown to be transmitted by ticks under natural or experimental conditions, and ticks remain likely vectors for other ehrlichiae, including *E. chafeensis*.

Canine ehrlichiosis. *E. canis*, the etiologic agent of canine ehrlichiosis, was 1st observed in 1935 in leucocytes of tick-infested dogs in Algeria. The disease has since been found in most regions of the world in which the primary vector (*R. sanguineus*) and its host, the domestic dog, are found. The disease was thought to be mild, but outbreaks in military working dogs during the Vietnam War resulted in hundreds of cases of morbidity and mortality. It is now known that the severity depends at least in part on the breed of dog infected; beagles, Alsatians, and German shepherds are especially susceptible. Dogs suffering the most severe form of canine ehrlichiosis (tropical canine pancytopenia) develop an initial, relatively mild illness from which they appear to recover. Within 2–3 months after infection, susceptible breeds develop pancytopenia, severe thrombocytopenia, hemorrhage (including severe nosebleeds), peripheral edema, and emaciation.

The European brown dog tick, *Rhipicephalus sanguineus*, transmits *E. canis* to domestic dogs; ticks, in turn, become infected by feeding on infected dogs. Transstadial transmission occurs in infected *R. sanguineus* but not transovarial transmission. Dogs are probably important as long-term reservoirs as well as amplification hosts. Dogs have been reported to remain infected with *E. canis* for at least 5 years (Weiss and Dasch 1981). The importance of other canid species in the ecology of *E. canis* is uncertain, but there is serological evidence suggesting that wild canids, such as coyotes and jackals, may be reservoirs of infection.

Canine granulocytic agent. The canine granulocytic agent, *E. ewingii*, was initially thought to be a form of *E. canis* but has since been described as a separate species. The resulting illness is less severe than that caused by *E. canis*, but a polyarthritis can occur in chronic cases. Little is known about the ecology of this agent, but *Amblyomma americanum* can be infected with *E. ewingii* and transmit the infection to dogs under experimental conditions.

Tick-borne fever. *Ehrlichia phagocytophila* causes a febrile illness in sheep and cattle in Europe. Infected animals suffer malaise, weight loss, and splenomegaly. This organism also has been reported to cause abortion in pregnant ewes. *Ixodes ricinus* is the vector of tick-borne fever and transmits *E. phagocytophila* transstadially but not transovarially. Both the tick and the vertebrate host appear to be reservoirs for the disease.

Human ehrlichiosis. The first identified case of human ehrlichiosis occurred in Arkansas in 1986 when a 51-year-old man became ill after being bitten by ticks (Walker and Fishbein 1991). Cases were initially identified on the basis of a 4-fold rise in titers to *E. canis* antigens in immunofluorescence assays. This led to speculation that the causative agent might be *E. canis*, but subsequent investigations resulted in isolation of a previously unrecognized ehrlichial organism that has been given the name *E. chafeensis* (Anderson et. al. 1991). Common symptoms of human ehrlichiosis include fever, headache, anorexia, rigors, thrombocytopenia, nausea, myalgia, and elevation of certain liver enzyme levels. Although ticks have not been definitely identified as vectors, most cases have a history that includes tick exposure, visiting rural areas, and onset during late spring and early summer. *Amblyomma americanum* appears to be a likely vector because the distribution of the majority of cases agrees well with the distribution of this tick.

Cowdria

Cowdria grow within membrane-bound vesicles, where they produce dense clusters of coccoid, ellipsoidal, or pleomorphic organisms. The only known species is *C. ruminantium*, which is the etiologic agent of "heartwater" disease. This severe disease causes high mortality in sheep, goats, and cattle in countries of sub-Saharan Africa and appears to have been introduced recently into the Caribbean (Kobold et al. 1992). *C. ruminantium* infects primarily the endothelium within the heart, brain, and spleen; however, lymphocytes and phagocytic cells can also be infected. Infected animals exhibit hydropericardium (heartwater); high fever; lacrimation; anorexia; depression; and signs of central nervous system involvement, including hypersensitivity to stimuli, exaggerated movements, and convulsions in severe cases. The primary vector is *Amblyomma hebraeum*, but other *Amblyomma* spp. have been demonstrated to be experimental vectors. Transstadial transmission of *C. ruminantium* occurs in ticks, but transovarial transmission is rare or nonexistent. An adult male *A. hebraeum* acquires *C. ruminantium* by feeding on an infected host, detaching from that host, and then reattaching shortly thereafter to another host, where it can transmit the infection (Andrew and Norval 1992). Domestic animals can be chronically infected and are potential reservoir hosts, but the primary reservoirs are thought to be wild ungulates. Recent advances in *Cowdria* research have been reviewed by Jongejan (1990).

Anaplasma

Anaplasma spp. are primarily tick-borne intracellular bacteria that infect a variety of wild and domestic ungulates (Kuttler 1984). These infections can result in severe disease (anaplasmosis) with mortality approaching 50% of infected individuals.

Chronic or subacute infections are also common. The most important species are *A. marginale*, *A. ovis*, and *A. centrale*. The primary target cell in the vertebrate host is the erythrocyte in which *Anaplasma* grows as small round inclusions. Development of *Anaplasma* in ticks has been described by Kocan (1986). Both transstadial and transovarial transmission occur. More than 20 different species of ixodid ticks from a number of genera are thought to be vectors for *Anaplasma*, including *Boophilus* and *Dermacentor*. Mechanical transmission by biting flies or contaminated fomites also occurs but is probably of less importance in nature than transmission by ticks. Adult male ticks may play a role in transmission. When adult male ticks feed on hosts infected with *Anaplasma marginale* they can become infected, detach from the initial host, and then reattach and transmit *Anaplasma* to another host.

Aegyptionella

Aegyptionella pullorum causes aegyptionellosis in domestic fowl and wild birds. Like *Anaplasma*, this organism infects erythrocytes and forms inclusion bodies composed of large numbers of initial bodies. The disease is most severe in chickens and can cause high mortality. *A. pullorum* is transmitted to birds by *Argas* ticks. Transstadial and transovarial transmission have been documented.

Coxiella

The etiologic agent of Q-fever, *Coxiella burnetii*, infects a wide variety of vertebrate species, including humans. Recent reviews of Q-fever include those by Aitken et al. (1987) and Sawyer et al. (1987). Wild and domestic ungulates are the primary reservoirs and sources of infection for humans. The acute infections exhibit fever, pneumonitis, hepatic and bone marrow granulomas, meningo-encephalitis, and endocarditis. The chronic form of the disease may cause glomerulonephritis, osteomyelitis, and severe, potentially life-threatening endocarditis. Despite these potential complications, many *C. burnetii* infections are asymptomatic or subclinical.

C. burnetii is a small, pleomorphic, coccobacillary organism that infects host cell macrophages, where it grows within the phagolysosome. These organisms differ from the other organisms discussed in their ability to survive in an inactive state for months or years in widely varying external environments. Most vertebrate hosts become infected through inhalation of infectious aerosols or contact with infectious vertebrate host materials, such as milk, urine, feces, birth products, or contaminated hides or wool. Arthropod vectors appear to be relatively unimportant as sources of infection. *C. burnetii* is included because it commonly infects ticks and can be passed indefinitely in these arthropods by transstadial and transovarial transmission. Feces of infected ticks can contain large numbers of organisms that remain viable for up to a year. Although ticks may play a reservoir role for *C. burnetii*, these arthropods are probably not essential reservoirs for maintaining the infection in nature.

Tularemia Bacteria

Tularemia was first identified during a rodent epizootic in 1911 in Tulare County, California, but has since been found throughout much of the Northern Hemisphere. The causative agent (*Francisella tularensis*) was isolated by George McCoy and C.W. Chapin the following year. Clinical cases in humans were identified in 1914, and the name "tularemia" was proposed in 1921 by Edward Francis to recognize the site of its original discovery. Symptoms include a flulike illness with nonspecific aches, headache, chills, and fever. Many forms of the disease have been described on the basis of the site of initial invasion of the tularemia organism. The ulceroglandular form is the most common (about 80% of cases). In this form of the disease an ulcer forms at the site of inoculation (often a vector bite or cut on the hands) and may persist for months. The infection then spreads via the lymphatics to regional lymph nodes, causing swelling and often necrosis. From 30–60% of cases are fatal; the most severe form of the disease is the systemic form of tularemia, which is characterized by septicemia, toxemia, severe headache, and high fever (Hopla and Hopla 1994).

The *F. tularensis* organism is a small, nonmotile, gram-negative coccobacillus. There are 2 recognized biovars that differ in geographic distribution and virulence. The Type A biovar is found only in North America and causes more severe forms of the disease— about 5% of untreated cases are fatal. Type B biovar strains have a holarctic distribution and generally produce milder illness. Tularemia is transmitted by arthropod vectors (fleas, biting flies, mites, and, most important, ticks), ingestion of contaminated food or water, contact with contaminated soil, water, or other materials and contact with infected animals.

A wide array of mammals and birds (and even amphibians and fish) have been reported to be infected. But the number of hosts that are truly important as reservoirs or sources of infection for arthropod vectors or other vertebrates, including humans, forms a much smaller list of species. Leporids (rabbits and hares), microtine rodents (voles, lemmings, and muskrats), beavers, sciurids (squirrel-like rodents), and domestic sheep are probably the most important mammalian hosts and have been associated with both large epizootics and human cases. Microtine rodents are especially interesting because they have been reported to be chronically infected and continuously shed viable *F. tularensis* in their urine (Bell and Stewart 1975). This results in contamination of water supplies and other materials and has been the source of extensive epidemics of tularemia in human populations; such epidemics are especially common in the Palearctic regions.

Ticks are important reservoirs and vectors for enzootic cycles of tularemia in both the Palearctic and Nearctic regions. Many species of *Amblyomma*, *Dermacentor*, *Haemaphysalis*, and *Ixodes* have been found to be naturally infected in both the Nearctic and Palearctic. Transstadial transmission occurs in ticks, but transovarial transmission is considered to be unimportant. There is some debate about the fate of tularemia

organisms in ticks. Most agree that *F. tularensis* multiplies within tick larvae, nymphs, and adults; some have reported that tularemia organisms can penetrate the gut of ticks, invade the hemocoel, and infect the salivary glands. Transmission to vertebrate hosts by ticks presumably occurs either through inoculation of *F. tularensis* along with tick saliva during feeding or through contamination of the feeding site with infective tick feces. Ticks are the most important means of transmission of tularemia to humans in areas such as the south central and Rocky Mountain regions of the United States, but are less important than biting flies in California, Utah, and Nevada. Tick-borne transmission of tularemia to humans in Palearctic regions is considered to be of secondary importance to other sources of exposure, such as contaminated water supplies (Hopla 1974; Jellison 1974; Stewart 1991).

Borrelia

Relapsing Fever

Relapsing fever spirochetes in the genus *Borrelia* have ravaged residents of Africa for centuries. Indeed, this scourge was first reported by David Livingstone in 1854 (Hoogstraal 1981). The agent of African tick-borne relapsing fever, *Borrelia duttoni* (as opposed to louse relapsing fever; *B. recurrentis*), is transmitted to humans by the Argasid tick *Ornithodoros moubata*. Humans are the sole reservoir of *B. duttoni*. Pigs can become involved in the ecology of relapsing fever in Africa by supporting populations of soft ticks in close proximity to human habitations (Walton 1964).

In North America, several species of relapsing fever spirochetes are transmitted by their respective soft tick vectors. *Ornithodoros hermsi* transmits *B. hermsi*, *O. turicata* transmits *B. turicatae*, and *O. parkeri* transmits *B. parkeri*. These relationships between vector and spirochete are quite specific. Attempts to infect 1 tick species with the spirochetes derived from another failed. The molecular basis for this specificity in the relapsing fever spirochete-vector relationship should prove an interesting topic for research.

Rodents are the reservoirs of North American relapsing fever. In the western United States infection occurs in spring or early summer when vacationing individuals return to recreational properties. During the winter, rodents often move into remote cabins not occupied by humans. The rodent-tick-rodent cycle is established as rodents nest in abandoned homes. When humans return, they are bitten by infected ticks. An interesting variation of this theme occurred at the North Rim of the Grand Canyon in 1973. The attic space of rustic tourist cabins provided the perfect habitat for the nests of chipmunks and pine squirrels. Within these pine cone heavens, populations of the soft tick *O. hermsi* became established. When a plague epizootic occurred, decimating these rodent populations, the ticks in the attics lost their principal hosts. Consequently, they headed downstairs and fed on the tourists. An outbreak of tick-borne relapsing fever resulted, with cases occurring in dozens of individuals (Boyer et al. 1977). A program of acaricidal spraying and rodent-proofing the cabins curtailed the epidemic.

The disease caused by relapsing fever spirochetes derives its name from alternating febrile (2–9 days) and afebrile (2–4 days) periods. The number of relapses ranges from 1–10, and spirochetemias coincide with the ability of the spirochetes to escape the humoral immune response. Relapsing fever spirochetes and African trypanosomes are similar in their ability to undergo antigenic variation. The ability of relapsing fever spirochetes to avoid the immune response is caused by a series of surface antigens (vmp) proteins. Apparently, a recombination event between an expression plasmid and a silent plasmid activates a new vmp gene, thus stimulating production of a new vmp protein (Barbour et al. 1991).

Lyme Disease

Until quite recently, *Borrelia* were thought to be primarily associated with Argasid ticks. A little-known *Borrelia* of cattle, *B. theileri*, had been reported to be transmitted by certain Ixodid ticks. But Dr. Willy Burgdorfer and colleagues revolutionized the study of *Borrelia* and the world of tick-borne diseases when they discovered spirochetes in the hard tick *Ixodes scapularis* in Shelter Island, New York (Burgdorfer et al. 1982). The *I. scapularis*–derived spirochetes proved to be a new spirochetal species, *Borrelia burgdorferi*. This new spirochete is now known to cause Lyme disease (or Lyme borreliosis), including the skin condition *erythema migrans*, arthritis, carditis, and neurologic disease (Steere 1989). Thousands of human cases of Lyme disease are reported annually in North America and Europe. Cases are also reported in Asia.

The principal vectors of *B. burgdorferi* are ticks in the *Ixodes ricinus* complex. In Europe, *I. ricinus* is the principal vector; in Asia, *I. persulcatus;* in the northeastern United States, *I. scapularis;* and in the western United States, *I. pacificus* (Lane et al. 1991). Rodents serve as the reservoirs of *B. burgdorferi*. Virtually all white-footed mice, *Peromyscus leucopus*, are infected with the Lyme disease spirochete in enzootic regions. Larval *I. scapularis* acquire the infection when feeding on an infected mouse, maintain the infection transstadially, and transmit the infection as nymphs. Although most infected nymphs feed on *P. leucopus*, thus maintaining the cycle, some nymphs feed on other hosts, including humans. Adult *I. scapularis* feed primarily on the white-tailed deer, *Odocoileus virginianus*. At the beginning of the 20th century, the white-tailed deer had been hunted almost to extinction in parts of North America and Europe. In addition, the removal of forested habitats through the expansion of agriculture caused the demise of North American and European deer populations. In the latter half of the 20th century, the reversion of agricultural lands to suburban forest and changes in hunting practices have caused an explosion of the deer population. The respective tick populations, *I. scapularis* in the northeastern United States and *I. ricinus* in Europe, have probably also increased. Economic and social changes associated with the industrial revolution and increasing human populations have increased the importance of tick-borne diseases near the end of the 20th century (Hoogstraal 1981).

Other Bacteria

For many years a tick-associated condition known as "lumpy wool" in sheep was thought to be caused by the fungus *Dermatophilus congolensis*. The etiologic agent is now classified as an Actinomycetales bacteria. A similar condition in cattle has been associated with the bite of *Amblyomma variegatum* (Matharon et al. 1989).

Viruses

A wide variety of viruses of humans and animals have been isolated from ticks. The principal tick-borne viruses causing human disease include tick-borne encephalitis (TBE), Crimean Congo hemorrhagic fever (CCHF), and Colorado tick fever (CTF). The primary tick-borne viruses causing disease in domestic animals include louping ill of sheep and African swine fever. In addition, various tick-borne viruses have been isolated from ticks associated with diverse wildlife (e.g., seabirds, cliff swallows, and camels).

Tick-Borne Encephalitis

TBE is caused by members of the Flavivirus family, transmitted in Europe by *I. ricinus* and in Asia by *I. persulcatus*. Previously, Russian spring summer encephalitis (RSSE), Omsk hemorrhagic fever (OMSK), central European encephalitis (CEE), Powassen encephalitis (POW), and Kyansur forest disease (KFD) were considered distinct entities but now are thought to be subtypes of TBE; the TBE complex consists of 12 viruses (Calisher 1988). Countries with high incidence rates of TBE include Russia, Austria, Germany, and Sweden.

To prevent potentially fatal TBE infections, a killed vaccine is administered to hundreds of thousands of individuals in Europe. The duration of immunity provided by this vaccine is limited; a ritual in endemic areas includes a boost of TBE vaccine prior to initiation of the summer holidays. The ecology and maintenance cycle of TBE are complicated and diverse; this diversity is a reflection of the vast territory in Eurasia over which TBE is endemic (Hoogstraal 1981).

Crimean Congo Hemorrhagic Fever

Crimean Congo hemorrhagic fever is caused by a virus in the family Bunyaviridae (Hoogstaal 1979). As the name suggests, the first record in modern times of this virus occurred in the Crimea during World War II. Changes in agriculture and hunting practices resulting from occupation allowed populations of hares and their associated tick *Hyalomma m. marginatum* to explode. The resultant epidemic affected about 200 people; 10% of the cases were fatal. Outbreaks of CCHF often occur during floods, wars, population movements, and agricultural changes, and are a reflection of human history during the 20th century (Hoogstraal 1981). The *H. marginatum* "complex" and *H. a. anatolicum* are of special importance as vectors to humans. Mammals are important as reservoirs, and birds are important as a source of blood for these ticks and as phoretic hosts, dispersing infected ticks to new areas.

Colorado Tick Fever

CTF is caused by a Coltivirus in the family Reoviridae. CTF virus exists in North America, and the closely related Eyach virus occurs in Europe. The classical vector of CTF is *Dermacentor andersoni*, which occurs in the Rocky Mountain area of the United States and Canada. In Colorado, the 2 principal reservoirs are the least chipmunk (*Tamias minimus*) and the golden-mantled ground squirrel (*Spermophilus lateralis*) (McLean et al. 1989). The illness caused by infection with CTF virus includes a distinct diphasic fever. The virus can be maintained in human erythrocytes for over 4 months postinfection. Five genotypes were found circulating in an enzootic area of Colorado (Brown et al. 1989).

Protozoa

The piroplasms are a group of protozoa transmitted by ticks. The 2 economocally important genera of piroplasms are *Babesia* and *Theileria*. The *Babesia* spp. undergo replication within vertebrate erythrocytes, whereas *Theileria* spp. are characterized by an exoerythrocytic cycle. Although piroplasms were thought to lack a sexual cycle in the tick, ultrastructural (Rudzinska et al. 1979) and genetic (Morzaria et al. 1992) evidence confirmed that piroplasms undergo a sexual cycle in the tick midgut. Piroplasms hold a special importance in vector-borne diseases. The first demonstration of transmission of a pathogen by an arthropod was the groundbreaking observation by Theobald Smith and F.L. Kilbourne (1893) that the etiologic agent of Texas cattle fever, *Babesia bigemina*, is transmitted by *Boophilus annulatus*.

Cattle Babesiosis

Babesia sporozoites transmitted by ticks directly enter cattle erythrocytes and replicate therein. The destruction of erythrocytes and resultant anemia are the primary pathology in cattle babesiosis; thus the name "redwater fever." The principal agents of cattle babesiosis include the large species *B. bigemina* and *B. major* as well as the small species *B. divergens* and *B. bovis*. Because the *Boophilus* vectors of cattle *Babesia* are 1-host ticks, meaning all 3 blood meals are taken on the same host, transovarial transmission of cattle *Babesia* within the tick is a prerequisite for survival of the pathogen. Larvae are infected transovarially, find a host, and molt to nymphs and adults on that animal. Both nymphs and adults transmit cattle *Babesia*. Curiously, young calves are more resistant to infection with cattle *Babesia* than are adult animals. The worst outbreaks of cattle babesiosis occur when older animals are moved from nonenzootic areas to tick-infested areas where the cycle is established. In Australia, animals are vaccinated at a young age with live *Babesia* organisms produced by passage through laboratory cattle. This expensive procedure could be avoided by the production of a subunit recombinant vaccine, which has been the target of recent study. In addition to cattle babesiosis, *Babesia* infecting equines, canines, caprines, and ovines is of concern to those in veterinary practice.

Human Babesiosis

Human babesiosis was thought to occur in isolated splenectomized individuals exposed to ticks infected with cattle *Babesia*; in the 1970s, however, individuals with intact spleens began to acquire infection from the rodent piroplasm *Babesia microti* (Spielman et al. 1985). The tick vector of human babesiosis proved to be the very same tick transmitting the Lyme disease spirochete, *I. scapularis*. Larval *I. scapularis* acquire piroplasms from infected rodents and subsequently transmit infection as nymphs to other rodents or people. Although some younger people have been infected with *B. microti*, older individuals are more at risk in endemic regions.

East Coast Fever (Theileriosis)

East Coast Cattle Fever is caused by infection with the piroplasm *Theileria parva*, and a principal tick vector in Africa is *Rhipicephalus appendiculatus*. *T. parva* is extremely pathogenic to cattle and has had a remarkable influence on the history of the development of the African continent. A total of 6 species of *Theileria* are recognized in African cattle, including *T. parva*, *T. annualta*, *T. mutans*, *T. taurotragi*, *T. velifera*, and *T. buffeli* (Young et al. 1992). The transmission cycles of *Theileria* depend on the species of African wildlife involved.

Filaria

Although ticks are not vectors of filarial nematodes of any medical or veterinary importance, tick-borne filaria have proven to be interesting animal models. The argasid tick *Ornithodoros tartakovskyi* transmits *Dipetalonema vitiae* to gerbils, a convenient laboratory host. In Europe, *I. ricinus* transmits the subcutaneous filaria *D. rugosicauda* to roe deer. In the United States, a microfilaria of exceptional size was found in *I. scapularis* from Shelter Island (Beaver and Burgdorfer 1984).

SUMMARY

Recent developments have brought tick-borne disease to the forefront in biomedical science. The discovery of new agents of human disease, for example, the Lyme disease spirochete and the agents of human ehrlichiosis and human babesiosi,s have provided tremendous energy and excitement to the field. As predicted by the recognized leading expert on tick-borne disease, the late Dr. Harry Hoogstraal, evolution of human society has caused dramatic changes in the landscape of tick-borne disease in the latter half of the 20th century. Modern molecular biologists and field-oriented classical biologists will find the field of tick biology and tick-borne disease a dynamic and fascinating topic for study.

REFERENCES

Aitken, I.D., K. Bogel, E. Cracea, E. Edlinger, D. Houwers, H. Krauss, M. Rady, J. Rehacek, H.G. Schiefer, I.V. Tarasevich, and G. Tringali. 1987. Q fever in Europe: Current aspects of aetiology, epidemiology, human infection, diagnosis, and therapy. *Infection* 15:323–327.

Anderson, B.E., J.E. Dawson, D.C. Jones, and K.H. Wilson. 1991. *Ehrlichia chafeensis*, a new species associated with human ehrlichiosis. *J. Clin. Microbiol.* 29:2838–2842.

Andrew, H.R., and R.A. Norval. 1989. The role of males of the bont tick (*Amblyomma hebraeum*) in the transmission of *Cowdria ruminantium* (heartwater). *Vet. Parasitol.* 34:15–23.

Barbour, A.M., C.J. Carter, N. Burman, C.S. Feitag, C.F. Garon, and S. Bergstrom. 1991. Tandem insertion sequence-like elements define the expression for variable antigen genes of *Borrelia hermsii*. *Infect. Immun.* 59:390–397.

Beati, L., J. Finidori, B. Gilot, and D. Raoult. 1992. Comparison of serologic typing, sodium dodecyl sulfate-polyacrylamide gel electrophoresis protein analysis, and genetic restriction fragment length polymorphism analysis for identification of rickettsiae: Characterization of two new rickettsial strains. *J. Clin. Microbiol.* 30:1922–1930.

Beaver, P.C., and W. Burgdorfer. 1984. A microfilaria of exceptional size from the Ixodid tick, *Ixodes dammini*, from Shelter Island, New York. *J. Parasitol.* 70:963–966.

Bell, J.F., and S.J. Stewart. 1975. Chronic shedding tularemia nephritis in rodents: possible relation to occurrence of *Francisella tularensis* in lotic waters. *J. Wildlife Dis.* 11:421–430.

Boyer, K.M., R.S. Munford, G.O. Maupin, C.P. Pattison, M.D. Fox, A.M. Barnes, W.L. Jones, and J.L. Maynard. 1977. Tick-borne relapsing fever: An interstate outbreak originating at Grand Canyon National Park. *Am. J. Epidemiol.* 105:469–479.

Bozeman, F.M., B.L. Elisberg, J.W. Humphries, K. Runcik, and D.B. Palmer Jr. 1970. Serologic evidence of *Rickettsia canada* infection of man. *J. Infect. Dis.* 121:367–371.

Brettman, L.R., S. Lewin, R.S. Holzman, W.D. Goldman, J.S. Marr, P. Kechijian, and R. Schinella. 1984. Rickettsialpox: Report of an outbreak and a contemporary review. *Medicine* 60:363–371.

Brown, S.E., B.R. Miller, R.G. McLean, and D.L. Knudsen. 1989. Co-circulation of multiple Colorado Tick Fever virus genotypes. *Am. J. Trop. Med. Hyg.* 40:94–101.

Burgdorfer, W., V.F. Newhouse, E.G. Pickens, and D.B. Lackman. 1962. Ecology of Rocky Mountain spotted fever in western Montana: 1. Isolation of *Rickettsia rickettsii* from wild mammals. *Am. J. Trop. Med. Hyg.* 76:293–301.

Burgdorfer, W., K.T. Friedhoff, and J.L. Lancaster Jr. 1966. Natural history of tick-borne spotted fever in the U.S.A. *Bull. WHO* 35:149–153.

Burgdorfer, W. 1968. Observations on *Rickettsia canada*, a recently described member of the typhus group rickettsiae. *J. Hyg. Epid. Microbiol. Immunol.* 12:26–31.

Burgdorfer, W. 1970. Hemolymph test: A technique for detection of rickettsiae in ticks. *Am. J. Trop. Med. Hyg.* 19:1010–1014.

Burgdorfer, W., and L.P. Brinton. 1975. Mechanisms of transovarial infection of spotted fever rickettsiae in ticks. *Ann. N. Y. Acad. Sci.* 266:61–72.

Burgdorfer, W. 1980. The spotted fever-group diseases. In: James Steele, editor, *CRC handbook series in Zoonoses*. Boca Raton, FL: CRC Press. pp. 279–301.

Burgdorfer, W., S.F. Hayes, and A.J. Mavros. 1981. Nonpathogenic rickettsiae in *Dermacentor andersoni*: A limiting factor for the distribution of *Rickettsia rickettsii*. In: W. Burgdorfer and R.L. Anacker, editors, *Rickettsiae and rickettsial diseases*. New York: Academic Press. pp. 585–594.

Burgdorfer, W., A.G. Barbour, S.F. Hayes, J.L. Benach, E. Grunwaldt, and J.P. Davis. 1982. Lyme disease—a tick-borne spirochetosis? *Science* 216:1317–1319.

Burgdorfer, W., A.G. Barbour, S.F. Hayes, O. Peter, and A. Aeschlimann. 1983. Erythema chronicum migrans—a tick-borne spirochetosis. *Acta Tropica* 40:79–83.

Burgdorfer, W., S.F. Hayes, and D. Corwin. 1989. Pathophysiology of the Lyme disease spirochete, *Borrelia burgdorferi*, in Ixodid ticks. *Rev. Infect. Dis.* 11:S1442-S1450.

Calisher, C.H. 1988. Antigenic classification and taxonomy of Flaviviruses (Family Flaviviridae) emphasizing a universal system for the taxonomy of viruses causing tick-borne encephalitis. *Acta Virol.* 32:469–478.

Evans, R., 3rd. 1992. Environmental control and immunotherapy for allergic disease. *J. Allergy Clin. Immunol.* 90:462–468.

Fishbein, D.B., and J.E. Dawson. Ehrlichiae. 1991. In: A. Balows, W.J. Hausler Jr., K.L. Herrman, H.D. Isenberg, and H.J. Shadomy, editors, *Manual of clinical microbiology*, 5th ed. Washington, DC: Amer. Soc. for Microbiol. pp. 1054–1058.

Gage, K.L., R.D. Gilmore, R.H. Karstens, and T.G. Schwan. 1992. Detection of *Rickettsia rickettsii* in saliva, hemolymph and triturated tissues of infected *Dermacentor andersoni* ticks by polymerase chain reaction. *Mol. Cell. Probes.* 6:333–341.

Gage, K.L., and D.H. Walker. 1992. Rickettsiae. In: D. Greenwood, R.C.B. Slack, and J.F. Peutherer, editors, *Medical microbiology*. New York: Churchhill Livingstone. pp. 447–457.

Gage, K.L., M.E. Schrumpf, R.H. Karstens, W. Burgdorfer, and T.G. Schwan. 1994. DNA typing of rickettsiae in naturally infected ticks using a PCR-RFPL typing system. *Am J. Trop. Med. Hyg.* 50:247–260.

Gothe, R., and A.W.H. Neitz. 1991. Tick paralyses: Pathogenesis and etiology. *Adv. Dis. Vector Res.* 8:177–204.

Hayes, S.F., W. Burgdorfer, and A. Aeschlimann. 1980. Sexual transmission of spotted fever group rickettsiae by infected male ticks: Detection of rickettsiae in immature spermatozoa of *Ixodes ricinus. Infect. Immun.* 27:638–642.

Hoogstraal, H. 1979. The epidemiology of tick-borne Crimean-Congo hemorrhagic fever in Asia, Europe, and Africa. *J. Med. Entomol.* 15:307–417.

Hoogstraal, H. 1981. Changing patterns of tickborne diseases in modern society. *Ann. Rev. Entomol.* 26:75–99.

Hoogstraal, H. 1985. *Argasid and Nuttallielid ticks as parasites and vectors.* Advanced Parasitology. London: Acad. Press. pp. 135–238.

Hopla, C.E. 1974. The ecology of tularemia. *Adv. Vet. Sci. Comp. Med.* 18:25–53.

Hopla, C.E., and A.K. Hoplea. 1994. Tularemia. In: G.W. Beran and J. H. Steele, editors, *Handbook of Zoonoses.* 2nd ed. Section A. Bacterial, Rickettsial, Chlamydial, and Mycotic Diseases. Boca Raton, FL: CRC Press. pp. 113–126.

Jellison, W.L. 1974. *Tularemia in North America.* Missoula, MT: Univ. Montana Foundation. 276 p.

Jongejan, F. 1990. *Tick/host interactions and disease transmission with special reference to Cowdria ruminantium (Rickettsiales).* Netherlands: University of Utrecht. 194 p.

Kelly, P.J., and P.R. Mason. 1990. Serological typing of spotted fever group rickettsia isolates from Zimbabwe. *J. Clin. Microbiol.* 28:2302–2304.

Kocan, K.M. 1986. Development of *Anaplasma marginale* Theiler in Ixodid ticks: Coordinated development of a rickettsial organism and its tick host. In: J.R. Sauer and J.A. Hair, editors, *Morphology, physiology, and behavioral biology of ticks.* Ellis Horwood series in acarology. Chichester: Ellis Horwood, Ltd. pp. 472–505.

Kocan, K.M., W.L. Goff, D. Stiller, W. Edwards, S.A. Ewing, P.L. Claypool, T.C. McGuire, J.A. Hair, and S.J. Barron. 1993. Development of *Anaplasma marginale* in salivary glands of male *Dermacentor andersoni. Amer. J. Vet. Res.* 54:107–112.

Krantz, G.W. 1978. *A manual of acarology.* 2nd ed. Corvallis: Oregon State University Book Stores.

Kuttler, K.L. 1984. *Anaplasma* infections in wild and domestic ruminants: A review. *J. Wildlife Dis.* 20:12–20.

Lackman, D.B. 1963. A review of information on rickettsialpox in the United States. *Clin. Pediatrics* 2:296–301.

Lane, R.S., J. Piesman, and W. Burgdorfer. 1991. Lyme Borreliosis: Relation of its causative agent to its tick vectors and hosts in North America and Europe. *Ann. Rev. Entomol.* 36:587–609.

Matharon, C., N. Barre, F. Rogar, B. Rogez, D. Martinez, and C. Shaikboudou. 1989. *Dermatophilus congolensis* bovine dermatophilosis in the French West Indies: 3. A comparison between infected and noninfected cattle. *Rev. Elev. Med. Vet. Pays. Trop.* 42:331–347.

McDade, J.E., and V.F. Newhouse. 1986. Natural history of *Rickettsia rickettsii. Ann. Rev. Microbiol.* 40:287–309.

McLean, R.G., R.B. Shriner, K.S. Pokorny, and G.S. Bowen. 1989. The ecology of Colorado tick fever in the Rocky Mountain National Park in 1974: 3. Habitats supporting the virus. *Am. J. Trop. Med. Hyg.* 40:86–93.

Morzaria, S.P., J.R. Young, P.R. Spooner, T.T. Dolan, A.S. Young, and R.R. Bishop. 1992. Evidence of sexual cycle in *Theileria parva* and characterization of the recombinants. In: U.G. Munderloh and T.J. Kurtti, editors, *First international conference on tick-borne pathogens at the host-vector interface: An agenda for research.* 15–18 September 1992. Saint Paul, Minnesota. Saint Paul, MN: University of Minnesota College of Agriculture. pp 71–74.

Oliver, J.H., Jr. 1989. Biology and systematics of ticks (Acari: Ixodidae) *Ann. Rev. Ecol. Syst.* 20:397–430.

Philip, R.N., E.A. Casper, W. Burgdorfer, R.K. Gerloff, L.E. Hughes, and E.J. Bell. 1978. Serological typing of rickettsiae of the spotted fever group by microimmunofluorescence. *J. Immunol.* 121:1961–1968.

Philip, R.N., and E.A. Casper. Serotypes of spotted fever group rickettsiae isolated from *Dermacentor andersoni* (Stiles) ticks in western Montana. *Am. J. Trop. Med. Hyg.* 30:230–238.

Philip, R.N., E.A. Casper, R.L. Anacker, M.G. Peacock, S.F. Hayes, and R.S. Lane. 1982. Identification of an isolate of *Rickettsia canada* from California. *Am. J. Trop. Med. Hyg.* 31:1216–1221.

Philip, R.N., E.A. Casper, R.L. Anacker, J. Cory, S.F. Hayes, W. Burgdorfer, and C.E. Yunker. 1983. *Rickettsia bellii* sp. nov.: a tick-borne rickettsia, widely distributed in the United States, that is distinct from the spotted fever and typhus biogroups. *Internat. J. Syst. Bacteriol.* 33:94–106.

Ristic, M., C.J. Holland, and M. Khondowe. 1991. An overview of research on ehrlichiosis: 4th international symposium on rickettsiae and rickettsial diseases. *Eur. J. Epid.* 7:246–252.

Regnery, R.L., C.L. Spruill, and B.D. Plikaytis. 1991. Genotypic identification of rickettsiae and estimation of intraspecies sequence divergence for portions of two rickettsial genes. *J. Bacteriol.* 173:1576–1589.

Rudzinska, M.A., A. Spielman, R.F. Riek, S.J. Lewengrub, and J. Piesman. 1979. Intraerythrocytic "gametocytes" of *Babesia microti* and their maturation in ticks. *Can. J. Zool.* 47:424–434.

Sauer, J.R., and J.A. Hair, eds. 1986. *Morphology, physiology, and behavioral biology of ticks.* Ellis Horwood series in acarology. Chichester: Ellis Horwood, Ltd. 510 p.

Sawyer, L.A., D.R. Fishbein, and J.E. McDade. 1987. Q fever: Current Concepts. *Rev. Infect. Dis.* 9:935–946.

Smith, T., and F.L. Kilbourne. 1893. Investigations into the nature, causation, and prevention of southern cattle fever. *US Dept. Agric. Bur. Anim. Ind. Bull.* 1:1–301.

Sonenshine, D.E. 1991. *Biology of Ticks, Volume 1.* New York: Oxford University Press. 447 p.

Spielman, A., M.L. Wilson, J.L. Levine, and J. Piesman. 1985. Ecology of *Ixodes dammini*-borne human babesiosis and Lyme disease. *Ann. Rev. Entomol.* 30:439–460.

Steere, A.C. 1989. Lyme Disease. *N. Engl. J. Med. 321*:586–596.

Stewart, S.J. 1991. *Francisella.* In: Balows, A., W.J. Hausler, K.L. Herrmann, H.D. Isenberg, and H.J. Shodomy, editors, *Manual of clinical microbiology.* Washington, D.C.: American Society for Microbiology. pp. 454–456.

Tamura, A., H. Urakami, and N. Osashi. 1991. *Rickettsia tsutsugamushi* and the other group of rickettsiae: 4th international symposium of rickettsiae and rickettsial diseases. *European J. Epid.* pp. 259–269.

Van Vliet, A.H., F. Jongehan, and B.A. van der Zeijst. 1992. Phylogenetic position of *Cowdria ruminantium* (Rickettsiales) determined by analysis of amplified 16S ribosomal DNA sequences. *Int. J. Syst. Bacteriol.* 42:494–498.

Walker, D.H., ed. 1988. *Biology of Rickettsial Diseases*, vols. 1 and 2. Boca Raton, FL: CRC Press.

Walker, D.H., and D.B. Fishbein. 1991. Epidemiology of rickettsial diseases: 4th international symposium on rickettsiae and rickettsial diseases. *Eur. J. Epid.* 7:237–245.

Walton, G.A. 1964. The *Ornithodoros "moubata"* group of ticks in Africa, control problems and implications. *J. Med. Entomol.* 1:53–64.

Weiss, E., and G.A. Dasch. 1981. The family Rickettsiaceae: Pathogens of domestic animals and invertebrates; nonpathogenic arthropod symbiotes. In: M.P. Starr, H. Stolp, H.G. Truper, A. Balows, and H.G. Schlegel, editors, *The prokaryotes.* Berlin and Heidelberg: Springer-Verlag. pp. 2161–2171.

Weiss, E. 1991. Rickettsiae and Chlamydiae: Taxonomy, Section 7. In: A. Balows, W.J. Hausler, K.L. Herrmann, H.D. Isenberg, and H.J. Shadomy, editors, *Manual of clinical microbiology,* 5th ed. Washington, D.C.: American Society for Microbiology. pp. 1033–1035.

Young, A.S., M.K. Shaw, H. Ochanda, S.P. Morzaria, and T.T. Dolan. 1992. Factors affecting the transmission of African *Theileria* species of cattle by Ixodid ticks. In: U.G. Munderloh and T.J.Kurtti, editors, *First international conference on tick-borne pathogens at the host-vector interface: An agenda for research.* 15–18 Sept. 1992. Saint Paul. Saint Paul: University of Minnesota College of Agriculture. pp. 65–70.

13. GENOME ORGANIZATION OF VECTORS

Dennis L. Knudson, Liangbiao Zheng, Scott W. Gordon,
Susan E. Brown, and Fotis C. Kafatos

INTRODUCTION

From Genes to Genomes: The Emergence of Genome Studies

In the latter half of the 20th century, the combination of genetics with biochemistry and crystallography revolutionized biology, facilitating our current understanding of life at the molecular level. The rapid accumulation of knowledge concerning the structure of biological molecules or molecular complexes has been assisted by genetic manipulations, and in turn, structural characterization has guided efforts to understand in vivo function through studying the phenotypic consequences of targeted mutations. This interdisciplinary dialectic for analyzing structure and function is called molecular genetics.

Whereas molecular genetics focused initially on the study of individual genes and gene products, a more global approach has emerged: genomic analysis. Technical advances have made it possible to rapidly construct genetic maps for the entire genome of even previously neglected or experimentally recalcitrant organisms. Other advances have made it possible to map genomes physically, by assigning cloned DNA sequences to specific chromosomes and chromosomal regions, or even ordering these sequences in a systematic manner according to their relative position. It is

now possible to contemplate carrying physical mapping to its ultimate resolution: sequencing an entire genome of an organism. Although only viral genomes have been sequenced to date, it is safe to predict that we will soon have the complete genomic sequences of several model organisms: prokaryotic (*Escherichia coli* and *Bacillus subtilis*) as well as eukaryotic (the yeast *Saccharomyces cerevisiae*, the nematode *Caenorhabditis elegans*, the fruit fly *Drosophila melanogaster*, and the plant *Arabidopsis thaliana*). The most ambitious projects of genomic analysis focus on the large and complex genomes of higher vertebrates—mice and humans. In every case, genome projects involve both genetic and physical mapping, and they aim at the integration of these maps with the ultimate primary sequence map, the linear order of all bases (Fig. 13.1). Availability of this global information will facilitate and guide our analysis of how organisms work, especially because the databases correlating structure and function are now becoming so extensive that the likely function of a protein can be inferred by examining the sequence of its gene.

Even with the accelerated advances in technology, the enormity of genome analysis projects should not be underestimated. The genomes of higher eukaryotes consist of roughly 10^8 to 10^{10} bp (base pairs) and probably encompass 10^4 to almost 10^6 genes, or protein-coding

175

units. Effective mapping of these genomes requires consistent, well-planned, and complementary efforts of many laboratories. If probes and data generated are to be useful, then they must be accessible through well-structured repositories and databases. The advanced, previously mentioned genome projects on model organisms are supplying the tools and approaches for effectively studying the genome organization of selected vectors, and rapid progress has been made in 2 mosquitoes, *Aedes aegypti* and *Anopheles gambiae*. Profound advances in our understanding of the biology of vectors will come from these molecular genetic studies.

Importance of Aedes aegypti *and* Anopheles gambiae

Aedes aegypti

Aedes aegypti has become the equivalent of the laboratory rat to the vector biologist because of the ease with which it can be colonized. Although *Ae. aegypti* is an important natural vector of dengue and yellow fever, it also supports the development of a wide variety of viruses, filarial nematodes, and avian malarial parasites, making it well suited as a model for laboratory studies (Chap. 6). Numerous researchers have examined the vector competence of *Ae. aegypti* from various geographic regions for arboviruses, such as, Chikungunya virus (217), dengue (74, 207) and yellow fever (2, 11, 205). *Aedes aegypti* has also served as a laboratory host for many filarial nematodes, including *Brugia malayi* (12, 173), *Brugia pahangi* (57, 58, 39, 121), *Dirofilaria immitis* (36, 166), *Dirofilaria repens* (89), and *Foleyella flexicauda* (211). Additionally, many of the avian malarias, including *Plasmodium gallinaceum*, develop readily in *Ae. aegypti* (102).

Anopheles gambiae

Anopheles gambiae was initially thought to be a single species, but now 6 sibling species, *An. arabiensis*, *An. gambiae*, *An. melas*, *An. merus*, *An. quadriannulatus*, and *An. bwambae*, are recognized based on apparent reproductive isolation (52, 53, 232) (Chap. 5). Analysis of nurse cell polytene chromosomes demonstrates that different sibling species have characteristic differences in banding patterns (47). These species range widely in Africa, with the exception of *An. bwambae*, which is found only in mineral spring water. *Anopheles merus* and *An. melas* are saltwater mosquitoes that inhabit the east and west coasts of Africa, respectively; both can be found in the same region as either *An. arabiensis* or *An. gambiae*. *Anopheles gambiae*, *An. arabiensis*, and *An. quadriannulatus* are freshwater mosquitoes. The first 2 are sympatric in sub-Saharan Africa, although *An. gambiae* tends to inhabit humid forest savannas and *An. arabiensis* predominates in arid savannas. *Anopheles quadriannulatus* can be sympatric with *An. arabiensis*. Among the 6 sibling species, only *An. gambiae* and *An. arabiensis* are important vectors for human malaria because the other taxa are predominantly zoophilic or have too limited a distribution to be medically significant vectors.

One area of research that promises to be fruitful in the development of new strategies for malaria control is the analysis of interactions between the parasite and infected vector (223). *Anopheles gambiae* provides an excellent system for such studies because of its small genome, high-quality polytene chromosomes, and because there is extensive knowledge of its ecology and population biology. Although there are difficulties in working with this vector in the laboratory—including difficulties in rearing and maintenance, in pair mating, and the lack of a large number of mutants—some of these limitations can be overcome using experimental approaches of modern molecular genetics and biology.

Scope and Purpose

This chapter focuses on the strategies taken, initial findings, and future prospects for mapping disease vector genomes. Progress made in identifying genetic elements and determining their genome organization is reviewed. Strategies for linkage and physical mapping of disease vector genomes are discussed, and an overview of these approaches is presented (Fig. 13.1.). Questions unique to disease vectors are raised, including vector competence, parasite-vector interaction, population and vector control, evolution, and speciation of vectors. The importance of constructing genome maps for insect species of economic and medical importance has been discussed elsewhere in reviews by Craig and Hickey (48), Kitzmiller (103),

Overview of Genome Mapping

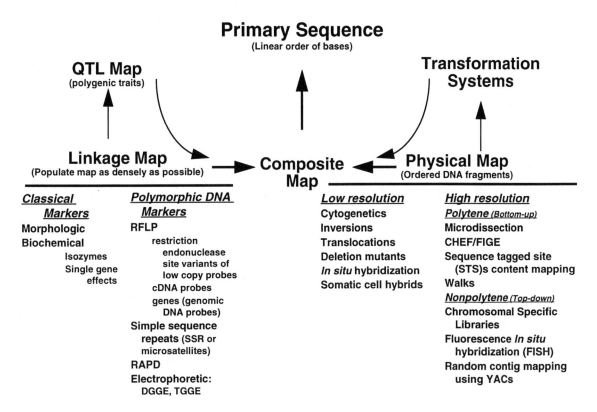

Primary Sequence
(Linear order of bases)

QTL Map
(polygenic traits)

Transformation Systems

Linkage Map
(Populate map as densely as possible)

Composite Map

Physical Map
(Ordered DNA fragments)

Classical Markers
Morphologic
Biochemical
   Isozymes
   Single gene effects

Polymorphic DNA Markers
RFLP
   restriction endonuclease site variants of low copy probes
   cDNA probes
   genes (genomic DNA probes)
Simple sequence repeats (SSR or microsatellites)
RAPD
Electrophoretic: DGGE, TGGE

Low resolution
Cytogenetics
Inversions
Translocations
Deletion mutants
In situ hybridization
Somatic cell hybrids

High resolution
Polytene (Bottom-up)
Microdissection
CHEF/FIGE
Sequence tagged site (STS)s content mapping
Walks
Nonpolytene (Top-down)
Chromosomal Specific Libraries
Fluorescence *In situ* hybridization (FISH)
Random contig mapping using YACs

13.1   Overview of genome mapping

Zraket et al. (242), Ashburner (6), and Heckel (78) and will not be reiterated here.

CYTOGENETIC ORGANIZATION

Genome Size and Other Physical Properties

Eukaryotic genomes are complex and consist of single copy, middle repetitive, and highly repetitive sequences. Genome size varies widely among organisms and reflects differences in the prevalence of these sequence classes. The mass of DNA in an unreplicated haploid genome, such as a sperm nucleus, is the genome size, or C-value. Nuclear genome size in eukaryotes is measured in picograms (10^{-12} g), where 1 picogram (pg) = 0.98×10^6 kb (kilobase) for double-stranded DNA (38). Although reassociation kinetics of denatured DNA strands is used frequently to determine genome size and composition (34), Feulgen cytophotometry is another commonly used method to determine genome size (59, 126).

Comparative studies of eukaryotic genomes indicate that there are 2 distinct types of genomes, according to the arrangement of repetitive DNA in relation to unique sequences. Short period interspersion describes a pattern in which single copy sequences, 1–2 kb in length, alternate with short (200–600 bp) or medium length (1–4 kb) repetitive sequences. This organization is characteristic of most higher eukaryotes, as typified by the frog *Xenopus* (26, 51). Genomes with long period interspersion consist of very long stretches (at least 13 kb) of effectively uninterrupted unique sequences bracketed by long usually >5 kb repetitive elements (127). This arrangement is characteristic of species with small (0.10–0.50 pg) genomes, such as *Drosophila* (127).

Cockburn and Mitchell (42) examined repetitive DNA interspersion patterns in several species of mosquitoes and other flies using recombinant libraries probed with genomic DNA. Five anopheline species showed a long period interspersion pattern similar to that described for *Drosophila melanogaster* (110) with about 18% of the genome composed of repetitive DNA. This figure is similar to that obtained by Black and Rai (26) for *An. quadrimaculatus*. Apparently, most of the anopheline repetitive DNA is not interspersed or is interspersed in less than 100 blocks per genome. In contrast, *Ae. aegypti* was found to have large amounts of interspersed repetitive DNA suggestive of the short period interspersion pattern (225). An intermediate pattern between short and long period interspersion types was observed in *Culex quinquefasciatus*. This genome consists of 20% unique and 80% repetitive sequences with little or no apparent interspersion of the 2 types (42), but Black and Rai (26) considered *Culex* to be of the short period type based on results using reassociation kinetics. The Culicidae represent the first example of a single taxonomic family with representatives of both long and short period genomic organization (26).

The genome size of disease vectors range from about 0.2–2 pg. The anopheline genomes are smaller generally than those of culicines (Table 13.1) and smaller genomes are associated with long period interspersion. The genome of some disease vectors are flexible, exhibiting variation in size within the same species, resulting from an increase of highly repetitive elements. For example, Rao and Rai (179) examined populations of *Aedes* species collected from various

locations around the world and found a 1.5-fold range of values. The 2 extreme strains of *Ae. albopictus* (Calcutta, 0.86 pg; Mauritius, 1.32 pg) showed differences in unique sequence content of only 2% (Calcutta, 36%; Mauritius, 34%). The genomic size differences were largely accounted for by the presence in the Mauritius strain of 1.5 times more foldback sequences and 2.7 times more highly repetitive sequences. In both strains, middle repetitive sequences were approximately equal.

Several studies have provided information on the DNA content of various species of mosquitoes and related Diptera (95, 179, 26, 107, 180) (Table 13.1). The lowest values were found in the subfamily Anophelinae ranging from 0.25 pg in *An. quadrimaculatus* to 0.34 pg in *An. freeborni*. Intermediate values were observed in the Toxorhynchitinae with 0.62 pg in *Toxorhynchites splendens*. The highest values and broadest variation occurred in the Culicinae, in which DNA content ranged from 0.54 pg in *Cx. quinquefasciatus* to 1.90 pg in *Ae. zoosophus*. Although little variation in genome size was observed between members of some genera (*Culiseta melanura*, 1.25 pg; *Cs. morsitans*, 1.21 pg), other genera showed significant differences. *Culex pipiens* was found to have nearly twice the DNA content as that of *Cx. quinquefasciatus*. In a study examining 23 species in the genus *Aedes*, DNA content ranged from a low of 0.59 pg in *Ae. pseudoscutellaris* to a high of 1.90 pg in *Ae. zoosophus* with the 2 highest values being found in the Protomacleaya subgenus (179). Among 7 species of the *scutellaris* taxonomic subgrouping, DNA content varied almost 2-fold from a low of 0.59 pg in *Ae. pseudoscutellaris* and *Ae. cooki* to a high of 1.28 pg in *Ae. katherinensis*. Size estimates of the *Ae. aegypti* genome range from 0.78 to 0.83 pg (179, 225).

Several studies have addressed intraspecific differences in the DNA content of *Aedes albopictus*, a recognized vector of dengue fever. This species is found on most of the islands in the Indian Ocean westward to Madagascar, almost all countries on mainland Asia, and most of the islands of the Pacific Ocean eastward to Hawaii. *Ae. albopictus* was recently introduced into the United States and quickly spread to become established in 20 states (76). Kumar and Rai (107) examined nuclear DNA content in 37 populations from

TABLE 13.1   Haploid genome size and complexity of disease vectors and others

Genus species	Strain	DNA pg	DNA Complexity Fold-back	Highly repeti-tive	Moder-ately repetitive	Unique	Reference
Aedes aegypti		0.81					(179)
Aedes aegypti	Bangkok	0.83		0.2	0.2	0.6	(225)
Aedes aegypti	Mos20 cell line	1.5		0.13	0.24	0.64	(225)
Aedes albopictus	8 strains	0.87–1.32					(179)
Aedes albopictus	Calcutta	0.86	0.1	0.17	0.37	0.36	(26)
Aedes albopictus	Mauritius	1.32	0.1	0.31	0.27	0.33	(26)
Aedes albopictus	37 strains	0.62–1.66					(108)
Aedes alcasidi		0.97					(179)
Aedes bahamensis		1.38					(179)
Aedes canadensis		0.90					(179)
Aedes caspius		0.99					(95)
Aedes cinereus		1.21					(179)
Aedes communis		1.01					(179)
Aedes cooki		0.59					(179)
Aedes excrucians		1.50					(179)
Aedes flavopictus		1.33					(179)
Aedes hebrideus		0.97					(179)
Aedes heischii		1.12					(179)
Aedes katherinensis		1.28					(179)
Aedes malayensis		0.94					(179)
Aedes metallicus		1.09					(179)
Aedes polynesiensis		0.73					(179)
Aedes pseudalbopictus		1.29					(179)
Aedes pseudoscutellaris		0.59					(179)
Aedes seatoi		0.97					(179)
Aedes stimulans		1.44					(179)
Aedes triseriatus		1.52					(179)
Aedes triseriatus		1.52	0.1	0.44	0.31	0.16	(26)
Aedes unilineatus		1.06					(179)

| Genus species | Strain | DNA pg | DNA Complexity | | | | Reference |
			Fold-back	Highly repeti-tive	Moder-ately repetitive	Unique	
Aedes zoosophus		1.90					(179)
Amblyomma americanum		1.08	0.04	0.18	0.42	0.36	(167)
Anopheles atroparvus		0.24					(95)
Anopheles freeborni		0.29					(95)
Anopheles gambiae	G3	0.27	0.06	0.33	0.33	0.6	(20)
Anopheles labranchiae		0.23					(95)
Anopheles quadrimaculatus		0.24	0.04	0.16		0.8	(26)
Anopheles quadrimaculatus		0.25					(180)
Anopheles stephensi		0.24					(95)
Armigeres subalbatus		1.24					(180)
Chaoborus americanus		0.40					(180)
Corethrella brakeleyi		0.47					(180)
Culex pipiens		1.02					(95)
Culex pipiens		0.54	0.11	0.38	0.29	0.22	(26)
Culex quinquefasciatus		0.54					(180)
Culex restuans		1.02					(180)
Culiseta litorea		1.06					(95)
Culiseta melanura		1.25					(180)
Culiseta morsitans		1.21					(180)
Haemagogus equinus		1.12					(180)
Mochonyx velutinus		0.58					(180)
Sabethes cyaneus		0.79					(180)
Toxorhynchites splendens		0.62					(180)
Wyeomyia smithii		0.86					(180)

Note: Genome sizes were determined by Feulgen cytophotometry in most references, except where genome complexity is reported, which was evaluated by reassociation kinetics.

around the world, including 12 recent introductions to the United States, and the populations were based upon the worldwide variation documented by Rao and Rai (179). There was no apparent correlation between geographic origin and nuclear DNA content even though a 3-fold variation in haploid DNA content was observed; populations from the same geographic areas often differed significantly from each other, whereas geographically separated populations were found to have similar DNA content. Populations from the most recently colonized regions, however, generally had higher DNA contents, and the highest values detected were from populations recently colonizing parts of the United States. Changes in nuclear DNA amounts can result from amplification of a preexisting sequence within the genome, transfer of a transposable element from another species, reverse transcription of an abundant RNA (retrotransposition), gene conversion, and unequal crossing over (42, 107, 130, 26). Kumar and Rai (107) theorized that each population has a DNA content that is imposed by the local microenvironment and that the variation observed in *Ae. albopictus* DNA content was a result of repetitive DNA sequences undergoing rapid change in response to that environment.

Chromosomal Organization

In most mosquitoes and nematocerous flies, the genome consists of 3 mostly metacentric chromosome pairs. With one exception, all species of Culicidae examined have a diploid chromosome number of 6 (2n = 6). (231, 78); however, in the anopheline *Chagasia bathana*, 2n = 8 (105). The usual chromosome arrangement is 2 sets of larger, metacentric or submetacentric autosomal chromosomes and 1 smaller set of metacentric sex-determining chromosomes. Among the 3 subfamilies of mosquitoes, only Anophelinae display sex chromosome dimorphism.

Rao and Rai (180) found a good correlation between chromosomal length and nuclear DNA content of 36 species of mosquitoes and members of closely related taxa. Total chromosome length was found to vary from 8.4 µm in *An. quadrimaculatus* to 38.3 µm in *Ae. zoosophus*, where an 8-fold difference in DNA content was accompanied by a 4.5-fold difference in chromosome

length. The increase in size was observed in all 3 chromosomes, and it was not confined to a particular set. Rai (176) studied mitotic chromosomes from numerous strains of *Ae. aegypti* and found the karyotype to be uniform. In laboratory-reared tsetse flies, there are supernumary chromosomes that are probably derived from 1 of 3 chromosome pairs. The function of these supernumary chromosomes is not clear.

The use of polytene chromosomes has been instrumental in studies of chromosomal aberrations and the localization of genes both by correlation of genetic and cytology and by molecular in situ hybridization of nucleic acid probes. Polytene chromosomes result from many rounds of DNA duplication without cytokinesisand are accompanied by alignment and condensation of the resulting DNA strands to form a specific pattern of bands and interbands. Polytene chromosomes can be found in many tissues, such as the salivary gland of larvae, midgut epithelium, Malpighian tubules, and nurse cells. Polytene chromosomes have been studied for many decades in *Drosophila* and have played a major role in the emergence of *D. melanogaster* as the genetically best-characterized higher eukaryote, having a well-correlated cytogenetic and genetic map. They have also played important roles in the study of population genetics and chromosomal evolution.

In anopheline mosquitoes, high quality squashes of polytene chromosomes can be obtained from the salivary glands of 4th instar larvae and from the nurse cells of half-gravid females (Fig. 13.2). A number of salivary gland chromosome maps for members of this genus have been published (103). The polytene chromosome banding patterns have been used extensively as markers for distinguishing species and ecotypes in the *An. gambiae* complex (47, 46).

In culicine mosquitoes, only *Cx. pipiens* has salivary gland polytene chromosomes, which are useful for mapping (212). Although large and well-banded polytene chromosomes can be found in tissues of several life stages of *Ae. aegypti*, attempts to manipulate them for cytogenetic examination have met with little success because they do not spread easily (48, 196a). This difficulty in preparing polytene chromosome spreads is due to ecoptic pairing, probably reflecting the existence of many regions of highly repetitive

Anopheles gambiae Polytene Chromosomes

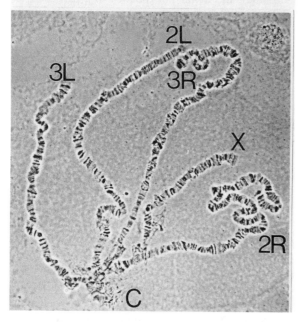

13.2 *Anopheles gambiae* polytene chromosomes. Polytene chromosomes of *Anopheles gambiae* (Karyotype: Xag, 2Rbc, 2La, 3R, 3L). The 5 arms are indicated, and C denotes the centromeres. Courtesy of Coluzzi.

DNA. Cytogenetic studies of aedine mosquitoes have been limited primarily to the metaphase chromosomes (Fig. 13.3) (141).

The centromere plays an important role in mediating attachment of a chromosome to spindle bodies during mitosis and meiosis, thus allowing the proper distribution of chromosomes into daughter cells. The centromeric structure of the yeast *Saccharomyces cerevisiae* is simple; the essential region consists of a core 125 bp fragment that is highly conserved in all the chromosomes (80). In contrast, the mammalian centromeres are highly complex, consisting of megabases of tandemly repetitive sequences. In humans, the centromeric DNA contains tandem repeats of a 170 bp core unit (230). Nothing is known about centromeres in disease vectors.

Telomeres are also important for chromosome integrity (146, 27). Chromosomes with broken ends are

Aedes aegypti Metaphase Chromosomes and FISH

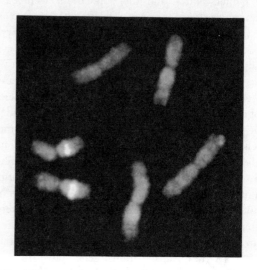

13.3 *Aedes aegypti* metaphase chromosomes and FISH. Digital imaging microscopy of *Ae. aegypti* metaphase chromosomes and FISH using a cosmid clone containing the rDNA cistron. Metaphase chromosomes were stained with propidium iodide (pi) and hybridized with the probe ck 1.21, which was labeled with biotin and detected with avidin-FTIC. The pi band in the q-terminus is seen in all similarly stained metaphase chromosomes, except where specific hybridization co-localizes with the pi band as seen here. Courtesy of Brown, Knudson, Menninger, and Ward.

unstable and tend to fuse to form dicentric chromosomes. In many organisms, the telomere consists of 6–8-bp sequence repeats, such as $(TTNGGG)_n$ in humans (139). A similar repeat sequence $(TTAGG)_n$ was found in *Bombyx mori* and other Lepidoptera (162). Neither the hexanucleotide nor the pentanucleotide repeats were found in *Drosophila* and other Diptera (162). In contrast, recent studies of certain chromosomes in *Drosophila* (22, 23, 116) have revealed 2 non-LTR (long terminal repeat) retrotransposons, with a poly(A) stretch at the end oriented proximal to the centromere. However, in situ hybridization with the cloned retrotransposon elements indicated that not all telomeres in *Drosophila* contain these elements, suggesting the presence of different telomere structures. Nothing is known about the telomere structure in disease vectors (116).

Sex

In most organisms, sex determination is controlled by nuclear genes although in a few cases it is determined by environmental factors such as temperature (81). Genetically controlled sex determination has been studied in some detail in model organisms, such as *C. elegans*, *D. melanogaster*, mouse, and humans, revealing different molecular mechanisms involved in sex determination and differentiation. In mouse and human, the male-determining Y chromosome has a dominant effect. In *Drosophila* and *C. elegans*, sex determination is controlled by the ratio of the sex chromosomes (X) to autosomes: A higher ratio, 2 X chromosomes to 2 sets of autosomes, leads to female development; a lower ratio, 1 X chromosome to 2 sets of autosomes, leads to male development.

The mechanism of sex determination in vectors is poorly understood. Culicine mosquitoes have a pair of chromosomes (chromosome I) that are similar in size but are distinguishable in many species by the presence in the (X) or absence in the (Y) of C-banding intercalary heterochromatin (156, 141, 142). Females are homogametic (XX); males, heterogametic (XY). Both sex chromosomes are genetically active, and thus sex appears to be inherited autosomally, by a single locus (131) or gene complex (48). The dominant, male-determining allele *(M)* is carried by the Y, whereas the recessive allele *(m)* is carried by the X.

Anopheline mosquitoes exhibit heteromorphic chromosomes, in that the X chromosome is longer than the Y. The Y chromosome consists mainly of heterochromatin and is not polytenized in the salivary glands. Because there is dimorphism between the male and female karyotype, the mechanism of sex determination appears to be comparable to that of mammals (78).

Mutations, such as the distorter gene *(d)* in *Aedes* and *Culex*, have been found to cause a deviation in the expected 1:1 sex ratio in the progeny, resulting in a preponderance of males (9, 79). The *d* locus was found to be tightly linked to but separate from the *M* locus (158). The phenotypic effect of the *d* mutation is similar to that of the meiotic drive mutation in *Drosophila* (125). The distortion is transmitted solely by the males and is not the result of postgametic mortality; there can be preferential fragmentation of the X chromosome during spermatogenesis (157, 201). The mechanisms of distortion in vectors are unknown. There is strong interest in distorter genes because of their potential utility in genetic control strategies.

Chromosome Evolution

Karyotypic analysis of many insect species has shown wide variations in chromosome numbers, although the number is strongly conserved within mosquitoes. The most definitive studies of chromosomal evolution have been performed in *Drosophila*, in which comparisons of polytene chromosome banding patterns suggest extensive conservation of large blocks of linked genes (synteny). Muller (146) proposed that pericentric inversions are extremely rare and that chromosomal arms (elements) retain their essential integrity, despite the occurrence of frequent paracentric inversions and occasional translocations. This interpretation has been confirmed by comparative studies of genetic linkage maps and by in situ hybridization of probes to polytene chromosomes.

Recent results suggest that synteny is widespread in cyclorrhaphous diptera. Mapping of cloned genes by in situ hybridization to polytene chromosomes demonstrated that there is linkage conservation of a block of genes encoding integrin, vitellogenin, and chorion proteins in both the Mediterranean fruit fly and *Drosophila* (239). Comparisons of genetic linkage maps of morphological markers suggested correspondence between chromosomes 2, 3, 4, 5, and 6 in blow fly; to 1, 3, 2, 4, and 5 in house fly; and to 2L, X, 3R, 3L, and 2R in *Drosophila melanogaster* (63). Synteny has also been observed in mammals. One extraordinary synteny between insects and mammals has been uncovered in the arrangement of homeo-box containing genes in *Drosophila*, the mouse, and humans. The order of these genes has not only been conserved, but the order of genes with similar anterior-posterior action domains has also been preserved (106). The prevalence of synteny is of considerable interest because it could permit localization of interesting genes in multiple species by virtue of their known location in a single model species. This possibility can now be explored in vector insects, as genome analysis progresses and provides tools for cross-species comparisons.

Comparative genome analysis in disease vectors has been limited in the past because of the lack of good genetic maps, with the obvious exception of *Ae. aegypti*. Comparison of genetic maps of isozymes among *Aedes*, *Culex*, and *Anopheles* spp. reveals instances of synteny (148, 129). There is a strong conservation of the 2 linkage groups, *Gpi-Odh-Hk* and *Pgm-Gpd-Had-Idh2*, among 6 species of *Aedes*. Such comparisons have also revealed shuffling of markers in different linkage groups. The linkage group I of *Ae. togoi* seems to be a composite of linkage groups I, II, and III of *Ae. aegypti* and linkage groups I and II of *Ae. triseriatus*. It has been suggested that whole-arm translocation might be responsible for the shuffling (129). The hypothesis, however, lacks supporting cytogenetic data. Another example of synteny has been observed in the clustering of 3 genes, *Dox1A1* encoding for diphenol oxidase, *Ddc* encoding for dopa decarboxylase, and *I2.37Cc* uncharacterized function, which are located on the right arm of the third chromosome in *An. gambiae* and on the right arm of the second chromosome in *D. melanogaster* (P. Romans, personal communication).

Comparative cytogenetic genome studies in anophelines have been possible because of the excellent polytene chromosomes found in nurse cell and larval salivary glands; the cytogenetic data on the *An. gambiae* complex are particularly extensive. Following the assumption, as in *Drosophila*, that cytologically indistinguishable inversions represent a single ancestral event, these studies have led to the suggestion that *An. quadriannulatus* has a primitive banding pattern and that ancient paracentric inversions are responsible for the differentiation of the banding patterns in different members of the complex. Intraspecific polytene chromosome inversions have also been observed. For example, *An. gambiae* Mopti differs from the Bamako strain by paracentric inversions in the right arm of the second chromosome. Although both types are sympatric and can interbreed easily in the laboratory, hybrids have not been observed in thousands of field-caught females (47, 46). It has been suggested that such inversions promote speciation and, by virtue of "locking in" blocks of gene-specific allelic combinations by suppressing recombination, can result in physiologically important variations of ecotypes, including their effective performance as disease carriers.

GENETIC ELEMENTS AND SEQUENCE LEVEL ORGANIZATION

Genes and Other Low Copy Sequences

Genes from disease vectors have been cloned, characterized, and sequenced. Genes of particular interest are those involved in vector competence, in olfaction, in host-seeking, in genes expressed in the midgut or hemocoel constitutively or induced by blood-feeding, and in genes expressed in the salivary gland.

Genes have been identified that encode polypeptides that are homologous with serine proteases from other organisms. In *An. gambiae*, at least 7 genes, encoding trypsin- and chymotrypsin-like proteins, are found clustered at a single genomic location (147). A similar family of genes encoding trypsin-like proteins have been reported in *Ae. aegypti* (7, 97), and 1 trypsin-like gene has also been cloned from the black fly *Simulium vittatum* (177).

Another family of genes encoding polypeptides that are homologous with maltases from yeast to *Drosophila* have been reported. Maltase, a member of the α-glucosidase family that breaks down maltose into glucose, can play an important role in digestion during sugar feeding. In *Ae. aegypti*, *MalI* encodes a polypeptide that is expressed exclusively in the salivary gland (88). In *An. gambiae*, 2 genes encoding maltase-like proteins have been characterized, but whether their expression is salivary gland–specific is not known (L. Zheng, unpublished results).

Moderate to Highly Repetitive Sequences

Moderately repetitive DNA represents sequences repeated from a dozen to several thousand times and often occurs either as dispersed within regions of otherwise unique sequence or in long blocks (33). Long, repetitive DNA blocks comprise from 5–15% of the total genomic DNA in many animals and include transcribed multigene families such as the ribosomal RNA genes, tRNA, and histone genes (67) as well as scrambled blocks of shorter sequences, or transposable elements.

Repetitive DNA accounts for between 20 and 84% of mosquito genomes and is probably responsible for a great deal of the observed intraspecific variations in genome size (26). In most cases, the number of copies of repetitive sequences found in mosquitoes was similar to observed values in other animals (26). Middle repetitive sequences occurred in 10–300 copies; highly repetitive elements were found in copy numbers ranging from 5000–15,000. The exception was strains of *Ae. albopictus*, in which highly repetitive sequences accounting for 17% of the Calcutta strain genome were present in copy numbers approaching 50,000, suggesting very few types of repeats, whereas highly repetitive sequences in the Mauritius strain had a copy number of only 2300 and accounted for over 30% of the genome.

Little is known about the chromosomal location of repetitive sequences in mosquitoes, with the exception of 4 satellite sequences mapped by in situ hybridization in *An. stephensi* (181). This information is necessary to understand the possible role of repetitive DNA in the structural organization of chromosomes as well as to develop useful probes for gene mapping. Recently, work on the human genome project has demonstrated that fluorescent in situ hybridization (FISH) is very effective for physically locating the chromosomal position of DNA sequences used as probes (224).

Microsatellites (Simple Sequence Repeats)

Microsatellite or simple sequence repeat (SSR) DNA consists of tandemly repeated copies of a core sequence such as $(dA)_n$, $(dG-dT)_n$, $(dC-dA-dC)_n$, or $(dG-dA-dT-dA)_n$ (209). Microsatellites are found widely dispersed throughout most of the genome in many eukaryotes and can occur as frequently as once every 10 kb (208). Usually they are located outside of the open-reading frame or transcribed region. Extensive length polymorphism occurs in microsatellite sequences, permitting their use for relationship studies of individuals within and between populations, and as a source of polymorphic DNA markers for genome mapping and linkage studies (208). The length polymorphisms can originate from unequal crossing-over,

unequal sister chromatid exchange, or slipped-strand mispairing during replication or repair (216).

Repeats such as $(dG-dT)_n$ have been found in all eukaryotic organisms, except yeast. In *An. gambiae*, conservative estimates suggest the presence of about 10,000 $(dG-dT)_n$ microsatellites in the haploid genome. In *Ae. aegypti*, the search for SSRs has not been as fruitful. For example, approximately 10^4 recombinant cosmids were screened with a $(dG-dT)_{15}$ probe, and microsatellites were detected at frequency of ~1 in 300 colonies screened (S.E. Brown, unpublished results). Since the average insert size was >30 kb, it appears that $(dG-dT)_n$ microsatellites are relatively infrequent in the *Ae. aegypti* genome. For comparison, in similar studies on the human genome yields, approximately 1 in 2 colonies examined are positive (122). The *Ae. aegypti* results have been duplicated by others, but 15 SSR markers have been identified and several have been found to exhibit Mendelian segregation (W.C. Black, personal communication). These findings emphasize the need to tailor the search for microsatellite sequences to repeats that occur frequently in the particular vector species. SSR markers distributed along the 3 *Aedes* chromosomes will be helpful in reconciling the linkage map with the physical map.

The function of microsatellite sequences is not known. Microsatellites such as $(dG-dT)_n$, however, have been found to be close to sites of DNA rearrangement (29). Furthermore, DNA fragments containing $(dG-dT)_n$ sequences might form Z-type DNA structure (75, 159). Recently, the expansion or contraction of certain trinucleotide repeats has been implicated in several human genetic disorders (66).

VNTR, or Minisatellite

Minisatellites are hypervariable, more complex regions of DNA, and they are found dispersed at numerous sites in the genome. They exhibit polymorphism due to a variable number of tandem repeats (VNTR) of a short 10–15-bp core sequence (91, 92). A hybridization probe consisting of the core sequence can detect many polymorphic minisatellite loci simultaneously to provide an individual organism's fingerprint; hence the synonymous term DNA fingerprinting. The use of multilocus minisatellite probes has become a standard tool for the establishment of associations or exclusions in criminal cases and for the determination of family relationships in paternity disputes (90). The same minisatellite loci used for human diagnostics were also found to be equally valuable in studying house sparrow demographics (229). Blanchetot (28) reported a tandemly repeated element from the house fly that created individual fingerprints when probed against genomic DNA. This element also cross hybridized with *Ae. aegypti* DNA. Other minisatellite sequences in Diptera have not been reported.

Transposable Elements

Another important category of interspersed, moderately repetitive DNA is the transposable elements. These are DNA sequences capable of moving from one place to another within the genome while retaining a copy at the original location; consequently, they appear in varying locations in different strains. Much of the current knowledge on transposable elements comes from research on *Drosophila*, in which these elements are responsible for many spontaneous mutations and chromosomal rearrangements. The proportion of a genome that consists of transposable elements varies from species to species but averages about 10% (61). There are 2 main types of transposable elements: transposons, which transpose directly from DNA to DNA; and retrotransposons, which transpose by an RNA intermediate and have structural features suggestive of such a transposition mechanism (30). Transposable elements are of great interest because they could be used to deliver foreign genes into an organism, to tag genes or promoter elements in mutagenesis experiments, or to spread a gene through a disease vector population (see Chap. 14).

P elements in *D. melanogaster* are an example of transposons (Chap. 14). A complete *P* element is 2.9 kb long and has 31 bp inverted terminal repeats. Intact *P* elements occur at a frequency of about 50 copies per genome and encode a transposase enzyme, which catalyzes its excision and transposition. Smaller elements resulting from internal deletions are incapable of transposing by themselves but can transpose when supplied with a functional transposase in *trans*

by an intact element (56). *P* and a related transposon, *hobo* (133, 200), have been used to develop reliable germ line transformation procedures in *D. melanogaster* (198); thus, the mechanisms controlling their transposition have been studied extensively (183). Recently, transformation has been accomplished with a third element, *Minos*, which was derived from *D. hydei* but absent from *D. melanogaster,* and which is related in sequence to the *Tc1* element of *C. elegans* (65, 64). *P* and *hobo* are present in some *D. melanogaster* strains but absent from others, and at least for *P*, strong evidence exists that it has spread in *D. melanogaster* populations across the world in a very brief period—approximately 50 years (100).

Another transposon is *mariner*, which was identified originally as an insertion element in the white gene of *D. mauritiana* (87). A *mariner*-like element has also been identified in the intron of the preprocecropin gene from the lepidopteran *Hyalophora cecropia* (120). It is a middle repetitive element with about 30–70 copies in *D. mauritiana* and about 100 in *H. cecropia*. The element is about 1.3 kb long and has inverted repeats (28 and 38 bp in *D. mauritiana* and *H. cecropia,* respectively) at the 2 ends.

Recently *mariner*-like elements have been found in 10 other insects, including 6 different orders (185, 186). Full-length clones were recovered from all of the species examined, including the mosquito *An. gambiae*. Interestingly, the majority of the *mariner* elements in *An. gambiae* shared high sequence similarity (>91% at the nucleotide level) with those from the horn fly. In light of the more than 200 Myr divergence between these 2 organisms, it has been suggested that a recent horizontal transfer of this subfamily element might have occurred. Another line of evidence for horizontal transfer of *mariner* element comes from the fact that *mariner* is present in both the lepidopteran *H. cecropia* and the higher dipteran *D. mauritiana*, but it is absent from a close relative of the latter, *D. melanogaster*. Horizontal transfer of transposable elements have also been suggested for *P* and *hobo,* and mites have been proposed to be the agent in the initial transfer of the *P* element to *D. melanogaster* (37, 101, 82).

Retrotransposons consist of 2 categories, the long terminal repeat (LTR) containing elements, which are similar in structure and function to retroviral proviruses of vertebrates, and the non-LTR retrotransposons (238). LTR elements range from 5–8.5 kb in length and have long, direct terminal repeats and short, imperfect inverted repeats at the terminal ends. The copia-like elements of *Drosophila* are an example of the LTR retrotransposons. The number of *copia* elements varies from 20–60 copies per genome. Examples of the non-LTR retrotransposons include the mammalian *LINE–1* elements and *Drosophila I* factors, *F* elements and *Jockey* (16), and *R1* and *R2* elements of *Bombyx mori* (35). They all lack inverted repeats (non-long terminal repeat elements) but have a poly(A) or (A)-rich tail at the 3' end. In each case, the full length element is about 4–6 kb, consisting of 2 open-reading frames. The 1st ORF contains cysteine-rich domains and the second shares homology with many reverse transcriptases.

Two classes of non-LTR elements have been described on the basis of target site insertion. The random elements appear to be distributed promiscuously throughout the host genome; a second group, the siteposons, insert into specific DNA sequences (4) and are exemplified by the *R1* and *R2* elements, which insert at the same location of the 28S rRNA gene in many insects (35, 238). Evidence for transposition of non-LTR elements through an RNA intermediate comes from their possession of ORFs encoding sequences similar to reverse transcriptases and nucleic acid binding domains of retroviral nucleocapsid proteins. These elements also terminate at the 3' end with an oligo (A) or (A)-rich tail, frequently preceded by a polyadenylation signal, and often have 5' end truncations attributable to incomplete reverse transcription. Pelisson et al. (172) provided direct evidence for retrotransposition of the *I* factor element in *Drosophila* by engineering an *I* factor bearing a special intron, thus demonstrating that transposition resulted in the accurate removal of the intron.

Besansky (18) described the *T1* family of retrotransposons from the *An. gambiae* complex. Full-length *T1* elements are 4.7 kb long, including 2 overlapping open-reading frames, one of which possesses structural motifs characteristic of reverse transcriptases. At the 3' end is an (A)-rich tail consisting of tandem repeats of TGAAA. *T1* occurs in approximately 100 dispersed copies belonging to 2 subtypes, *T1α* and *T1β*. Although both subtypes are present in all 5 sibling species examined, *T1α* seems to be absent in *An. merus* (17).

Two site-specific retrotransposon families, *RT1* and *RT2*, have also been identified from *An. gambiae* complex. Both compete for an identical insertion site in the coding region of the 28S rRNA gene (19), which is 634 bp 3' from the typical site of *R1* insertions in other insects but are also present outside of the rDNA repeats from a few to about 100 copies. Among the sibling species of the complex, *An. merus* seems to be devoid of *RT1* and *RT2* whereas *An. quadriannulatus* lacks *RT1*.

Mouches et al. (145) described a highly repetitive element, *Juan*, from *Cx. pipiens quinquefasciatus* and *Cx. tarsalis*. Sequencing of 3 different copies revealed similarities to the *Drosophila I, Jockey*, and *F* elements. All copies examined appeared to be truncated at the 5' end and carry only degenerate ORFs (143). Recently, full-length (4.7 kb) *Juan-A* elements were shown to be widely dispersed in about 200 copies throughout the genomes of *Ae. aegypti, Ae. albopictus, Ae. polynesiensis, Cx. tarsalis, An. gambiae*, and an agricultural pest, *Ceratitis capitata* (144). Both examples that were sequenced were flanked by direct 11-bp repeats, probably representing target site duplication during transposition. Although examples of *Juan-A* elements truncated at the 5' end were identified, approximately 80% of all copies were estimated to be full length. This element is very similar in 3 nonsibling *Aedes* species, which might suggest horizontal transfer.

Identification and characterization of additional transposable elements in mosquitoes will be an important first step in any future genetic control strategies designed to interrupt vector-borne disease cycles. A key goal is to identify potentially exploitable transposable elements that can be used for the development of transformation vectors capable of directing the integration of recombinant genes into the mosquito genome.

rDNA Cistrons

In most disease vectors, the rDNA is usually found at 1 cytogenetic location, for example, near the centromere of the X chromosome in *An. gambiae* and *An.*

arabienses and in chromosome I in *Ae. aegypti* and *Cx. quinquefasciatus* (107, 127a). However, rDNA can be found at 2 positions in *An. quadriannulatus*, *An. melas*, and *An. merus*; in *An quadimanulatus*, it is present in the Y chromosome as well as the X. In *Ae. triseriatus*, rDNA can be found in chromosomes I and III (41).

As in many other eukaryotes, the rDNA is arranged as head-to-tail tandem repeats and is present in 100–1000 copies in most vectors. There are about 250 copies in *An. gambiae* (44) and about 500 in *Ae. aegypti* and *Ae. albopictus;* the average length of the *Ae. aegypti* repeat unit is about 9.0 kb (68, 107). The number of repeats increases to about 1200 in adult *Ae. aegypti* (169). A typical rDNA repeat consists of an intergenic spacer (IGS), followed by the transcribed region, which is posttranscriptionally processed to form the 18S, 5.8S, 28Sα, and 28Sβ rRNAs. Preceding the 18S coding sequence is the external transcribed spacer (ETS), and surrounding the 5.8S rDNA are 2 internal transcribed spacers (ITS).

Genetic variation within and between mosquito populations has been examined by studying rDNA sequence variation. Black et al. (25) found extensive and continuous variation in the nontranscribed spacer regions of *Ae. albopictus* with little evidence of conservation within each of 17 populations from around the world. Although IGS sequences in the *An. gambiae* complex show both intra- and interspecies variation, resulting in part from the presence of small repeat sequences, the IGS sequences near the coding units show a species-specific restriction pattern. Species-diagnostic IGS probes have been developed to distinguish the morphologically similar taxa of the *An. gambiae* complex (210).

Highly Repetitive Elements

Highly repetitive DNA is usually present in tens of thousand, to millions of copies and is often arranged in long tandem repeats of relatively simple sequences. It can have a G + C content different from that of unique sequence DNA and consequently gives distinct bands in CsCl gradients, thus the term "satellite DNA" (33). Clustered highly repetitive satellite DNAs have been studied extensively in the mouse and *Drosophila* (155). Many of these sequences are present in centromeric and telomeric heterochromatin and are not normally transcribed (93); they are possibly directly related to the physical maintenance, replication, and transmission of the chromosomes. Repetitive scaffold sequences seem to be involved in the attachment of nucleosomes and other higher order structures to the nuclear membrane (78). Simple sequence $(dG-dT)_n$ repeats can contribute to packaging and condensing DNA into chromosomes as well as to determining what distinguishes constitutive heterochromatin from euchromatin, or facultative heterochromatin (199). Other repetitive sequences that constitute so-called selfish DNA, including transposable elements, have no function other than to maintain themselves (165).

GENETIC MAPPING

A genetic map is the order and distance in recombination units of all markers on the chromosomes. Considerable effort has gone into the generation of genetic maps with morphological and isozyme markers for the mosquitoes *Ae. togoi*, *Ae. triseriatus*, *Ae. aegypti*, *An. albimanus*, *An. quadrimaculatus*, and, to a lesser extent, *An. gambiae* (160, 161). These efforts have been extremely productive, especially for *Ae. aegypti*. The number of such markers for most disease vectors, however, has not increased dramatically since the late 1970s (160, 161), primarily because of the difficulty in generating and maintaining the genetic stocks that contain individual markers. Recently, RFLPs, restriction fragment length polymorphism, and microsatellite polymorphic DNA markers, which can be maintained together in a few stocks and can be scored easily in multifactorial crosses, have revitalized genetic analysis of disease vectors and have allowed the generation of reasonably dense genetic maps for both *Ae. aegypti* and *An. gambiae*. Construction of these maps has been facilitated by simultaneous analysis of many highly polymorphic markers using computers.

Genetic linkage describes the fundamental observation that 2 genes located near one another on the same chromosome are not inherited independently. If the loci are very close together, they will almost invariably be inherited together. If the loci are further apart, crossing over between homologous chromosomes during meiosis can create new combinations of alleles.

The recombination frequency increases with the distance between loci. The probability of recombinant and parental (nonrecombinant) combinations is equal (or 0.5) when loci are far apart, just as when loci are unlinked (present on different chromosomes). The study of recombination events along a chromosome populated by numerous genetic markers makes possible the localization of a gene of interest to within a fairly narrow length of DNA (184). Genetic linkage maps are available currently for 27 species of insects, of which mosquitoes account for one-third (Table 13.2)(78). The *Drosophila melanogaster* map has over 3,700 loci, whereas most linkage maps for mosquitoes are in the range of 10–80 loci (6). Thus, the resolution of genetic maps is low for most insects, and markers are relatively long distances apart; consequently, map-based cloning strategies to isolate genes are ineffective (234). The availability of a genetic map with many closely spaced markers in the region of interest becomes a necessity because the greater the resolution of the map the greater the likelihood of finding the gene of interest. When linked molecular markers are identified and mapped to positions flanking a gene of interest, then new, even more closely located markers and probes can be isolated from the region between the flanking markers as a prelude to physical map construction and chromosomal walks to the gene. Clearly, the point of genetic linkage mapping is to provide markers that will segregate with a phenotypic trait of interest. If the trait segregates in a simple Mendelian manner, then this is straightforward and is only limited by our ability to have many easily scored polymorphic markers. If the trait exhibits continuous variation, resulting from the segregation of multiple genetic factors, some of which can be modified by environmental factors, then the segregation results must be explained using the theory of quantitative inheritance, which invokes what are termed quantitative trait loci (QTL) (112).

In modern practice, multipoint linkage analysis of polymorphic markers is used to construct a maximum likelihood map (8, 111). Although this analysis can handle family pedigree as well as F_2 intercrosses and F_2 backcrosses, the F_2 data collection offers distinct advantages because it is compatible with QTL analysis. The F_2 intercross requires homozygous parentals, resulting in heterozygous F_1; the F_1 are allowed to interbreed and the progeny, the F_2 intercross, are examined for the marker. In the case of the backcross, both parents need not be homozygous, and the F_2 backcross is generated by F1 x Parent. Both procedures rely on being able to score the individual progeny for the loci in question.

Sufficient genetic variability must be present in the vector population to allow the development of an adequate number of polymorphic markers. In this connection, it should be emphasized that mapping projects and population studies are highly synergistic. Examining genetic variation within and among populations of disease vectors provides information useful on systematic and taxonomic relationships, migration patterns, vector competency, and insecticide resistance. Not only is this information of value to medical entomologists, epidemiologists, and other public health professionals (particularly those involved with surveillance and control of vector-borne diseases), but it also provides the basis of markers for genetic mapping. Conversely, the markers developed for mapping purposes are powerful tools for population studies.

Weir (227) lists 5 types of data that can be used to examine genetic variation: phenotypic data (dominant and codominant markers), allozyme data, protein sequence data, restriction fragment data, and DNA sequence data (Fig. 13.1). Recently developed molecular techniques have allowed great advances to be made in the field of population genetics. Earlier, only morphological characters and allozymes were available for mapping studies; now an entire battery of molecular techniques allows the investigation of genetic differences at the DNA level. Each of these techniques has advantages and disadvantages for use in the analysis of genetic variability, and ultimately the choice of which techniques to employ will be influenced by the laboratory resources available and the question posed.

Morphological and Resistance Markers

A number of simple mutations exhibiting Mendelian segregation have been identified in various mosquitoes kept in the laboratory (103). These mutations are indicated in recent linkage map compilations (160, 161).

Eye color mutations are common and useful because of the ease of their scoring. The most common

TABLE 13.2   Linkage maps of disease vectors

Genus species	Pairs of autosomes	Sex determination mechanism	Linkage groups correlated to chromosomes	Mapped locia		Reference
				Number	Type	
Aedes aegypti	3	autosomal	Yes	77	mer	(151, 149)
				53	RFLP	(194)
				26	RFLP	Severson, personal communication
				33	RAPD	(71)
				70	RAPD-SSCP	Bosio and Black, personal communication
Aedes togoi	3	autosomal	No	23	me	(206)
Aedes triseriatus	3	autosomal	Yes	30	em	(128, 150)
Anopheles albimanus	2	XX/XY	Yes	34	mer	(153)
Anopheles culicifacies	2	XX/XY	No	17	mre	(190)
Anopheles gambiae	2	XX/XY	Partly	11	me	(152, 85)
				120	SSR	(240) and Zheng, personal communication
				13	RAPD	Dimopoylos and Louis, personal communication
Anopheles quadrimaculatus	2	XX/XY	Yes	22	mer	(154)
Anopheles stephensi	2	XX/XY	No	18	mre	(171)
Culex pipiens	3	autosomal	Yes	19	mer	(10, 115, 54)
Glossina morsitans	2	XX/XY	Partly	12	em	(69)

Adapted from a recent review (78); minor additions and modifications have been made. All species listed are dipterans. Haploid number of chromosomes for all species is n = 3, and the number of linkage groups is also 3. Abbreviations for type include: m = morphological mutants, e = enzyme polymorphism, r = resistance to insecticides, SSR = simple sequence repeats microsatellites, RFLP and RAPD = DNA markers. The order of m, e, and r is taken from the original review and indicates the more numerous marker by order (78).

eye color mutation, white eye *(w)*, has been observed in *An. gambiae, An. albimanus, Ae. togoi, Ae. aegypti, Cx. pipiens,* and other mosquitoes. This phenotype is usually linked to loci on the sex chromosomes, chromosome I in culicines, or X in anophelines, with the exception of *Ae. togoi,* in which it maps to chromosome II (206). It is not known whether these mutations occur in homologous genes in different mosquitoes; in general, mutations in many genes can generate the same eye color phenotype. Recent cloning and mapping data on *An. gambiae,* however, indicated that the *w* locus of this species is a homologue of the *Drosophila w* gene (N. Besansky, personal communication). Other eye color mutations have also been observed and described, such as the *An. gambiae* pink eye *(p)* mutation; and a few eye morphology mutations have also been observed.

Other common morphological mutations described in anophelines mosquitoes are collarless and lunate *(l)*, and *l* has been mapped to the second chromosome in *An. gambiae, An. albimanus,* and *An. quadrimaculatus* (L. Zheng, unpublished results). In culicines, yellow larvae *(y)* is a common morphological mutation that maps to chromosome II in *Ae. triseriatus* and *Ae. aegypti.*

The genetics of insecticide resistance has attracted considerable attention, largely because of the practical implications for vector control. Consequently, a large body of work has accumulated on resistance to DDT, dieldrin, malathion, and pyrethroids. Mutations in 1 of 2 loci on chromosomes II and III can give rise to resistance to DDT or malathion. Amplification of esterase genes results in resistance to DDT and malathion. The dieldrin resistance mutation *(Dl)* has been mapped to the second chromosome in *An. gambiae, An. quadrimaculatus,* and *Ae. aegypti,* but in *An. albimanus,* it maps to chromosome III. Recent findings indicate that resistance to dieldrin is caused by the same amino acid substitution, from alanine to serine, in the GABA receptor/chloride ion channel gene in *Ae. aegypti, D. melanogaster,* and other insects (213, 60, 214).

So far only 2 lethal mutations in *Ae. triseriatus* (both on the 2nd chromosome) and 3 in *Ae. aegypti* (all on chromosome I) have been described. Lethal mutations can be used in balancer chromosomes, an important tool that suppresses recombination and therefore maintains mutant chromosomes intact, including those that bear deletion mutations. Clearly, more lethal mutations are needed in *Aedes, Culex,* and *Anopheles* if effective tools for dissecting gene function via deletion mapping are to be developed.

Biochemical Markers

Allozyme analysis uses electrophoretic variation detected in common enzymes to infer genetic variability in natural populations. When subjected to electrophoresis, enzymes of the same size and shape move through a gel at a rate largely determined by the ratio of positively to negatively charged amino acids. If an enzyme has an amino acid replacement that leads to a difference in overall charge, the result will be a change in electrophoretic mobility.

A major problem with allozymes is that fewer than 2% of the enzymes recognized by the Enzyme Commission can be analyzed by staining gels, and many of those are electrophoretically monomorphic (6). This limits the total number of loci that can be examined in a given population and the amount of data that can be collected. Allozymes may not provide a true estimate of the variation that actually exists in a population. For example, a single nucleotide substitution in a protein coding sequence can be a silent substitution and not result in any detectable change in the electrophoretic pattern. Similarly, amino acid replacements that do not result in a net change in ionic charge are often not detected. Despite these apparent drawbacks, allozyme analysis continues to be used in a wide variety of organisms with great success.

Populations of *Ae. aegypti* are characterized by a tremendous amount of genetic variability, and the most widely used approach to detect this variation has been the use of allozymes (202). Allozyme studies have been used to identify the regional origin of a population (174), distinguish subspecies (204, 203), examine differences in genetic heterogeneity between populations (222), and correlate susceptibility to infection with yellow fever virus with genetic-geographic regions (205). Allozyme markers constitute a major proportion of the mapped loci on mosquito linkage maps (Table 13.2).

Polymorphic DNA Markers

Polymorphic DNA markers are based on variations in the DNA sequence. There are 5 basic types of useful polymorphisms: RFLP; VNTR, variable number tandem repeat polymorphism; RAPD, randomly amplified polymorphic DNA; SSR, simple sequence repeat (microsatellite) polymorphism; and SSCP, single strand conformation polymorphism (175). The utility of these markers is not limited to mapping because they are also extremely useful in population studies.

RFLP and VNTR polymorphisms are detected by Southern blot hybridization, in which a DNA probe is hybridized to a membrane containing genomic DNA that has been restriction digested, electrophoresed, and transferred to that membrane (197). RFLP indicate changes in fragment length that result from the loss (or gain) of a restriction site. VNTR polymorphism is the result of different alleles carrying a different number of a short core repeat (10 bp to >100 bp). RAPD and SSR polymorphisms rely on the technique called polymerase chain reaction (PCR), in which a DNA fragment can be amplified manyfold by repeated denaturation and DNA replication with a pair of primers flanking the DNA target (189). RAPD-PCR amplification uses an arbitrary primer (often 10 bases) and genomic DNA as the template. It generates a set of bands representing loci in which the primer sequence is found in inverted orientation twice, separated by other sequences not exceeding the length (approximately 3 kb) that can be amplified by PCR; some of these bands are polymorphic. SSR, or microsatellite polymorphism, results from variations in the number of tandemly arrayed di- , tri- , or even tetranucleotide repeats. PCR amplification of microsatellite markers requires the usage of a pair of unique primers that flank the repeat array. SSCP results from a variation in sequence that leads to a conformational change in the single-stranded DNA. Although SSCP can detect a single base change in sequence that is undetectable by any of the other methods, less routine electrophoretic techniques, such as nondenaturing gradient gels, are required for genotype determination. So far only RFLP, RAPD, RAPD-SSCP, and microsatellite markers have been used as genetic markers in disease vectors. RAPD and microsatellite markers are important because they are produced by PCR and require minute amounts of sample DNA; thus, they permit the scoring of single individuals for a very large number of markers.

RFLP

Restriction enzyme digestion of genomic DNA from different individuals, followed by Southern blot hybridization with cloned probes of known or unknown sequence, often yields detectable polymorphisms in the size of DNA fragments produced, or RFLPs. The individual to individual variation in the observed hybridization patterns is caused by underlying differences in the target DNA sequence, such as base substitutions that create or abolish restriction sites, or DNA insertions or deletions in the region encompassed between the restriction sites. RFLPs are dispersed widely throughout the genome, and they are often inherited as codominant, Mendelian markers. Any cloned DNA fragment can potentially detect polymorphism and serve as an RFLP marker; thus, significant regions of the genome can be saturated with RFLP markers. RFLP markers have been used for map construction for both plants and animals.

RFLP analysis is limited because it can only monitor a portion of the genome containing the restriction sites under examination. In cases in which a comparison between 2 closely related individuals is required, RFLP may not provide sufficient markers that are discriminating (13). Another drawback to the use of RFLP analysis with mosquitoes is that only limited quantities of DNA can be isolated from a single mosquito (0.5–3 µg), and most of this genomic DNA is required for the blot, as compared to 5 ng (or less) of DNA required for PCR-based polymorphism analysis. In addition, the time required to complete an experiment and the reliance on radioactively labeled probes for greatest sensitivity are also drawbacks, especially when multiple assays are required from each sample. Some RFLP-based markers of short length could be converted to PCR-based assays when DNA sequences external to the 2 pertinent restriction sites are known. The genomic DNA is used as template for the PCR amplification with 2 opposing oligonucleotide primers that flank the RFLP region. After electrophoresis and band isolation, the purified band can be cut using restriction endonucleases and analyzed by gel electrophoresis (3).

RFLP markers from *Ae. aegypti* have been used to examine genetic diversity among 10 laboratory populations of *Ae. aegypti* and 9 populations representing 4 *Cx. pipiens* subspecies (196). Many of the *Ae. aegypti* markers cross hybridize under conditions of high stringency with other genera of the subfamily Culicinae and to a lesser extent with a member of the Anophelinae. In contrast, examination of mitochondrial DNA (mtDNA) RFLPs in 17 populations of *Ae. albopictus* revealed extremely low levels of variation; over 99% of all fragments identified were shared in all populations (98). When used to examine the relationships of 7 species of the *Ae. scutellaris* subgroup and 4 of the *Ae. albopictus* subgroup, restriction fragment analysis of mtDNA revealed a great deal of polymorphism among the species. These data, however, yielded conflicting results in phylogenetic analysis when compared with the available morphology and allozyme data (99).

RAPD

A relatively recent development in detecting DNA polymorphisms involves the use of the polymerase chain reaction to amplify arbitrary regions of the genome using a single primer (236, 228). This technique, referred to as RAPD-PCR, uses a single 10-base primer to produce a genotype-specific collection of amplified DNA fragments. By altering only a single base in the primer, an entirely different pattern of amplified DNA can be obtained (236). Increased numbers of polymorphisms were reported through the use of multiple 10-base primers in a single reaction (104). DNA polymorphisms detected by RAPD-PCR probably arise by several means. A mutation, insertion, or deletion resulting in the creation or destruction of a priming site can account for polymorphisms. Additionally, DNA polymorphisms can result from an insertion between 2 priming sites, rendering them too distant for successful amplification (loss of a band), or from an insertion or deletion between 2 priming sites, which alters the length of the amplified fragment without affecting amplification. The technique works regardless of genome size or organization as demonstrated by studies involving bacteria, fungi, plants, invertebrates, and vertebrates (236).

RAPD markers are almost always dominant markers. Heterozygous individuals with a single copy of an amplifiable sequence are indistinguishable from homozygotes with 2 copies. Codominant markers, resulting in different size fragments amplified from the same locus, have been reported but are uncommon (236). Since RAPD markers are randomly generated, they can represent either single copy or repetitive sequences. The latter case can create a problem if the marker is to be used as an anchor for physical mapping or chromosome walking. Nearly 50% of *Arabidopsis* RAPD markers cloned for use as probes hybridized to repetitive DNA (236, 182). Seven of 8 RAPD markers identified from *Fusarium* were found to be of low copy number, suggesting that the percentage of RAPD markers representing repetitive sequences is related to the size and complexity of the genome being analyzed (50).

RAPD markers have been used in a variety of applications. RAPD-PCR was found to reveal genetic variability in several species in which other techniques such as allozyme analysis had been unsuccessful (24). In several studies, the density of markers on a linkage map in regions only sparsely populated by RFLP markers was substantially increased in a short period of time through the addition of RAPD markers (168, 182). RAPD markers have been used successfully to distinguish members of cryptic species complexes (235), to identify cultivars (84) and hybrids (5), and to distinguish between fungal pathotypes (70). RAPD markers can also be of use in identifying traditional RFLPs. When cloned *Arabidopsis* RAPD markers were used as probes for hybridization, 16 of 18 clones identified an RFLP (182). Segregation patterns of RFLPs detected with RAPD markers as probes were identical to those of the original RAPD markers (236).

There are several advantages to the use of RAPD-PCR to detect DNA polymorphisms over other molecular-based assays. No nucleotide sequence information concerning the target DNA is required for successful amplification, and only a single random primer is needed for the reaction. The process requires small amounts of DNA, which permits samples to be split for other diagnostic procedures. RAPD-PCR can also be completed from start to finish in less than 24 hours without the use of radioactive materials or hybridizations; the observed pattern of bands is sensitive to the conditions of the experiment and reproducible conditions are mandatory for consistent results.

SSR, or Microsatellite

Simple sequence repeats (SSR, or microsatellite sequences), such as $(dG-dT)_n$ have proven to be excellent markers in linkage analysis because they are highly polymorphic, widely distributed in the genome, and codominant (226, 14). Litt and Luty (122) reported codominant Mendelian inheritance of $(dT-dG)_n$ repeat fragments in 3 different human families, confirming the usefulness of microsatellites for linkage analysis. Identification of microsatellites from random genomic libraries can be accomplished easily by screening with labeled synthetic probes complementary to the microsatellite target. Positive clones are sequenced, and knowledge of the unique sequence flanking the SSR array permits the design of primers for PCR-based assays. These assays allow rapid detection of microsatellites from small quantities of target DNA without the need for blotting and hybridization (226).

Linkage Disequilibrium

When 2 genetic loci are physically close together, little recombination can occur between them. Consequently, in a population in which recombination normally randomizes the arrangement of alleles for most linked genes, certain alleles at such tightly linked loci occur together more frequently than expected. This linkage disequilibrium has been used for finding markers that are tightly linked (within about 100 kb) to disease genes in humans. In *An. gambiae*, linkage disequilibrium was found for an esterase phenotype allele and the encapsulation of *Plasmodium* parasites in the midgut (45, 220, 221). With a high density of polymorphic DNA markers, the whole genome can be surveyed for linkage disequilibrium of a particular DNA marker with a qualitative trait of interest. RAPD or RFLP markers that show linkage disequilibrium with a particular trait can also be found. Such analysis, termed bulk segregant analysis, compares the unique differences between 2 bulked DNA samples taken from 2 pools of individuals with contrasting phenotypes (136). Linkage disequilibrium promises to be a useful approach to identify DNA markers that are tightly linked to a gene of interest, and bulk segregant analysis provides an approach to identify such a DNA marker.

Quantitative Trait Loci Mapping

Unlike a qualitative trait, such as eye color, some traits can only be evaluated through quantitative measurement, and these traits are often controlled by multiple genetic loci. If the locations of the genes controlling such a trait are unknown, then the entire genome must be surveyed in an attempt to find Mendelian genetic markers that contribute to the trait. This analysis is quantitative trait loci (QTL) mapping.

The concept of phenotypes resulting from the interplay of multiple genetic loci, which can be modified by environmental factors, was first suggested in the early 20th century. Since then, attempts have been made to identify the major and minor genes that contribute to a quantitative trait in question. Although the methodology for QTL mapping was proposed earlier (237), only recently has detailed QTL mapping become feasible, due to the development of polymorphic DNA markers spread throughout the genome. The traditional approach to mapping QTLs involves a genetic marker taken one at a time. There are a number of disadvantages in this approach because phenotypic effects of QTLs are underestimated, QTL map locations can be ambiguous as distant linkage cannot be discerned from a small phenotypic effect, and the number of progeny required in testing is large (112). An alternative approach combines interval mapping with selective genotyping, thereby reducing the number of progeny to be genotyped. Although selective genotyping requires a larger population, it genotypes only those individuals whose phenotypes deviate significantly from the mean. In addition, environmental noise and genetic noise can be reduced by progeny testing and studying several regions, respectively (112). Lander and Botstein (112) have improved the genetic linkage map through a combination of interval mapping, that is, mapping with multiple loci within a region, and statistical analysis. Complex traits, such as fruit mass and plant yield and hypertension in mammals, have been dissected (55,

86). In rats 1 locus (*Bp1*), for example, was found to control about 20% of the variance of hypertension whereas another locus (*Bp2*) contributed significantly less (86).

The Aedes aegypti *Linkage Map*

Craig and Hickey (48) provided the first comprehensive overview of *Ae. aegypti* genetics including a linkage map. They placed 29 markers, including morphological mutants, insecticide resistance, filarial susceptibility, and sex, into 3 linkage groups covering a total map distance of 110 units. McDonald and Rai (132) published the first reported correlation between linkage groups and chromosomes in *Ae. aegypti*. Their work resulted in renumbering the chromosomes from Rai's (176) original system (I = the shortest, III = the longest) to correspond to the linkage groups. Under the new nomenclature, the designations of chromosomes II and III were switched so that the largest chromosome was now numbered II. An ever-increasing number of genetic markers generated through the research efforts of many investigators necessitated the integration of available data into a new map (151, 149). The most recent integrated map includes a total of 77 markers, consisting of morphological, enzyme, physiological, and lethal markers, and it covers 171 map units. This map has been referred to as the *Ae. aegypti* classical genetic linkage map (Fig. 13.4).

Recently, an *Ae. aegypti* RFLP linkage map has been constructed (194). This map (Fig. 13.4) consists of 50 DNA markers that identify 53 loci covering 134 map units across the *Ae. aegypti* genome and representing 60% of the genome based on the estimate of a total genetic distance of 228. Determination of linkage associations between RFLP markers and several morphological marker loci allowed for partial integration of the RFLP markers into the classical genetic linkage map. Linkage associations for an additional 26 DNA markers also have been determined recently (D. Severson, personal communication). Most of these RFLP markers consist of random cDNA clones obtained from an *Ae. aegypti* Liverpool strain cDNA library; however, several represent clones of known genes. The 79 RFLP loci identified to date cover the entire *Ae.*

aegypti genome at an average spacing of about 2 map units between markers.

RAPD DNA markers have also been evaluated for use as a tool in constructing a linkage map of *Ae. aegypti* (71). Seven primers were selected to analyze 2 backcross families from F_1 females and backcross males. PCR products were analyzed, and each family was scored for the presence or absence of selected RAPD markers. Seven primers yielded a total of 80 markers in the 2 families of which only 33 were scored and placed in linkage groups. Recently, 70 RAPD-SSCP markers have been placed on the genetic linkage map relative to loci *blt, re, s,* and sex (C.F. Bosio and W.C. Black, personal communication).

A maximum genetic map length has been calculated for *Ae. aegypti* based on a model of chiasmata crossover frequencies (233). The average number of chiasma per cell was found to be 4.56 (1.52 / bivalent × 3), and the total map length was estimated by multiplying the average number of chiasmata per cell by 50 to yield 228 map units, based on the assumption that rates of crossover and chiasmata were equivalent (219). Chiasmata were also assumed to be distributed proportionally to chromosome length, resulting in the assignment of map lengths of 62 units, 86 units, and 80 units to chromosomes I, II, and III, respectively, in the classical linkage map (151). Considering the genome size to be about 780 Mb (179), each cM corresponds to 3 Mb. Unfortunately, markers are not uniformly distributed. For example, 18 markers span only 32 units of a predicted 80-unit map in linkage group III. This implies that either markers have not yet been found that delimit the ends of linkage group III or chiasmata occur in this chromosome at a lower rate than the model predicts. A similar situation exists in linkage groups I and II, in which the majority of markers are located in a central cluster; however, markers have been mapped at the extremes in both of these linkage groups. McDonald and Rai (132) previously suggested that recombination is not uniform throughout the length of the chromosomes in this species. Areas of the chromosomes that do not crossover much, such as heterochromatic regions, thus would be underrepresented on the map.

Aedes aegypti Linkage Maps

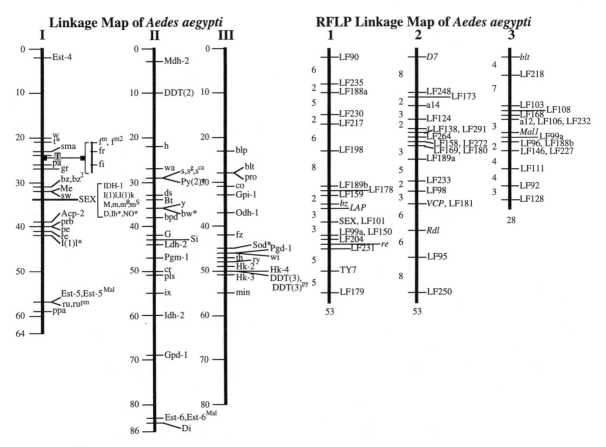

13.4 *Aedes aegypti* linkage maps. Classical and RFLP genetic linkage maps of *Aedes aegypti* chromosomes are represented. Map positions of a variety of markers are denoted, including morphologic, allozyme, and filarial susceptibility at 24 map units (151, 149). RFLP genetic linkage map data represents cDNA clones as probes as RFLP markers (194). Courtesy of Knudson.

Another problem with linkage mapping is that the actual placement of 1 marker in relation to another might be incorrect. Munstermann and Craig (151) listed several possible sources of error that could contribute to misplacement of markers. First, exaggerated crossover values can be obtained when markers are not fully penetrant or are difficult to score. Second, the distance between markers could be underestimated when loci are on opposite arms of a chromosome and double crossovers cannot be scored. Finally, large differences in crossovers between given markers from 1 strain to the next can be due to inversions or other factors influencing crossover rates. Crossover values can be extremely variable in *Aedes*, even in lines with supposedly identical genetic backgrounds reared under controlled environmental conditions (103). Experimental factors including rearing temperature, age, and sex of mosquitoes have also been shown to influence cross-over rates (48). Although markers are positioned relative to one another in the linkage group, their actual location or orientation within the chromosome has not been determined.

The detailed RFLP linkage map for *Ae. aegypti* is a powerful tool that has assisted initial efforts to resolve a complex phenotypic trait, such as filarial worm susceptibility, into its discrete genetic components (194). Three independent trials involving F_2 populations of females resulting from crosses between strains of *Ae. aegypti* susceptible and refractory to *Brugia malayi* have been conducted (195). Females were exposed to blood meals infected with *B. malayi* and subsequently dissected to determine the number of infective stage (L3) larvae that had successfully developed. DNA was extracted from each mosquito carcass and used to prepare Southern blots. These blots were screened with a series of RFLP markers that covered the entire *Ae. aegypti* RFLP linkage map. The data were then analyzed to evaluate correlation with different RFLP marker combinations and select the set that explained the most phenotypic variance with the least number of markers. A set of 2 RFLP DNA markers explained a significant portion of the observed phenotypic variance for filarial worm susceptibility in each of their trials. One marker, *LF178*, resided within a 10 cM interval on chromosome, mapping to the general genome location reported for the f^m locus (134), and it appears to be linked with a simple recessive character. A second marker, *LF98*, is located on chromosome II, and it resides within a 9 cM interval, which exhibits an additive effect to filarial susceptibility, and its effect was dependent upon the genetic background of the mosquito strain (Fig. 13.4). These results indicate that at least 2 genes (defined by 2 QTL) are involved in determining *B. malayi* susceptibility (195, 193).

The Anopheles gambiae *Linkage Map*

The principal malaria vector in Africa, *An. gambiae*, has not been studied extensively by classical genetic linkage mapping because only a few mutations resulting in an observable morphological phenotype have been described and there is great difficulty in doing genetic crosses by pair mating. Nevertheless, major progress in mapping has been made using microsatellite markers that have been identified easily from an *An. gambiae* genomic library (240). Microsatellites that contain as few as 6 consecutive arrays of the dinucleotide $(dG-dT)_n$ proved polymorphic, and more than 85% of the microsatellite markers isolated were found to be polymorphic within and between different strains. Mass matings were performed between female Suakoko (wild type) and male WE (carrying a sex-linked white eye, *w*, mutation) mosquitoes. Five families were generated with a total of 248 offspring from the backcross of the heterozygous females to WE male. The eye phenotype of each offspring and the genotypes of the parents and each offspring at 40 microsatellite markers were determined (Figs. 13.5 and 13.6.) A detailed genetic map was constructed for the X chromosome, covering a total of 44 cM and an average distance of less than 2 cM between markers (Fig. 13.7). The map covers about 90% of the X chromosome based on a estimate of 50 cM total for the X chromosome. The linkage map was integrated with the polytene chromosome map because many of the microsatellites were derived from libraries of DNA from specific chromosomal divisions, and other markers were located on the polytene chromosomes by in situ hybridization. The *w* mutation was localized between 2 flanking markers that are about 1 cM on either side. Cytogenetic mapping of these 2 microsatellite markers predicted that the *w* gene is between nurse cell polytene chromosome bands 2C and 1A. Recent cloning of a cytogenetic homologue of the *Drosophila w* gene at 2A is consistent with these genetic mapping results. The same families of genetic crosses were also used for the construction of a genetic map for the 2 autosomes. Backcrosses were also done between heterozygous females at lunate *(l)*, Dieldrin resistance *(Dild)*, red eye *(r)*, and homozygous recessive males to map these autosomal genetic markers. The *l* and *Dild* genes were placed on the second chromosome, and *r* on the third (L. Zheng, unpublished results).

Thirty-seven RAPD markers from *An. gambiae* have been identified and characterized (H.G. Dimopoylos and C. Louis, personal communication). Thirteen were found to be inherited as dominant

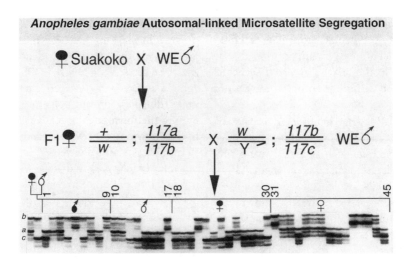

13.5 *Anopheles gambiae* autosomal-linked microsatellite segregation. Pattern of inheritance of autosomal-linked microsatellite markers in a 3-generation cross. The phenotype of eye color and genotype at microsatellite *AG2H117* (shortened to *117*) were determined for both parent and their 45 offspring, family A (240). There are approximately equal number offspring with *w 117a* and + *117a* (16 versus 14); and with *w 117b* and + *117b* (8 versus 7). Hence, they are inherited independently, *AG2H117* on the 2nd chromosome, *w* on the X chromosome. Courtesy of Zheng and Kafatos.

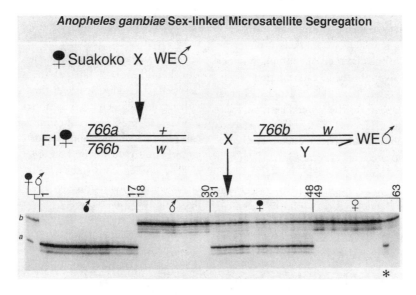

13.6 *Anopheles gambiae* sex-linked microsatellite segregation. Pattern of inheritance of X chromosome linked microsatellite markers in similar generation crosses, family B (240). The phenotype of eye color and the genotype at microsatellite *AGXH766* (shortened to *766*) were determined for both parents and their 63 offspring. From the preponderance of *w 766b* and + *776a* offspring, it is clear that *766a* is on the same chromosome with +, whereas *766b* is with *w* in the female parent. Only 1 recombinant between *766* and *w* were observed (asterisks). Courtesy of Zheng and Kafatos.

markers in genetic crosses. These markers have been integrated into the genetic map of *An. gambiae* based on microsatellite markers. The majority of the RAPD

Anopheles gambiae
X Chromosome Linkage Map

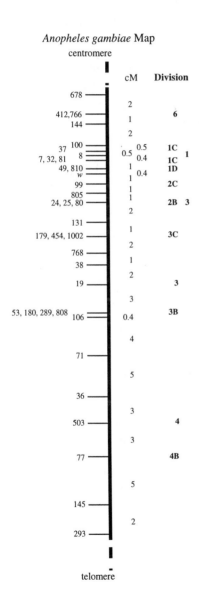

Anopheles gambiae Map

bands have also been cloned and sequenced; some contain repetitive elements, whereas many contained unique sequences.

The current map has 120 microsatellite markers, 42 on the X, 53 on the 2nd, and 25 on the 3rd chromosome (L. Zheng, unpublished results). Thirteen RAPD markers have also been integrated into this map, so that the total number of markers mapped is about 125. Assuming a total genetic map of 250 cM, the current map has an average resolution of about 2 cM, and some of these markers have also been localized cytogenetically by in situ hybridization to polytene chromosomes.

RFLP markers have been produced for *An. gambiae* (P. Romans, personal communication). Some of these markers have been localized cytogenetically to nurse cell polytene chromosomes, and linkage mapping has also been performed. In one case an RFLP marker at the diphenol oxidase coding locus *(Dox)* segregated independently from a gene encoding an esterase *(EstA/C)*. These data are consistent with the cytogenetic locations of these 2 genes, with *Dox* on the right arm of the 3rd chromosome and *EstA/C* on the left arm of the 2nd chromosome (187).

Laboratory strains and field collected mosquitoes exhibit variations in their response to *Plasmodium* infection. Some mosquitoes block the development of *Plasmodium* by encapsulating the oocyst in the midgut, thus preventing the formation of sporozoites. Genetic selection with the *An. gambiae* G3 strain has generated phenotypically pure lines that are refractory to the simian parasite, *P. cynomolgi* B. These lines also encapsulate other *Plasmodium* spp., although certain *P. falciparum*

13.7 *Anopheles gambiae* X chromosome linkage map. Current genetic map of the X chromosome of *Anopheles gambiae* consists of a total of 36 markers, including the *white eye* (*w*) mutation. Microsatellite markers are indicated with distance from neighbors expressed in cM and correlated with polytene chromosome divisions where known. The prefix *AGXH* was omitted for simplicity. The map covers a total of 44 cM, with an average of 1.5 cM between markers. The actual distance between markers (in cM) and their cytogenetic locations (on nurse cell polytene chromosome) is also shown. Courtesy of Zheng and Kafatos.

strains from Africa are not encapsulated efficiently (45, 220, 221). Genetic analysis shows that the encapsulation of *P. cynomolgi* B is controlled primarily by a single locus, *Pif-B*, and that susceptibility is dominant over refractoriness. Further analysis suggests that encapsulation is generally associated with the esterase phenotype *EstA/A* and with chromosome karyotype, 2La+, which is the wild-type arrangement of polytene bands, on the left arm of the 2nd chromosome. The susceptibility phenotype is associated with another esterase phenotype *EstC/C* and karyotype 2La, which is an inversion of divisions 22–26 on the left arm of the 2nd chromosome. Another locus, *Pif-C*, seems to play an important part in the encapsulation of *P. cynomolgi* Ceylon (220, 221). Recent work demonstrated that the esterase A or C phenotype results from the product of 2 genes, both located in the 2La inversion (49).

PHYSICAL MAPPING

Although the genomic content of an organism is ordered into a linear array of genetic elements that are organized into chromosomes, the sheer size of the chromosomal DNA prohibits its direct manipulation. Historically, cytogenetic approaches have provided important mapping information, and it is here where the value of polytene chromosomes is most apparent. Nevertheless, this type of physical mapping is inherently low resolution by molecular standards. More recently, physical mapping strategies have been developed to create random recombinant libraries, which contain smaller fragments of the genome, and then to order these manageable fragments to provide a physical map of contiguous fragments (contigs) representing the genome (Fig. 13.1). It is ironic that we begin with ordered information (chromosomes), break them into smaller unordered fragments, and finally reorder those fragments. This reductionist approach, however, is not without benefits because it provides the tools for gene identification or isolation and ultimately for primary DNA sequence determination.

Low-Resolution Mapping

In mosquitoes, most physical mapping done to date has utilized the banding patterns displayed in polytene chromosomes of *Anopheles* in which inversions,

translocations, and deletions have been identified. In addition, numerous cloned DNA fragments have been mapped to their chromosomal location with a reasonable degree of accuracy using in situ hybridization (V. Kumar, F. Collins, P. Romans, and others, unpublished observations). This latter approach has been applied to mapping fragments to aedine metaphase chromosomes (107, 109). Somatic cell hybrids have not been developed for disease vector genomes.

High-Resolution Mapping

High-resolution mapping approaches have blossomed in recent years due in large part to the explosive growth in genome programs. These approaches can be divided generally into "bottom-up" or "top-down" (short-range or long-range) mapping strategies, based upon the scale of the mapping or starting materials, although the overlap in these 2 approaches can be considerable. Chromosome specific libraries, contig mapping, electrophoretic techniques, and DNA sequencing strategies are bottom-up approaches; whereas random contig mapping using large fragments and fluorescence in situ hybridization (FISH) are top-down approaches. FISH is an example of an approach that now overlaps these distinctions because it is being applied in short- and long-range mapping projects.

Chromosome Specific Libraries and Contig Mapping

The development of chromosome specific libraries has been driven in large part by the desire to minimize the random nature of library production and subsequent contig assembly. Although a number of approaches have been employed, including chromosome sorting using a fluorescent-activated cell sorter, microdissection approaches have been the most productive. *Drosophila* with its polytene chromosomes represents the paradigm for this fine-scale mapping strategy. Briefly, a chromosomal division is dissected digested with *Sau*3A, and linkers are added to the fragments. The linkers are used as PCR primers for the amplification of the fragments, providing a continual source of division specific probes (190a). This approach is not limited to those organisms that exhibit polytene chromosomes; it has been applied to metaphase chromosomes of humans as well (123, 124). The divisional libraries can be used as a source of clones to identify coarsely mapped genes or to assign the location of other independently cloned sequences. Conversely, they can be used as probes to isolate large clones, such as cosmids and yeast artificial chromosomes (YACs), derived from a region of the genome; these are then ordered by determining their molecular overlaps, resulting in a collection of contiguous or clustered clones called contigs (96). Contigs can also be assembled from total genomic libraries but with greater difficulty.

Electrophoretic Techniques

Pulsed field gel electrophoresis and its derivatives are relatively recent developments that allow the separation of DNA in the Mb size ranges (21). When these tools are used in conjunction with restriction endonuclease enzymes that rarely cut the DNA, direct physical mapping of cloned sequences onto large pieces of genomic DNA is possible. These tools are particularly important in the characterization of YAC libraries and in the verification of contig maps.

Sequence Tagged Site Content Mapping

A unique sequence is the best landmark in the ultimate genomic map, the complete DNA sequence of an organism. It can also be used as a landmark during the process of its development, that is, physical mapping. Sequence tagged sites (STS) are markers that have proven exceedingly useful in physical mapping of the human genome (164). They are short, unique genomic regions that are easily detected by PCR amplification (189). The presence of the target sequence delineated by the primer sites can be evaluated using PCR on virtually any complex DNA source, including genomic DNA, genomic libraries (YAC, cosmid, phage, plasmid), cDNA libraries, and individual clones. STS markers have been used routinely to systematically screen human genome YAC libraries by PCR of successively smaller DNA pools derived from a given library (77, 72, 73, 192, 191, 137). The final result is the development of an ordered, linear arrangement of overlapping YAC DNA clones. This approach has yielded contig maps for human chromosomes (40, 62).

STS markers also have been generated successfully from human cDNA sequences (1).

Fluorescence In Situ Hybridization (FISH)

The challenge in genomic mapping is to map a large number of clones at regularly spaced intervals spanning the region of interest and to accomplish the task rapidly and efficiently (224). Recent advances in FISH and digital imaging microscopy have had a profound impact on high resolution physical mapping and gene identification (113, 114, 31, 118, 117, 224, 94, 135, 32, 83, 218). FISH is the most direct method to assign a probe to a specific chromosome and determine its regional location (224). The technique involves labeling a DNA probe sequence with a reporter molecule such as biotin (215). The probe and target metaphase chromosome spreads or interphase nuclei are denatured, and the complementary probe and target are allowed to reanneal. After washing to remove unhybridized and mismatched probe, samples are incubated with a fluorescent tagged affinity reagent such as avidin or antibiotin. Examination by fluorescence microscopy reveals a discrete fluorescent signal visible at the site of probe-chromosome hybridization. The map coordinates of hybridized probes can be expressed in terms of their fractional length distance from a chromosomal reference point, such as the terminus of the p arm ($p$ter), relative to the total length of the chromosome (117). Map coordinates are then referred to in terms of the fractional length of the chromosome from the p terminus, or FL$p$ter. The technique has been successful using probe sequences contained in plasmid, phage, cosmid, and yeast artificial chromosome YAC vectors without having to remove the insert prior to hybridization. When probe sequences contain repetitive DNA, a suppression hybridization is required to allow the interspersed unique sequences to be mapped (119).

The genetic resolution level of FISH and digital imaging microscopy, that is, the ability to resolve 2 signals (probes), depends upon the material examined (135, 224, 83). Probes are mapped initially to metaphase chromosomes, where the resolution is approximately 1 Mb. When the density of probes mapped to a particular region is so great that the signals appear co-localized, then interphase nuclei are examined. The resolution of interphase nuclei mapping is 50–100 kb, and the relationship between kb versus distance measured between signals in interphase nuclei is essentially linear up to 2 Mb (218). The 3rd level is termed extended chromatin mapping (or DIRVISH— direct visual hybridization), in which FISH is done on decondensed DNA. This increases resolution between signals from 1–2 kb (74a, 170). DIRVISH is used for extremely fine ordering of probes, and it shows promise in many mapping applications. Using probes in combinations is an extremely powerful approach to FISH mapping because multiple probes can be mapped concurrently, and it is the method of choice in interphase nuclei mapping.

Random Contig Mapping Using Large Fragments

Although YAC, bacterial artificial chromosomes, and the P1 phage cloning system are capable of cloning large fragments, the YAC cloning system is capable of producing recombinants that contain genomic inserts in the Mb size range. There are real advantages in being able to clone large genomic fragments; the most obvious is that fewer clones are required to cover the genome. For genome size of 780 Mb, only 3,590 clones with 1 Mb inserts would cover at a 99% percent probability, compared to 35,918 clones needed when the inserts are 100 kb in size.

In random contig mapping with YAC libraries, insert-specific fingerprints are generated, and these data are used to assemble contigs that can be assigned to chromosomes via FISH mapping (15, 40). This approach has been extremely productive in the human genome projects in which a 1st generation physical map of YAC contigs for all chromosomes has been reported (43). Contigs were constructed by probing the restricted YACs with moderately repetitive elements such as *L1* and *THE*, resulting in YAC insert-specific fingerprints. As more data are generated, the fingerprints coalesced into larger and larger contigs. Using the YAC cloning system is not for the faint of heart—it is as challenging to establish the technology in the laboratory as it is useful.

The Aedes aegypti *Physical Map*

Studies are under way currently using FISH in the construction of a physical map of the *Ae. aegypti* genome (34a). Briefly, cosmid and YAC probes used in FISH experiments of metaphase chromosomes have yielded paired signals, one on each arm of the sister chromatids, and they have been ordered along the chromosomes. More than 40 different probes have been mapped to the 3 chromosomes of *Ae. aegypti*, and these included 28 to chromosome I, 6 to chromosome II, and 6 to chromosome III (Fig. 13.8). In addition, the ribosomal rDNA cistron has been identified and mapped to chromosome I (Fig. 13.3). The latter was identified as an intense signal, readily detectable by several cosmids and YAC probes by FISH. This finding refines the reported map location of the rDNA cistron on chromosome I to 66.5% FL*p*ter (107, 127a). The rDNA cistron has been placed on the genetic linkage map as the nucleolar-organizer *(NO)* locus (Figs. 13.4, 13.8).

FISH mapping of metaphase chromosomes requires high-quality chromosome preparations that exhibit high mitotic indices, and protocols have been developed that consistently yield high quality chromosomes using mosquito cell lines (34a). Using cell lines as a source of mapping materials has a number of other benefits, including their continuous availability, consistency in preparations and genetic background, high mitotic indices that allow fine-scale mapping, and their availability to any laboratory from the American Type Culture Collection. As the physical map resolves, it will be necessary to compare cell line chromosomal map locations with chromosomes prepared from the whole mosquitos whose chromosomes are usable for FISH (S.E. Brown and D.L. Knudson, unpublished data) when prepared following Rai's basic procedures (176, 178).

The Anopheles gambiae *Physical Map*

Unlike *Ae. aegypti*, the actively studied malarial vector mosquito *An. gambiae* exhibits excellent, well-spread polytene chromosomes. The polytene chromosomes in *An. gambiae* have permitted a microdissection approach for physical mapping, which was pioneered with *Drosophila*. A low-resolution, *An. gambiae* physical map was constructed by this procedure (241). In

Aedes aegypti Composite Map of Chromosome I

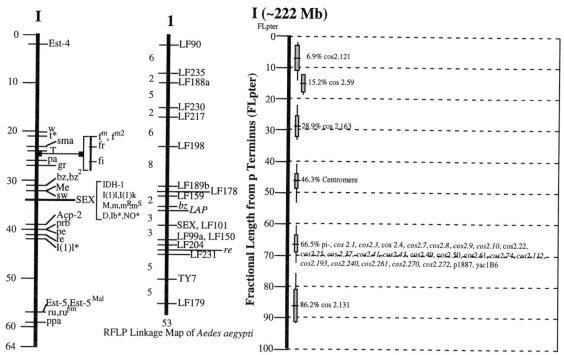

13.8 *Aedes aegypti* composite map of chromosome I. Physical map of *Ae. aegypti* chromosome I compared with the genetic linkage maps. The FISH-mapped probes are placed on the physical map as a fractional length from the *p* (smallest arm) terminus. Courtesy of Brown and Knudson.

this study, 54 distinct divisions of the polytene chromosomes, each encompassing approximately 4 Mb, were microdissected, restriction enzyme digested, ligated to synthetic primers, and PCR amplified to create pools of divisional probes. Dot blot filters of all the probes arranged in numerical order were prepared and screened with previously prepared cloned sequences of known chromosomal location. The dot blots served to identify the correct chromosomal location of cloned DNA fragments. This type of system could be of great value to quickly map genes and other molecular markers such as restriction fragment length polymorphisms and random amplified polymorphic

DNA. Furthermore, this system can be useful for identifying genes by homology. Many cloned genes from *Drosophila* are available and could be used to screen the dot blot library for the homologous mosquito genes. The libraries can also be used to select cosmid, P1, or YAC clones from a chromosomal region of interest, which then can be assembled into contigs, as is done in *Drosophila* (96).

Transformation Systems in Mapping

Once a target gene is isolated to approximately 2 Mb or less fragment, efforts to identify and isolate the gene itself begin. The simplest approach is to transform mosquitoes with a YAC that covers the locus. Mosquito transformation systems are currently being examined (4, 140, 138). Unfortunately, mosquito transformation systems are not yet available that are useful for mapping genes. Given the realities of today's mosquito transformation systems and the lack of deletion mutant mosquito strains, either the transformation systems need continued support or an alternative strategy must be developed.

Correlation of Genetic and Physical Maps

The physical maps should be integrated with linkage map data. The 2 maps can be reconciled using STS markers, developed for individual polymorphic DNA markers, to identify large genomic clones for placement on the physical map via FISH. After clones containing STS are identified, they can be mapped physically via FISH, providing an extremely rapid integration of the linkage and physical maps, sensitive enough to detect variations in the map units/Mb ratio along the chromosome as has been reported in yeast chromosome III (163). Although in theory cDNAs can be used directly as probes for FISH mapping (188), in practice, they have not proven to be useful due in part to the size of their intron sequences or gene complexity. When polytene chromosomes are available, the correlation of the 2 maps is straightforward, using in situ hybridization techniques similar to those used with the *An. gambiae*.

CONCLUSION

Considering the number and the impact of the infectious diseases transmitted by *Ae. aegypti* and *An. gambiae*, it is not surprising that they have emerged as the organisms whose genomic organizations are being studied actively. Although much has been accomplished in understanding their genomic organization, much still remains.

Aedes aegypti and *An. gambiae* are important models for genomic mapping, and their maps need to be developed for many reasons. *Culicinae*, which includes *Aedes* mosquitoes, is composed of approximately 1,600 species and accounts taxonomically for the largest group of mosquito species. *Anophelinae* and *Toxorhynchitinae* have approximately 325 and 60 species, respectively. The mapping models for these 2 species are representative for a large number of dipteran species. They vector a number of debilitating and lethal pathogens of humans and other vertebrates, and as such, they are models for both viral and parasite susceptibility, because mosquito strains exhibit different vector competency for these pathogens. Their genetic linkage maps are advanced compared to other mosquito maps, making them the best genetically characterized mosquito species, and these maps will be essential to uncover the genetic basis for phenotypic characters unique to disease vector biology. The methodological approaches being used in physically mapping their genomes utilize the best of the technology that has been developed in other more advanced mapping projects, and these approaches have capitalized on the unique characteristics of each. For example, FISH and digital imaging microscopy make physical mapping of *Ae. aegypti* a practical and feasible undertaking. Similarly, the polytene chromosomes of *An. gambiae* have provided powerful tools for mapping this mosquito species. Because there are basic differences in these 2 mosquito species, comparative studies of their respective maps should also prove instructive.

Finally, genetic and physical mapping studies will yield reagents useful in biologic, developmental, and physiologic studies. Chromosome maps developed will be essential in gene identification for simple and quantitative traits. These mapping projects are exciting developments that will contribute to our understanding of mosquito genetics, provide a foundation upon which to build our understanding of mosquito physiology and vector competency, and aid in attaining our goal of developing new strategies for the control of vector-borne diseases.

ACKNOWLEDGMENTS

We acknowledge the support from the John D. and Catherine T. MacArthur Foundation, TDR/WHO, and the Colorado Agricultural Experiment Station. Our colleagues, many of whom are cited herein, willingly shared their data and are acknowledged for their responsiveness to our many inquiries. Susan Wood is also acknowledged for her assistance with the literature cited.

REFERENCES

1. Adams, M.D., J.M. Kelley, J.D. Gocayne, M. Dubnick, M.H. Polymeropoulos, H. Xiao, C.R. Merril, A. Wu, B. Olde, R.F. Moreno, A.R. Kerlavage, W.R. McCombie, and J.C. Venter. 1991. Complementary DNA sequencing: Expressed sequence tags and human genome project. *Science* 252:1651–1656.

2. Aitken, T.H.G., W.G. Downs, and R.E. Shope. 1977. *Aedes aegypti* strain fitness for yellow fever virus transmission. *Am. J. Trop. Med. Hyg.* 26:985–989.

3. Akopyanz, N., N.O. Bukanov, T.U. Westblom, and D.E. Berg. 1992. PCR-based RFLP analysis of DNA sequence diversity in the gastric pathogen *Helicobacter pylori. Nucleic Acids Res.* 20:6221–6225.

4. Aksoy, S. 1991. Site-specific retroposons of the trypanosomatid Protozoa. *Parasit. Today* 7:281–285.

5. Arnold, M.L., C.M. Buckner, and J.J. Robinson. 1991. Pollen-mediated introgression and hybrid speciation in Louisiana irises. *Proc. Natl. Acad. Sci. USA* 88:1398–1402.

6. Ashburner, M. 1992. Mapping insect genomes. In: J.M. Crampton and P. Eggleston, editors, *Insect molecular science.* San Diego: Academic Press. pp. 51–71.

7. Barillas-Mury, C., R. Graf, H.H. Hagedorn, and M.A. Wells. 1991. cDNA and deduced amino acid sequence of a blood meal-induced trypsin from the mosquito, *Aedes aegypti. Insect Biochem.* 21:825–831.

8. Barker, D., P. Green, R. Knowlton, J. Schumm, E. Lander, A. Oliphant, H. Willard, G. Akots, V. Brown, T. Gravius, C. Helms, C. Nelson, C. Parker, K. Rediker, M. Rising, D. Watt, B. Weiffenbach, and H. Donis-Keller. 1987. Genetic linkage map of human chromosome 7 with 63 DNA markers. *Proc. Natl. Acad. Sci. USA* 84:8006–8010.

9. Barr, A.R. 1969. Divided-eye, a sex linked mutation in *Culex pipiens* L. *J. Med. Ent.* 6:393–397.

10. Barr, A.R. 1975. Culex. In: R.C. King, editors, *Handbook of genetics: Invertebrates of genetic interest,* Vol. 3. London: Plenum Press. pp. 347–376.

11. Beaty, B.J., and T.H.G. Aitken. 1979. *In vitro* transmission of yellow fever virus by geographic strains of *Aedes aegypti. Mosq. News* 39:232–238.

12. Beckett, E.B. 1971. Histological changes in mosquito flight muscle fibres associated with parasitization by filarial larvae. *Parasitol.* 63:365–372.

13. Beckmann, J.S. 1988. Oligonucleotide polymorphisms: a new tool for genomic genetics. *Biotechnology* 6:1061–1064.

14. Beckmann, J.S., and J.L. Weber. 1992. Survey of human and rat microsatellites. *Genomics* 12:627–631.

15. Bellanné-Chantelot, C., B. Lacroix, P. Ougen, A. Billault, S. Beaufils, S. Bertrand, I. Georges, F. Gilbert, I. Gros, G. Lucotte, L. Susini, J. Codani, P. Gesnouin, S. Pook, G. Vaysseix, J. Lu-Kuo, T. Ried, D. Ward, I. Chumakov, D. Le Paslier, E. Barrilot, and D. Cohen. 1992. Mapping the whole human genome by fingerprinting yeast artificial chromosomes. *Cell* 70:1059–1068.

16. Berg, D.E., and M.M. Howe, editors 1989. Mobile DNA. Washington, D.C.: American Society for Microbiology. 972 p.

17. Besansky, N.J. 1990. Evolution of the T1 retroposon family in the *Anopheles gambiae* complex. *Molecular Biology and Evolution* 7:229–246.

18. Besansky, N.J. 1990. A retrotransposable element from the mosquito *Anopholes gambiae. Mol. Cell. Biol* 10:863–871.

19. Besansky, N.J., S.M. Paskewitz, D.M. Hamm, and F.H. Collins. 1992. Distinct families of site-specific retrotransposons occupy indentical postions in the rRNA genes of *Anopheles gambiae. Mol. Cell. Biol* (1211) 5102–5110.

20. Besansky, N.J., and J.R. Powell. 1992. Reassociation kinetics of *Anopheles gambiae* Diptera: Culicidae. DNA. *Entomological Society of America* 29:125–128.

21. Bickmore, W. 1992. Analysis of genomic DNAs by pulsed-field gel electrophoresis. In: R. Anand, editors, *Techniques for the analysis of complex genomes* chap. 2. London: Academic Press, Harcourt Brace Jovanovich. pp. 19–38.

22. Biessmann, H., L.E. Champion, M. O'Hair, K. Ikenaga, B. Kasravi, and J.M. Mason. 1992. Frequent transpositions of *Drosophila melanogaster* HeT-A transposable elements to receding chromosome ends. *Eur. Mol. Biol. Org. J.* 11:4459–4469.

23. Biessmann, H., K. Valgeirsdottir, A. Lofsky, C. Chin, B. Ginther, R.W. Levis, and M. Pardue 1992. HeT-A, a transposable element specifically involved in "healing" broken chromosome ends in *Drosophila melanogaster. Mol. Cell. Biol* 12:3910–3918.

24. Black, W.C., IV, N.M. DuTeau, G.J. Puterka, J.R. Nechols, and J.M. Pettorini. 1992. Use of random amplified polymorphic DNA polymerase chain reaction RAPD-PCR to defect DNA polymorphisms in aphids (Homoptera: Aphididae). *Bull. Ent. Res.* 82:151–159.

25. Black, W.C., IV, D.K. McLain, and K.S. Rai. 1989. Patterns of variation in the rDNA cistron within and among world populations of a mosquito, *Aedes albopictus* (Skuse). *Genetics* 121:539–550.

26. Black, W.C. IV, and K.S. Rai. 1988. Genome evolution in mosquitoes: Intraspecific and interspecific variation in repetitive DNA amounts and organization. *Genetic Research* 51:185–196.

27. Blackburn, E.H. 1991. Structure and function of telomeres. *Nature* 350:569–573.

28. Blanchetot, A. 1989. Detection of highly polymorphic regions in insect genomes. *Nucleic Acids Res.* 17:3313.

29. Boehm, T., L. Mengle-Gaw, U.R. Kees, N. Spurr, I. Lavenir, A. Forster, and T.H. Rabbitts. 1989. Alternating purine-pyrimidine tracts may promote chromososmal translocation seen in a variety of human lymphoid tumours. *Eur. Mol. Biol. Org. J.* 8:2621–2631.

30. Boeke, J.D., and V.G. Corces. 1989. Transcription and reverse transcription of retrotransposons. *Ann. Rev. of Microbiol.* 43:403–434.

31. Boyle, A.L., S.G. Ballard, and D.C. Ward. 1990. Differential distribution of long and short interspersed element sequences in the mouse genome: Chromosome karyotyping by fluorescence in situ hybridization. *Proc. Natl. Acad. Sci. USA* 87:7757–7761.

32. Boyle, A.L., D.M. Feltquite, N.C. Dracopoli, D.E. Housman, and D.C. Ward. 1992. Rapid physical mapping of cloned DNA on banded mouse chromosomes by fluorescence *in situ* hybridization. *Genomics* 12:106–115.

33. Britten, R.J., and E.H. Davidson. 1971. Repetitive and nonrepetitive DNA sequences and a speculation on the origins of evolutionary novelty. *Quart. Rev. Biol.* 46:111–137.

34. Britten, R.J., D.E. Graham, and B.R. Neufeld. 1974. Analysis of repeating DNA sequences by reassociation. *Meth. Enzymol.* 29:363–418.

34a. Brown, S.E.J. Menninger, M. Difillipantonio, B.J. Beaty, D.C. Ward, and D.L. Knudson. 1995. Toward a physical map of *Aedes aegypti*. *Insect Mol. Biol.* 4:161–167.

35. Burke, W.D., D.G. Eickbush, X. Yue, J. Jakubczak, and T.H. Eickbush. 1993. Sequence relationship of retrotransposable elements R1 and R2 within and between divergent insect species. *Molec. Biol. Evol.* 10:163–185.

36. Buxton, B.A., and G.R. Mullen. 1981. Comparative susceptibility of four strains of *Aedes aegypti* (Diptera: Culicidae) to infection with *Dirofilaria immitis*. *J. Med. Ent.* 18:434–440.

37. Calvi, B.R., T.J. Hong, S.D. Findley, and W.M. Gelbart. 1991. Evidence for a common evolutionay origin of inverted repeat transposons in Drosophila and plants: Hobo, Activator, and Tam3. *Cell* 66:465–471.

38. Cavalier-Smith, T. 1985. Introduction: the evolutionary significance of genome size. In: T. Cavalier-Smith, editors, *The Evolution of Genome Size*. London: John Wiley & Sons. pp. 1–36.

39. Christensen, B.M., and D.R. Sutherland. 1984. *Brugia pahangi*: Exsheathment and midgut penetration in *Aedes aegypti*. *Trans. Amer. Microbiol. Soc.* 103:423–433.

40. Chumakov, I., P. Rigault, S. Guillou, P. Ougen, A. Billaut, G. Guasconi, P. Gervy, I. LeGall, P. Soularue, L. Grinas, L. Bougueleret, C. Bellanné-Chantelot, B. Lacrois, E. Barillot, P. Gesnouin, S. Pook, G. Vaysseix, G. Frelat, A. Schmitz, J. Sambucy, A. Bosch, X. Estivill, J. Weissenbach, A. Vignal, H. Riethman, D. Cox, D. Patterson, K. Gardiner, M. Hattori, Y. Sakaki, H. Ichikawa, M. Ohki, D. Le Paslier, R. Heilig, S. Antonarakis, and D. Cohen. 1992. Continuum of overlapping clones spanning the entire human chromosome 21q. *Nature* 359:380–387.

41. Clements, A.N. 1992. The biology of mosquitoes. Vol. 1. London: Chapman and Hall. 595 p.

42. Cockburn, A.F., and S.E. Mitchell. 1989. Repetitive DNA interspersion patterns in diptera. *Arch. Insect Biochem. Physiol.* 10:105–113.

43. Cohen, D., I. Chumakov, and J. Weissenbach. 1993. A first-generation physical map of the human genome. *Nature* 366:698–701.

44. Collins, F.H., S.M. Paskewitz, and V. Finnerty. 1989. Ribosomal RNA genes of the *Anopheles gambiae* species complex. In: *Advances in Disease Vector Research*, Vol. 6. New York: Springer-Verlag. pp. 1–28.

45. Collins, F.H., R.K. Sakai, K.D. Vernick, S. Paskewitz, D.C. Seeley, L.H. Miller, W.E. Collins, C.C. Campbell, and R.W. Gwadz. 1986. Genetic selection of a *Plasmodium*-refractory strain of the malaria vector *Anopheles gambiae*. *Science* 234:607–610.

46. Coluzzi, M., V. Petrarca, and M.A. Di Deco. 1985. Chromosomal inversion intergradation and incipient speciation in *Anopheles gambiae*. *Bollettino di Zoologia* 52:45–63.

47. Coluzzi, M., A. Sabatini, V. Petrarca, and M.A. Di Deco. 1979. Chromosomal differentiation and adaptation to human environments in the *Anopheles gambiae* complex. *Trans. Roy. Soc. Trop. Med. Hyg.* 73:483–497.

48. Craig, G.B., Jr. and W.A. Hickey. 1967. Genetics of *Aedes aegypti*. In: J.W. Wright and R. Pal, editors, *Genetics of Insect Vectors of Disease*, chap. 3. Amsterdam: Elsevier Publishing. pp. 67–131.

49. Crews-Oyen, A.E., V. Kumar, and F.H. Collins. 1993. Association of two esterase genes, a chromosomal inversion, and susceptibility to *Plasmodium cynomolgi* in the African malaria vector *Anopheles gambiae*. *Am. J. Trop. Med. Hyg.* 49:341–347.

50. Crowhurst, R.N., B.T. Hawthorne, E.H.A. Rikkerink, and M.D. Templeton. 1991. Differentiation of *Fusarium solani* f. sp. *cucurbitae* races 1 and 2 by random amplification of polymorphic DNA. *Cur. Gen.* 20:391–396.

51. Davidson, E.H., B.R. Hough, W.H. Klein, and R.J. Britten. 1975. Structural genes adjacent to interspersed repetitive DNA sequences. *Cell* 4:217–238.

52. Davidson, G. 1962. *Anopheles gambiae* complex. *Nature* 196:907.

53. Davidson, G. 1964. The five mating types in the *Anopheles gambiae* complex. *Riv. di Malariol.* 43:167–183.

54. Dennhöfer, L. 1975. Genlokalisation auf den larvalen Speicheldrüsenchromosomen der Stechmücke *Culex pipiens* L. *Theor. Appl. Genet.* 45:279–289.

55. Edwards, M.E., C.W. Stuber, and J.F. Wendel. 1987. Molecular-maker-facilitated investigations of quantitative-trait loci in Maize. I. Numbers, genomic distribution and types of gene action. *Genetics* 116:113–125.

56. Eggleston, P. 1991. The control of insect-borne disease through recombinant DNA technology. *Heredity* 66:161–172.

57. Ewert, A. 1965. Comparative migration of microfilariae and development of *Brugia pahangi* in various mosquitoes. *Am. J. Trop. Med. Hyg.* 14:254–259.

58. Ewert, A. 1965. Exsheathment of the microfilariae of *Brugia pahangi* in susceptible and refractory mosquitoes. *Am. J. Trop. Med. Hyg.* 14:260–262.

59. Feulgen, R., and H. Rossenbeck. 1924. Microskopisch-chemischer Nachweis einer Nucleinsaure von Typus der Thymonucleinsaure und die darauf beruhende selective Farbung von Zellkerner in mikroskopischen Praparaten. *Z. Physiol. Chem.* 135:203.

60. ffrench-Constant, R.H., T.A. Rocheleau, J.C. Steichen, and A.E. Chalmers. 1993. A point mutation in a *Drosophila* GABA receptor confers insecticide resistance. *Nature* 363:449–451.

61. Finnegan, D.J. 1992. Transposable elements and their biological consequences in *Drosophila* and other insects. In: J.M. Crampton and P. Eggleston, editors, *Insect Mol. Science*. London: Academic Press. pp. 35–46.

62. Foote, S., D. Vollrath, A. Hilton, and D.C. Page. 1992. The human Y chromosome: Overlapping DNA clones spanning the euchromatic region. *Science* 258:60–66.

63. Foster, G.G., M.J. Whitten, C. Konovalov, J.T.A. Arnold, and G. Maffi. 1981. Autosomal genetic maps of the Australian sheep blow fly *Lucilia cuprina dorsalis* R.-D. (Diptera: Calliphoridae) and possible correlations with linkage maps of *Musca domestica* L. and *Drosophila melanogaster* (Mg.). *Gen. Res.* 37:55–69.

64. Franz, G., T.G. Loukeris, G. Dialektaki, C.R.L. Thompson, and C. Savakis. 1994. Mobile *Minos* elements from *Drosophila hydei* encode a two-exon transposase with similarity to the paired DNA-binding domain. *Proc. Natl. Acad. Sci. USA*. 91:4746–4750.

65. Franz, G. and C. Savakis. 1991. *Minos*, a new transposable elements from *Drosophila hydei*, is a member of the Tc1-like family of transposons. *Nucleic Acids Res.* 19:6646.

66. Fu, Y.H., D.P.A. Kuhl, A. Pizzuti, M. Pieretti, J.S. Sutcliffe, S. Richards, A.J.M.H. Verkerk, J.J.A. Holden, R.G. Fenwick Jr., S.T. Warren, B.A. Oostra, D.L. Nelson, and C.T. Caskey. 1991. Variation of the CGG repeats at the fragile X site results in genetic instability: Resolution of the Sherman paradox. *Cell* 67:1047–1058.

67. Galau, G.A., M.E. Chamberlain, B.R. Hough, R.J. Britten, and E.H. Davidson. 1976. Evolution of repetitive and nonrepetitive DNA. In: F.J. Ayala, editors, *Molecular evolution*. Sunderland, MA: Sinauer Associates, Inc. pp. 200–224.

68. Gale, K., and J. Crampton. 1989. The ribosomal genes of the mosquito, *Aedes aegypti*. *Europ. J. Biochem.* 185:311–317.

69. Gooding, R.H. 1984. Genetics of *Glossina morsitans morsitans* (Diptera: Glossinidae): 9. Definition of linkage group III and further mapping of linkage groups I and II. *Can. J. Gen. Cytol.* 26:253–257.

70. Goodwin, P.H., and S.L. Annis. 1991. Rapid identification of genetic variation and pathotype of *Leptosphaeria maculans* by random amplified polymorphic DNA assay. *Appl. Environ. Microbiol.* 57:2482–2486.

71. Gordon, S.W. 1993. Molecular Genetics of *Aedes aegypti*. Ph.D., Colorado State University, Fort Collins. 238 p.

72. Green, E.D., and M.V. Olson. 1990. Systematic screening of yeast artificial-chromosome libraries by use of the polymerase chain reaction. *Proc. Natl. Acad. Sci. USA* 87:1213–1217.

73. Green, E.D., H.C. Riethman, J.E. Dutchik, and M.V. Olson. 1991. Detection and characterization of chimeric yeast artificial-chromosome clones. *Genomics* 11:658–669.

74. Gubler, D.J., S. Nalim, R. Tan, H. Saipan, and J.S. Saroso. 1979. Variation in susceptibility to oral infection with dengue viruses among geographic strains of *Aedes aegypti*. *Am. J. Trop. Med. Hyg.* 28:1045–1052.

74a. Haaf, T., and D.C. Ward. 1994. Structural analysis of (α-satellite DNA and centromere proteins using extended chromatin and chromasomes. *Human Mol. Gen.* 3:697–709.

75. Haniford, D.B., and D.E. Pulleyblank. 1983. Facile transition of poly (d(TG).d(CA)) into a left-handed helix in physiological conditions. *Nature* 302:632–634.

76. Hawley, W.A. 1988. The biology of *Aedes albopictus*. *J. Amer. Mosq. Contr. Assoc.* Suppl. 4:1–40.

77. Heard, E., B. Davies, S. Feo, and M. Fried. 1989. An improved method for screening of YAC libraries. *Nucleic Acids Res.* 17:5861.

78. Heckel, D.G. 1993. Comparative genetic linkage mapping in insects. *Ann. Rev. Entomol.* 38:381–408.

79. Hickey, W.A., and G.B. Craig Jr. 1966. Genetic distortion of sex ratio in a mosquito, *Aedes aegypti*. *Genetics* 53: 1177–1196.

80. Hieter, P., D. Pridmore, J.H. Hegemann, M. Thomas, R.W. Davis, and P. Philippsen. 1985. Functional selection and analysis of yeast centromeric DNA. *Cell* 42:913–921.

81. Hodgkin, J. 1992. Genetic sex determination mechanisms and evolution. *BioEssays* 14:253–261.

82. Houck, M.A., J.B. Clark, K.R. Peterson, and M.G. Kidwell. 1991. Possible horizontal transfer of *Drosophila* genes by the mite *Proctolaelaps regalis*. *Science* 253:1125–1129.

83. Hozier, J.C., and L.M. Davis. 1992. Cytogenetic approaches to genome mapping. *Anal. Biochem.* 200:205–217.

84. Hu, J., and C.F. Quiros. 1991. Identification of broccoli and cauliflower cultivars with RAPD markers. *Plant Cell Reports* 10:505–511.

85. Hunt, R.H. 1987. Location of genes on chromosome arms in the *Anopheles gambiae* group of species and their correlation to linkage data for other anopheline mosquitoes. *Med. Vet. Entomol.* 1:81–88.

86. Jacob, H.J., K. Lindpaintner, S.E. Lincoln, K. Kusumi, R.K. Bunker, Y.P. Mao, D. Ganten, V.J. Dzau, and E.S. Lander. 1991. Genetic mapping of a gene causing hypertension in the stroke-prone spontaneously hypertensive rat. *Cell* 67:213–234.

87. Jacobson, J.W., M.M. Medhora, and D.L. Hartl. 1986. Molecular structure of a somatically unstable transposable element in *Drosophila*. *Proc. Natl. Acad. Sci. USA* 83:8684–8688.

88. James, A.A., K. Blackmer, and J.V. Racioppi. 1989. A salivary gland-specific, maltase-like gene of the vector mosquito *Aedes aegypti*. *Gene* 75:73–83.

89. Javadian, E., and W.M. MacDonald. 1974. The effect of infection with *Brugia pahangi* and *Dirofilaria repens* on the egg-production of *Aedes aegypti*. *Ann. Trop. Med. Parasitol.* 684.:477–481.

90. Jeffreys, A.J., M. Turner, and P. Debenham. 1991. The efficiency of multilocus DNA fingerprint probes for individualization and establishment of family relationships, determined from extensive casework. *Am. J. Hum. Genet.* 48:824–840.

91. Jeffreys, A.J., V. Wilson, and S.L. Thein. 1985. Hypervariable 'minisatellite' regions in human DNA. *Nature* 314:67–73.

92. Jeffreys, A.J., V. Wilson, and S.L. Thein. 1985. Individual-specific 'fingerprints' of human DNA. *Nature* 316:76–79.

93. Jelnick, W.R., and C.W. Schmid. 1982. Repetitive sequences in eukaryotic DNA and their expression. *Ann. Rev. Biochem.* 51:813–844.

94. Johnson, C.V., J.A. McNeil, K.C. Carter, and J.B. Lawrence. 1991. A simple, rapid technique for precise mapping of multiple sequences in two colors using a single optical filter set. *Genet. Anal. Tech. Appl.* 8:75–76.

95. Jost, E., and M. Mameli. 1972. DNA content of nine species of Nematocera with special reference to the sibling species of the *Anopheles maculipennis* group and the *Culex pipiens* group. *Chromosoma* 37:201–208.

96. Kafatos, F.C., C. Louis, C. Savakis, D.M. Glover, M. Ashburner, A.J. Link, I. Sidén-Kiamos, and R.D.C. Saunders. 1991. Integrated maps of the *Drosophila* genome: Progress and prospects. *Trends in Genetics* 7:155–161.

97. Kalhok, S.E., L.M. Tabak, D.E. Prosser, W. Brook, A.E.R. Downe, and B.N. White. 1993. Isolation, sequencing and characterization of two cDNA clones coding for trypsin-like enzymes from the midgut of *Aedes aegypti*. *Insect. Mol. Biol* 2:71–79.

98. Kambhampati, S., and K.S. Rai. 1991. Mitochondrial DNA variation within and among populations of the mosquito *Aedes albopictus*. *Genome* 34:288–292.

99. Kambhampati, S., and K.S. Rai. 1991. Variation in mitochondrial DNA of *Aedes* species (Diptera: Culicidae). *Evolution* 45:120–129.

100. Kidwell, M.G. 1983. Evolution of hybrid dysgenesis determinants in *Drosophila melanogaster*. *Proc. Natl. Acad. Sci. USA* 80:1655–1659.

101. Kidwell, M.G. 1992. Horizontal Transfer. *Current Opinion in Genetics and Development* 2:868–873.

102. Kilama, W.L., and G.B. Craig Jr. 1969. Monofactorial inheritance of susceptibility to *Plasmodium gallinaceum* in *Aedes aegypti*. *Ann. Trop. Med. Parasitol.* 63:419–432.

103. Kitzmiller, J.B. 1976. Genetics, cytogenetics, and evolution of mosquitoes. *Adv. Gen.* 18:315–433.

104. Klein-Lankhorst, R.M., A. Vermunt, R. Weide, T. Liharska, and P. Zabel. 1991. Isolation of molecular markers for the tomato (*L. esculentum*) using random amplified polymorphic DNA (RAPD). *Theor. Appl. Genet.* 83:108–114.

105. Kreutzer, R.D. 1978. A mosquito with eight chromosomes: *Chagasia bathana* Dyar. *Mosq. News* 38:554–558.

106. Krumlauf, R. 1992. Evolution of the vertebrate *Hox* homeobox genes. *BioEssays* 14:245–252.

107. Kumar, A., and K.S. Rai. 1990. Chromosomal localization and copy number of 18S + 26S ribosomal RNA genes in evolutionarily diverse mosquitoes (Diptera, Culicidae). *Hereditas* 113:277–289.

108. Kumar, A., and K.S. Rai. 1990. Intraspecific variation in nuclear DNA content among world populations of a mosquito, *Aedes albopictus* (Skuse). *Theor. Appl. Genet.* 79:748–752.

109. Kumar, A., and K.S. Rai. 1991. Organization of a cloned repetitive DNA fragment in mosquito genomes (Diptera: Culicidae). *Genome* 34:998–1006.

110. Laird, C.D., and B.J. McCarthy. 1969. Molecular characterization of the *Drosophila* genome. *Genetics* 63:865–882.

111. Lander, E.S., and D. Botstein. 1986. Mapping complex genetic traits in humans: New methods using a complete RFLP linkage map. *Cold Spring Harbor Symposia on Quantitative Biology* 51:49–62.

112. Lander, E.S., and D. Botstein. 1989. Mapping Mendelian factors underlying quantitative traits using RFLP linkage maps. *Genetics* 121:185–199.

113. Langer, P.R., A.A. Waldrop, and D.C. Ward. 1981. Enzymatic synthesis of biotin-labeled polynucleotides: Novel nucleic acid affinity probes. *Proc. Natl. Acad. Sci. USA* 78:6633–6637.

114. Langer-Safer, P., M. Levine, and D.C. Ward. 1982. Immunological method for mapping genes on Drosophila polytene chromosomes. *Proc. Natl. Acad. Sci. USA* 79:4381–4385.

115. Laven, H. 1967. Formal genetics of *Culex pipiens*. In: J.W. Wright and R. Pal, editors, *Genetics of insect vectors of disease*. Amsterdam: Elsevier. pp. 17–66.

116. Levis, R.W., R. Ganesan, K. Houtchens, L.A. Tolar, and F.M. Sheen. 1993. Transposons in place of telomeric repeats at a *Drosophila* telomere. *Cell* 75:1083–1093.

117. Lichter, P., A.L. Boyle, T. Cremer, and D.C. Ward. 1991. Analysis of genes and chromosomes by nonisotopic *in situ* hybridization. *Genet. Anal. Tech. Appl.* 81.:24–35.

118. Lichter, P., C.C. Tang, K. Call, G. Hermanson, G.A. Evans, D. Housman, and D.C. Ward. 1990. High-resolution mapping of human chromosome 11 by *in situ* hybridization with cosmid clones. *Science* 247:64–69.

119. Lichter, P., and D.C. Ward. 1990. Is nonisotopic *in situ* hybridization finally coming of age? *Nature* 345:93–95.

120. Lidholm, D.A., G.H. Gudmundsson, and H.G. Boman. 1991. A highly repetitive, *mariner*-like element in the genome of *Hyalophora cecropia*. *J. Biol. Chem.* 266:11518–11521.

121. Lindsay, S.W., and D.A. Denham. 1986. The ability of *Aedes aegypti* mosquitoes to survive and transmit infective larvae of *Brugia pahangi* over successive blood meals. *J. Helminthol.* 60:159–168.

122. Litt, M., and J.A. Luty. 1989. A hypervariable microsatellite revealed by in vitro amplication of a dinucleotide repeat within the cardiac muscle actin gene. *Am. J. Hum. Genet.* 44:397–401.

123. Lüdecke, H.J., G. Senger, U. Claussen, and B. Horsthemke. 1989. Cloning defined regions of the human genome by microdissection of banded chromosomes and enzymatic amplification. *Nature* 338:348–350.

124. Lüdecke, H.J., G. Senger, U. Claussen, and B. Horsthemke. 1992. Generation of region-specific probes by microdissection and universal enzymatic DNA amplification. In: R. Anand, editors, *Techniques for the analysis of complex genomes*. London: Academic Press, Harcourt Brace Jovanovich. pp. 214–229.

125. Lyttle, T.W. 1993. Cheaters sometimes prosper: Distortion of mendelian segregation by meiotic drive. *Trends in Genetics* 9:205–210.

126. Macgregor, H.C., and J.M. Varley. 1983. *Working with animal chromosomes.* New York: J. Wiley and Sons. 250 p.

127. Manning, J.E., L.W. Schmid, and E.H. Davidson. 1975. Interspersion of repetitive and nonrepetitive DNA sequences in the *Drospohila melanogaster* genome. *Cell* 4:144–155.

127a. Marchi, A. and E. Pili. 1994. Ribosomal RNA genes in mosquitoes: Localization by fluorescence *in situ* hybridization (FISH). *Heredity.* 72:599–605.

128. Matthews, T.C., and L.E. Munstermann. 1990. Linkage maps for 20 enzyme loci in *Aedes triseriatus. J. Heredity* 81:101–106.

129. Matthews, T.C., and L.E. Munstermann. 1994. Chromosomal repatterning and linkage group conservation in mosquito karyotic evolution. *Evolution* 48:146–154.

130. McClain, D.K., K.S. Rai, and M.J. Frazer. 1986. Interspecific variation in the abundance of highly repeated DNA sequences in the *Aedes scutellaris* (Diptera: Culicidae) subgroup. *Ann. Entomol. Soc. Amer.* 79:784–791.

131. McClelland, G.A.H. 1962. Sex linkage in *Aedes aegypti. Trans. Roy. Soc. Trop. Med. Hyg.* 56:4.

132. McDonald, P.T., and K.S. Rai. 1970. Correlation of linkage groups with chromosomes in the mosquito, *Aedes aegypti. Genetics* 66:475–485.

133. McGinnis, W., A.W. Shermoen, and S.K. Beckendorf. 1983. A transposable element inserted just 5' to a Drosophila glue protein gene alters gene expression and chromatin structure. *Cell* 34:75–84.

134. McGreevy, P.B., G.A.H. McClelland, and M.M.J. Lavoipierre. 1974. Inheritance of susceptibility to *Dirofilaria immitis* infection in *Aedes aegypti. Ann. Trop. Med. Parasitol.* 68(1):97–109.

135. McNeil, J.A., C.V. Johnson, K.C. Carter, R.H. Singer, and J.B. Lawrence. 1991. Localizing DNA and RNA within nuclei and chromosomes by fluorescence *in situ* hybridization. *Genet. Anal. Tech. Appl.* 8:41–58.

136. Michelmore, R.W., I. Paran, and R.V. Kesseli. 1991. Identification of markers linked to disease-resistance genes by bulked segregant analysis: A rapid method to detect markers in specific genomic regions by using segregating populations. *Proc. Natl. Acad. Sci. USA* 88:9828–9832.

137. Moir, D.T., T.E. Dorman, A.P. Smyth, and D.R. Smith. 1993. A human genome YAC library in a selectable high-copy-number vector. *Gene* 125:229–232.

138. Monroe, T.J., M.C. Muhlmann-Diaz, M.J. Kovach, J.O. Carlson, J.S. Bedford, and B.J. Beaty. 1992. Stable transformation of a mosquito cell line results in extraordinarily high copy numbers of the plasmid. *Proc. Natl. Acad. Sci. USA* 89:5725–5729.

139. Morin, G.B. 1989. The human telomere terminal transferase enzyme is a ribonucleoprotein that synthesizes TTAGGG repeats. *Cell* 59:521–529.

140. Morris, A.C., T.L. Schaub, and A.A. James. 1991. FLP-mediated recombination in the vector mosquito, *Aedes aegypti. Nucleic Acids Res.* 19:5895–5900.

141. Motara, M.A., and K.S. Rai. 1977. Chromosomal differentiation in two species of *Aedes* and their hybrids revealed by Giemsa C-banding. *Chromosoma* 64:125–132.

142. Motara, M.A., and K.S. Rai. 1978. Giemsa C-banding patterns in *Aedes (Stegomyia)* mosquitoes. *Chromosoma* 70:51–58.

143. Mouchès, C., M. Agarwal, K. Campbell, L. Lemieux, and M. Abadon. 1991. Sequence of a truncated *LINE*-like retroposon dispersed in the genome of *Culex* mosquitoes. *Gene* 106:279–280.

144. Mouchès, C., N. Bensaadi, and J.C. Salvado. 1992. Characterization of a *LINE* retroposon dispersed in the genome of three nonsibling *Aedes* mosquito species. *Gene* 120:183–190.

145. Mouchès, C., Y. Pauplin, M. Agarwal, L. Lemieux, M. Herzog, M. Abadon, V. Beyssat-Arnaouty, O. Hyrien, B.R. de Saint Vincent, G.P. Georghiou, and N. Pasteur. 1990. Characterization of amplification core and esterase *B1* gene responsible for insecticide resistance in *Culex. Proc. Natl. Acad. Sci. USA* 87:2574–2578.

146. Muller, H.J. 1941. Induced mutations in *Drosophila*. In: *Cold Spring Harbor Symposia on Quantitative Biology*, Vol. 9, Cold Spring Harbor, NY: Cold Spring Harbor Press. pp. 151–167.

147. Müller, H.M., J.M. Crampton, A. della Torre, R. Sinden, and A. Crisanti. 1993. Members of a trypsin gene family in *Anopheles gambiae* are induced in the gut by blood meal. *Eur. Mol. Biol. Org. J.* 12:2891–2900.

148. Munstermann, L.E. 1981. Enzyme linkage maps for tracing chromosomal evolution in *Aedes* mosquitoes. In: M.W. Stock, editors, *Application of genetics and cytology in insect systematics and evolution.* Proceedings of the symposium of the national meeting of the Entomological Society of America; December 1–2, 1980; Atlanta. Moscow: Forest, Wildlife, and Range Experiment Station, University of Idaho. pp. 129–140.

149. Munstermann, L.E. 1990. Gene map of the yellow fever mosquito (*Aedes [Stegomyia] aegypti*) (2N=6). In: S.J. O'Brien, editor, *Genetic maps: Locus maps of complex genomes: Lower eukaryotes*, 5th ed., Vol. 3. Cold Spring Harbor: Cold Spring Harbor Laboratory Press. pp. 179–183.

150. Munstermann, L.E. 1990. Gene map of the eastern North American tree hole mosquito *Aedes triseriatus*. In: S.J. O'Brien, editor, *Genetic maps: Locus maps of complex genomes.*, 5th ed., Vol. 3. Cold Spring Harbor: Cold Spring Harbor Laboratory Press. pp. 184–187.

151. Munstermann, L.E., and G.B. Craig Jr. 1979. Genetics of *Aedes aegypti*: Updating the linkage map. *J. Heredity* 70:291–296.

152. Narang, S., and J.A. Seawright. 1982. Linkage relationships and genetic mapping in *Culex* and *Anopheles*. In: W.W.M. Steiner, W.J. Tabachnick, K.S. Rai, and S. Narang, editors, *Recent developments in the genetics of insect disease vectors: A symposium proceedings*. Champaign, IL: Stipes Publishing Co. pp. 231–289.

153. Narang, S.K., and J.A. Seawright. 1990. Linkage map of the mosquito *Anopheles albimanus*. In: S.J. O'Brien, editor, *Genetic maps: Locus maps of complex genomes.*, 5th ed., Vol. 3. Cold Spring Harbor: Cold Spring Harbor Laboratory Press. pp. 190–193.

154. Narang, S.K., J.A. Seawright, and S.E. Mitchell. 1990. Linkage map of the mosquito *Anopheles quadrimaculatus* species A. In: S.J. O'Brien, editor, *Genetic maps: Locus maps of complex genomes*, 5th ed., Vol. 3. Cold Spring Harbor: Cold Spring Harbor Laboratory Press. pp. 194–197.

155. Nei, M. 1987. *Molecular evolutionary genetics*. New York: Columbia University Press. 512 p.

156. Newton, M.E., D.I. Southern, and R.J. Wood. 1974. X and Y chromosomes of *Aedes aegypti* (L.) distinguished by Giemsa C-banding. *Chromosoma* 49:44–49.

157. Newton, M.E., R.J. Wood, and D.I. Southern. 1976. A cytogenetic analysis of meiotic drive in the mosquito, *Aedes aegypti* (L.). *Genetica* 46:297–318.

158. Newton, M.E., R.J. Wood, and D.I. Southern. 1978. Cytological mapping of the M and D loci in the mosquito, *Aedes aegypti* (L.). *Genetica* 48:137–143.

159. Nordheim, A., and A. Rich. 1983. The sequence (dC-dA)$_n$.(dG-dT)$_n$ forms left-handed Z-DNA in negatively supercoiled plasmids. *Proc. Natl. Acad. Sci. USA* 80:1821–1825.

160. O'Brien, S.J., editor. 1990. *Genetic maps: Locus maps of complex genomes: Lower eukaryotes*. 5th ed., Vol. 3. Cold Spring Harbor: Cold Spring Harbor Laboratory Press. 201 p.

161. O'Brien, S.J., ed. 1993. *Genetic maps: Locus maps of complex genomes: Lower eukaryotes* (33 maps). 6th ed., Vol. 3. Cold Spring Harbor: Cold Spring Harbor Laboratory Press. 318 p.

162. Okazaki, S., K. Tsuchida, H. Maekawa, H. Ishikawa, and H. Fujiwara. 1993. Identification of a pentanucleotide telomeric sequence, (TTAGG)$_n$, in the silkworm *Bombyx mori* and in other insects. *Mol. Cell. Biol.* 13:1424–1432.

163. Oliver, S.G., et al. 1992. The complete DNA sequence of yeast chromosome: 3. *Nature* 357:38–46.

164. Olson, M., L. Hood, C. Cantor, and D. Botstein. 1989. A common language for physical mapping of the human genome. *Science* 245:1434–1435.

165. Orgel, L.E., F.H.C. Crick, and C. Sapienza. 1980. Selfish DNA. *Nature* 288:645–646.

166. Palmer, C.A., D.D. Wittrock, and B.M. Christensen. 1986. Ultrastructure of Malpighian tubules of *Aedes aegypti* infected with *Dirofilaria immitis*. *J. Invertebr. Path.* 48:310–317.

167. Palmer, M.J., J.A. Bantle, X. Guo, and W.S. Fargo. 1994. Genome size and organization in the Ixodid tick, *Amblyomma americanum* (L.). *Insect. Mol. Biol* 3:57–62.

168. Paran, I., R. Kesseli, and R. Michelmore. 1991. Identification of restriction fragment length polymorphism and random amplified polymorphic DNA markers linked to downy mildew resistance genes in lettuce, using near-isogenic lines. *Genome* 34:1021–1027.

169. Park, Y.J., and A.M. Fallon. 1990. Mosquito ribosomal RNA genes: Characterization of gene structure and evidence for changes in copy number during development. *Insect Biochem.* 20:1–11.

170. Parra, I., and B. Windle. 1993. High resolution visual mapping of stretched DNA by fluorescent hybridization. *Nature Genetics* 5:17–21.

171. Parvez, S.D., K. Akhtar, and R.K. Sakai. 1985. Two new mutations and a linkage map of *Anopheles stephensi*. *J. Heredity* 76:205–207.

172. Pelisson, A., D.J. Finnegan, and A. Bucheton. 1991. Evidence for retrotransposition of the *I* factor, a *LINE* element of *Drosophila melanogaster*. *Proc. Natl. Acad. Sci. USA* 88:4907–4910.

173. Perrone, J.B., and A. Spielman. 1986. Microfilarial perforation of the midgut of a mosquito. *J. Parasitol.* 72(5):723–727.

174. Powell, J.R., and W.J. Tabachnick. 1980. Genetics and the origin of a vector population: *Aedes aegypti*, a case study. *Science* 208:1385–1387.

175. Rafalski, J.A., and S.V. Tingey. 1993. Genetic diagnostics in plant breeding: RAPDs, microsatellites and machines. *Trends in Genetics* 9:275–280.

176. Rai, K.S. 1963. A comparative study of mosquito karyotypes. *Ann. Entomol. Soc. Amer.* 56:160–170.

177. Ramos, A., A. Mahowald, and M. Jacobs-Lorena. 1993. Gut-specific genes from the black fly *Similium vittatum* encoding trypsin-like and carboxypeptidase-like proteins. *Insect. Mol. Biol.* 2:149–163.

178. Rao, P.N., and K.S. Rai. 1987. Comparative karyotpes and chromosomal evolution in some genera of nematocerous (Diptera: Nematocera) families. *Ann. Entomol. Soc. Amer.* 80:321–332.

179. Rao, P.N., and K.S. Rai. 1987. Inter- and intraspecific variation in nuclear DNA content in *Aedes* mosquitoes. *Heredity* 59:253–258.

180. Rao, P.N., and K.S. Rai. 1990. Genome evolution in the mosquitoes and other closely related members of superfamily Culicoidea. *Hereditas* 113:139–144.

181. Redfern, C.P.F. 1981. Satellite DNA of *Anopheles stephensi* Liston (Diptera: Culicidae). *Chromosoma* 82:561–581.

182. Reiter, R.S., J.G.K. Williams, K.A. Feldmann, J.A. Rafalski, S.V. Tingey, and P.A. Scolnik. 1992. Global and local genome mapping in *Arabidopsis thaliana* by using recombinant inbred lines and random amplified polymorphic DNAs. *Proc. Natl. Acad. Sci. USA* 89:1477–1481.

183. Rio, D.C. 1990. Molecular mechanism regulating *Drosophila P* element transposition. *Ann. Rev. Gen.* 24:543–578.

184. Risch, N. 1992. Genetic linkage: Interpreting LOD scores. *Science* 255:803–804.

185. Robertson, H.M. 1993. The *mariner* transposable element is widespread in insects. *Nature* 362:241–245.

186. Robertson, H.M., and E.G. MacLeod. 1993. Five major subfamilies of *mariner* transposable elements in insects, including the Mediterranean fly, and related arthropods. *Insect. Mol. Biol.* 2:125–139.

187. Romans, P., D.C. Seeley, Y. Kew, and R.W. Gwadz. 1991. Use of a restriction fragment length polymorphism (RFLP) as a genetic marker in crosses of *Anopheles gambiae* (Diptera: Culicidae): Independent assortment of a diphenol oxidase RFLP and an esterase locus. *J. Med. Ent.* 28:147–151.

188. Rudy, B., K. Sen, E. Vega-Saenz de Miera, D. Lau, T. Ried, and D.C. Ward. 1991. Cloning of a human cDNA expressing a high voltage-activating, TEA-sensitive, type-A K+ channel which maps to chromosome 1 band p21. *J. Neuro. Res.* 29:401–412.

189. Saiki, R.K., D.H. Gelfand, S. Stoffel, S.J. Scharf, R. Higuchi, G.T. Horn, K.B. Mullis, and H.A. Erlich. 1988. Primer-directed enzymatic amplication of DNA with a thermostable DNA polymerase. *Science* 239:487–491.

190. Sakai, R.K., K. Akhtar, and C.J. Dubash. 1985. Four new mutations and a linkage map of species A of *Anopheles culicifacies. J. Heredity* 76:140–141.

190a. Saunders, R.D.C., D.M. Glover, M. Ashburner, I. Siden-Kiamos, C. Louis, M. Monastirioti, C. Savakis, and F. Kafatos. 1989. PCR amplification of DNA microdissected from a single polytene chromosome band: A comparison with conventional microcloning. *Nucleic Acids Res.* 17:9027–9037.

191. Selleri, L., J.H. Eubanks, M. Giovannini, G.G. Hermanson, A. Romo, M. Djabali, S. Maurer, D.L. McElligott, M.W. Smith, and G.A. Evans. 1992. Detection and characterization of "chimeric" yeast artificial chromosome clones by fluorescent *in situ* suppression hybridization. *Genomics* 14:536–541.

192. Selleri, L., G.G. Hermanson, J.H. Eubanks, and G.A. Evans. 1991. Chromosomal *in situ* hybridization using yeast artificial chromosomes. *Genet. Anal. Tech. Appl.* 8:59–61.

193. Severson, D.W. 1994. Applications of molecular marker analysis to mosquito vector competence. *Parasit. Today* 10:336–340.

194. Severson, D.W., A. Mori, Y. Zhang, and B.M. Christensen. 1993. Linkage map for *Aedes aegypti* using restriction fragment length polymorphisms. *J. Heredity* 84:241–247.

195. Severson, D.W., A. Mori, Y. Zhang, and B.M. Christensen. 1994. Chromosomal mapping of two loci affecting filarial worm susceptibility in *Aedes aegypti. Insect. Mol. Biol.* 3:67–72.

196. Severson, D.W., A. Mori, Y. Zhang, and B.M. Christensen. 1994. The suitability of restriction fragment length polymorphism markers for evaluating genetic diversity among and synteny between mosquito species. *Am. J. Trop. Med. Hyg.* 50:425–432.

196a. Sharma, G.P., O.P. Mittal, S. Chaudhry, and V. Pal. 1978. A preliminary map of the salivary gland chromosomes of *Aedes (stegomyia) aegypti* (Culicadae, Diptera). *Cytobios* 22:169–178.

197. Southern, E.M. 1975. Detection of specific sequences among DNA fragments separated by gel electrophoresis. *J. Mol. Biol.* 98:503.

198. Spradling, A.C., and G.M. Rubin. 1983. The effect of chromosomal position on the expression of the Drosophila xanthine dehydrogenase gene. *Cell* 34:47–57.

199. Stallings, R.L., A.F. Ford, D. Nelson, D.C. Torney, C.E. Hildebrand, and R.K. Moyzis. 1991. Evolution and distribution of $(GT)_n$ repetitive sequences in mammalian genomes. *Genomics* 10:807–815.

200. Streck, R.D., J.E. MacGaffey, and S.K. Beckendorf. 1986. The structure of *hobo* elements and their insertion sites. *Eur. Mol. Biol. Org. J.* 5:3615–3623.

201. Sweeny, T.L., and A.R. Barr. 1978. Sex ratio distortion caused by meiotic drive in a mosquito, *Culex pipiens* L. *Genetics* 88:427–446.

202. Tabachnick, W.J. 1991. Evolutionary genetics and arthropod-borne disease: The yellow fever mosquito. *Amer. Ent.* 37:14–24.

203. Tabachnick, W.J., L.E. Munstermann, and J.R. Powell. 1979. Genetic distinctness of sympatric forms of *Aedes aegypti* in East Africa. *Evol.* 33:287–295.

204. Tabachnick, W.J., and J.R. Powell. 1979. A world-wide survey of genetic variation in the yellow fever mosquito, *Aedes aegypti*. *Gen. Res.* 34:215–229.

205. Tabachnick, W.J., G.P. Wallis, T.H.G. Aitken, B.R. Miller, G.D. Amato, L. Lorenz, J.R. Powell, and B.J. Beaty. 1985. Oral infection of *Aedes aegypti* with yellow fever virus: Geographic variation and genetic considerations. *Am. J. Trop. Med. Hyg.* 34:1219–1224.

206. Tadano, T. 1984. A genetic linkage map of the mosquito *Aedes togoi*. *Jap. J. Gen.* 59:165–176.

207. Tardieux, I., O. Poupel, L. Lapchin, and F. Rodhain. 1990. Variation among strains of *Aedes aegypti* in susceptibility to oral infection with dengue virus type 2. *Am. J. Trop. Med. Hyg.* 43:308–313.

208. Tautz, D. 1989. Hypervariability of simple sequences as a general source for polymorphic DNA markers. *Nucleic Acids Res.* 17:6463–6471.

209. Tautz, D., and M. Renz. 1984. Simple sequence repeats are ubiquitous repetitive components of eukaryotic genomes. *Nucleic Acids Res.* 12:4127–4138.

210. Taylor, K.A., S.M. Paskewitz, R.S. Copeland, J. Koros, R.F. Beach, J.I. Githure, and F.C. Collins. 1993. Comparison of two ribosomal DNA-based methods for differentiating members of the *Anopheles gambiae* complex (Diptera: Culicidae). *J. Med. Ent.* 30:457–461.

211. Terwedow, H.A., and G.B. Craig Jr. 1977. *Waltonella flexicauda*: Development controlled by a genetic factor in *Aedes aegypti*. *Exp. Parasit.* 41:272–282.

212. Tewfik, H.R., and A.R. Barr. 1974. The salivary gland chromosomes of *Culex pipiens* L. *Mosq. News* 34:47–54.

213. Thompson, M., F. Shotkoski, and R. ffrench-Constant. 1993. Cloning and sequencing of the cyclodiene insecticide resistance gene from the yellow fever mosquito *Aedes aegypti*: Conservation of the gene and resistance associated mutation with *Drosophila*. *Federation of European Biological Societies Letters* 325:187–190.

214. Thompson, M., J.C. Steichen, and R.H. ffrench-Constant. 1993. Conservation of cyclodiene insecticide resistance-associated mutations in insects. *Insect. Mol. Biol.* 2:149–154.

215. Trask, B.J. 1991. Fluorescence *in situ* hybridization: Applications in cytogenetics and gene mapping. *Trends in Genetics* 7:149–154.

216. Traut, W., J.T. Epplen, D. Weichenhan, and J. Rohwedel. 1992. Inheritance and mutation of hypervariable (GATA)n microsatellite loci in a moth, *Ephestia kuehniella*. *Genome* 35:659–666.

217. Turell, M.J., J.R. Beaman, and R.F. Tammariello. 1992. Susceptibility of selected strains of *Aedes aegypti* and *Aedes albopictus* (Diptera: Culicidae) to Chikungunya virus. *J. Med. Ent.* 29:49–53.

218. van den Engh, G., R. Sachs, and B.J. Trask. 1992. Estimating genomic distance from DNA sequence location in cell nuclei by a random walk model. *Science* 257:1410–1412.

219. Ved Brat, S., and K.S. Rai. 1973. An analysis of chiasmata frequencies in *Aedes aegypti*. *The Nucleus* 16:184–193.

220. Vernick, K.D., and F.H. Collins. 1989. Association of a *Plasmodium*-refractory phenotype with an esterase locus in *Anopheles gambiae*. *Am. J. Trop. Med. Hyg.* 40:593–597.

221. Vernick, K.D., F.H. Collins, and R.W. Gwadz. 1989. A general system of resistance to malaria infection in *Anopheles gambiae* controlled by two main genetic loci. *Am. J. Trop. Med. Hyg.* 40:585–592.

222. Wallis, G.P., W.J. Tabachnick, and J.R. Powell. 1984. Genetic heterogeneity among Caribbean populations of *Aedes aegypti. Am. J. Trop. Med. Hyg.* 33(3):492–498.

223. Warburg, A., and L.H. Miller. 1991. Critical stages in the development of *Plasmodium* in mosquitoes. *Parasit. Today* 7:179–181.

224. Ward, D.C., P. Lichter, A. Boyle, A. Baldini, J. Menninger, and S.G. Ballard. 1991. Gene mapping by fluorescent in situ hybridization and digital imaging microscopy. In: J. Lindsten and U. Pettersson, editors, *Etiology of Human Disease at the DNA Level.* New York: Raven Press. pp. 291–303.

225. Warren, A.M., and J.M. Crampton. 1991. The *Aedes aegypti* genome: Complexity and organization. *Gen. Res.* 58:225–232.

226. Weber, J.L., and P.E. May. 1989. Abundant class of human DNA polymorphisms which can be typed using the polymerase chain reaction. *Am. J. Hum. Genet.* 44:388–396.

227. Weir, B.S. 1990. *Genetic data analysis.* Sunderland, MA: Sinauer Associates. 377 p.

228. Welsh, J., and M. McClelland. 1990. Fingerprinting genomes using PCR with arbitrary primers. *Nucleic Acids Res.* 18:7213–7218.

229. Wetton, J.H., R.E. Carter, D.T. Parkin, and D. Walters. 1987. Demographic study of a wild house sparrow population by DNA fingerprinting. *Nature* 327:147–149.

230. Wevrick, R., and H. Willard. 1991. Physical map of the centromeic region of human chromosome 7: Relationship between two distinct alpha satellite arrays. *Nucleic Acid Res.* 19:2295–2301.

231. White, G.B. 1980. Academic and applied genetics aspects of mosquito cytogenetics. In: R.L. Blackman, G.M. Hewitt, and M. Ashburner, editors, *Insect cytogenetics.* Oxford: Blackwell Scientific Publications. pp. 245–274.

232. White, G.B. 1985. *Anopheles bwambae* sp.n., a malaria vector in the Semliki Valley, Uganda, and its relationships with other sibling species of the *An. gambiae* complex (Diptera: Culicidae). *Syst. Ent.* 10:501–522.

233. White, M.J.D. 1973. *Animal cytology and evolution.* Cambridge: Cambridge Unversity Press.

234. Wicking, C., and B. Williamson. 1991. From linked marker to gene. *Trends in Genetics* 7:288–293.

235. Wilkerson, R.C., T.J. Parsons, D.G. Albright, T.A. Klein, and M.J. Braun. 1993. Random amplified polymorphic DNA (RAPD) markers readily distingush cryptic mosquito species (Diptera: Culicidae: *Anopheles*). *Insect Mol. Biol.* 1:205–211.

236. Williams, J.G.K., A.R. Kubelik, K.J. Livak, J.A. Rafalski, and S.V. Tingey. 1990. DNA polymorphisms amplified by arbitrary primers are useful as genetic markers. *Nucleic Acids Res.* 18:6531–6535.

237. Wright, S. 1968. *Evolution and the genetics of populations.* Vol. 1. Genetic and biometric foundations. Chicago: University of Chicago Press. 469 p.

238. Xiong, Y., and T.H. Eickbush. 1990. Origin and evolution of retroelements based upon their reverse transcriptase sequences. *Eur. Mol. Biol. Org. J.* 9:3353–3362.

239. Zacharopoulou, A., M. Frisardi, C. Savakis, A.S. Robinson, P. Tolias, M. Konsolaki, K. Komitopoulou, and F.C. Kafatos. 1992. The genome of the Mediterranean fruit fly *Ceratitis capitata*: Localization of molecular markers by *in situ* hybridization to salivary gland polytene chromosomes. *Chromosoma* 101:448–455.

240. Zheng, L., F.H. Collins, V. Kumar, and F.C. Kafatos. 1993. A detailed genetic map for the X chromosome of the malaria vector, *Anopheles gambiae. Science* 261:605–608.

241. Zheng, L., R.D.C. Saunders, D. Fortini, A. della Torre, M. Coluzzi, D.M. Glover, and F.C. Kafatos. 1991. Low-resolution genome map of the malaria mosquito *Anopheles gambiae. Proc. Natl. Acad. Sci. USA* 88:11187–11191.

242. Zraket, C.A., J.L. Barth, D.G. Heckel, and A.G. Abbott. 1990. Genetic linkage mapping with restriction fragment length polymorphisms in the tobacco budworm *Heliothis virescens.* In: H.H. Hagedorn, J.G. Hildebrand, J.H. Kidwell, and J.H. Law, editors, *Insect molecular science.* New York: Plenum Press. pp. 13–20.

14. MOLECULAR GENETIC MANIPULATION OF VECTORS

Jonathan O. Carlson

INTRODUCTION

The ability to introduce recombinant DNA constructions into the genomes of organisms has been extremely valuable for investigating the molecular biology of several species. Much has been learned regarding the influence of various genes on the life processes of these organisms through the use of so-called reverse genetics. In this process, mutations are introduced into a gene by recombinant DNA techniques, and these modified genes are then introduced to see what effect the mutation has.

The application of such approaches to vector biology would be particularly interesting not only for the study of the vector organisms themselves but also for the investigation of vector-parasite interactions. As more becomes known regarding the genetic factors that affect vector competence, genes associated with competence will likely be identified and isolated. Reverse genetic approaches will be invaluable in elucidating the molecular bases of vector competence and in defining the structure-function relationships that affect interactions between the vector and the parasite that it transmits.

It is not yet possible to routinely do such experiments with vector insects; however, it seems likely that techniques will be developed that will make this feasible. If sufficient knowledge is gained from such studies, it might be possible to genetically engineer insects that are refractory to infection by parasites or at least incapable of transmitting them to other hosts. Whether such an organism could be released and effectively compete with natural populations is problematic, both scientifically and politically. However, recent invasions of wild *Drosophila melanogaster* populations with transposable elements such as the *P* element and the spread of cytoplasmic incompatibility in natural populations suggest that there might be some hope for introduction of genes into populations in the future.

In this chapter, the approaches that have been used to manipulate other organisms are reviewed first. Subsequently, work done with vector insects is reviewed, and finally strategies that might be used to genetically engineer mosquitoes that are incapable of transmitting arboviruses are presented.

Throughout this chapter the term "transformation" describes the introduction of DNA into the genome of a cell or organism such that it is stably propagated during cell division to subsequent generations. The term "transgenic" indicates that the construct is stably incorporated into the germ line of an organism and is transmitted to the offspring.

EFFECTIVE TRANSFORMATION SYSTEMS

In developing a strategy for transformation of vector insects, it is instructive to examine the nature of other successful transformation systems to see whether similar approaches might be followed. There are two different systems that are routinely used to produce transgenic animals. These systems serve to illustrate the variety of strategies that have been successfully exploited and can serve to guide efforts to develop routine transformation of vector insects.

Drosophila

The transposable element *P* of *Drosophila melanogaster* was discovered as a cause of hybrid dysgenesis. This term is used to describe mutations induced when males from a *P* strain (containing *P* elements) were mated with females from an M strain (lacking *P* elements). These mutations result from insertions of the *P* element DNA randomly into the genome of the offspring during early embryogenesis (Rubin et al. 1982).

Transformation of *Drosophila* is generally accomplished by injection of DNA molecules that carry derivatives of the *P* transposable element into early embryos (Rubin and Spradling 1982; Ashburner 1989). Under the proper conditions the *P* element will transpose from the injected DNA molecule to a chromosomal site where it will be stably maintained during cell division. If it is incorporated into the germ line, it will be passed on to subsequent generations. The embryo must be injected with the DNA at the early cleavage stage when nuclei are actively replicating but prior to the formation of cellular membranes. This presumably facilitates the entry of the *P* element DNA into the nuclei where it can be transposed into the genome.

The organization of the *P* element is typical of many transposons (Chap. 13). The ends of the element are defined by 31 bp (base pairs) inverted repeats. These flank a 2.8 kb (kilobase) gene encoding the transposase protein, which mediates the integration of the *P* element DNA into the *Drosophila* genome. Expression of the transposase protein is restricted to the germ line by tissue-specific RNA splicing (Rio 1990). The third intron in the primary transcript precursor of the transposase mRNA is only spliced out of the RNA in the germ line tissue. For this reason the DNA must be injected into the pole plasm at the posterior end of the embryo where pole cells are subsequently formed. These pole cells ultimately become

the germ line of the organism. Thus incorporation of *P* element DNA into the germ line is relatively frequent and efficient.

A number of sophisticated vectors have been developed from the *P* element that allow the incorporation of recombinant gene constructs between the inverted repeat ends of the transposon (Ashburner 1989). The transposase protein is capable of working in *trans*, which has allowed the development of binary vector systems in which transposase expressed from one DNA molecule can mediate transposition of a recombinant transposon from another DNA molecule into the genome. This has allowed the stable insertion of many recombinant gene constructs into the *Drosophila* genome. The recombination event is of the illegitimate type, meaning that there is no requirement for sequence homology between the *P* element DNA and the site of insertion. Thus, as with most transposons, the *P* element is able to insert at many sites distributed randomly throughout the genome. The site of insertion can have a significant effect on the expression of the gene both in terms of level and tissue specificity of expression. This presumably reflects the proximity of enhancers and other regulatory sequences to the insertion site. At the present time there is no general way of targeting a gene construct to a particular site in the genome of *Drosophila*. Thus although it is relatively easy to generate transgenic *Drosophila*, the site of insertion might not be appropriate for the required analysis.

The Drosophila transformation system was developed as a result of detailed knowledge of the molecular genetics of the *P* element. Although similar transposons have not yet been described in vector insects, it is reasonable to expect that they exist and, once found, might be amenable to exploitation along similar lines to the *P* element.

The Mouse

Transgenic mice can be produced in several ways. The 1st to be developed was microinjection of DNA into the pronuclei of fertilized eggs (Palmiter and Brinster 1986). This usually results in the integration of variable numbers of copies of the DNA into random sites in the genome via illegitimate recombination. Unfortunately, there is no way to control either the copy number or the site of integration into the mouse genome. Thus wide variation in expression of the inserted gene is observed.

A 2nd method for production of transgenic mice is to infect mouse embryos with recombinant retroviruses that carry the gene of interest (Jaenisch 1988). This also results in incorporation of the gene at random sites in the genome via the retroviral integration mechanism, which is very similar to the transposition mechanism outlined for the *P* element.

The 3rd method allows the generation of transgenic mice with more precisely defined mutations and represents a significant advance in transgenic technology. Embryonic stem (ES) cells can be cultured from mouse embryos. These retain the ability to differentiate into essentially any cell type if reintroduced into blastocyst stage embryos. The ability to culture these cells allows powerful techniques developed for genetic manipulation of cultured cells to be applied before reintroducing them into the embryo (Capecchi 1989). If these genetically engineered ES cells become part of the germ line, the offspring of the mouse will carry the recombinant DNA construct. One particularly important application of this technology has been the production of "knockout mice." In these mice, mutations that inactivate, the gene of interest are incorporated into the mouse genome by homologous recombination. These events are relatively rare compared to the random integrations by illegitimate recombination; however, selection for such events is possible in cell culture (Capecchi 1989). The ability to use homologous recombination to integrate the recombinant DNA constructs enables scientists to inactivate or otherwise modify a gene of interest and thus solve problems associated with position effects resulting from insertion at inappropriate sites. This technology has allowed unprecedented application of reverse genetic methodology to a higher eukaryote. The critical step of this technology was to develop methods for in vitro culture and genetic manipulation of the pluripotent ES cells. Whether similar methodology can be developed for equivalent insect cells (for example, pole cells) has not been investigated, although the ability to do so would be invaluable.

TRANSFORMATION OF VECTOR INSECTS

Attempts to transform non-Drosophilid insects have been considerably less successful than the systems reviewed above. Most of these have attempted to adapt the *P* element system as developed in *Drosophila* to other insects. Thus far, transformation of 3 species of mosquito has been reported.

All of the mosquito transformations used the *P* element vector pUChsneo (Stellar and Pirrotta 1985), which carries the bacterial gene for neomycin resistance as a selectable marker (Fig. 14.1). G418 (Geneticin) is

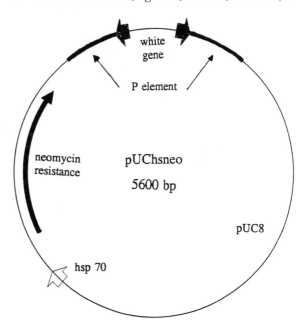

14.1   The *P* element vector pUChsneo. The plasmid is based on the cloning vector pUC8 and contains a plasmid replication origin and ampicillin resistance gene that allow growth and selection in *E. coli*. Genetic elements relevant to its use in *Drosophila* are the *Drosophila* hsp70 promoter (open broad arrowhead), the neomycin phosphotransferase (G418 resistance) gene (solid arrow), and the *P* element inverted repeats and adjacent regions (filled arrowheads and thick lines). The region designated white gene is outside of the *P* element and comes from an insertion in the *Drosophila* white gene upon which the contruct was based. (Figure from Margaret Kovach.)

an aminoglycoside antibiotic that is toxic to most eukaryotes. It is inactivated by phosphorylation by the enzyme neomycin phosphotransferase encoded by the *neo* gene of the bacterial transposon *Tn5*. Resistance to G418 has been used to select transformed tissue culture cells from many species. It has been used to select transformed *Drosophila* larvae (Stellar and Pirrotta 1985). In pUChsneo the *neo* gene is transcribed from the *Drosophila* hsp70 heat-shock promoter, which has been shown to be active in a wide variety of eukaryotic cells, including mosquito cells. pUChsneo has been injected into mosquito embryos along with a suitable helper plasmid that provided the *P* transposase. Offspring of surviving mosquitoes were raised in water containing G418, and resistant mosquitoes were recovered. At least some of these carried pUChsneo DNA when assayed by Southern blot hybridization. This basic experiment has been done with *Anopheles gambiae* (Miller et al. 1987), *Aedes triseriatus* (McGrane et al. 1988), and *Aedes aegypti* (Morris et al. 1989). One line of transgenic *Anopheles gambiae* has been characterized in considerable detail. The integration was shown to have occurred near the telomere of 1 of the chromosomes (Graziosi et al. 1990). Unfortunately, the frequency with which transformed mosquitoes were recovered was low, and none of the mosquitoes had DNA integrated as a result of the *P* element transposase activity. The low frequency of detection of plasmid insertions and the relative instability from generation to generation have prevented the routine production of transgenic mosquitoes.

Although the generation of transgenic mosquitoes has been difficult, introduction of DNA constructs into mosquito cells is readily accomplished. Both transient transfection and stable transformation of *Aedes albopictus* and *Aedes aegypti* cell lines have been possible (Monroe et al. 1992; Shotkoski and Fallon 1993; Lycett and Crampton 1993). Stable transformants of *Aedes albopictus* C6/36 cells containing anywhere from 1–50,000 copies of plasmid DNA per cell have been isolated (Monroe et al. 1992). Thus, manipulation of the mosquito genome in these cells is relatively routine. This should facilitate the investigation of gene expression in these cells from various transfected promoter-gene constructs.

Although not useful for achieving stable transformation, the Sindbis virus expression system shows considerable promise as a transient gene expression system in both mosquito cells and whole mosquitoes (Fig. 14.2). Sindbis virus (an alphavirus) has an RNA genome and infects both mammalian and insect cells. An infectious clone of the Sindbis virus genome has been modified to allow insertion of foreign genes (Xiong et al. 1989; Hahn et al. 1992). Transfection of in vitro transcribed RNA from this clone into mammalian cells results in production of high titers of infectious recombinant Sindbis virus. This virus can infect either mosquito cells or mosquitoes. Sindbis virus infection is not cytopathic in insect cells; instead it establishes a persistent infection. This allows relatively long-term expression of the gene in the infected cells over a period of a few days to a few weeks (Olson et al. 1992; Higgs et al. 1993). Thus, the consequences of expression of a gene of interest can be studied without the development of transformed cells or transgenic animals.

REQUIREMENTS FOR AN EFFICIENT TRANSFORMATION SYSTEM

To develop an efficient transformation system for an organism such as a mosquito, several characteristics must be incorporated to facilitate success. At a minimum the following things must be addressed: (1) an effective means of delivering the genetic construct into the target cell, (2) some mechanism for distinguishing transformed individuals from nontransformed individuals, (3) some mechanism for ensuring the stable maintenance of the genetic construct from generation to generation, and (4) genetic elements that allow the appropriate expression of genes of interest. These 4 points will be reviewed in the context of mosquitoes.

Methods for Delivery of DNA

The majority of attempts to generate transgenic insects have relied upon microinjection of DNA into eggs as is done with *Drosophila*. For this to be effective in other insects, considerable time should be spent optimizing protocols for microinjection. Egg-laying behavior, kinetics of chorion hardening, and kinetics of pole cell

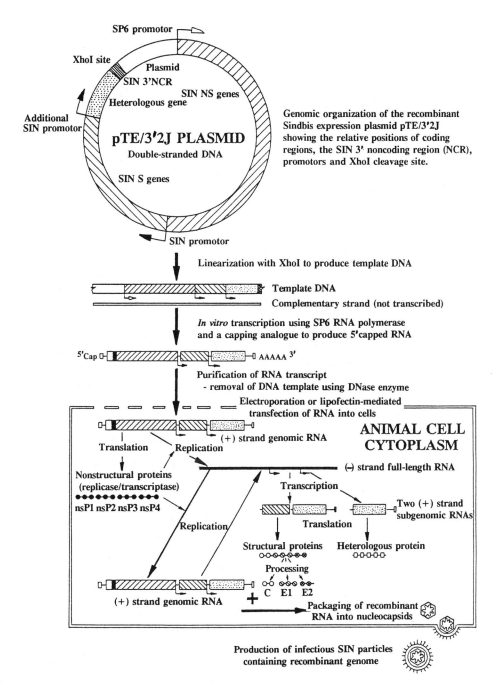

14.2 The Sindbis virus expression system. (From S. Higgs, A. M. Powers, and K. E. Olson. 1993. "Alphavirus Expression Systems: Applications to Mosquito Vector Studies," *Parasitology Today* 9:444–452. Elsevier Trends Journals, Cambridge. With permission.)

formation are among the factors that must be considered. The rate of survival of the embryo after injection will vary depending on the insect and the skill of the experimenter. For *Aedes triseriatus*, a survival rate of 6–10% (as measured by percent of adults resulting from injected eggs) is typical (data from >7000 eggs). The experimental procedure is rather tedious, and injecting a large number of embryos can be logistically difficult.

Thus, development of alternate methods of DNA delivery is desirable. Expression of reporter gene constructs in *Anopheles gambiae* embryos after introduction by microprojectile bombardment has been reported (Mialhe and Miller 1994). Evaluation of cationic liposomes as delivery systems is in progress. Success in either of these methods will greatly facilitate this research.

An attractive alternative is to use viruses as gene delivery vehicles. Transduction (the packaging of genes into virus particles and their subsequent delivery to cells by the infectious process) has been very successful in the genetic manipulation of mammalian cells and organisms; various gene therapy strategies based upon viruses are currently being developed (Mulligan 1993). However, with the conspicuous exception of the baculoviruses of Lepidopterans, this method of gene delivery has not been exploited in insects. This method of gene delivery is attractive because the natural infectious process is used to deliver the gene construct to the cell, which should be considerably more efficient than the artificial procedures described. The Sindbis virus system described in the previous section is an excellent example of this because it is possible to infect and detect expression of exogenous genes in nearly 100% of cells after infection with recombinant virus. In order for this process to be useful in transformation, the recombinant virus must have a DNA genome or pass through a DNA phase during infection as in the case of retroviruses. Recombinant retroviruses, adenoviruses, parvoviruses, papovaviruses, herpesviruses, and poxviruses have all proven useful for expression under a variety of situations in mammalian systems. Unfortunately the DNA viruses of vector insects are poorly characterized.

One exception to this is a parvovirus of *Aedes mosquitoes* (the *Aedes* densonucleosis virus) (Butchatsky 1989). The genome of this virus has been cloned and sequenced (Afanasiev et al. 1991). A full-length infectious clone has been constructed. The gene for *E. coli* B-galactosidase has been cloned downstream from 3 putative promoters, and after transfection into mosquito cells, expression of B-galactosidase was detected from all 3 constructs. Replication and packaging of the recombinant viral genomes in tissue culture cells has been demonstrated, and experiments to demonstrate transduction in mosquitoes are in progress (Afanasiev et al. 1994). Thus a DNA viral vector for *Aedes* mosquitoes seems possible.

Another potentially attractive approach would be to introduce intact genetically altered cells into embryos, for example, in the ES cells of mice. Pole cells from *Drosophila* have been removed from 1 embryo and successfully transplanted into a 2nd embryo, where the cells became incorporated into the germ line (Illmensee and Mahowald 1974). Thus, the possibility exists that the pole cells could be genetically manipulated before they are reintroduced. Unfortunately, nothing is known regarding whether these pole cells can be cultured and remain pluripotent and transplantable. Experiments along these lines could result in a powerful system such as the ES cell technology for generating transgenic insects.

Methods for Detecting Transformants

Transgenic *Drosophila* are generally detected by including a gene for a visible marker in the recombinant DNA construct that is introduced into the embryo. This is readily accomplished in *Drosophila* because a number of eye color mutants have been described, and the genes that code for the wild-type alleles have been isolated and sequenced. These genes have been incorporated into many of the *P* element vectors. Thus, by simple examination of the offspring of injected embryos it is possible to determine if they have incorporated the gene construct. Similar eye color mutations have been described for several species of mosquitoes, and work to isolate the genes for pigment synthesism is in progress. Whether the *Drosophila* genes would complement mosquito mutations is unknown.

Dominant selectable markers such as genes that confer resistance to antibiotics have been used extensively in tissue culture. The *neo* gene that inactivates G418 and the *hyg* gene that inactivates hygromycin are both bacterial genes for antibiotic resistance. The *neo* gene has been incorporated into a *P* element vector (pUChsneo) and has been used to select transformed *Drosophila*. Mosquitoes have also been transformed at much lower frequency as described earlier with this plasmid. A similar plasmid, pUChshyg, that contains the *hyg* has also been constructed (Monroe et al. 1992) and has been used to routinely transform mosquito tissue culture cells.

The dihydrofolate reductase *(DHFR)* gene has recently been isolated from a line of *Aedes albopictus* tissue culture cells in which the gene had been amplified about 1200-fold during selection for methotrexate resistance (Shotkoski and Fallon 1991). This gene can be used as a dominant selectable marker in tissue culture to select for clones that are resistant to high levels of methotrexate (Shotkaski and Fallon 1993). Whether it can be used in whole mosquitoes is unknown.

Other potentially useful selectable markers in insects are genes conferring resistance to various insecticides. A bacterial gene encoding a phosphotriesterase that hydrolyzes organophosphate insecticides has been inserted into *Drosophila melanogaster* by *P* element transformation. These flies are resistant to levels of paraoxon that are lethal to nontransformed flies (Benedict et al. 1994). Resistance to organophosphate insecticides in *Culex pipiens* results from the amplification of a chromosomal gene for an esterase protein that detoxifies the insecticide (Mouches et al. 1986; Raymond et al. 1991). A gene mediating resistance to the cyclodiene dieldrin has recently been cloned from *Aedes aegypti* (Thompson et al. 1993). These genes could provide convenient selectable markers at the whole organismal level similar to the *DHFR*-methotrexate resistance system described.

Of course, if a transformation system that is very efficient could be developed, there would be no need for a selectable marker. One could simply screen organisms for the presence of the genetic construct by suitable nucleic acid detection techniques such as the polymerase chain reaction (PCR). Unfortunately, the small amount of DNA in most vector insects severely limits the types of analysis that can be done (e.g., Southern blots) on individuals. Nevertheless, a leg removed from a mosquito, for example, provides sufficient DNA to detect a gene construct by PCR.

Stable Maintenance of the Genetic Construct

There are 2 possible ways for a recombinant DNA construct to be maintained in an organism from generation to generation. One of these is to become integrated into the genome by recombination. The 2nd way is for the construct to be maintained as a separate self-replicating entity that faithfully replicates and segregates from generation to generation.

Integration

Integration requires that a recombination event occur between the DNA construct and the cellular genome. Illegitimate recombination seems to be the predominant type of recombination in mammalian cells when DNA is introduced into them. For example, if a gene construct carrying sequences homologous to a gene in the mouse genome is introduced into mouse cells, it is 10–1000 times more likely to be integrated at sites other than the homologous gene (Capecchi 1989). This is in contrast to lower eukaryotes such as yeast in which homologous recombination is more frequent than illegitimate recombination. The relative frequency in insect cells is unknown. As mentioned earlier in the chapter, integration by illegitimate recombination does not allow control of either the copy number or the site of integration, and this can result in considerable variation in the expression of the gene construct in the transformed cells.

Integration by Homologous Recombination

Although the number of illegitimate recombination events generally exceeds the number of homologous recombination events in mammalian cells, it has been possible to select for homologous events by including both positive and negative selectable markers in the transfecting plasmid DNA (Capecchi 1989). A positive selectable marker such as *neo* is cloned within a region of homology with the cellular genome. A negative selectable marker that can be selected against, such as the herpes simplex virus thymidine kinase *(TK)* gene, is also included in the plasmid outside of the region of homology. Gancyclovir, an antiherpes drug that is a nucleoside analogue, is phosphorylated by the herpes *TK* but not by the cellular *TK* to form a toxic product. After transfection, cells that have the plasmid inserted into the genome by homologous recombination can be selected by resistance to G418 *(neo⁺)* and gancyclovir *(TK⁻)*. Gancyclovir resistance therefore implies that the herpes *TK* gene is not incorporated during the integration event, but G418 resistance implies that the *neo* gene is incorporated. The most common way for this to be accomplished is by recombination between the cellular sequences that flank the *neo* gene in the plasmid and the homologous sequences in the genome. Thus, the infrequent homologous recombinants can be selected against the background of random integrants that are resistant to gancyclovir *(neo⁺)* and sensitive to gancyclovis *(TK+)*. If cells that have undergone these homologous recombination events are capable of subsequent differentiation, as in the case of mouse ES cells, it is possible to generate animals with the recombinant gene as described.

Integration by Transposition

The integration of transposable elements also takes place by illegitimate recombination. However, the recombination event is mediated by the transposase that acts on the ends of the transposable element. This generally results in only a single copy integrated per site without rearrangement of the genes carried on the transposon. Thus, although it is not possible to direct integration to a given site in the genome, it is an improvement over nontransposase-mediated random insertions. Since the *Drosophila P* element hasn't transposed in non-Drosophilids, efforts to find alternate transposable elements have intensified. Another *Drosophila* transposon, *hobo*, has also been developed into a transformation system in *Drosophila*. *Hobo* seems to be clearly related to the *Ac* transposon in maize and the *Tam3* transposon in snapdragon (Calvi et al. 1991). The *Drosophila hobo* can be mobilized in houseflies, and an endogenous *hobo*-like element known as *Hermes* has been found in the house fly

genome (Atkinson et al. 1993; Warren et al. 1994). A similar situation exists for the *mariner* transposon from *Drosophila mauritiana*. A *mariner*-based vector has been used for transformation of *Drosophila melanogaster* (Lidholm et al. 1993). Sequences closely related to *mariner* have also been found in many insects, including *Anopheles* mosquitoes (Robertson 1993). Thus it might be that *hobo* or *mariner* have a broader host range and will be able to transpose in organisms other than *Drosophila* such as mosquitoes (Warren and Crampton 1994).

Transposons that transpose via an RNA intermediate are known as retrotransposons or retroposons. Some of these are closely related to retroviruses and code for gene products having sequence homology with reverse transcriptase. Among the best characterized of these are the *Ty* family of transposons in yeast, which have been shown to have a viruslike particle transposition intermediate (Boeke et al. 1985; Garfinkel et al. 1985). These retrotransposons can thus be thought of as retroviruses that have lost the ability to have an extracellular phase; alternatively, retroviruses can be thought of as retrotransposons that have gained an extracellular phase. The *Ty* elements have been very useful in genetic manipulation in yeast, and retroviruses have been extensively used in mammals for applications such as gene therapy. Retrotransposons/retroposons have been isolated from several insects, including *Drosophila* (Ashburner 1989) and mosquitoes (Besansky 1989; Besansky et al. 1994). Nevertheless, little has been done to develop them as transformation vectors along the lines of retroviral vectors. Recently, recombinant mammalian retroviral vectors have been pseudotyped with vesicular stomatitis virus G glycoprotein as the envelope protein (Burns et al. 1993). These vectors have a very broad host range, including nonmammalian species such as the zebra fish. Approaches such as these should have considerable potential for insects as well.

Integration by Site-Specific Recombination

The development of site-specific recombination systems for transformation of insect cells may also be possible. In site-specific recombination, a specific enzyme, a recombinase, mediates the recombination between DNA molecules that contain specific target sequences (typically 20–40 bp long). Several of these systems have been described in bacteria and 1 in yeast. The FLP-FRT system from yeast and the cre-lox system from bacteriophage P1 have been used to introduce genes into the genomes of eukaryotic tissue culture cells (O'Gorman et al. 1991; Fukushige and Sauer 1992). In each of these systems the recombinase (FLP or cre) protein efficiently catalyzes recombination between pairs specific sites (FRT or lox) on either the same or different DNA molecules. Plasmids containing FRT sites have been introduced into mosquito embryos by microinjection along with a plasmid that expresses the FLP recombinase protein (Morris et al. 1991). Both intramolecular and intermolecular recombination between FRT sites have been detected. Similarly, cre-mediated recombination between lox sites on plasmids has been demonstrated in mosquito embryos (Carlson et al. 1995). Thus, the introduction of a lox or FRT site into the mosquito genome could permit the introduction of other constructs into that site by site-specific recombination. This would allow reproducible introduction of various genes at the same site in the mosquito genome and would remove potential problems associated with position effects on gene expression. This has been effectively demonstrated with independent lox mediated insertions into the genome of mammalian tissue culture cells (Fukushige and Sauer 1992).

Stable Extrachromosomal Elements

An alternative strategy for stable maintenance of a genetic construct is to introduce the construct on a DNA molecule that is maintained extrachromosomally in the cell. This mode of existence is common in prokaryotic organisms because many if not most bacteria carry plasmids. Plasmids are also found in yeast but do not seem common in higher eukaryotes, although viruses such as Epstein-Barr virus or papillomaviruses are maintained as plasmids in mammalian cells.

Work with yeast artificial chromosomes (YACs) has helped to define elements that are necessary for stability of extrachromosomal elements. At a minimum, stable extrachromosomal existence implies that the DNA molecule carries an origin of replication and some

mechanism to assure that the plasmid segregates to both daughter cells during cell division. An autonomously replicating sequence (ARS) serves as a replication origin to assure that the YAC is replicated during the cell cycle. Second, a centromere sequence (CEN) assures that the YAC will interact with the mitotic spindle and that 1 copy will end up in each daughter cell after division. Finally, addition of telomeres at the ends of the DNA molecules is necessary for the stable maintenance of linear DNA molecules in cells. As long as these elements are present DNA molecules of $20,000–10^6$ bp can be stably maintained in yeast cells. Are similar constructions possible in higher eukaryotes? Interestingly, transformants of *Aedes albopictus* C6/36 cells occasionally contain large arrays of up to 60,000 copies of the transforming plasmid that resemble chromosomes (Fig. 14.3), and these arrays are maintained stably from generation to generation (Monroe et al. 1992). Thus, we postulate that sequences that function as the elements described above are present on these arrays. Attempts to identify these elements are under way; the eventual goal is to use them to generate mosquito artificial chromosomes (MACs) for use in transformation of mosquito cells and mosquitoes.

Expression of Genes on Recombinant DNA Constructs

Expression of genes contained on the constructs introduced into mosquito cells depends upon the availability of suitable transcriptional promoters, terminators, RNA processing signals, translational control sequences, and so on. Few of these have been identified from mosquitoes and even fewer have been functionally characterized. Fortunately, a large number have been isolated and characterized from *Drosophila*. Several constructs in which various reporter genes have been cloned downstream of the *Drosophila* heat-shock and metallothionein promoters have been introduced into mosquito tissue culture cells (Durbin and Fallon 1985; Kovach et al. 1992). In both transient transfection and stable transformation, expression can be detected from these promoters and at least in some cases expression is inducible by either heat shock or metal ions.

Thus it seems reasonable to be optimistic that many if not most promoters isolated from *Drosophila* will be active in mosquito cells. In fact many of the signals that control various aspects of gene expression, such as RNA processing and initiation and termination of translation, are conserved throughout eukaryotes, and these would be expected to function in mosquitoes regardless of their origin.

Nevertheless, the isolation and characterization of mosquito gene control sequences should be actively pursued. The fine tuning of appropriate tissue-specific expression and temporal control of gene expression could very well be governed by species-specific elements. For instance, the control of genes induced by blood-feeding might involve control elements unique to mosquitoes.

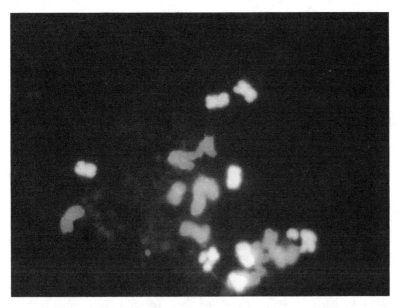

14.3 Mosquito artificial chromosomes (MACs). The metaphase chromosomes are from a C6/36 *Aedes albopictus* cell stably transformed with approximately 20,000 copies of the plasmid pMT2 (Kovach et al. 1992). The chromosomes were hybridized in situ with pMT2 DNA labeled with biotin. Hybrids were visualized with fluorescein-conjugated avidin. The MACs fluoresce brightly. The mosquito chromosomes stained with propidium diiodide are dimmer. (Photograph from Margaret Kovach.)

STRATEGIES THAT INTERFERE WITH ARBOVIRUS INFECTION OF ARTHROPODS

Assuming that efficient routine transformation of mosquitoes can be achieved, what genes would we introduce into them? Genes that affect vector competence have not yet been isolated or characterized. Nevertheless, it is still possible to devise strategies based upon work in other systems that could be expected to reduce the ability of the mosquito to support a viral infection. Because viruses are obligate intracellular parasites, it is reasonable to introduce genes that would interfere with the various steps of viral reproduction inside the cell. This approach has been termed intracellular immunization. Considerable success has been achieved in the development of plants that are resistant to various plant viruses by using these strategies. There are also a few examples of transgenic animals and many of genetically modified animal cells that have been rendered resistant to infection.

One prominent strategy has been to express the genes for various viral structural proteins in the cell or organism. For example, expression of the coat protein of tobacco mosaic virus (TMV) in tobacco plants resulted in virus resistant plants (Powell et al. 1986). Similarly, transgenic chickens engineered to express the envelope glycoprotein of avian retroviruses are resistant to infection by retroviruses of the same type (Federspiel et al. 1989; Salter and Crittenden 1989). The mechanism by which this interference takes place differs from virus to virus. For example, the coat-protein-mediated interference for TMV can be bypassed by transfecting cells with naked RNA or even with partially disrupted virus particles (Register and Beachy 1988). This suggests that the endogenously expressed coat protein interferes with an early event in the infection perhaps involved in the uncoating process. This contrasts with coat-protein-mediated interference in potato virus X, which is effective against naked RNA (Hemenway et al. 1988). Interference to retroviral infection by envelope glycoprotein expression seems to be caused by interaction of the protein with the receptor, resulting in a lack of free receptors on the cell surface to allow binding of virus (Federspiel et al. 1989; Salter and Crittenden 1989). Thus, many different steps in a virus infection could be interrupted by expression of the viral structural protein.

Expression of nonstructural proteins can also result in interference. These proteins generally are involved in the replication of the nucleic acid or regulation of viral gene expression. Sometimes dominant mutant forms of these proteins can be created that compete effectively with the wild type and thereby prevent the normal course of an infection. For example, mutant viral RNA dependent RNA polymerases have been described that can bind to RNA template but are incapable of RNA synthesis (Inokuchi and Hirashima 1987). Expression of these mutant proteins prevents normal viral replication. Another example involves the herpes virus transcription transactivator *VP16*. A *VP16* gene that encodes a truncated version that lacks an activating domain but retains the nucleic acid binding domain has been constructed, and expression of this protein interferes with herpes infection (Friedman et al. 1988).

Another general strategy for interference with viral infection is to express antisense RNA. This is RNA that is complementary to sense RNA, such as viral messenger RNA or genomic RNA, and this antisense RNA presumably binds to form a double helical RNA. Mechanisms of inhibition by antisense RNA could include interference with the proper folding of the sense RNA into a critical secondary structure or prevention of translation of mRNA by binding to a ribosome binding site. Although used with some success in the development of virus resistant plants (Powell et al. 1989; deHaan et al. 1992), an even more striking example is provided by data from our laboratory. A recombinant Sindbis virus was constructed that expresses an antisense RNA to the LaCrosse virus small RNA segment (Fig. 14.4). When mosquito cells were persistently infected with this Sindbis virus and subsequently challenged with LaCrosse, very little LaCrosse virus was produced (Powers et al. 1994). Thus antisense RNA is a potentially valuable strategy for interfering with a productive viral infection.

Other more novel approaches could be exploited. Ribozymes are catalytic RNA molecules that have enzyme activity. The ribozymes that are capable of sequence-specific cleavage of RNA molecules (Forster and Symons 1987; Hazeloff and Gerlach 1988; Uhlenbeck 1987; Hampel and Tritz 1989) have been extensively studied. These ribozymes are based upon naturally occuring self-cleaving RNAs. The specificity of the cleavage reaction is determined by including nucleotide sequences complementary to the target sequences adjacent to the active site domain of the ribozyme molecule. The use of ribozymes designed to cleave viral genomic RNA (Sarver et al. 1990; Sullenger and Cech, 1993) is an attractive method of intracellular immunization against arboviruses because there is potential for highly specific catalytic destruction of the viral genome. Other strategies based on decoy RNA molecules that bind to critical viral proteins are possible. For example, through the use of PCR and protein binding selection, it has been possible to develop RNA molecules having a pseudoknot configuration that bind and inhibit the HIV reverse transcriptase (Tuerk et al. 1992). It should be possible to develop similar inhibitor molecules for arbovirus polymerases as well.

The approaches mentioned are not an exhaustive list of strategies for intracellular immunization. Rather, they are intended to illustrate that knowledge of the molecular virology of a virus can contribute to the development of strategies that disrupt the infection cycle. Similarly, when more is known about the determinants of vectorial capacity in the insect, other strategies based upon physiological and behavioral factors could also be formulated.

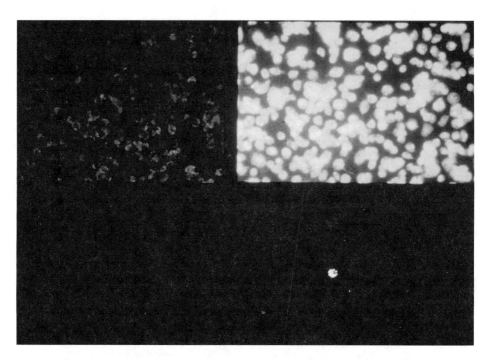

14.4   Intracellular interference to LaCrosse virus infection. All 4 panels contain approximately equal numbers of C6/36 *Aedes albopictus* cells. In A, cells were infected with wild type Sindbis virus at a multiplicity of infection (moi) of 50. Sindbis antigen was visualized by immunofluorescence with antiserum to Sindbis virus. Essentially all cells were infected with Sindbis virus. In B, cells were infected with wild type Sindbis virus at moi 50 and challenged 48 hours later with LaCrosse virus at moi 0.1. LaCrosse antigen was detected 48 hours later by immunofluorescence using a monoclonal antibody to the nucleocapsid protein. Essentially all cells were infected with LaCrosse, demonstrating that Sindbis virus does not interfere with LaCrosse virus. In C and D, cells were infected with recombinant Sindbis virus that expresses antisense RNA to the LaCrosse nucleocapsid protein gene at moi 50. The cells were challenged 48 hr later with LaCrosse virus at moi 0.1. LaCrosse antigen was detected 48 hours later by immunofluorescence using either a monoclonal antibody to the nucleocapsid protein (C) or a monoclonal antibody to the envelope glycoprotein (D). Little antigen was detected with either antibody, demonstrating that expression of antisense RNA to the nucleocapsid gene prevents LaCrosse virus replication in cells. (Photograph from Ann Powers.)

REFERENCES

Afanasiev, B.N., E.E. Galyov, L.P. Buchatsky, and Y.V. Kozlov. 1991. Nucleotide sequence and genomic organization of Aedes densonucleosis virus. *Virology* 185:323–336.

Afanasiev, B.N., Y.V. Kozlov, J.O. Carlson, and B.J. Beaty. 1994. Densovirus of *Aedes aegypti* as an expression vector in mosquito cells. *Exper. Parasit.* 79:322–339.

Ashburner, M. 1989. Drosophila: *A laboratory handbook.* Cold Spring Harbor, NY: Cold Spring Harbor Press.

Atkinson, P.W., W.D. Warren, and D.A. O'Brochta. 1993. The hobo transposable element of Drosophila can be crossed-mobilized in houseflies and excises like the AC element of maize. *Proc. Natl. Acad. Sci. USA* 90:9693–9697.

Benedict, M.Q., J.A. Scott, and A.F. Cockburn. 1994. High-level expression of the bacterial *opd* gene in *Drosophila melanogaster:* Improved inducible insecticide resistance. *Insect Mol. Biol.* 3:247–252.

Besansky, N.J. 1990. A retrotransposable element from the mosquito *Anopheles gambiae. Mol. Cell Biol.* 10:863–871.

Boeke, J.D., D.J. Garfinkel, C.D. Styles, and G.R. Fink. 1985. Ty elements transpose through an RNA intermediate. *Cell* 40:491–500.

Buchatsky, L.P. 1989. Densonucleosis virus of bloodsucking mosquitoes. *Dis. of Aquat. Org.* 6:145–150.

Burns, J.C., T. Friedmann, W. Driever, M. Burrasiano, and J.K. Yee. 1993. Vesicular stomatitis virus G glycoprotein pseudotyped retroviral vectors: Concentration to very high titer and efficient gene transfer into mammalian and nonmammalian cells. *Proc. Natl. Acad. Sci. USA* 90:8033–8037.

Calvi, B.R., T.J. Hong, S.D. Findley, and W.M. Gelbart. 1991. Evidence for a common evolutionary origin of inverted repeat transposons in *Drosophila* and plants: hobo, activator and tam3. *Cell* 66:465–471.

Capecchi, M.R. 1989. Altering the genome by homologous recombination. *Science* 244:1288–1292.

Carlson, J., K. Olson, S. Higgs, and B. Beaty. 1995. Molecular genetic manipulation of mosquito vectors. *Ann. Rev. Entomol.* 40:359–388.

deHaan, P., J.J.L. Gielen, M. Rains, I.G. Wijkamp, A. van Schepen, D. Peters, M.Q.J.M. van Grinsven, and R. Goldbach. 1991. Characterization of RNA-mediated resistance to tomato spotted wilt virus in transgenic tobacco plants. *Bio. Tech.* 10:1133–1137.

Durbin, J.E., and A.M. Fallon. 1985. Transient expression of the chloramphenical acetyl transferase gene in cultured mosquito cells. *Gene* 36:173–178.

Federspiel, M.J., L.B. Crittenden, and S.H. Hughes. 1989. Expression of avian reticuloendotheliosis virus envelope confers host resistance. *Virology* 173:167–177.

Forster, A.C., and R.H. Symons. 1987. Self cleavage of plus and minus RNAs of a virusoid and a structural model for the active sites. *Cell* 49:211–220.

Friedman, A.D., A.J. Trizenberg, and S.L. McKnight. 1988. Expression of a truncated viral trans-activator selectively impedes lytic infection by its cognate virus. *Nature* 335:452–454.

Fukushige, S., and B. Sauer. 1992. Genomic targeting with a positive-selection lox integration vector allows highly reproducible gene expression in mammalian cells. *Proc. Natl. Acad. Sci. USA* 89:7905–7909.

Garfinkel, D.J., J.D. Boeke, and G.R. Fink. 1985. Ty element transposition: Reverse transcriptase and virus-like particles. *Cell* 45:507–517.

Graziosi, C., R.K. Sakai, and P. Romans. 1990. Method for in situ hybridization to polytome chromosomes from ovarian nurse cells of Anopheles gambiae (Diptera: Culicidae). *J. Med. Ent.* 27:905–912.

Hampel, A., and R. Tritz. 1989. RNA catalytic properties of the minimum (-)TRSV sequence. *Biochemistry* 28:4929–4933.

Haseloff, J., and W.L. Gerlach. 1988. Simple RNA enzymes with new and highly specific endoribonuclease activities. *Nature* 334:585–591.

Hemenway, C., R.X. Fang, W.K. Kaniewski, N.H. Chua, and N.E. Tauer. 1988. Analysis of the mechanism of protection in transgenic plants expressing potato virus X coat protein or its antisense RNA. *EMBO Jour.* 7:1273–1280.

Higgs, S., A.M. Powers, and K.E. Olson. 1993. Alphavirus expression systems: Applications to mosquito vector studies. *Parasit. Today* 9:444–452.

Illmensee, K., and A.P. Mahowald. 1974. Transplantation of posterior polar plasm in *Drosophila*. Induction of germ cells at the anterior pole of the egg. *Proc. Natl. Acad. Sci. USA* 71:85, 97, 98, 1016–1020.

Inokuchi, Y., and A. Hirashima. 1987. Interference with viral infection by defective viral replicase. *J. Virol.* 61:3946–3949.

Jaenisch, R. 1988. Transgenic animals. *Science* 240:1468–1474.

Kovach, M.J., J.O. Carlson, and B.J. Beaty. 1992. A *Drosophila* metallothionein promoter is inducible in mosquito cells. *Insect Mol. Biol.* 1:37–43.

Lidholm, D.A., A.R. Lohe, and D.L. Hartl. 1993. The transposable element *mariner* mediates germline transformation in *Drosophila melanogaster*. *Genetics* 134:859–868.

Lycett, G.J., and J.M. Crampton. 1993. Stable transformation of mosquito cell lines using a hsp70::*neo* fusion gene. *Gene* 136:129–136.

McGrane, V., J.O. Carlson, B.R. Miller, and B.J. Beaty. 1988. Microinjection of DNA into *Aedes triseriatus* ova and detection of integration. *Am. J. Trop. Med. Hyg.* 39:502–510.

Mialhe, E., and L.H. Miller. 1994. Biolistic techniques for transfection of mosquito embryos *(Anopheles gambiae)*. *Biotechniques* 16:924–932.

Miller, L.H., R.K. Sakai, P. Romans, R.W. Gwadz, P. Kantoff, and H.G. Coon. 1987. Stable integration and expression of a bacterial gene in the mosquito *Anopheles gambiae*. *Science* 237:779–781.

Monroe, T., M.C. Muhlmann-Diaz, M.J. Kovach, J.O. Carlson, J.A. Bedford, and B.J. Beaty. 1992. Stable transformation of a mosquito cell line results in extraordinarily high copy numbers of the plasmid. *Proc. Natl. Acad. Sci. USA* 89:5725–5729.

Morris, A.C., P. Eggleston, and J. M. Crampton. 1989. Genetic transformation of the mosquito *Aedes aegypti* by microinjection of DNA. *Med. Vet. Ent.* 3:1–7.

Morris, A., T. Schaub, and A. James. 1991. FLP-mediated recombination in the vector mosquito, *Aedes aegypti*. *Nucleic Acids Res.* 19:5895–59.

Mouches, C., N. Pasteur, J.B. Berge, O. Hyrien, M. Raymond, B.R. De Saint Vincent, M. De Silvestri, and G.P. Georghiou. 1986. Amplification of an esterase gene is responsible for insecticide resistance in a California *Culex* mosquito. *Science* 233:778–780.

Mulligan, R.C. 1993. The basic science of gene therapy. *Science* 260:926–932.

O'Gorman, A., D.T. Fox, and G.M. Wohl. 1991. Recombinase-mediated activation and site specific integration in mammalian cells. *Science* 251:1351–1355.

Olson, K.E., J.O. Carlson, and B.J. Beaty. 1992. Expression of the chlorphemicol acetyltransferase gene in *Aedes albopictus* (C6/36) cells using a noninfectious Sindbis virus expression vector. *Insect Mol. Biol.* 1:49–52.

Olson, K.E., S. Higgs, C.S. Hahn, C.M. Rice, J.O. Carlson, and B.J. Beaty. 1994. Expression of chloramphenicol acetyltransferase in *Aedes albopictus* (C6/36) cells and *Aedes triseriatus* mosquitoes using double subgenomic Sindbis virus vectors. *Insect Biochem. Mol. Biol.* 24:39–48.

Palmiter, R.D., and R.L. Brinster. 1986. Germ-line transformation of mice. *Ann. Rev. Gen.* 20:465–499.

Powell, P.A., R.S. Nelson, B. De, N. Hoffman, S.G. Rogers, R.T. Fraley, and R.N. Beachy. 1986. Delay of disease development in transgenic plants that express the tobacco mosaic virus coat protein gene. *Science* 232:738–743.

Powell, P.A., D.M. Stark, P.R. Sanders, and R.N. Beachy. 1989. Protection against tobacco mosaic virus in transgenic plants that express tobacco mosaic virus antisense RNA. *Proc. Natl. Acad. Sci. USA* 86:6949–6952.

Powers, A.M., K.E. Olson, S. Higgs, J.O. Carlson, and B.J. Beaty. 1994. Antiviral intracellular immunization using a recombinant Sindbis virus vector. *Virus Res.* 32:57–67.

Raymond, M., A. Collaghan, P. Fort, and N. Pasteur. 1991. Worldwide migration of amplified insecticide resistance genes in mosquitoes. *Nature* 350:151–153.

Register, J.C. III, and R.N. Beachy. 1988. Resistance to TMV in transgenic plants results from interference with an early event in infection. *Virology* 166:524–532.

Rio, D.C. 1990. Molecular mechanisms regulating *Drosophila P* element transposition. *Ann. Rev. Gen.* 24:543–578.

Robertson, H.M. 1993. The mariner transposable element is widespread in insects. *Nature* 362:241–244.

Rubin, G.M., M.G. Kidwell, and R.M. Bingham. 1982. The molecular basis of P-M hybrid drysgenesis: The nature of induced mutations. *Cell* 29:987–994.

Rubin, G.M., and A.C. Spradling. 1982. Genetic transformation of *Drosophila* with transposable element vectors. *Science* 218:348–353.

Salter, D.W., and L.B. Crittenden. 1989. Artificial insertion of a dominant gene for resistance to avian leukosis virus into the germ line of the chicken. *Theo. App. Gen.* 77:457–461.

Sarver, N., E.M. Cantin, P.S. Chang, J.A. Zola, P.A. Ladne, D.A. Stephens, and J.J. Rossi. 1990. Ribozymes as potential anti-HIV–1 therapeutic agents. *Science* 247:1222–1225.

Shotkoski, F.A., and A.M. Fallon. 1993. The mosquito dihydrofolate reductose gene functions as a dominant selectable marker in transfected cells. *Insect Biochem. Mol. Biol.* 23:883–893.

Stellar, H., and V. Pirrotta. 1985. A transposable P vector that confers selectable G418 resistance to *Drosophila* larvae. *EMBO Jour.* 4:167–171.

Sullenger, B.A., and T.R. Cech. 1993. Tethering ribozymes to a retroviral packaging signal for destruction of viral RNA. *Science* 262:1566–1569.

Thompson, M., F. Shotkoski, and R.H. ffrench-Constant. 1993. Cloning and sequencing of the cyclodiene insecticide resistance gene from the yellow fever mosquito *Aedes aegypti:* Conservation of the gene and the resistance associated mutation. *FEBS Letters* 325:187–190.

Tuerk, C., S. MacDougal, and L. Gold. 1992. RNA pseudoknots that inhibit human immunodeficiency virus type 1 reverse transcriptase. *Proc. Natl. Acad. Sci. USA* 89:6988–6992.

Uhlenbeck, O.C. 1987. A small catalytic oligoribonucleotide. *Nature* 328:596–600.

Warren, A.M., and J.M. Crampton. 1994. Mariner: Its prospects as a DNA vector for the genetic manipulation of medically important insects. *Parasit. Today* 10:58–63.

Warren, W.D., P.W. Atkinson, and D.A. O'Brochta. 1994. The *Hermes* transposable element from the house fly, *Musca domestica*, is a short inverted repeat-type element of the *hobo, Ac, Tam3(hAT)* element family. *Gen. Res. Camb.* 64:87–97.

15. GENE EXPRESSION IN VECTORS

Anthony A. James and Ann Marie Fallon

INTRODUCTION

Current interest in control of insect-borne disease by genetic manipulation (Chaps. 14 and 33) has resulted in the use of molecular techniques that may extend to vector species, genetic capabilities now available only for the fruit fly, *Drosophila melanogaster*. With *D. melanogaster* as well as with other model organisms, such as the bacterium *Escherichia coli* and the budding yeast *Saccharomyces cerevisiae*, efforts to study gene expression began even before the structure of the DNA double helix was known. These first analyses identified changes in phenotype that could be correlated with a biochemical difference that reflects activity of a gene product. Mutational analysis of genes provided the first evidence for distinct control regions, such as promoters, that regulate expression of contiguous coding regions "in cis" (i.e., linked regulatory elements and coding sequences present on the same DNA molecule). The phenotypes of organisms with multiple mutations provided further evidence that some aspects of gene expression are regulated "in trans" by the products of other genes. This chapter discusses the analysis of gene expression in vector arthropods, which presents a particular challenge because the classical genetic information that has accumulated over many decades with *Drosophila* is not available for vector species.

In this chapter we emphasize molecular approaches that have been used to facilitate analysis of gene structure and expression in vector arthropods. We focus on mosquitoes, for which studies on vector competence and insecticide resistance have begun to stimulate interest in detailed molecular analysis of physiological processes that might be manipulated in transgenic strains. Methods for isolating genes from vector species, characterizing these cloned genes, and analyzing their expression are outlined to provide a broad overview of this rapidly growing field. Examples of the application of these analyses are given as well as a description of efforts toward development of the gene transfer technologies that are fundamental to genetic manipulation of vector species.

WHAT IS MEANT BY GENE EXPRESSION?

Depending on the context in which it is used, gene expression has several meanings. In its more limited definition, gene expression refers specifically to the transcription of RNA from a gene and, if appropriate, its subsequent translation into a protein. From this perspective, gene expression encompasses the mechanistic analysis of transcriptional and translational control at the molecular level. Such studies may be descriptive, comparative, qualitative, or quantitative; they seek to identify "what" specific factors regulate expression of a gene, and "how" this regulation is achieved. These studies are particularly advanced in those species that have now become model organisms, for example, *E. coli*, *Saccharomyces cerevisiae*, *Caenorhabditis*, and *Drosophila*.

In the context of the material presented in this chapter, the term "gene expression" extends beyond the precise definition to include the biological background within which the gene functions. For example, many arthropods require rapid accumulation of large quantities of a particular gene product during a critical developmental stage. This can be accomplished by transcriptional and/or translational control, potentially facilitated by multiple gene copies in polytene or polyploid chromosomes in specific, differentiated cells. DNA units smaller than a chromosome may also occur in multiple copies. For example, developmentally regulated amplification of chorion protein genes in ovarian follicle cells facilitates rapid deposition of the eggshell (chorion) proteins in *Drosophila*. As we shall see, in vector mosquitoes, selective amplification of esterase genes is associated with some forms of insecticide resistance.

An important aspect of gene expression is the coordinate regulation of groups of individual genes that are physically separated on multiple chromosomes. At the level of the organism, this coordinate gene expression is often regulated by endocrine factors. In particular, application of gene transfer technologies to vector insects will likely draw upon molecular aspects of coordinate gene expression that facilitate the physiological interactions that have coevolved specifically within the insect vector and the pathogen it transmits.

GENE EXPRESSION IN VECTOR INSECTS: SPECIAL CONSIDERATIONS

Vector arthropods share many properties with their nonvector relatives. Least likely to change are those genetic and physiological processes that occur during early development, specifically in embryogenesis (Chap. 16), and subsequent metamorphosis of the immature stages. For example, some of the similarities between mosquitoes and *Drosophila* have begun to be exploited in transformation strategies. Because the precision with which genetic studies can be undertaken with *Drosophila* is not available for any vector species, a particular challenge to vector biologists is the choice of which genes to study. Metabolic processes with potential to be manipulated without compromising the biological "fitness" of the vector that

also interface with pathogen acquisition, maintenance, or transmission are largely undefined. Even for those vector species that have suitable polytene chromosomes, little emphasis has been placed on the classical mutational analyses that have been so useful in *Drosophila* in identifying distinct regulatory elements, coding regions, and their interactions. Most of the classic genetic analyses undertaken with vector species have been limited to such visible mutations as eye color. It is anticipated that the study of genetic variation among vector populations with regard to physiologically important processes such as hematophagy, vector competence, and some types of insecticide resistance will provide at least a limited insight into the possible genetic complexity that might be manipulated in transgenic organisms.

Hematophagy

The evolution of blood-feeding has allowed vector arthropods to exploit a widely available nutritional source (Chap. 2). Blood is much richer in protein than the majority of plant products available to phytophagous arthropods. Some vectors, notably ticks and triatomine bugs, feed exclusively on blood throughout their life cycle; blood provides the nutrients for growth and metamorphosis. In some insects, such as the tsetse fly, both adult males and females feed on blood. More common, however, is the model represented by the mosquito, in which only the adult female takes a blood meal, and the amino acids recovered following blood digestion provide precursors for the synthesis of large amounts of yolk proteins that are deposited in eggs. In these species, the number of eggs produced is directly correlated with the amount of blood ingested in the previous blood meal; however, there are indications that females of these species in nature also feed on blood for short-term nutrition.

The independent evolutionary origin of blood-feeding in the various taxa must be considered when gene similarities are compared in tissues such as salivary glands and midgut (Chap. 20). For example, all hematophagous arthropods have a platelet antiaggregating factor, the enzyme apyrase, that helps them feed efficiently. Although the specific activities and biochemical profiles vary for apyrases, it is believed that they all belong to the same general family of nucleoti-dases. In contrast, analysis of mosquito salivary gland antihemostatic activities suggests that some evolution-ary adjustments to blood-feeding were still in progress as the recognized mosquito subfamilies were being established. Different types of vasodilatory molecules, and therefore genes, occur among species. In *Ae. aegypti*, a tachykinin-like molecule, sialokinin, is present; in *An. albimanus*, a catechol oxidase/peroxi-dase functions as a vasodilator.

Thus in mosquitoes a common solution to platelet aggregation, the production of apyrase, is present, and separate solutions to vasodilatory activities have evolved (Chap. 20). This suggests that in the evolution of blood-feeding, selection of genes or members of gene families to fill specific functions was not opti-mized before the separation of the anopheline from the culicine mosquitoes (Chap. 20). Further molecular analyses should shed light on the evolution of other functions (genes) related to hematophagy, such as the enzymes involved in blood digestion.

The molecular analyses of hematophagy have focused on 4 major tissues: salivary gland, midgut, fat body, and ovaries. These studies encompass important aspects of blood-feeding, including the uptake, diges-tion, and utilization of the blood meal. Vector arthro-pods have evolved a number of salivary gland activities that counteract the host response to injury during feeding. Insects and ticks have been shown to salivate antihemostatic, antiinflammatory, and antiimmune activities, which are the products of genes expressed specifically in the salivary glands. In the midgut, molecular events initiated by blood-feeding include the rapid synthesis of proteases and the production of a peritrophic matrix that surrounds the ingested blood bolus (Chaps. 18 and 20). It has been known for some time that midgut-expressed trypsins and chymo-trypsins play an important role in blood digestion (Chap. 18). An important process of long-standing interest in mosquitoes is the synthesis of yolk proteins by the fat body and their uptake by developing oocytes. These proteins include the abundantly synthesized yolk protein, vitellin, and a number of other proteins expressed at lower levels. The yolk protein and related genes are developmentally regulated; in anautogenous mosquitoes, they are expressed only in adult females following blood ingestion, and they are expressed prin-cipally in a specific tissue, the fat body. The major yolk protein is expressed as a precursor, vitellogenin, that is processed before it ends up in the egg as vitellin. In *Ae. aegypti*, the fat body also expresses a protein of about 50 kDa called vitellogenic carboxypeptidase. Its expression is similar to that of the vitellogenins and, like vitellogenins, the protein is transported to the developing oocyte, where it is thought to be involved in protein hydrolysis during embryogenesis. An addi-tional gene encoding a cathepsin D-like protein has also been isolated, and its involvement in vitellogenesis or embryogenesis has yet to be determined. Finally, we note that the uptake of the various proteins into the developing oocyte is the result of a highly specific and efficient process. The analysis of the receptor-ligand interactions that take place promises to reveal ways in which it might be possible to introduce exogenous proteins and other macromolecules into the eggs as a basis for various vector and disease-transmission con-trol strategies.

Vector Competence

Hematophagy enables the transmission of pathogens, and the wound made during feeding is often the princi-pal site for entry of pathogens into the vertebrate host. However, it is clear that the vector is more than just a "flying syringe" in the infection process because highly specific interrelations have evolved between vectors and the pathogens they transmit. The ability of a vector to support the development and propagation of a patho-gen is called vector competence (Chap. 4). From genetic studies of many different vector species, it has been demonstrated that even 1 gene can profoundly affect vector competence. For example, in *Ae. aegypti* loci have been identified that make the mosquito refractory to infection by pathogens that cause filariasis and avian malaria. Strains of *An. gambiae* and *An. stephensi* have been selected that are refractory to vari-ous *Plasmodium* species. For the molecular biologist, the identification and mapping of such genes is a first step toward their cloning and characterization. It is anticipated that the characterization of genes involved in vector competence will reveal novel host-parasite interactions that can be exploited to control the transmission of diseases.

Genes associated with vector competence, in which mutations may confer a parasite-refractory phenotype, are likely to encode products essential for parasite growth or development. This absence of a vital gene product is characteristic of recessive mutations, which are difficult to study because investigators are looking for the *absence* of infection (or the destruction of parasites) as the phenotype. When screening the progeny of crosses between refractory and susceptible animals, the gene being studied is only 1 of many possible causes for an animal not being infected. Given these limitations, it is not surprising that no naturally arising refractory gene has yet been characterized at the molecular level. To overcome the problem of working with recessive mutations, linked marker genes that encode a more easily scored phenotype, such as an enzyme variant or DNA polymorphism, are being sought. With such a marker, whose expression is tightly linked to the refractory phenotype, genetic analysis and chromosomal location studies could be done using the marker gene for reference. For example, in *An. gambiae* a tightly linked esterase variant that allows a relatively straightforward genetic analysis has been effectively used to focus on a gene that confers resistance to strains of *Plasmodium falciparum*. This analysis has shown that there are other unlinked genes that also have an effect on the phenotype. Multiple gene effects may be predominant among endogenously derived refractory genes.

Although characterization of the natural bases for vector competence might provide important insights for vector control, present efforts with transgenic organisms would be facilitated by the availability of a refractory gene with a dominant phenotype that is completely penetrant and that shows no variable expression. Such genes confer resistance to the parasite. In addition, because 1 of the goals of manipulating genes involved in vector competence is to increase the prevalence of the gene in wild populations, a parasite resistance gene should have no deleterious effects on the organism. Because no existing gene exhibits all these desirable properties, several investigators have proposed the synthesis of genes with antiparasite activities. Cloning techniques would be used to link the control elements from an appropriate endogenous gene to an exogenous coding region so that when it is expressed it interferes with parasite maintenance, replication, or transmission (Chap. 14). Possible antiparasite coding regions include antisense RNAs to target viral pathogens and cloned genes that express antiparasite antibodies.

Insecticide Resistance

More accessible than resistance genes conferring parasite-refractory phenotypes are the genes that confer resistance to inexpensive and relatively safe insecticides. With the development of 2nd-generation insecticides in the late 1930s, ambitious attempts to reduce or eliminate mosquito-borne disease were undertaken, initially with spectacular success (Chap. 29). DDT was cheap, safe, and effective. In the 1950s and 1960s, vector populations were reduced dramatically, and disease diminished. However, the environmental impact of DDT and other chlorinated hydrocarbons was not recognized until some time after their worldwide use became common, and the rate at which mosquitoes and other insects developed resistance to chemical insecticides was unanticipated.

Efforts to understand insecticide resistance (Chap. 30) and the potential utility of these genes in selection schemes for transgenic organisms have provided an important stimulus for extension of gene expression studies to vector arthropods. Characterization of the genes involved has thus far revealed 3 genetic bases for resistance: DNA amplification, changes in regulatory elements, and point mutations. In *Culex quinquefasciatus*, amplification of a gene encoding the esterase B1 activity results in high levels of esterase protein that confer resistance to a variety of organophosphate insecticides. Interestingly, although this type of resistance is found nearly worldwide in *Cx. quinquefasciatus*, it appears to have arisen only 1 or a few times and yet has spread through global populations. In *An. stephensi*, increased expression from a cytochrome *P-450* gene is implicated in pyrethrin resistance. It appears that elevated expression of the protein from a single gene is sufficient to produce the resistant phenotype. Whether this changed expression is caused by new regulatory elements or alterations in preexisting elements remains to be determined. Resistance to dieldrin and other cyclodienes results from an amino acid change in 1 of the proteins that forms the GABA receptor. The gene was first characterized in *D. melanogaster* but has also been shown to exist in *Ae. aegypti*. That the nature of the mutation in the receptor seems to be the same in a number of different species is remarkable.

These examples of insecticide resistance genes illustrate the diversity of molecular responses that a vector may exhibit to a selective pressure. It is conceivable that with sufficient understanding of their modes of resistance, these various genes may be exploited in genetic control strategies. For example, cyclodiene resistance or cytochrome *P-450* genes could provide useful selective markers in transformation protocols. Manipulation of a single gene associated with resistance should be fairly straightforward, especially if the gene has an effect in the heterozygous animal. The use of phenotypes produced by amplified genes would be complex because of potential variability of the phenotype and the difficulty of handling large amplified regions of repetitive genes.

Insect Vector–Pathogenic Agent Interactions

The extent to which *Drosophila* can provide models for genetic control of disease transmission is limited because *Drosophila* does not feed on blood and is not a vector of pathogens. Unique to each vector insect is the precise interaction between its own physiology and the life cycle of the pathogenic agent that it transmits. Many processes are also unique between vector and disease agent and thus should be examined.

Studies on the viral, protozoan, and filarial agents transmitted by mosquitoes have progressed largely in their own arenas. For example, using cloning technologies, the flaviviruses, including the yellow fever virus vectored by *Ae. aegypti*, have been genetically mapped, sequenced, and details of their gene expression investigated. Similarly, Sindbis virus, a typical member of the alphaviridae, has been modified to express transiently foreign genes in mosquitoes (Chap. 14). The molecular biology of malaria parasites, *Plasmodium* spp., has been extensively studied and substantial success with technologies for maintaining these parasites in vitro

has been achieved. In addition, transformation procedures have been developed for many of the protozoan parasites. Finally, specific aspects of mosquito-filarial worm interactions are being uncovered, including the induction of a mosquito immunity protein by *Brugia malayi*.

An essential aspect of these largely independent studies is their extension to include molecular infrastructure of vector-agent interactions that maintain disease transmission cycles. Here, unfortunately, with the exception of continuous cell lines that have been used to investigate viral replication, genetically tractable systems for mosquitoes and other medically important insects are limited.

Thus, with vectors the current state-of-the-art focuses principally on accumulation of the molecular repertoire of cloned genes, regulatory elements, and transformation procedures that will support implementation of genetic control strategies. From this perspective, it is useful to draw on the extensive and detailed information already available for *Drosophila* to evaluate how it can best be utilized to advance work with vector species, preferably without having to duplicate for each species the genetic infrastructure available for *Drosophila*. For example, studies with *P* element–transformed *Drosophila* already provide gene probes and conceptual approaches that serve as important models for eventual manipulation of the mosquito, given a suitable transposable element.

ISOLATION OF GENES FROM VECTOR SPECIES

In many cases efforts to understand gene expression in vector species are natural extensions of earlier physiological studies, which provided a framework for the application of new molecular techniques as they became available. For example, the abundance of vitellin protein in mosquito eggs led to the physiological analysis of the hormonal regulation of its synthesis, production of antibodies against egg yolk proteins, biochemical characterization of vitellogenin subunits, cloning of the corresponding genes, analysis of their expression using hybridization techniques, and sequencing of regulatory elements.

In other cases it was the development of molecular tools that made it feasible to work with small quantities of material available from insect tissues. For example, arthropod salivary glands encode functions whose genetic manipulation provides approaches for disruption of disease transmission. The ability to clone directly and characterize these genes bypasses the standard physiological analyses that were done prior to the cloning of the vitellogenin gene. Similar efforts to those used to isolate genes expressed in the mosquito salivary glands have been undertaken with major organ systems in many vector species.

Current strategies for studying gene expression typically begin with the physical isolation of the gene itself and the subsequent use of hybridization or amplification technologies to monitor its expression in the insect. Laboratory techniques for isolating specific genes and examining the details of their expression in vivo and in vitro are highly developed. In an ever increasing number of cases, researchers can plan with confidence the isolation of many genes, particularly if a suitable probe is available.

Although gene isolation strategies are straightforward, they can be labor intensive. Isolating a specific gene can be extremely difficult because of the genome size relative to the number of possible genes. It is important to note that the size of a genome does not necessarily reflect its complexity (amount of unique sequence DNA) or the subjective evolutionary status of the organism. The mosquito *Aedes aegypti* has a genome size of approximately 8×10^8 bp (base pairs). Thus it is a fairly large genome, approximately one-third the size of the human genome and 3 times larger than that of *D. melanogaster*. However, if the average gene extends over $2–4 \times 10^3$ bp of DNA sequence, the *Ae. aegypti* genome contains sufficient DNA to encode as many as 400,000 genes. Given an estimated gene number of 100,000 in metazoans, it can be inferred that about 75% of the mosquito genome consists of noncoding sequence. Finding a single specific gene in this background could prove difficult. Thus, gene isolation protocols are typically designed to minimize random searching by incorporating methods that specifically identify a given gene or select for a class of genes with the proper characteristics.

Genomic and cDNA Libraries

In most cases, it is difficult to purify a single gene or fragment of DNA from a eukaryotic organism in sufficient quantity for study. Mitochondrial DNA and ribosomal RNA (rRNA) genes, which are exceptional because they occur in multiple copies and have distinct physical properties that allow them to be differentiated from the rest of the genomic DNA, were some of the first genes isolated and characterized using nonrecombinant technology. For example, in *D. melanogaster*, electron microscopic analysis of genomic DNA enriched for rRNA genes provided the initial documentation of intervening sequences, which are more familiarly termed introns when they occur within protein coding regions. These analyses are the exception. Even with multicopy genes, most isolation protocols today take advantage of the increased ease of manipulation of specially designed plasmid and bacteriophage cloning vectors and the exploitation of restriction endonucleases and other purified enzymes to construct DNA libraries. These libraries allow individual DNA fragments to be quantitatively isolated and replicated to usable quantities in bacteria.

Two general classes of libraries based on genomic DNA and cDNA are used in gene isolation studies, each of which offers specific and complementary advantages. In planning a cloning strategy, it is best to decide what types of probes will be available for subsequent screening and whether it will be more productive to screen a genomic or cDNA library. Properly constructed genomic libraries should contain the gene but require more work to identify and characterize coding regions. cDNA libraries can contain multiple copies of a target gene (if it is abundantly expressed) and therefore can be easier to screen; however, cDNAs corresponding to poorly expressed or low abundance mRNAs can be difficult to identify.

A genomic library is a collection of individual bacteriophage or plasmid DNAs, usually several hundred thousand, each containing a unique fragment of the insect genome inserted by cloning techniques. Ideally the library should be large enough to represent the total genome of the insect. To this end, bacteriophage or cosmid libraries are usually preferred because individual recombinants can accommodate larger fragments of

DNA than can plasmids. In theory genomic libraries contain all sequences, coding and noncoding, and generally are the only sources of DNA that have a regulatory function.

Many popular cloning manuals provide the details of library construction and screening. Briefly, genomic libraries are made by generating from purified total DNA a collection of individual, double-stranded DNA fragments produced by digestion with a commercially available restriction endonuclease. These fragments are inserted by ligation into a bacteriophage or plasmid DNA molecule, called the cloning vector. Individual fragments are propagated by amplifying the cloning vector (which contains an origin of DNA replication) in appropriate host bacteria. The libraries can be plated out at densities that allow the screening and recovery of single pure clones or plaques. Replicates of the plated libraries are transferred to filters (filter lifts) for screening procedures. Genomic libraries for many of the major vector species exist already and are readily obtainable from colleagues. Alternatively, it is not difficult to construct or contract the construction of libraries for any new species or strain.

A cDNA library is made from copy, or complementary, DNA that is synthesized in vitro from cellular RNA transcripts using the retroviral enzyme, reverse transcriptase. After synthesis of first-strand cDNA using reverse transcriptase, the RNA template is removed using RNAse H, which specifically degrades the RNA strand of an RNA/DNA heteroduplex. The first-strand cDNA is then used as the template to produce a double-stranded cDNA molecule that can be ligated into a cloning vector. Alternatively, polymerase chain reaction (PCR) amplification techniques can be used to produce the cDNA. One property of cDNA libraries is that in vitro synthesis can result in less than full-length products; therefore, special measures are taken during first-strand synthesis to maximize full-length synthesis. Despite these precautions, cDNA clones are often incomplete at their 5'-ends (first-strand synthesis begins at the 3'-end of the RNA). Additionally, secondary structure in the RNA template can also affect the length of the cDNA. Finally, genes that encode alternative mRNAs generated by differential splicing may correspond to multiple different cDNA clones.

Because cDNA libraries are made from an RNA template, they represent genes that are being expressed in the tissue that was the source of the RNA. cDNA libraries are less complex than genomic libraries (contain fewer *different* types of sequences) and are often enriched for those sequences that are the objects of the study. For example, a study of gene expression in the fat body or salivary gland of a mosquito begins with the construction of a cDNA library from RNA isolated from dissected fat body or salivary gland tissue, respectively. Such libraries would contain cDNAs for all genes being expressed in the tissue at the time the RNA was isolated. Genes expressed more abundantly are correspondingly represented in the library, i.e., more cDNAs are synthesized from the more abundant mRNA. Thus, the vitellogenin gene is represented among the cDNA clones from fat body tissue of blood-fed mosquitoes; likewise, salivary gland protein genes but not the vitellogenin gene are represented in clones from salivary gland. cDNA libraries are thus easier to screen, but the cloned DNA corresponds to coding sequence only. Regulatory sequences, introns, and nonexpressed genes are absent from cDNA libraries. To obtain these sequences, a cDNA clone is often used secondarily to screen a genomic DNA library.

Library Screening

Techniques for library screening are available in many laboratory manuals; by carefully following the protocols, a gene of interest can be selected from a library of several hundred thousand independent clones. Depending on the type of library and choice of cloning vector, various protocols are available for purification of large amounts of the clone containing the desired DNA sequence. With some techniques it is possible to obtain several hundred micrograms of purified DNA.

Identifying and isolating the proper recombinant clone from a library requires a probe. Nucleic acid probes can be either DNA or RNA, a synthetic oligonucleotide based on known or predicted sequence, or the product of PCR. In particular, PCR technology has greatly facilitated the isolation of genes for which some sequence information is known. Heterologous screening, in which DNA probes from 1 organism are used to isolate the corresponding gene from another, can vary in their success depending on the amount of conserved nucleotide sequence between the 2 species. When possible, PCR primers should be based on regions known to be conserved among families of genes and to reflect the codon bias of the target organism.

Specificity of the probe depends on its ability to form a duplex between itself and the target DNA. Thus, probes can be so specific as to be absolutely complementary to the target DNA or can be degenerate with some mismatching in base composition. DNA fragments used as probes can be labeled by a number of techniques, the most common being variations of a protocol called random priming. A mixture of random sequence, single-strand hexanucleotides is annealed to denatured probe DNA. The random primers provide the free 3'-OH of a deoxyribonucleoside required by DNA polymerase to initiate synthesis, generating many short strands of sequence complementary to the template. Inclusion of radioactive deoxyribonucleoside triphosphates provides a simple means of making a labeled probe. Alternatively, radiolabeling is rapidly being replaced by chemiluminescent labeling techniques that do not require isotope.

Hybridization conditions are typically adjusted to favor formation of a duplex molecule between the probe and the homologous sequence represented in the library. Under ideal incubation conditions, probes will hybridize specifically to the complementary target DNA. In practice, various probes give differing degrees of cross hybridization with both cloning vector DNA and with partially homologous genomic DNA (i.e., an expressed, intron-containing gene and corresponding processed pseudogenes are typically detected by the same cDNA probe), making unambiguous identification of the desired clone dependent on more than hybridization criteria. Optimization of hybridization conditions (temperature, salts, and other factors that affect stringency) and/or substitution of an RNA probe can be essential to finding the correct clone, particularly when it corresponds to a single-copy gene. Specific hybridization can be revealed by a number of detection protocols adapted to reveal the location of radiolabeled or nonradiolabeled probes and therefore

the complementary clone containing the DNA fragment of interest.

Cloning vectors are available for constructing cDNA expression libraries. Expression libraries facilitate isolation of a cDNA that encodes a protein or epitope for which antibodies are available. In these vectors, the cDNAs are cloned with their coding sequence in-frame with an existing gene. Upon induction, a fusion protein consisting of a portion of the existing gene linked to the protein encoded by the cDNA is produced. When a complete library is induced, several hundred thousand fusion proteins are expressed. Individual plaques expressing fusion proteins can be transferred to membrane or filter supports, screened with antibodies against the target protein, the plaque isolated, and the cDNA recovered. For example, a mammalian host responds to salivary secretions from ticks and insects by making antibodies. Polyclonal sera can be used to screen for those components of saliva (and for their genes) involved in inducing this immune response. This approach has been used to characterize a gene encoding a protein secreted from tick salivary glands shortly after attachment to the host. This protein acts as a glue to cement the tick to the vertebrate host. Some of the difficulty of removing ticks is caused by this salivary cement.

A gene of interest can also be cloned using an approach that involves first isolating and partially sequencing the protein. The gene encoding a potent erythema-inducing factor (EIF) expressed in the salivary glands of the sand fly, *Lutzomyia longipalpes*, was cloned using this approach (Chap. 20). Sufficient amounts of EIF were purified such that an amino acid sequence could be derived by Edman degradation protocols. The amino acid sequence provided the basis for synthesizing oligonucleotides that were used to PCR amplify a DNA fragment that was then used to isolate the corresponding gene.

Using antibodies and PCR amplification with probes made to conserved regions, trypsin cDNAs and genes have been isolated from *Ae. aegypti* and *An. gambiae*. The molecular analysis of these genes has confirmed earlier biochemical studies indicating that 2 distinct phases of trypsin synthesis follow blood-feeding in *Ae. aegypti*. An early phase is characterized by the brief expression of trypsins that have an approximate Mr (relative molecular weight) of 32 and 36 kDa. These are replaced later in digestion by a 30 kDa late trypsin, which is the principal digestive enzyme in the midgut and is a product of a separate gene from those expressing the early trypsins. It has been proposed that the early trypsins digest a small part of the blood meal, releasing products that directly or indirectly stimulate the synthesis of the more abundant late trypsin. These putative breakdown products remain to be identified.

The complexity of digestion of blood meal proteins by trypsin in the mosquito has been supported by analysis of one of the early and the late trypsin cDNAs, which have been cloned and sequenced. At the primary sequence level, the early gene appears to be more related to other insect trypsin genes than does the late; however, the molecular analysis confirmed that these trypsin genes belong to a multigene family, of which several members are expressed in the midgut. The cDNA and genomic clones corresponding to as many as 7 different trypsin genes were isolated during a PCR-based screen of *An. gambiae*.

Specialized Screening Protocols

Because they represent only those genes that are expressed, cDNA libraries can be screened by differential or subtractive protocols, which are particularly powerful when analyzing a single tissue or a biological system with a characteristic developmental or gene expression profile. These techniques rely on being able to separate the cDNA products of genes expressed in 1 tissue from those in all other tissues. A typical differential screen involves plating out a cDNA library and making duplicate filter lifts. One set of filters is hybridized with an RNA or cDNA probe made from the tissue or stage of development of interest, and the other set is hybridized with a probe from some other tissue or stage. Comparison of the signals on the duplicate filters reveals several interesting features. The cDNAs from genes expressed throughout the animal show signal on both copies of a duplicate set of filters. Such cDNAs are thought to encode "housekeeping," or vital cellular genes, or other genes with constitutive expression. In addition, some cDNAs only have signal on 1 of a set of duplicate filters. These represent

cDNAs that are complementary to genes expressed specifically in the tissue that served as the source for the probe. Furthermore, the intensity of the signal is proportional to the representation of that particular gene product in the probe. Differential screening therefore affords a straightforward method for isolating cDNAs complementary to genes expressed specifically and relatively abundantly in a particular tissue.

The initial work to identify genes expressed specifically in the salivary glands of *Ae. aegypti* was based on differential screening. The differential screen relied on 2 probes, 1 made from RNA isolated from salivary glands and the other from RNA isolated from the carcass (every tissue but the glands). The probe was labeled by partially hydrolyzing the RNA in a basic solution and then end-labeling the RNA with (^{32}P-ATP and polynucleotide kinase. The labeled probe was hybridized to duplicate filters, and those clones that hybridized only with the salivary gland RNA probe were further characterized. Screening in this manner yielded cDNAs homologous to genes that are expressed abundantly and specifically in the adult salivary glands.

Similarly, genes encoding 2 midgut proteases of the black fly, *Simulium vittatum*, have been isolated and characterized by differential screening of a genomic library. One of the proteases is a trypsin similar to the family described in *An. gambiae* and the early trypsins of *Ae. aegypti*. The 2nd protease, a carboxypeptidase, is the 1st example of a midgut carboxypeptidase cloned from insects. The gene sequence and its conceptual translation shows that it has similarity to a yolk-associated serine carboxypeptidase in *Ae. aegypti*. Interestingly, the black fly protease has been immunologically localized to the peritrophic matrix. The function of this matrix has been the subject of much speculation, and the association of proteases with the matrix possibly indicates that it has a role in digestion, perhaps serving as a solid support for the enzymes, preventing their loss as digestion proceeds.

Midgut gene expression has been exploited in the development of antivector vaccines against ticks in which successful feeding requires that they overcome the host immune response (Chap. 34). By immunizing cattle with tick midgut extracts, researchers are able to prevent ticks from remaining attached. This strategy works because the vertebrates are immunized against antigens they normally would not encounter, and the ticks have not evolved an appropriate response. When the tick ingests the antibody-laden blood meal from an immunized host, its midgut is attacked by components of the host immune system present in the blood meal and damaged sufficiently to cause death. The major antigen conferring this protection is a midgut membrane protein, whose corresponding gene has been cloned and evaluated as a recombinant vaccine. Similar strategies are currently being explored for the production of antiflea and antimosquito vaccines.

Differential screening with 1st-strand cDNA probes made from RNA isolated from post–blood-fed females (females were staged so that they had completed trypsin and other midgut gene expression and were synthesizing yolk and other proteins necessary to oogenesis) were used to screen genomic libraries of *Ae. aegypti* and *An. gambiae* for vitellogenin genes. The differential probes were prepared from male RNA or unfed female RNA for *Ae. aegypti* and *An. gambiae*, respectively. In *Ae. aegypti*, 2 separate and distinct clones were isolated and characterized by restriction mapping and sequencing. Genomic Southern blots using cDNAs as probes indicated that there can be as many as 5 different vitellogenin genes in *Ae. aegypti*, but it is not known how many of these are expressed. At least 5 genes were discovered in *An. gambiae*, 4 of which map to the right arm of chromosome 2 in a tandem array. Sequence information from the *An. gambiae* genes shows that they share with *D. melanogaster* vitellogenin genes common features, including putative hormone responsive elements as well as fat body and ovarian enhancer-like sequences.

A variation on the theme of differential screening is subtractive hybridization, which removes common or overlapping cDNAs from a preparation by differential binding of single-stranded versus double-stranded nucleic acid on materials such as hydroxyapatite (HAP). The procedure involves making the 1st strand of cDNA from RNA isolated from the tissue of interest. This cDNA is hybridized with a 5– 10-fold excess of RNA of another tissue. The cDNA/RNA hybrids are loaded on a column of HAP and rinsed with a low concentration phosphate buffer. The duplex material binds to the column, whereas single-stranded material washes through. The flow-through is hybridized again in excess of RNA and the cycle repeated. This procedure yields a highly purified cDNA fraction complementary to those genes expressed only in the target tissue. The cDNA can then be made double-stranded and cloned or used as a probe for library screening. The use of PCR to amplify rare cDNAs has made possible the isolation of genes expressed in as few as 1 cell using subtractive hybridization techniques.

Recently a technique for identifying and displaying tissue- and stage-specific gene expression has been developed using PCR and either polyacrylamide or agarose gel electrophoresis. In this protocol, mRNA prepared from 2 different sources, 1 from the stage and tissue of interest and the other from a control stage or tissue, are subjected to RT-PCR. RT-PCR is a protocol in which a primer is used in a reverse transcriptase reaction to produce single-strand cDNA. This is followed by the addition of a 2nd primer to the reaction and subsequent PCR amplification. In this way, rare mRNAs can be amplified to the point of detection. The key to this procedure is the use of an oligo-dT primer with a random dinucleotide on the 3'-end. This dinucleotide limits the number of possible mRNAs to which the oligo-dT can anneal and makes the subsequent analysis easier. The 2nd primer is an arbitrary, short 6–7 base primer that can anneal randomly to the single-strand cDNA. Subsequent rounds of amplification produce segments of cDNA unique to each population of mRNAs. The cDNAs are visualized on acrylamide or agarose gels as a differnetial display. Bands can be excised and reamplified as probes or cloned directly. By altering the dinucleotide on the oligo-dT primer and the sequence of the short primer, it is possible to identify cDNAs that represent the majority of genes showing stage- and tissue-specific expression. This technique provides a powerful method of analyzing populations of hormone-responsive genes, tissue-specific gene expression in the nervous system, and other genes that produce low abundant mRNAs.

Gene Characterization

The degree to which a specific gene is characterized depends on the ultimate goal of the research. Studies of the mechanistic aspects of transcriptional control often require a detailed knowledge of primary genomic sequences of regulatory regions, coding regions, and introns. Although control regions may be located both upstream and downstream as well as within introns of a given gene, most analyses begin with the 500- to 1000-bp sequence immediately adjacent to the transcription start site. Alternatively, initial efforts to genetically engineer a cell line or an organism may simply require knowing that a particular DNA fragment encodes an activity of interest.

Characterization of positive clones typically begins with restriction analysis of 1 or more (potentially overlapping) isolates and generation of a classical restriction enzyme map. These studies often provide initial information on the complexity of the gene and help in the design of probes for other studies. Typical questions asked about a cloned gene include: How many copies of the gene are present in the genome? What are the patterns of the gene's expression? What are the nucleic acid sequences of the gene and deduced amino acid sequences of its protein product(s)? How well are these sequences conserved among species? How do specific regulatory elements control gene expression? In the following section, we review general approaches to these questions.

Copy Number and Genomic Organization

Various hybridization techniques typified by Southern blotting, Northern blotting, and "dot" blotting have been developed to facilitate structural characterization of a gene and analysis of its expression. Gene copy number, for example, is commonly evaluated by Southern or dot blot analyses. For Southern analysis, genomic DNA is digested to completion independently with several different restriction enzymes, usually those with a 6-bp recognition sequence. Digestion fragments are separated according to size by agarose gel electrophoresis and transferred to a membrane, and the membrane is incubated with a labeled probe corresponding to the gene of interest. Following detection procedures, the presence of 1 or 2 bands in each individual digest

suggests that the gene is present as a single-copy (or 2 alleles per diploid) genome. Such is the case for the L8, L14, and L31 ribosomal protein genes from *Ae. albopictus*. Similarly, a simple banding pattern results when multicopy genes are arranged in tandemly repeating units, such as the rRNA cistrons, amplified dihydrofolate reductase genes in methotrexate-resistant mosquito cells, and amplified esterase genes in organophosphate-resistant *Culex*.

When Southern blotting reveals multiple bands in a number of different digests, the gene is likely to be a member of a multigene family. Quantitation of multicopy genes is routinely accomplished using dot-blotting techniques, in which a dot containing a known amount of genomic DNA on a filter is compared to a standard curve based on a known single-copy gene. Under properly controlled conditions in which the concentrations of genomic DNA and cloned DNA standards corresponding to the probe are known, comparison of the hybridization signal intensity indicates the copy number of the gene. For example, this approach was used to determine that the dihydrofolate reductase gene can be amplified to 1200 copies per haploid genome in *Ae. albopictus* cells.

The most rigorous and accurate estimate of copy number involves isolation and mapping all possible members of the gene family from a complete genomic library. Differences in restriction patterns in the DNA flanking a gene (restriction fragment length polymorphisms, or RFLPs) indicate unique localization of the sequence in the genome. This type of approach (along with genomic Southerns) was used to estimate the copy number of midgut trypsin genes in *An. gambiae*. A more stringent method for determining copy number of a gene is to sequence portions of the flanking DNA of all putative members of the family. Demonstrating that each gene is surrounded by a different region of the genome will establish it as unique. However, this analysis involves significant investment in labor and time, and restriction fragment maps usually suffice for most studies.

Analysis of the genomic and chromosomal organization of a gene can reveal features that influence its expression. For example, genes that exist as members of gene families are likely to share a common progenitor gene. Variations in expression and utilization of individual members of the family presumably evolve through changes in the DNA associated with the controlling and protein encoding regions. Thus, comparisons between promoter regions of different members of the same family can identify putative DNA sequences associated with tissue- or stage-specific expression. When making interspecific comparisons, it is important to know whether a gene belongs to a multigene family because accurate evaluation of interspecific differences should be based on genes that are strictly homologous.

In the long term, mapping the chromosomal location of known and cloned genes can be potentially useful. For example, as unknown genes with phenotypes associated with vector competence are explored, they can be mapped with respect to known genes. Furthermore, the analysis of synteny may provide data upon which to base studies of the evolution of the various vector species. Meiotic and physical maps now exist for *Ae. aegypti* and *An. gambiae*, and these maps will help in the isolation and characterization of genes involved in vector competence. Specific mapping techniques are discussed elsewhere (Chap. 26).

DNA Sequencing

Methods for sequencing genes have improved significantly since the 1st reports from the laboratories of F. Sanger and W. Gilbert. Many investigators now have access to automated sequencing equipment or to sequencing facilities that provide the service for them. The results of sequencing efforts often are submitted to databases independently of their publication status, and many journals require such submission before accepting manuscripts reporting sequence information.

The primary sequence of a gene or a cDNA can provide a wealth of information. The sequence of a cDNA should have an open-reading frame (ORF, a region that is free of termination codons when conceptually translated into protein) that usually extends over most of its length. There may be several ORFs, but the longest one usually corresponds to the reading frame that specifies the sequence of the protein encoded by the gene. The ORF also determines the 5'- and 3'-ends of the cDNA and defines the sense and antisense strands of the cDNA. Note that RNAs and single-strand DNAs have

a directionality imposed by the phosphodiester linkage. The 5'-end is the 5'-carbon on the sugar, which is phosphorylated to form the nucleotide precursors. The 3'-end is the 3'-carbon of the sugar, which is hydroxylated. The 5'-end of an mRNA encodes the amino-terminus of the protein product, and the 3'-end, the carboxy-terminus. By convention, figures and diagrams designate the genomic sequence of a gene by the strand that is identical to the mRNA, with T replacing U, the 5'-end of which is oriented at the left; the 3'-end is at the right. Additionally, when the locations of various features in the primary sequence are described, upstream identifies sequences on the 5'-end, and downstream identifies sequences on the 3'-end of a particular fragment or sequence feature.

The conceptual (or deduced) translation product is predicted by consecutive triplet codons in an ORF, and if a homologous gene has been characterized, its sequence can provide insight into the identity of the gene. Large databases exist against which any newly derived protein sequence can be compared. Amino acid sequence matched with known proteins or characterized domains of proteins often provide clues to the type and function of the protein.

The sequence of a cDNA often includes 1 or more generally ubiquitous eukaryotic signal sequences. For example, a polyadenylation signal sequence of the general form AATAAA is often found near the 3'-end of the coding region. At the 5'-end, a methionine initiation codon (ATG in the cDNA, AUG in the RNA) is often observed. This codon is the 1st one translated in the majority of mRNAs and therefore can be a reliable marker for the start of the coding region. The cDNA sequence usually corresponds to a mature mRNA sequence from which the introns have been spliced. In addition, cDNA sequences have shown that some mRNAs contain long 5'- or 3'-end untranslated regions, which may measure several hundred nucleotides in length. Interestingly, more of these long untranslated regions are found in the cDNAs of *An. gambiae* than in *Ae. aegypti*, although direct comparisons of homologous cDNAs are limited.

Comparison of a cDNA sequence with a genomic sequence of the corresponding gene can reveal details about the structure of the gene. Because cDNAs typically lack introns, direct alignment of the cDNA sequence with the genomic sequence easily reveals the positions and sizes of introns. Furthermore, comparison of the 5'-end of the cDNA with the genomic sequence can help delineate the upstream, noncoding region of the gene and set limits on the area likely to contain the transcription initiation site. By comparing genomic DNA with cDNA sequence and by primer-extension or S1-nuclease analyses, a fairly complete picture can be obtained of the nascent and fully processed, posttranscriptionally modified mRNA product.

Examination of the genomic sequence should help identify other features of eukaryotic genes such as a TATA sequence that binds a transcription factor, TFIID (necessary for the initiation of transcription by RNA polymerase II), that is located upstream of the transcription initiation site. Other 5'-end features can include a CAAT box and a GC-rich region, both involved in transcription regulation. Additionally, short, tandem, or inverted repeated DNA sequences sometimes can be found in the region upstream from the transcription initiation region. Such sequences could have regulatory roles in tissue- and stage-specific expression. Collectively, all these sequences define the promoter of the gene, that discrete region capable of initiating transcription.

Analysis of Transcription

The analysis of transcription builds upon the structural characterization of a gene by defining when, where, and how much of a particular RNA is expressed. Methods for detecting specific transcription products involve the quantitative isolation of mRNA, hybridization of a probe to the specific mRNA, and a sensitive means of detecting the hybridization. Common protocols include Northern analysis, RNAse or other nuclease protection analyses, primer extension and DNA polymerase stop analyses, RT-PCR amplification, and hybridization of a probe in situ to mRNA in tissue sections. Once the profile of expression is established, a more rigorous analysis includes experiments that will identify the cis- and trans-acting factors that regulate expression.

In vector arthropods, differential gene expression characterizes the succession of developmental phases that accompany embryogenesis, metamorphosis, and reproduction in sexually competent adults. These stages are clearly demarcated in mosquitoes, sand flies, and other Diptera that undergo a complete metamorphosis. In these vectors, only the adult stage can transmit disease, and this ability is often restricted to adult females. In contrast, insects that undergo incomplete metamorphosis, such as triatomines, can transmit disease in the blood-feeding, immature stages.

Superimposed on the developmental changes in gene expression are physiological and behavioral changes in the adult that also require specific gene expression. Mosquitoes, for example, undergo a consistent pattern of changes following adult emergence (Chaps. 5 and 6). Recently emerged females do not feed on blood for the first few days. Once the ovaries and fat body have become competent to respond to reproductive hormones, female mosquitoes enter an aggressive behavior pattern of searching for an appropriate host. After successful feeding, digestion of the blood meal in the midgut is accompanied by the transcription of yolk protein (vitellogenin) genes in the fat body. After secretion into the hemolymph, vitellogenins are actively taken up by maturing oocytes. Mature eggs are fertilized and deposited before a 2nd reproductive cycle begins with another blood meal.

During each of these phases, specific gene expression occurs in a variety of tissues. For example, recently emerged female mosquitoes actively synthesize salivary gland proteins, and the respective genes appear fully expressed. Once a blood meal has been taken, the midgut synthesizes an abundance of the digestive enzyme, trypsin. As digestion proceeds, the yolk protein genes are abundantly transcribed under the control of 20-hydroxyecdysone. The housekeeping genes encoding ribosomal proteins appear to be regulated at the levels of transcription and translation respectively during pre- and post–blood-feeding phases of the female reproductive cycle.

Techniques to define precisely when and where a gene is transcriptionally active depend on detecting the RNA transcript corresponding to the specific gene of interest. Several different approaches are available depending on the precision of staging required. Most procedures involve the isolation of total or poly-adenylated (poly-A$^+$) mRNA and detection of the appropriate transcript within the sample. It is generally assumed that the presence of a particular mRNA is an indication of the active expression of its corresponding gene. This is likely true for an mRNA with a short half-life, on the order of 30 minutes, which has been documented especially during early insect development; however, eukaryotic mRNAs can be fairly stable with typical half-lives varying between 6 and 24 hr. Furthermore, most half-life estimates are based on the detection of hybridizable mRNA, and they give no indication of whether the mRNA is actually being translated into protein or even if it is sufficiently intact to be translated. Therefore, detecting the presence of an mRNA, for example, on Northern or dot blots, does not necessarily imply that the gene was undergoing active transcription when the RNA was obtained, or that the mRNA was being translated.

Although the precision afforded by detecting the presence of a specific mRNA is sufficient for most purposes, techniques involving run-off transcription, in which a labeled precursor ribonucleoside triphosphate incubated with isolated nuclei is incorporated into mRNA transcripts that were in the process of elongation when the nuclei were isolated, can facilitate discrimination between transcriptional and translational control of gene expression. However, techniques for isolating nuclei from most insect tissues remain to be established, and the earliest uses of these approaches are likely to be undertaken with cultured cells.

Sequence analysis often identifies specific regulatory elements in the vicinity of the transcription start site that function as the promoter. However, elements known as enhancers located in the general proximity (same chromosome, within several kb distance) of the coding region often have specific effects on the amount and/or tissue-specificity of transcription and often are not evident by knowing the primary sequence. Unlike promoters located at the 5'-end of the coding regions, enhancers may function on either side of a gene in either orientation, and sometimes even in introns. Enhancers are identified principally by their activity in functional assays. Furthermore, gene expression studies have pushed the level of analysis back an additional step by characterizing the proteins that bind to specific promoter and enhancer elements.

TRANSFORMATION

Among the most powerful techniques for evaluating control of gene expression are transformation procedures that allow the investigator to manipulate a cloned gene in the test tube, reintroduce it into cultured cells (or organisms), and evaluate the effect of the manipulation on gene expression (Chap. 14). The ability to mimic, disrupt, or restore expression by manipulating control elements will provide important tools for genetic engineering of mosquitoes; the development of such techniques is an absolute requirement for the advancement of this field. However, the initial outcome of the application of these approaches will be new basic information on control of those aspects of gene expression that facilitate maintenance of pathogenic agents. Because transformation procedures circumvent some of the classical genetic techniques that have facilitated analysis of gene expression in *Drosophila*, considerable emphasis has been placed on developing this technology for vector species.

Organism-Level Transformation

The substantial successes with organism-level transformation of *Drosophila* were made possible by the discovery of a naturally occurring transposable element, *P* (Chap. 14). The *P* element has been cloned, sequenced, characterized, and successfully implemented as a vector for introduction of cloned DNA into the *Drosophila* genome. Direct adaptation of *P* element transformation technologies to mosquitoes and other arthropod vectors by embryo microinjection has been unsuccessful. Experiments with *P* elements resulted in few transformants being recovered, and these were the result of illegitimate recombination rather than *P*-mediated transposition. Several laboratories are in the process of examining whether heterologous transposable elements, such as *hobo*, *mariner*, and the FLP-FRT recombinase from yeast, might be adapted to transform mosquito embryos. Other laboratories are seeking to identify and characterize endogenous mosquito transposable elements that may function in the vector species. Along these same lines, efforts are under way to explore potential genetic manipulation of vector arthropods using naturally occurring symbionts, retroviruses, RNA viruses such as Sindbis, and DNA densonucleosis viruses (Chap. 14).

Movable genetic elements that function effectively in the mosquito would provide the solution for transformation for some disease control strategies based on the genetic manipulation of the vector. In addition, the further utility of such elements is illustrated by the use of "enhancer traps" to identify new classes of developmentally regulated or tissue-specific genes in *D. melanogaster*. Enhancer traps are *P*-element constructs containing a promoter-reporter module consisting of a weak promoter controlling the expression of an easily assayed reporter gene, such as the bacterial ß-galactosidase gene (*ß-gal*). In *Drosophila*, *P*-element transposition mediates integration of the plasmid into the genome. Because the weak promoter alone allows only minimal expression of the reporter gene, strong *ß-gal* expression occurs only when random incorporation of the enhancer trap occurred near a strong enhancer; that is, expression of the reporter gene reflects the activity of another closely linked gene. After transformed animals are evaluated for the tissues and stages that express *ß-gal,* the transposable element along with flanking chromosomal DNA can be recovered, and the linked gene identified. This technique has proven to be powerful in the analysis of the nervous system of *Drosophila*. Currently, there are no constructs of this type that function in mosquitoes; however, the discovery of transposable elements or other integrating nucleic acid vectors could lead to similar applications.

Effective germ-line transformation procedures will have to produce transgenic animals at a frequency sufficiently high that transformed individuals can be recovered in numbers adequate for genetic characterization. Moreover, the spread of transferred genes at the population level will require mobilization facilities similar to those of the *Drosophila P* element, which has naturally invaded *Drosophila melanogaster* without compromising biological fitness at the level of the population. Finally, suitable selectable marker genes, such as the insecticide resistance genes described earlier, will be needed to simplify recovery of transformants, and containment facilities will be required to test strategies for genetic disruption of disease transmission in the laboratory. Although these technical requirements are substantial, the modest progress thus far reported encourages further efforts.

Cis-Acting Elements: Transfection of Cultured Cells

Because organism-level transformation in *Drosophila* is so efficient, relatively little work has been done in vitro with *Drosophila* cell culture systems. In contrast, the challenge to organism-level transformation in mosquitoes leaves cell culture as 1 of the more promising avenues for advancing the design and testing of strategies that will be of ultimate value for embryo manipulation.

Several mosquito cell lines from a variety of species are available; among the best characterized is the *Ae. albopictus* line of Singh. The subclones of this line in current use include LT-C7, C6-36, and C7-10. Largely through the efforts of Victor Stollar and associates, the techniques of vertebrate somatic cell genetics have been applied to *Ae. albopictus* cells. Procedures have been developed for mutagenesis, selection, and characterization of mutant clones, somatic cell fusion, and DNA-mediated gene transfer. Methods for transforming mosquito cells include use of various chemical agents, including lipofectin, polybrene, and calcium phosphate. A variety of mutant cell lines are available, including cells resistant to methotrexate in which the dihydrofolate reductase gene is amplified. Thymidine kinase-deficient lines, selected on the basis of their resistance to 5-bromodeoxyuridine, have been used to extend suicide selection techniques to mosquito cells. These techniques have been used productively in mice in which the herpes simplex virus thymidine kinase coding region, expressed from a tissue-specific promoter, has been used to ablate specific tissues. Vectors that function as dominant selectable marker genes in transformed mosquito cells include the hygromycin phosphotransferase gene and the mosquito dihydrofolate reductase gene, which allow for recovery of stably transformed clones containing multiple DNA copies. Given the success of transformation in cell culture, it is unfortunate that the pole cells of the blastoderm (Chap. 16), which might be considered the equivalent of mammalian embryonic stem cells, have not been adapted to tissue culture.

Identification of cis-acting elements, which are required to be on the same piece of DNA and often in a specific orientation with respect to the gene, is typically done in transiently transfected cells, provided the transformation efficiency is high enough to detect promoter activity. In these expression assays, activity of putative control elements is typically monitored using a reporter gene whose transcription or translation directly reflects the activity of the regulatory elements under study (Chap. 14). A reporter gene is chosen because it has a straightforward and sensitive assay and minimal background activity of a corresponding endogenous gene. Useful reporter genes for vector analyses include the bacterial genes encoding *ß-gal* and chloramphenicol acetyl transferase *(CAT)*, and the firefly luciferase gene. Of these, the luciferase gene affords the most sensitivity and is linearly quantifiable over the greatest range of activity.

Based on insect genes thus characterized, principally from *Drosophila*, reasonable estimates can be made of the amount of genomic sequence required for transcriptional control. With the possible exception of enhancers, control elements usually occur within 1000 nucleotides of the start of transcription, with the most significant sequences being within a few hundred nucleotides. Cis-acting elements are identified in these assays by comparing reporter gene expression from a series of constructs in which putative promoter regions are systematically deleted. Deletions of negative regulatory elements should lead to increased activity of the reporter gene, whereas deletions of positive regulatory elements should produce the opposite result. When generating deletions, it is essential to consider the spacing of putative regulatory elements. For an element that requires a fixed distance from the start of transcription, a deletion that affects this distance may change reporter gene activity as a secondary effect. Regulatory elements may also occur downstream of the transcription start site, for example in the 1st intron, as has been shown with vertebrate ribosomal protein and dihydrofolate reductase genes. The potential presence of such elements should also be taken into account when reporter gene constructs are designed. Finally, enhancers often fail to meet this rigorous definition of a control element because they can be active in a number of locations and orientations.

Arthropod cell cultures are derived principally from embryos or early larvae and are thought to arise from an undifferentiated population of dividing cells. These cells clearly express certain classes of genes, such as the members of the heat-shock protein family, genes inducible by exogenous stimuli such as the metallothionein genes, or genes that encode such proteins as actin, expected to function in all cells. Thus, for genes that are expressed in any tissue, these functional analyses are similar to classical complementation analysis. However, for cloned genes whose expression is controlled by tissue- or stage-specific regulatory elements, continuous cell lines may lack essential transcription factors that regulate gene expression in vivo. Although many cell lines synthesize, for example, ecdysone-inducible proteins, the functions of these hormone-inducible proteins from cells, their potential expression in the organism, and the extent to which hormone-responsive cell lines will be appropriate for detailed analysis of tissue-specific genes (such as the mosquito vitellogenin gene) remain to be carefully evaluated. Finally, stable transformation technologies allow the production of cells with specific phenotypes that can have important applications in gene transfer. For example, stably transformed cells that express a hormone receptor gene under the control of an inducible heat-shock promoter are possible.

Given these considerations, it is not surprising that when expression of the tissue- and stage-specific alcohol dehydrogenase gene was assayed in nuclear preparations from embryonic *D. melanogaster*, the results suggested that correct expression of some genes requires their specific target tissue. By far the optimal situation for assaying promoters would incorporate transgenic animals, in which the gene occurs in the tissue from which it was derived, to complement studies in cell culture. Ideally this would involve stable germ-line transformation, with the incorporation of the test gene into the genome, preferably at the correct site by homologous recombination. Unfortunately, development of efficient techniques for stable transformation of vector arthropods at the level of the organism remains an essential but unrealized priority. We note, however, that control elements of the chorion protein genes from the silkworm *Bombyx mori* have been shown to function in a tissue- and stage-specific manner when introduced into *D. melanogaster* via *P*-element mediated transformation. If this observation extends to other insect genes, the functional evaluation of mosquito genes in transformed *Drosophila* could provide an important tool for characterization of regulatory elements while the appropriate technologies are being developed for direct studies in vector species.

Transient expression assays in dissected tissues or embryos can meet some of the immediate requirements for gene analysis at the level of the organism. In these protocols, gene constructs are introduced into a tissue or embryo, and the activity of the construct is assayed following an appropriate incubation period. As with transfection in cell culture, success of these protocols depends on introduction of the DNA into the cells, uptake of the DNA into the nucleus, expression of the gene, and a sensitive assay for its expression. In some cases, there is the additional requirement that the introduced DNA persist for several days in order to be expressed. By removing the basement membrane, it has been possible to use lipofection reagents to introduce DNA into differentiated adult mosquito salivary glands. Considerable expression was observed from an inducible promoter, the *D. melanogaster* heat-shock 70 gene, controlling the expression of the luciferase gene.

Trans-Acting Elements: DNA Binding Proteins

Trans-acting elements are usually proteins that bind to a specific sequence near a gene. These proteins quantitatively or qualitatively regulate gene expression. DNA sequences that bind these proteins are revealed indirectly by observing the change in expression in cells transfected with deletion constructs. Because these proteins bind DNA, transfection studies are typically extended by gel retardation (band shift) analysis, which detects the decreased electrophoretic mobility of a DNA fragment bound to protein. Similarly, various "footprinting" assays, in which bound protein protects DNA from DNAse digestion, or chemical modification (usually methylation) allow specific identification of DNA-protein binding interactions. The protected protein-DNA complexes can be visualized on sequencing gels. Finally, once a DNA domain that binds a protein is identified, the purified DNA fragment can be incorporated into an affinity column for purification of the protein and subsequent isolation of the gene encoding the trans-acting protein.

SUMMARY

The techniques of molecular biology have provided important new tools for analysis of gene expression in vector arthropods. Drawing upon basic studies with *Drosophila*, vector biologists hope eventually to develop transgenic strategies for control of disease transmission. Vector-borne diseases are currently increasing, resulting from a combination of factors, including insecticide resistance, resistance of pathogenic agents to chemotherapeutic drugs, and complex sociological and economic factors accompanying human population growth and manipulation of the environment. It is clear that increased basic understanding of vector biology and new approaches to control arthropod-borne disease are an important priority for the developing world.

FURTHER READING

Besansky, N., V. Finnerty, and F.H. Collins. 1992. Molecular perspectives on the genetics of mosquitoes. *Adv. Gen.* 30:123–184.

Carlson, J., K. Olson, S. Higgs, and B. Beaty. 1995. Molecular genetic manipulation of mosquito vectors. *Ann Rev. Entom.* 40:359–388.

Clements, A.N. 1992. *The biology of mosquitoes.* Vol. 1. London: Chapman and Hall.

Fallon, A.M. 1991. DNA-mediated gene transfer: Applications to mosquitoes. *Nature* 352:828–829.

Hagedorn, H.H., J.G. Hildebrand, M.G. Kidwell, and J.H. Law, editors. 1990. *Molecular insect science.* New York: Plenum Press.

James, A.A. 1994. Molecular and biochemical analyses of the salivary glands of vector mosquitoes. *Bull. de l'Institut Pasteur* 92:113–150.

Law, J.H., editor. 1987. *Molecular entomology.* UCLA Symposia on Molecular and Cellular Biology New Series, vol. 49. New York: Alan R. Liss.

Law, J.H., J.M. Ribeiro, and M.A. Wells. 1992. Biochemical insights derived from insect diversity. *Ann. Rev. Entom.* 40:359–388.

Lewin, B. 1994. *Genes V.* New York: Oxford University Press.

16. EMBRYONIC DEVELOPMENT

E.W. Cupp and Marcelo Jacobs-Lorena

INTRODUCTION

Arthropod embryology has been described in scientific literature since the late 1880s. In this literature there are many detailed accounts at the class and order levels; thus, embryological descriptions of medically important species are widely scattered. To provide sufficient background on arthropods of medical importance, this chapter first gives a general account of insect embryogenesis using selected aspects from the reviews of Anderson (1972, 1972a) and Sander et al. (1985) and then describes specific embryogenic details for representative vector taxa. The chapter concludes by presenting current knowledge of the cellular/molecular biology of pattern formation in arthropod embryos, using *Drosophila* as an example.

GENERAL MORPHOLOGY OF THE REPRODUCTIVE SYSTEM

The reproductive biology of arthropod vectors follows the division of labor pattern typical of the Metazoa, i.e., the male of the species produces spermatozoa in the testes and the female produces oocytes in the ovaries. Males also secrete a seminal fluid that is produced by specialized accessory glands. This biochemically complex material protects the sperm as they are conveyed to the female during mating and then nourishes them once inside the female.

The mechanical process of sperm transfer requires the use of copulatory organs (genitalia, or terminalia, in insects; chelicerae in ticks and gamasid mites), which vary in structure by species. With few exceptions, the newly inseminated female receives the sperm into a genital chamber (the bursa copulatrix) and stores them in a specialized structure (the spermatheca) from which they are released during oviposition to fertilize the eggs as they pass along the oviduct. Members of the Cimicidae are an exception: spermatozoa are deposited into the hemocoel via a specialized organ (organ of Berlese). In this case, a sharp portion of the male terminalia penetrates the abdominal cuticle while a 2nd part deposits the sperm, or semen mixture, into the organ of Berlese. Sperm then travel out of the specialized organ through the hemocoel to the ovaries, where fertilization occurs.

Two general types of ovaries have been described in insects on the basis of internal architecture and function. In the 1st, the panoistic ovary, all oogonia eventually become oocytes. This type of ovary is typical of the more primitive orders of insects; however, panoistic ovaries can occur among certain species of the Siphonaptera (fleas), an order of highly evolved ectoparasites. The 2nd type of ovary, the meroistic ovary, is characterized by the development of oogonia to both oocytes and nurse cells. In this case, the nurse cells and oocyte may be organized within an ovariole in an alternate fashion (polytrophic) or the nurse cells are restricted to the germarium (telotrophic). For example, the Hemiptera have telotrophic meroistic ovaries whereas the Diptera exhibit polytrophic meroistic ovaries. In this latter group, the ovary is subdivided into tubelike ovarioles that lie parallel to each other and are loosely bound together by a thin membrane. The ovariole is subdivided into follicles that serve as the basic reproductive units.

Oogenesis is characterized by differentiation of oocytes from a terminal germarium. These female cells then accumulate yolk and pass through to oviducts where, en route to the exterior, fertilization occurs. Thus, in most cases, embryogenesis is completed outside of the body. Viviparous insects, represented by *Glossina* spp., are an exception.

GENERAL EMBRYOLOGICAL PATTERNS OF DEVELOPMENT

The overall pattern of development of arthropod embryos may differ significantly, and therefore they are useful for comparing evolutionary relationships. This strategy has been taken to compare fate maps." A fate map is "an interpretive extraction from the blastula or blastoderm . . . for the epitomization of a whole developmental sequence" of arthropods representing a number of diverse taxa (Anderson 1979). On the basis of those embryological data and other morphological comparisons, scientists have concluded that the phylum Arthropoda is polyphyletic and could be divided into 3 phyla—Crustacea, Uniramia (insects and their allies), and Chelicerata (spiders, ticks, mites, etc.). At the genus and species level, fate maps also assist in defining where progenitor cells for various body parts are located during this early phase of embryogeny (see Fig. 16.8). Mapping of specific cell types and variation can therefore reveal different types of eggs on the basis of developmental potential. These morphogenetic differences, which are sometimes striking, should be borne in mind when considering general descriptions of arthropod embryogenesis. The specialty literature should be referred to for in-depth details of the particular arthropod group of interest.

Within the Insecta, the eggs of hemimetabolous and holometabolous species differ in several general ways. In the Hemimetabola, the eggs are usually long and ovoid, have thickened chorions, and contain large amounts of yolk with little cytoplasm. The nucleus, which is surrounded by a small quantity of cytoplasm, is centrally located. Development of some species may be lengthy, often requiring weeks. In contrast, eggs of holometabolous orders commonly have less yolk and are smaller than those of the Hemimetabola. Development is therefore relatively rapid because there is less yolk.

Early Embryogenesis

The unfertilized egg normally has a characteristic shape and size based on the morphological traits of the species (Fig. 16.1). It is encased in a multilayered shell that protects the developing embryo from a variety of environmental hazards, particularly desiccation. This complex structure usually includes a chorion, composed of endochorion and exochorion; a wax layer; and a nonliving vitelline membrane. The micropyle, which

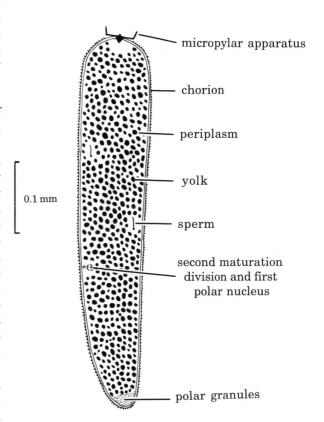

0.1 mm

micropylar apparatus

chorion

periplasm

yolk

sperm

second maturation division and first polar nucleus

polar granules

16.1 *Culex quinquefasciatus.* Sagittal section through an oocyte undergoing the second maturation division. Redrawn from Clements 1992; based on Davis 1967, *Austral. J. Zool.* 15:547–579.

is located at one end of the egg, serves as the entry point for the sperm.

The egg is typically large in relation to the body size of the female and has both longitudinal and ventrolateral axes that can be ascertained before or shortly after the initiation of embryonic development. In Diptera, the posterior of the egg can often be recognized by the presence of polar granules, which accumulate in the polar plasm of the oocyte, stain positively for RNA, and are instrumental in the formation of pole cells. Dorsoventral orientation is more problematic but can be determined early in development by noting that the median line of symmetry of the thickened embryonic primordium marks the ventral midline of the egg (Sander et al. 1985). Overall egg shape can also be useful. For example, in nematocerous Diptera such as mosquitoes, the anteroposterior axis is elongated, and the egg is ovoid to cylindrical.

Initiation of meiotic division (and the production of an egg pronucleus) signals activation. When oviposition is initiated, the egg nucleus is in the metaphase of the 1st maturation division. Division continues and produces an egg pronucleus (and 3 polar bodies). The egg pronucleus, which migrates into the interior of the egg, then pairs with that of the sperm to form the zygote nucleus, which is surrounded by a halo of cytoplasm; synchronous mitotic division (cleavage divisions) follows without cell division. The result of these and subsequent mitoses is the creation of numerous nuclei, each of which is surrounded by small, stellate masses of cytoplasm (cytoplasmic islands) that lack a limiting membrane. However, there is no corresponding division of the egg as a whole. These nucleated cytoplasmic aggregations are called energids. Through this division process, hundreds of nuclei are created that move throughout the yolk and ultimately migrate to the surface of the egg. Typically, the rate of cleavage is more rapid in holometabolous insects than in hemimetabolous species. The egg can have a conspicuous cytoplasmic reticulum that merges peripherally with a yolk-free periplasm. This reticulum network links the cleavage energids during early division with each other and with the periplasm.

The Blastoderm

As the cleavage energids migrate to the surface, the periplasm eventually becomes uniformly populated with nuclei. This process results in the formation of the syncytial blastoderm. Following migration, the peripheral nuclei then undergo synchronous mitotic divisions that result in a doubling of the nuclear population at each replicative cycle. As nuclear division continues, cytoplasm moves from the interior of the yolk mass into the periplasm so that the syncytial blastoderm thickens (Fig. 16.2). Migration of cytoplasm continues, and a 2nd layer forms under the nucleated peripheral layer.

When mitosis of the peripheral nuclei is completed, membranes form from the surface of the syncytium and penetrate radially into the interior of the egg, thereby

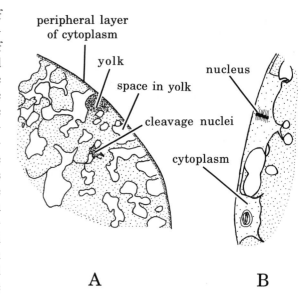

A   B

16.2 *Rhodnius prolixus*. (A) Cleavage nuclei at 16–32 stage after 24 hr of incubation. (B) Early blastoderm formation. Cleavage nuclei have reached peripheral layer of the cytoplasm (periplasm). One nucleus shows division. Reprinted from "The early embryonic development of *Rhodnius prolixus*." *Q.J. Microsc. Sci.* 78:71–91, by permission of The Company of Biologists Ltd.

enwrapping the nuclei to form cells (Fig. 16.3). The length of membrane penetration extends to the central yolk mass so that individual cells are demarcated and a continuous plasma membrane forms that separates the cell layer from the yolk. Prior to cellularization, the nuclei also change in shape, becoming ovoid and developing nucleoli. This entire process results in the formation of a peripheral, uniform cellular blastoderm that encircles a core yolk system (yolk sac).

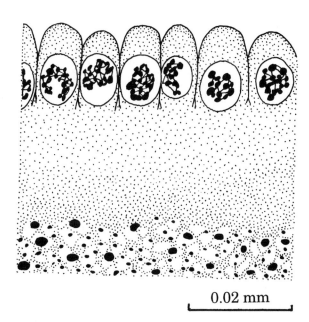

0.02 mm

16.3 *Glossina tachinoides*. Late blastoderm formation showing the penetration of lateral membranes into the interior of the egg to complete cellularization. Redrawn from Hagan 1951. "The early embryonic development of *Rhodnius prolixus*." *Q. J. Microsc. Sci.* 78:71–91. Used with permission of The Company of Biologists Ltd.

Not all cleavage energids migrate to the periplasm; some remain within the interior to digest yolk. These are referred to as vitellophages, and their role is to make the yolk constituents available as nutrients for the developing tissues. Their classification is based on origin and/or location. Primary vitellophages are linked by the cytoplasmic reticulum network and are found in the interior of the yolk. Secondary vitellophages invade the yolk mass from their peripheral position either in the syncytial or cellular blastoderm. In some species (particularly among nematocerous Diptera), primary vitellophages may be lacking entirely so that the secondary vitellophages are the 1st to enter the yolk. Tertiary vitellophages have been described in a few species of cyclorrhaphous Diptera; these cells develop from anterior and posterior rudiments of the midgut and bud into the yolk mass (Anderson 1972a).

The Differentiated Blastoderm

Several important changes occur in the uniform cellular blastoderm, resulting in the formation of 2 important components: the thickened embryonic primordium (also referred to as the embryonic rudiment, anlage, or germ band when it becomes clearly delimited) and the extra-embryonic blastoderm, which is involved in membrane formation. With the exception of certain species of Diptera, the general basis for differentiation is similar between hemimetabolous and holometabolous insects.

Embryonic Primordium

Ventral to ventrolateral cells of the blastoderm, which will form the embryonic primordium, aggregate and begin to increase in number by mitosis. As a result, this primordium consists of a broad ventral band of columnar cells that expands anteriorly to become a pair of rounded head lobes (sometimes referred to as the protocephalon) (Anderson 1972). The general dimensions (length and shape) of the primordium vary by species, but at this stage, holometabolous embryos are longer than hemimetabolous taxa.

As the embryonic primordium grows longer, it becomes a distinctive germ band that eventually is externally segmented. A sequential process of segment delineation takes place in which "growth zones" occur and determine the direction (anterior-to-posterior or vice versa) along the longitudinal axis in which differentiation will proceed. Thus, as growth and segmentation occurs, limb buds develop on the head, thorax, and abdomen in a linear, sequential fashion from which antennal, gnathal, and thoracic segments appear (Fig. 16.4).

Following the appearance of the head lobes, the stomodaeum is formed by an invagination in the midline

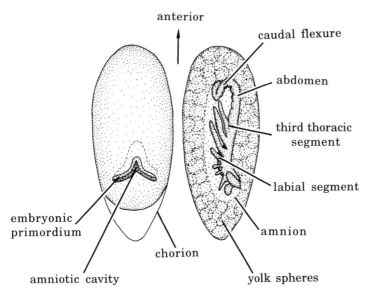

anterior

caudal flexure

abdomen

third thoracic segment

labial segment

embryonic primordium

amnion

chorion

amniotic cavity

yolk spheres

16.4 *Haematopinus eurysternus.* (A) The germ band shortly after the onset of elongation (ventral view). (B) The segmented germ band stage of this sucking louse (lateral view). From S.J. Counce and C.H. Waddington, eds., *Developmental Systems: Insectes, Vol. 1*, by permission of Academic Press Ltd.

between these structures. This occurrence usually precedes the invagination of the proctodaeum at the posterior end of the germ band, which occurs after most of the abdominal segments have been formed (see the section on gastrulation).

The direction of movement of the segmenting germ band in relation to the yolk mass varies and indicates the particular arthropod taxa. Thus, the germ band of some species penetrates into the interior whereas in others it extends along the surface of the yolk mass. For example, in the Dictyoptera (cockroaches and related forms), the germ band grows in a posterior direction along the ventral surface of the yolk; in nematocerous Diptera, the germ band extends along the dorsal surface of the yolk mass.

Complete penetration into the yolk sac with subsequent movements is evident among certain hemimetabolous groups and involves several distinctive steps which, collectively, are termed blastokinesis. In the preliminary phase, "anatrepsis," the germ band moves into and becomes completely immersed in the yolk sac.

Katatrepsis, which occurs later during embryogenesis in concert with the rupture of the embryonic membranes, is the active migration of the embryo to reposition itself in the egg.

Extra-Embryonic Blastoderm

The remainder of the blastoderm not involved with formation of the embryonic primordium is called the extra-embryonic blastoderm (or extra-embryonic ectoderm). It spreads over the yolk and with the embryonic primordium forms the serosa, an embryonic membrane.

Germ Cell Formation

In Insecta, the formation of primordial germ cells (which are formed in the embryo and eventually become the gametes in the adult) is an early event that, in holometabolous insects, sometimes precedes blastoderm formation. In Diptera determination of primordial germ cells (called pole cells) is controlled by polar granules. These organelles accumulate in the polar plasm during oogenesis and are found continuously throughout the life cycle of the germ line. During the early phase of oogenesis, the granules contain RNA (mRNA and others). After fertilization, they acquire polysomes and disperse into the posterior polar plasm, where, after pole cell formation, they associate with the outer nuclear envelope (Mahowald 1992).

Pole cells are characteristically spherical and contain nuclei that are larger than the epithelial cells of the embryonic primordium. They occur in clusters beneath the posterior end of the primordium, and the numbers vary by species (Fig. 16.5). Movement from this location to the embryonic gonads then occurs at a later time in embryogenesis. Because of attempts to introduce foreign DNA into developing vector embryos to produce transformed progeny, knowledge of the spatial and temporal aspects of pole cell formation and the times for migration into the embryo is critical.

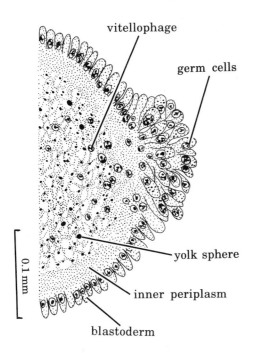

vitellophage

germ cells

yolk sphere

inner periplasm

blastoderm

0.1 mm

16.5 *Glossina tachinoides.* Sagittal section of posterior end of egg showing the position of the primordial germ cells (pole cells) projecting beyond the blastoderm. Redrawn from Hagan

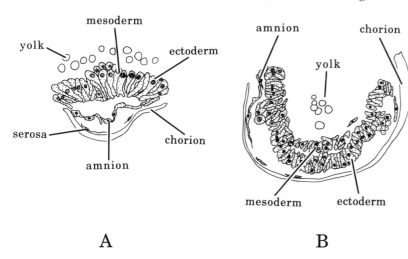

mesoderm

yolk

ectoderm

serosa

chorion

amnion

A

amnion

chorion

yolk

mesoderm

ectoderm

B

16.6 *Simulium pictipes.* (A) Transverse section through the anterior end of the embryo showing the beginning of gastrulation. The cells in the midline are elongating and pushing up in the absence of a gastral groove. (B) Formation of the mesoderm (inner layer). From "The Embryology of the black fly, *Simulium pictipes,*" Hagen. *Ann. Ent. Soc. Am.* 26:641–671, by permission of the publisher.

Gastrulation

Gastrulation is an intricate step in insect embryogenesis in which the architecture of the embryonic primordium changes from that of a single layer of epithelial cells to a bilayer by invagination (or migration) of cells along the midline. This change occurs while the embryonic primordium grows in length. The route of invagination is demarcated along the ventral midline, often by a transient gastral groove, as cells first elongate and then move toward the interior to come into contact with the yolk; they then proliferate and spread as a single layer of cuboidal cells beneath the outer columnar layer (Fig. 16.6). The creation of 2 cell strata by this method thus defines 2 distinctive layers. The outer layer is the ectoderm; the newly created inner layer is the mesoderm. The cells of the outer layer then invaginate anteriorly and posteriorly at the points of closure of the gastral groove to produce the stomodaeum and proctodaeum, respectively (Fig. 16.7). The remainder of the outer layer is referred to as the embryonic ectoderm.

During gastrulation, the inner layer of cells at the center of the anterior cell mass, which form the anterior midgut rudiment, are carried inward as the stomodaeum is formed. Conversely, while the proctodaeum is formed by invagination of the posterior end of the germ band, the inner layer of cells at the center of the posterior cell mass are also carried inward to form the posterior midgut rudiment. The remainder of the inner layer forms the mesoderm.

The occurrence and origin of a distinctive 3rd layer associated with gut formation—the endoderm—is somewhat controversial. This layer was earlier thought to form the midgut of the digestive tract by cellular proliferation that begins at each end of the inner layer and ends by growth around the yolk. However, in this chapter we will

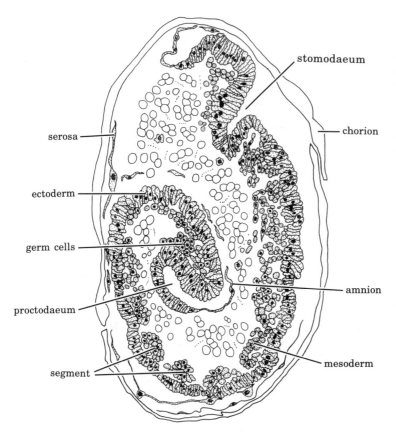

serosa

ectoderm

germ cells

proctodaeum

segment

stomodaeum

chorion

amnion

mesoderm

16.7 *Simulium pictipes.* Longitudinal section of 36-hr embryo demonstrating the formation of the stomodaeum and proctodaeum. From "The Embryology of the black fly, *Simulium pictipes,*" Hagen. *Ann. Ent. Soc. Am.* 26:641–671, by permission of the publisher.

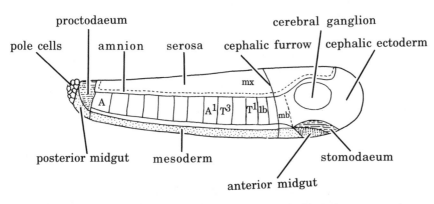

proctodaeum

pole cells

amnion

serosa

cerebral ganglion

cephalic furrow

cephalic ectoderm

mx

A

A¹ T³ T¹ lb

mb

posterior midgut

mesoderm

anterior midgut

stomodaeum

16.8 *Culex quinquefasciatus.* Fate map of this mosquito at the blastoderm stage indicating the zones of development. Redrawn from Anderson 1972; based on Davis 1967, *Austral. J. Zool.* 15:547–579.

not call this 1 layer but separate it into 2, the anterior and posterior midgut rudiments. In the earlier literature, these areas were also referred to as the mesenteron rudiments.

Gastrulation in the Insecta is variable and illustrates fundamental differences in embryogenesis. For example, in the Diptera, the ventral groove is deep and closure occurs by the rapid movement of ectodermal cells (Anderson 1972a). In certain nematocerans, the mesoderm spreads rapidly underneath the ectoderm as closure occurs, but formation of the anterior and posterior midgut rudiments is delayed until completion of the stomodaeum and proctodeum. This process differs in the Cyclorrhapha, in which both anterior and posterior midgut rudiments can be identified as soon as gastrulation begins. Following gastrulation, it is possible to outline a basic pattern of the embryonic primordium of the differentiated blastoderm leading to the formation of groups of cells that constitute presumptive areas of development (Fig. 16.8).

Membranes

As noted earlier, the chorion and vitelline membrane surround the space in which embryogenesis occurs and maintain the physical integrity of the egg prior to embryonation. However, during development, other membranes are formed to protect the embryo. The process in hemimetabolous and holometabolous species is similar, except for the cyclorrhaphous Diptera, which will be discussed later.

Shortly after differentiation of the uniform cellular blastoderm and during elongation, the margins of the embryonic primordium begin to curl ventrally (first seen at the posterior end) and eventually produce the amniotic folds that encase the ventral surface of the germ band (Fig. 16.7). This folding process also creates a fluid-filled space, the amniotic cavity, on the venter of the germ band. As development continues, this membrane stretches around the developing embryo. A second membrane, the serosa, is formed by the extra-embryonic blastoderm and forms an outer embryonic membrane that surrounds the amnion and the yolk mass.

In most hemimetabolous insects, both membranes are ruptured at the anterior end of the embryo during katatrepsis, the active, complex migratory movement that repositions the segmented germ band within the egg space. Katatrepsis relocates the embryo so that further growth and differentiation can occur. This phenomenon, as reviewed by Anderson (1972), is preceded by anatrepsis, i.e., the movement of the germ band over the posterior pole of the yolk mass followed by migration along the ventral surface until the posterior end of the germ band reaches the posterior pole of the egg. The embryos of some species may also rotate during this migratory step so that the head returns to the anterior end of the egg but is facing dorsally. Simultaneously with katatrepsis, the amnion moves back over the surface of the yolk, and the serosa contracts in a dorsal position.

The embryonic membranes and amniotic space are vestigial or eliminated in cyclorrhaphous Diptera presumably because of the relatively large size of the embryonic primordium and its rapid growth. The serosa is absent but may be represented by an ephemeral dorsal epithelium that is eliminated.

Pole Cell Migration and Early Embryogenesis

The formation and movement of pole cells is crucial in creating the internal architecture of the embryonic gonads of many types of vector insects. In many species, the pole cells move into and cluster as a group in proximity to the embryonic rudiment before gastrulation begins (Fig. 16.5). In some Nematocera, the blastoderm forms prior to migration so that the pole cells are externally located and must traverse this structure. Regardless of their initial location and subsequent movement into the interior, at some later time these cells move into the interior of the developing embryo, separate bilaterally into 2 groups, and are enveloped by the gonadal mesodermal sheaths.

Gross Definition of the Embryo

During germ band development, several morphogenetic events occur that define the exterior appearance of the body and give rise to appendages. Limb buds emerge on the thorax and abdomen. The labrum appears on the putative head as a single or paired lobe in the median line anterior to the stomodaeum. Its appearance coincides with that of the antennal rudiments. Segmentation, which defines the somites or individual units of the body, occurs, partitioning and delineating the ectodermal or mesodermal layers. Through cell thickening and separation, mesodermal tissue "blocks" develop as paired, hollow somites along a longitudinal axis. The somites become body segments. Coelomic cavities in the segments form by internal splitting of the mesoderm within the blocks; the peripheral mesodermal layers also split into layers (somatic and splanchnic) that line the body wall and subsequently form muscles, fat body, or enwrap organs.

Dorsal Closure

The ventral portion of the embryonic body is established following completion of germ band elongation and segmentation. The lateral and dorsal portions of the body then form from cellular strips along the margin of the germ band as each border extends over the yolk until they join at the dorsal midline (dorsal closure). The mechanics of the process are associated with the fusion, rupture, and retraction of the embryonic membranes which, depending on the species, can create a dorsal organ by the serosa and a temporary ("provisional") dorsal closure over the surface of the yolk mass by the amnion. The germ band simultaneously contracts in length so that the posterior end returns to the posterior pole of the egg. Growth of the margins then occurs, and partial or complete closure results so that a tubular embryo is formed.

As reviewed by Anderson (1972a), dorsal closure varies between orders with certain medically important taxa exhibiting distinct specializations. In the Siphonaptera (fleas), when the germ band shortens, the serosa ruptures and withdraws dorsally but the amnion remains intact. However, after the dorsal organ is formed, the amnion spreads above it, ruptures ventrally, and then contracts dorsally to provide provisional closure prior to growth by the margins of the germ band. In nematocerous Diptera, fusion, rupture, and retraction of the amnion and serosa occur as described, or only the amnion ruptures and withdraws. In cyclorrhaphous Diptera, the extra-embryonic ectoderm or its derivative membranes provide the temporary structure for dorsal closure as the germ band shortens.

Organogenesis and Histogenesis

As the general form of the embryo is being established, a 2nd process, organogenesis, is initiated during the late germ band stage. This series of developmental steps leads to the creation of organs and related structures from the ectodermal and mesodermal layers. Thus, during organogenesis, the ectoderm generates sense organs and the nervous system, the tracheae and the basic skeletal structure, the foregut, salivary glands, hindgut, Malpighian tubules, and peripheral portions of the reproductive tract. The mesoderm forms the gut musculature, hemocytes, the dorsal heart and related muscles and cells, segmental musculature and fat body, and gonadal sheath and ducts. The mesoderm from the walls of the cephalic somites produces the stomodaeal muscles and segmental muscles in the head whereas the mesoderm in the proctodeum forms the proctodaeal musculature.

Histogenesis is the transformation of embryonic cells into tissue-specific cell types. This prolonged process occurs after organogenesis and assists in the development of the larva or nymph. However, in some cases, histogenesis is evident at the early germ band stage when neuroblasts give rise to neuron progenitor cells (Sander et al. 1985).

The Head

The formation of the embryonic head is generally similar in both hemimetabolous and holometabolous insects. This composite structure basically develops from 5 postoral segments—the antennal, premandibular, and 3 gnathal segments (mandibular, maxillary, labial)—and possibly a preantennal segment. As ectodermal proliferation ensues, the antennal and premandibular segments migrate anteriorly to a preoral position (Fig. 16.9). The mesoderm within each somite gives rise to the necessary musculature for the appendages of the respective segments.

The antennae, which develop from ectodermal evaginations, grow longer during extension of the segmented germ band so that they trail ventrally beneath the embryo. The labrum, which demarcates the anterio-medial part of the head, also grows during this time as do the maxillary and labial ectodermal buds, which form the respective palps of both those structures.

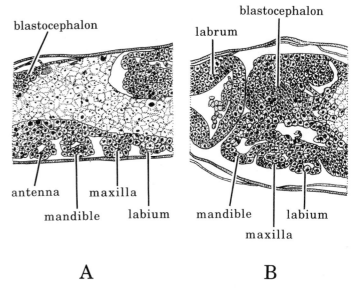

16.9 *Aedes aegypti.* (A) Longitudinal section of a 30-hr egg showing mouthparts in the process of anterior migration. (B) Egg at 35 hr showing mouthparts after migration. Reprinted from *Int. J. Insect Morph. and Embryol.* 7, Raminani and Cupp, "Embryology of *Aedes aegypti* (L.) Diptera (Culicidae): Organogenesis," 273–296, © 1978, with kind permission from Elsevier Science Ltd., The Boulevard, Langford Lane, Kidlington OX5 1GB, UK.

Ectodermal invaginations produce the tentorium and cephalic apodemes (which strengthen the head capsule) and the corpus allatum, the neurosecretory gland that is critical in growth and development because of its production of juvenile hormone (JH). The corpus allatum, which arises from dual lateral ectodermal invaginations in the mandibular-maxillary region of the head, migrates to a dorsal position on the stomodaeum. The salivary glands, which are also formed from ectoderm, begin in the labial region as invaginations that subsequently grow posteriorly beneath the stomodaeum into the thorax where they differentiate into both gland and ducts. The ducts ultimately connect medially to the hypopharynx, which is formed from the sternal region of several gnathal segments.

Embryos of certain cyclorrhaphous Diptera may be "acephalic" maggots (larvae) as a result of head involution. This developmental process involves the invagination of the gnathal and related cephalic segments into the thoracic area of the embryo shortly after dorsal closure. The mouthparts develop from the ectodermal lining of the walls of the deep cavity that is formed.

The Nervous System and Brain

The basic architecture of the ventral nervous system is established in both hemimetabolous and holometabolous insects during the early stages of germ band segmentation when portions of the ectoderm move into the interior to form paired, lateral, neural ridges along a central neural groove. The ridges are produced by 3–5 rows of blast cells that first proliferate and then bud inward to construct ganglion cells (Fig. 16.10). A median strand of ectoderm forms the floor of the neural groove and, depending upon species, ultimately aids the development of the neurilemma. Neuroblast cell activity continues, eventually becoming restricted within each twosome of somites to form paired segmental ganglia (Anderson 1972).

As the ganglia increasingly thicken and move proximally, a neuropile with axonic outgrowths forms. These outgrowths continue to develop so that each segment 1st becomes linked longitudinally by axons and then by lateral (transverse) commissures. Most insects have 3 pairs of gnathal ganglia, 3 thoracic pairs, and 10 abdominal pairs. The tripartite brain is formed from the paired lateral ganglia initially located both in front and back of the stomodaeum. Specifically, these are the premandibular ganglia (tritocerebrum, posterior to the stomodaeum), the antennal ganglia (deuto-cerebrum, peripheral to the stomodaeum), and the protocerebral ganglia (anterior to the stomodaeum). In the course of development, the tritocerebral and deutocerebral ganglia move forward into a preoral position; however, the tritocerebral commissure remains postoral. The stomatogastric nervous system, which lies ventral to the brain, evolves from 3 distinct ectodermal evaginations located dorso-medially on the stomodaeum. These cells produce the frontal, hypocerebral, and ventricular ganglia of that system.

Eye discs develop from the ectodermal surface of the lateral optic ganglia. These normally differentiate into compound eyes and are partially or completely connected to the protocerebrum by lateral optic ganglia.

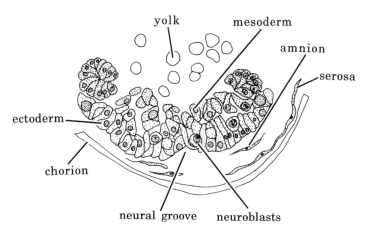

16.10 *Simulium pictipes.* Transverse section through the abdominal region of a 24-hr embryo showing neural groove and neuroblasts. From "The Embryology of the black fly, *Simulium pictipes*," Hagen. *Ann. Ent. Soc. Am.* 26:641–671, by permission of the publisher.

The Gut and Malpighian Tubules

The developmental outline for the gut is established during elongation of the germ band with the formation of the stomodaeum (anterior) and proctodaeum (posterior). This process creates 2 cylindrical invaginations that are lined with ectodermally derived epithelium. The middle portion (midgut) is formed from the anterior and posterior midgut rudiments, which are histologically distinct tissues. In the stomodaeum, which forms the foregut, the anterior portion of the tube bends backward on itself to form the proventricular region while the remaining part of the tract develops into the esophagus. The proctodaeum grows inward to form the hindgut; its distal portion develops rudimentary outgrowths that protrude into the hemocoel and ultimately give rise to the Malpighian tubules.

The midgut is formed by proliferation of cells from both the anterior and posterior midgut rudiments (see the section on gastrulation). Strands of cells emanate from these ventro-lateral rudiments so that the remaining yolk mass is eventually encompassed and an ovoid, protracted midgut is formed that connects the fore- and hindguts. Resorption of the yolk mass is then initiated. As the yolk is digested, the midgut epithelium develops in many species and is instrumental in this process. In some species of Diptera, the vitellophages migrate to the yolk's surface and form a temporary epithelial template for the formation of the definitive midgut epithelium. However, with rare exception the vitellophages are digested with the yolk. In certain higher Diptera, pole cells may also contribute to gut development via formation of portions of the midgut and hindgut epithelium.

The Gonads

Gonadal development varies in hemimetabolous and holometabolous insects (Anderson 1972, 1972a). The patterns of development for the hemimetabolous orders are: (a) primordial germ cells can first be seen within the mesodermal walls of the abdominal segments and eventually proliferate to form bilateral strands of cells that become the gonads; (b) primordial germ cells differentiate during blastoderm formation and are carried into the yolk during elongation of the germ band, where they separate into 2 bilateral groups to form the gonads; and (c) primordial germ cells differentiate during early gastrulation, migrate to the mesodermal walls of the abdominal somites, and continue to develop as described for (a). The interior portions of the ducts are derived from the mesoderm, whereas the exterior portions and accessory glands are ectodermal in origin.

Gonad formation in the Holometabola generally follows the scheme noted for (b). Primordial germ cells migrate into the interior of the blastoderm, divide into 2 groups, and then move through the yolk to enter the mesodermal sheaths of the 5th and 6th abdominal segments. Ducts and accessory glands develop after hatching from both mesodermal and ectodermal layers as noted.

The Respiratory System

The tracheal rudiments in both hemi- and holometabolous insects are formed from bilateral pairs of ectodermal invaginations located on each segment from the 2nd thoracic to the 8th abdominal segment. These invaginations bifurcate, join longitudinally, and then branch throughout the embryo to form a diffuse system of hollow tubes that promote gaseous exchange. The tracheae eventually become lined with a cuticle, and their lateral openings give rise to the spiracles, the valves that control the flow of gases into and out of the system. In some holometabolous species, one or more of the spiracular openings may be permanently closed. For example, in the cyclorrhaphous Diptera all except the 1st and last pair of spiracles are sealed. Oenocytes (secretory cells that are found in the larval/nymphal epidermis) also arise from groups of cells adjacent to the abdominal tracheal invaginations.

Imaginal Discs

Holometabolous insects possess groups of cells, or imaginal discs, that are initially set apart during embryogenesis and, during metamorphosis, will form many of the adult structures. Thus, the embryo in the Holometabola is organized as a dual system consisting of both larval and "adult" (imaginal) cells. The cells are set apart during organogensis; thus, specific adult rudiments can be identified and followed during both embryogenesis and postembryonic metamorphosis.

Embryogeny of the Acari

The embryology of medically important acari (particularly mites) is generally lacking compared to that of other major vector groups. This paucity is due largely to technical and biological problems, e.g., the small size and the centrolecithal structure of the eggs of many species, which has slowed preparation (fixation, sectioning), examination, and description. However, an overview of the embryology of *Ornithodoros moubata* is available that not only provides excellent comparative details (Aeschlimann 1958; Aeschlimann and Hess 1984) but also describes the major differences in embryogenesis between the acari and insects. Currently, these include differences in formation of the embryonic primordium, the extra-embryonic membranes, and the mechanisms associated with blastokinesis.

The acarine egg is encased by an exterior chorion and an interior vitelline membrane. The egg is normally centrolecithal (yolk is concentrated in the center of the egg) with a distinct periplasm. The oocyte nucleus is surrounded by cytoplasm that connects to the exterior by a cytoplasmic reticulum. In *O. moubata*, following fertilization nuclear division occurs in synchronous waves as the nuclei (and their attendant cytoplasm) migrate to the surface of the egg. A uniform cellular blastoderm is formed that surrounds the yolk sac; primary vitellophages remain in the yolk. In ticks, the blastoderm is often referred to as a periblastula, and the yolk-filled cavity, the blastocoel. Aeschlimann (1958) suggested that the primary vitellophages remain intact during embryogenesis and contribute to the formation of the gut epithelium.

Certain cells along the blastoderm form a distinct aggregation of cells (germinal primordium) that will form the ventral portion of the embryo. This mass proliferates into the yolk and is called the germ disc; it demarcates the telson (posterior) of the embryo. The appearance and backward migration of this disc indicates gastrulation. Developmentally, this cellular aggregation represents the inner layer (mesoderm) whereas the remaining exterior blastoderm cells form the ectoderm. Cellular proliferation occurs anteriorly so that a cephalic lobe (acron) is formed. The acron and the telson continue to grow and eventually reach the dorsal side of the putative embryo. Primary vitellophages and an endodermal layer (derived from the germ disc as internal proliferating cells) possibly play a part in the formation of the midgut.

Segmentation begins anteriorly and forms the prosoma (the locomotory portion of the body). Initially, 3 ambulatory segments are delineated followed by the pedipalpal and secondary ambulatory segments. The cheliceral segment completes the formation of the prosoma, a composite of 6 segments. As segmentation continues, 5 abdominal segments emerge and join with the telson to complete the formation of the opisthosoma. Formation of the ventral nerve cord is similar to that in insects and begins in the germ band stage along a central neural groove (sulcus ventralis).

At this point blastokinesis begins, and the germ band contracts longitudinally (Aeschlimann and Hess 1984). The germ band moves onto the surface of the yolk mass and leads to the developmental outline of the 6-legged larva. Part of this process involves the failure of the "buds" of the 4th pair of legs to develop in the embryo. Instead, in many acarine species this terminal pair of legs appears at the molt of the hexapod larva to the octopod nymph.

The major body parts of the acari differ generally from that of insects but can also be divided into 3 units—gnathosoma, prosoma, and opisthosoma (Chap. 1). The last 2 are often merged into a single functional unit—the idiosoma. The gnathosoma bears the mouthparts and cephalic sensory structures and is functionally equivalent to the insect head. However, these trophic units are not homologous as evidenced by their differing embryological origins and their striking morphological differences. As described by Aeschlimann and Hess (1984) the chelicerae arise posterior to the stomodaeum but migrate forward to a preoral position where they then undergo a 90° rotation; the pedipalps also migrate to a position postero-lateral to the stomodaeum. The hypostome, previously thought to arise from the coxal lobes of the pedipalps, probably has its origin in the ventral poststomodaeal lips.

Very little else is known about acarine embryology except the formation of the rectal sac and Malpighian tubules from the proctodeum. These excretory structures function in the developing embryo and accumulate guanine crystals.

Embryogeny of **Rhodnius prolixus**

The architecture and developmental pattern of the egg of this bloodsucking bug is typical of the more highly evolved Hemimetabola. Embryogenesis takes 26–29 days at 21° and 90% relative humidity (Mellanby 1936; 1937). Cleavage of energids begins at 12 hr after fertilization, and a uniform blastoderm is formed by 55–60 hr. The embryonic primordium is formed ventro-laterally from cuboidal cells. Germ cells bud off of the posterior pole of the blastoderm between 66–76 hr after fertilization and, with invagination of the germ band, are carried forward through the yolk where they come to lie at the extreme posterior end of the developing embryo. Invagination and anatrepsis of the germ band begins at 76–86 hours and pushes the ventral part of the embryonic primordium toward the dorsal posterior of the egg space so that most of the germ band ultimately is located within the yolk. Formation of the amnion and serosa follows the usual method, and their growth also pulls the anterior end of the germ band into a more superficial position at the posterior end of the egg space. The mesoderm arises from the central portion of the invaginated embryonic primordium and the ectoderm from the peripheral outer layer. Differentiation of organs and tissues begins.

At day 12, the second stage of blastokinesis begins and is completed within 48 hr. This process reorients the embryo so that the thorax and abdomen rotate through 180° while the head moves forward to the anterior part of the egg. This movement allows sufficient space for the growth of the appendages. On the putative head, the labrum grows midventrally and the mandibular, maxillary, and labial segments begin development. The legs grow posteriorly and extend beyond the tip of the abdomen, where they bend around the embryo. Dorsal closure is initiated on day 13 and is completed within 3 days, thereby completely enclosing the yolk. The external appearance of the embryo changes very little from this point until eclosion.

Development of internal organs is generally typical of hemimetabolous insects. The ventral nervous system, corpora allata, subesophageal nerve mass, and dorsal heart are well developed by day 12. Gonadal development is completed by days 19–21 as the germ cells form continuous longitudinal strands through abdominal segments 6–8. Formation of the gut requires more time due to differentiation and growth of the midgut, but by 26 days the entire tract is virtually complete as are the salivary glands, stylet-like mouthparts, and Malpighian tubules.

Embryogeny of the Culicidae

Embryological descriptions are available for 4 genera of mosquitoes representing 6 species. These accounts, reviewed by Clements (1992), include the 3 genera of major medical importance (*Anopheles*, *Culex*, *Aedes*) and also span the phylogenetic spectrum of the family. With few exceptions, these reports indicate a general similarity of embryogenesis among the species examined and demonstrate that development within the Culicidae is typical of the Holometabola.

Early Embryology

Nuclear division following fertilization is so rapid that the first mitotic cycle in some species may be completed within 15–20 minutes. In *Culex pipiens*, migration of energids to the periplasm begins after the 7th division, with some of the cleavage nuclei entering the posterior pole to bind polar granules; by 2–3 hr after oviposition, distinct pole cells are evident. In *Aedes aegypti*, pole cell formation begins at hour 3 and is completed an hour later. Numbers of pole cells formed range from 12–16 in *Cx. pipiens* to 20–30 in *An. maculipennis*.

A syncytial blastoderm is formed in *Cx. pipiens* within 4–5 hr with uniform cellularization occurring about an hour later. This process occurs at hours 8–9 in *Ae. aegypti*. Following this step, secondary vitellophages migrate from both the posterior and anterior ends of the blastoderm to join their primary counterparts in the yolk.

Delineation of the embryonic primordium and the extra-embryonic membranes also occurs at this time. In *Ae. aegypti*, the ventral columnar blastodermal cells form the embryo proper while those cells located at the ventrolateral portion of the blastoderm form the amnion. Development of this membrane begins at hour 14, and over the next 3 hr a thin layer of cells is produced that covers the entire germ band. Cells of the extreme lateral and dorsal blastoderm form the serosa, a thin membrane that adheres closely to the amnion but encloses the entire egg contents.

Pole cells of both *Ae. aegypti* and *Ae. vexans* enter the blastoderm by the end of hour 11 by way of the blastoderm nuclei and then migrate anteriorly. In so doing, they locate on the tip of the germ band. This process differs from that of *Cx. fatigans* (*Cx. quinquefasciatus*), in which the pole cells do not enter the blastoderm but sink into the presumptive posterior midgut and proctodaeal invagination and migrate in those rudiments.

Gastrulation with midventral mesoderm formation occurs at hour 12 in *Ae. aegypti*. Unlike *Culex* and *Anopheles* species, a gastral groove does not form in *Aedes*—the presumptive mesodermal cells simply elongate and migrate as an irregular, scattered group. Segmentation of the germ band begins by hour 15 so that 17 well-defined somites (1 blastocephalon, 3 gnathal, 3 thoracic, and 10 abdominal) are present by hour 19. Stomodaeal and proctodaeal invaginations also occur at this time.

Organogenesis

To depict organogenesis in the Culicidae, *Aedes aegypti* will be used as an example; for complete details, see the description by Raminani and Cupp (1978).

The Head

The rudiments of the mouthparts and antennae appear early in development and can be traced separately. By hour 25, the antennae, mandibles, and maxillae begin to form; these structures migrate anteriorly so that the mouthpart rudiments eventually are located on the ventral side of the blastocephalon whereas the antennal rudiments retain a dorsal position. By hour 35, the labrum is demarcated as a separate lobed area on the blastocephalon. At this time, the lateral walls of this area undergo compression, buckle inward, and thicken. Slender cytoplasmic processes arise from the outer ends of the ectodermal cells along the walls and develop into feeding brushes. Other parts of the labrum subsequently transform into the palatum and hairs of the oral brushes so that by hour 60 two large beds of feeding brushes are present.

After mouthpart migration, the mandibles and maxillae are recognizable at hour 25 as ectodermal buds. These 2 paired structures form the floor of the larval mouth. At hour 45, the outer ectodermal cells of the mandibles secrete a thin cuticular layer that gradually thickens over the course of embryogeny. Palps arise from the anterior end of the maxillae by hour 35. Labial rudiments are noticeable by hour 30 as 2 ectodermal lobes located posterior to the maxillae. The lobes fuse, migrate anteriorly, and form the posterior portion of the larval mouth.

The antennal rudiments originate from the posterior margins of the blastocephalon and are noticeable by hour 25 after fertilization as ectodermal buds immediately posterior to the stomodaeal invagination. These rudiments migrate anteriorly, between the junction of the labral lobe and the blastocephalon, and by 65 hours these sensory structures become 3-segmented.

The Gut and Malpighian Tubules

The fore- and hindgut rudiments are formed at hour 19 as ectodermal invaginations, and the midgut eventually forms from cells derived at the tips of these infoldings. Differentiation of the stomodaeum into the foregut, pharynx, esophagus, and proventriculus is complete by hour 65. At this point, a concentration of yolk cells can be seen at the tip of the proventriculus. Mesodermal cells form a thin layer around the stomodaeal invagination, which subsequently differentiates into the musculature covering the foregut.

Ectodermal cells of the terminal unit (segment 17) elongate and migrate anteriorly to form the proctodaeal invagination. Mesodermal cells in the posterior part of the segment then generate a thin layer around this pocket and enclose the pole cells. The invaginating cells then undergo a series of divisions at the rim of the invagination. Cells at the rear form the posterior portion of the midgut whereas those at its base differentiate into the proctodaeum. Cellular division continues followed by migration so that the invagination eventually protrudes vertically into the yolk mass as a rounded structure with the pole cells at the tip.

The proctodaeum begins differentiation at hour 45; within 5 hours its anterior end has widened to form the eventual junction with the midgut, the pyloric ampulla. This area differentiates posteriorly to form the hindgut, which consists of the ileum and colon; a rectum is not formed in the embryo. By hour 65, epithelial cells secrete a chitinous intima that lines the hindgut.

The Malpighian tubules arise as 5 short tubular ectodermal projections from the free end of the proctodaeum. By hour 40, following completion of germ band shortening, the tubules occupy their usual position at the junction of the hindgut and midgut. Each layer consists of a single layer of ectodermal cells with a narrow cavity.

The presumptive anterior and posterior midgut gives rise to 2 ventro-lateral ribbons of cells at hours 30–35 that grow toward each other over a period of 5–10 hours and eventually fuse. During this process, the midgut cords reach the inner layer of mesodermal cells of the trunk segments; this lamina splits off to form the splanchnic mesodermal layer, which differentiates into the midgut musculature. After fusion, the cords grow ventrad and dorsad to contribute to the formation of the ventral portion of the midgut and dorsal closure of the embryo. By hour 60, the midgut is a closed tube, completely surrounding the yolk mass. At hour 70, the gastric caeca arise as tubular outgrowths from the midgut at its junction with the foregut. Eventually 8 caeca are formed in this location.

The Nervous System and Fat Body

Formation of the ventral nerve cord begins at hour 15 when neuroblasts from both sides of the thoracic and abdominal segments migrate inward and come to lie between the ectodermal and mesodermal layers. Following migration, a longitudinal neural groove develops and acts as a mold for the formation of the ventral nerve cord. Neural cells collect on both sides of the groove and form 2 ganglionic lobes in each segment. Nerve fibers, derived from cells along the medial margin of each lobe, extend across and fuse by hour 40 to form a single ganglion per body segment.

Ectodermal cells in the posterior region of the blastocephalon begin to proliferate bilaterally at hour 35 to form 2 large cellular masses. These presumptive neuroblasts differentiate to form the tripartite brain, which is located between the pharynx and the posterior margin of the blastocephalon. Differentiation of the neuropile begins at 40 hr. Cells along the medial margins form axons; by hour 45 the neural filaments from the

proto- and deutocerebral lobes of the brain extend medially and fuse over the esophagus to form the supraesophageal ganglion. The trisegmental subesophageal ganglion is formed by hour 65 from masses of neural cells located at the posterior part of each gnathal segment (mandible, maxillae, labium). A few cells along the medial margins of each mass form axons, and by hour 45 differentiation of the neuropile takes place.

The retrocerebral complex is formed from 2 unequal masses of ectodermal cells that proliferate from the middle region of the blastocephalon at hour 45 and migrate posteriorly. The larger dorsal aggregation differentiates into the corpus cardiacum, and the smaller ventral mass gives rise to the corpus allatum. The former consists of 2 layers of oval cells with a central neuropile; the corpus allatum appears as a concentric collection of 4–5 cells with a central cavity. The rudiments of these glands are interconnected by nerve fibers.

The frontal ganglion of the stomodaeal nervous system (stomatogastric) begins to form at hour 45 from the anterior migration of the ectodermal cells along the medial margin of the pharynx. The lateral margins of the ganglion elongate so that by hour 60 they connect to axonic projections from the tritocerebrum. A prominent recurrent nerve is also formed that extends posteriorly along the dorsal surface of the pharynx and esophagus; it gives rise to 2 nerves that innervate the esophagus. The outer layer of somatic mesodermal cells forms the fat body. These cells are evident in the 50-hour embryo.

Gonads

By 30 hours, the pole cells are located in the tip of the proctodaeal invagination. As shortening of the germ band progresses, this invagination with its enclosed pole cells is gradually pulled posteriorly. By hour 35, it reaches the level of the 6th and 7th abdominal segments, where the pole cells divide into 2 groups and migrate bilaterally, forming the gonadal rudiments. The number of pole cells in each rudiment varies between 4–6, and at this point the polar granules are attached to the nuclear membranes. A layer of flattened mesodermal cells, which later differentiates into the gonadal epithelium, surrounds each rudiment.

Embryogeny of *Glossina tachinoides*

Glossina spp. (tsetse) are a group of highly evolved cyclorrhaphous Diptera that are important vectors of African trypanosomes (Chap. 10). Both adult sexes are completely dependent on blood for nutrition, feeding once a day on a variety of large mammals. The female flies are also viviparous, i.e., the egg is retained internally until embryogeny is complete; the larva, which remains inside the female, is nourished beyond the embryonic stage by means of paired milk glands. The female subsequently gives "birth" to a fully formed larva that quickly burrows into the ground and pupates. This mode of viviparity is referred to as adenotrophic because the egg contains sufficient yolk to nourish the embryo until it hatches, and specialized maternal organs are present to feed the larva in utero. Embryogenesis in this group of flies is quite rapid, often requiring only 24–36 hours. A brief but detailed account of early embryonic development is available for *Glossina tachinoides* and is summarized here (Hagan 1951).

Cleavage and Blastoderm Formation

Cleavage is rapid, and early nuclear migration results in both clumps and scattered individual nuclei in the yolk and superficial periplasm, suggesting that not all nuclei reach the outer surface simultaneously. A uniform stratum of nuclei is formed, and the thin periplasm becomes distinctly granular, forming a 2nd inner layer. Cellularization occurs as furrows form between nuclei and move toward the interior of the egg, penetrating the outer periplasm to establish cell membranes. The cells produced are uniform columnar epithelium and are slightly more than twice as tall as they are wide. Primordial germ cells (pole cells) can be seen in the posterior portion of the egg; these cells are formed from cleavage nuclei that migrate into this region. The pole cells are located dorsolaterally and protrude well above the cells of the blastoderm proper.

Germ Band Formation and Embryo Definition

Formation of the embryonic primordium (germ band) is initiated along the ventral portion of the blastoderm. Several rows of cells on either side of the midline grow noticeably taller whereas the remaining cells of the blastoderm decrease in height. This initial process differentiates the embryonic primordium from the remainder of the dorsal blastoderm as well as the ectoderm from the mesoderm. The area of cellular differentiation continues from the anterior to the posterior poles, and the embryonic primordium ultimately extends over the yolk so that its 2 distal portions are recurved at the extremities; the anterior portion, which will form the cephalic portion, is therefore directed back over the top while the posterior end points anteriorly (Fig. 16.11). The amnion, which covers the entire embryo or its ventral surface in most insect species, is either highly transitory or nonexistent in *Glossina* spp. A medial neural groove is formed by elongated ectodermal cells, and nerve cords are formed in the late germ band stage. The latter are

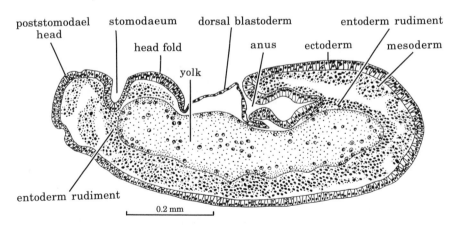

16.11 *Glossina tachinoides*. Sagittal sections showing composite picture of germ band with stomodaeal and proctodaeal invaginations and initiation of head formation. Redrawn from Hagan 1951.

derived from the 2 strands of cells that lie on either side of the neural groove.

The proctodaeal invagination precedes formation of the stomodaeum and, topographically, is located slightly anterior to the germ band. This invagination defines the area that will be the embryonic abdomen and gives rise to the rudiments of the hindgut and the Malpighian tubules. The invaginating ectoderm of the stomodaeum forms a large, round depression that gives rise to the foregut. The point of indentation begins at the center of the anterior end of the germ band, which is dorsal in position. The head region of the larva is evident near the antero-lateral thickening of cells of the germ band ectoderm.

Mesodermal Derivatives

The developmental process leading to the formation of the midgut is generally similar to that described for *Rhodnius prolixus* and *Aedes aegypti*. A bilayer of mesodermal cells extends in both directions from the anterior and posterior midgut rudiments as thin strands to gradually encompass the yolk. These cells migrate laterally and dorsally as a single layer of epithelium. A thin layer of mesoderm from the segment walls produces a weak musculature around the digestive tract. This layer also produces the heart muscles and fat body, which are dispersed both dorsoventrally and antero-posteriorly. The utilization of this layer thus leaves a large hemocoelomic space within the embryo.

The Gonads

In embryos that have just completed the formation of the midgut, the pole cells can been recognized as 2 irregular masses that extend from the penultimate abdominal segment forward over the last third of the yolk. In more advanced embryos, these cell masses are drawn forward so that they come to lie in segments 9–11; they are surrounded by mesodermal cells that form a thin sheath. Thin strands of cells then infiltrate between groups of germ cells to form several chambers.

Tracheae

Ectodermal invaginations leading to trachea formation can be detected at the beginning of katatrepsis. These appear as a series of paired lateral openings with the exception of a single posterior pair that open near the upper margin of the terminal part of the germ band. In *Glossina tachinoides*, there are 11 pairs. Through a process of invagination, lumen formation, and branching, 2 main tracheal trunks are formed ventrally and dorsally. A thin cuticula eventually surrounds the embryo and lines the longitudinal tracheal trunks as well.

MOLECULAR GENETICS OF *DROSOPHILA* EMBRYONIC DEVELOPMENT AND PATTERN FORMATION

Drosophila spp. are the best characterized arthropods from a genetic and developmental point of view. In this section we compare and contrast the use of experimental genetic systems in *Drosophila* and other insects. We also outline some of the molecular principles that guide the establishment of the *Drosophila* embryonic body plan. Finally, the potential benefits that can be derived from this knowledge for the study of vectors are briefly discussed.

Drosophila and Insect Vectors as Experimental Systems

Morphological aspects of arthropod embryonic development are relatively well understood. However, only *Drosophila* has been extensively studied at the molecular level. Advantages such as ease of rearing and short generation time have made *Drosophila* the best genetically characterized multicellular organisms.

Rearing

Drosophila stocks are kept at room temperature in small vials containing a cornmeal/molasses/yeast–based food. To perpetuate the stock the flies are transferred to a new vial every 2–3 weeks (less often if the stock is maintained at a lower temperature of 18°C). The generation time at 25°C is 10 days, slightly shorter than that of *Aedes aegypti*. About 25–30 generations can be obtained annually, an important consideration when classic genetic experiments are performed. In comparison, only about 3 generations per year can be obtained with the mouse, which is the best genetically characterized mammal. Although several mosquito species also have a short generation time and have been used for more genetic studies than any other insect vector, it is much more laborious to maintain mosquitoes than *Drosophila*. Other insect disease vectors are even more difficult to rear. For example, black fly larvae grow in streams and must be reared in the laboratory in flowing water at controlled temperatures and with periodic, timed feedings.

Genetics

The well-characterized genetics of *Drosophila* translates into thousands of different characterized mutations, most of which are mapped to chromosome locations and kept in stock centers. In contrast, fewer than 100 loci have been identified for *Ae. aegypti* (Munstermann 1990), and a number of the strains have been lost. Obviously, the ability to keep frozen stocks of different insect strains and mutants would be extremely helpful, especially considering the difficulties of maintaining the insects. Such methods have been available for keeping mammalian embryos, but curiously, it has been much more difficult to implement similar freezing methods for insects. Recently, methods have been developed to store frozen *Drosophila* stocks (Mazur et al. 1992) and scientists hope that similar technologies will become available for insect vectors. The ability to keep frozen stocks will ease genetic studies and provide more sophisticated genetics. Thus, numerous and important issues such as the characterization of resistance genes that render vectors unsuitable hosts for pathogens could be addressed.

Tools to Study Drosophila

Since Morgan first identified the famous *Drosophila* *white* mutant in 1910, significant technological advances have contributed to the recent explosion of knowledge, and genetics has played a crucial role. Sophisticated balancer chromosomes have been created that greatly facilitate genetic studies.[1] A major landmark in the genetics of *Drosophila* embryonic development was established by the classic paper of Nusslein-Volhard and Wieschaus (1980). Their approach was disarmingly simple considering its fundamental importance. Nusslein-Volhard and Wieschaus systematically mutated each of the 3 major *Drosophila* chromosomes and screened mutant larvae

for specific body pattern defects. For the screen, larvae homozygous for each of the new mutations were examined microscopically to determine whether specific pattern elements were defective. The rationale was that inactivation of genes required for general cell maintenance and metabolism (e.g., housekeeping genes) would result in a nondescript dead-embryo phenotype. In contrast, they hypothesized that mutations in genes with specific roles in the formation of pattern elements would yield larvae defective only in those elements. As a result of their massive undertaking, these investigators found a number of genes that are required for the differentiation of specific structures in the embryo. This study, and others that followed, were critical for our present understanding of *Drosophila* embryogenesis.

The advent of gene cloning and nucleic acid technology, including DNA sequencing, provided major technological breakthroughs. In situ hybridization to polytene chromosomes of salivary glands provided a "meeting point" between genetics and molecular biology because both mutations and cloned DNA could be localized to specific positions on polytene chromosomes. In situ hybridization is also helpful in the determination of the direction of "chromosome walks." Moreover, in situ hybridization of nucleic acid probes to tissue sections or whole-mount embryos and the localization of proteins with antibodies by similar techniques allow the identification of specialized cells that are morphologically indistinguishable from their neighbors early in development. For instance, in situ hybridization with DNA from a pair rule class gene, resulting in the now well-known 7-stripe "zebra" pattern, demonstrated that nuclei in the early syncytial blastoderm embryo are already expressing regionally specialized products (Hafen et al. 1984).

Another landmark was the discovery by Rubin and Spradling (1982) of *P* element–mediated transformation. *P* elements (Chaps. 13 and 14) are transposable elements that encode a transposase, which is an enzyme that promotes integration into the genome of any sequence flanked by the *P* element terminal repeats. Usually a gene encoding a selectable marker (for example, the *white* gene) and the gene under study are placed between the repeats and injected into the posterior part (where pole cells form) of embryos mutant for the *white* gene. A certain proportion of the progeny of the injected embryos will carry the construct in their chromosome. These flies can be identified by their colored eyes (as opposed to the white eyes of nontransformed flies).

P element transformation has numerous uses. For example, it can be used to confirm that a cloned gene is affected in a given mutant by rescue of the mutant phenotype. It can also be used to study the effects of gene misexpression by combining the coding part of a gene with a heterologous promoter (for example, a heat-shock promoter). Functional analysis of different domains of the gene can be done by transforming genes with altered or missing sequences. *P* element transformation is relatively simple and does not require sophisticated equipment. If similar technology could be developed for other insects, transformation with the appropriate gene could be used to alter the biology of vectors (e.g., resistance to a parasite or microbial pathogen). Unfortunately, *P* elements are genus-specific and do not integrate into nondrosophilid insects. Although transformation of mosquitoes has been achieved (Crampton et al. 1990), it has not yet been accomplished on a routine basis. The development of efficient transformation methods for vectors is currently an active area of research.

Drosophila *Development*

The *Drosophila* egg is approximately 0.5 mm long and 0.14 mm in diameter. It stores vast quantities of nutrients, ribosomes, and enzymes, most of which are in quantities sufficient to support full embryonic development. Most of these materials are synthesized during oogenesis by 15 highly polyploid nurse cells and transported to the oocyte through cytoplasmic bridges. A 3rd type of cell, the follicle cell, surrounds the oocyte and nurse cells, forming the egg chamber (see top of Fig. 16.16). The follicle cells synthesize the eggshell, the vitelline membrane, and as will be pointed out later, molecules crucial for the proper differentiation of the embryo. The large DNA content of the nurse cells allows oogenesis to proceed very rapidly. The youngest stage egg chamber develops into a mature oocyte in only a little over 3 days. Fertilization

occurs in the oviduct while the egg is being laid. Fertilization triggers the completion of meiosis and a very rapid series of 9 nuclear divisions in a common cytoplasm (Fig. 16.12A). At about 1.5 hours of development, most nuclei migrate to the egg periphery. The pole cells are formed at this time (Fig. 16.12B). The nuclei divide 4 more times and at about 3 hours of development membranes are formed around each nucleus, producing the cellular blastoderm (Fig. 16.12C). Gastrulation starts immediately after completion of cellularization. Posterior cells migrate dorso-anteriorly, resulting in the "extended germ band" embryo at about 6 hours of development (Fig.

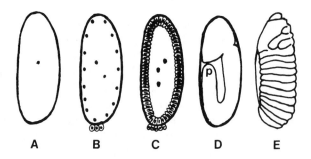

16.12 Stages of early *Drosophila* development. Ventral is to the right and anterior is up for all illustrations in this figure. (A) Embryo at fertilization. (B) Embryo at ~1.5 hr of development. After about 9 nuclear divisions in a common cytoplasm, most of the nuclei move to the cortex of the egg. At this stage, a few cells (pole cells) form only at the posterior end. (C) Embryo at ~3 hr of development. After 13 nuclear divisions, the resulting ~6,000 nuclei around the entire cortex are incorporated into cells. Immediately thereafter, gastrulation begins with a series of invaginations (not shown). (D) Embryo at ~6 hr of development. Gastrulation and germ-band elongation produce an embryo with cells most posterior lying behind the developing head region (p = posterior end of germ band). Segmentation starts at this stage (not shown). (E) Embryo at ~10 hr of development. After the germ band shortens, the lobed head segments, 3 thoracic segments, the 8 abdominal segments, and the caudal region are visible. Organogenesis ensues, and the larva hatches at about 22 hr of development. Reproduced, with permission, from the *Annual Review of Cell Biology, Vol. 2*, © 1986, by Annual Reviews, Inc.

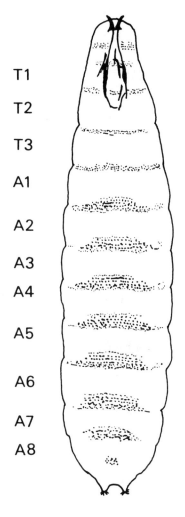

T1
T2
T3
A1
A2
A3
A4
A5
A6
A7
A8

16.13 Ventral view of a fully formed larva. The denticle belts provide clear landmarks for the segmented pattern. T1–T3: thoracic segments 1–3; A1–A8: abdominal segments 1–8. Reproduced from R. Ransom, ed., *A handbook of Drosophila development.* New York: Elsevier Biomedical Press, 1982.

16.12D). This is followed by "shortening" of the germ band (completed by about 10 hours of development), a process that results in the transformation of the embryo from U-shaped to rod-shaped (Fig. 16.12E). Segmentation of the embryo occurs concomitantly (Fig. 16.12E). Organogenesis follows, and the larva hatches at about 22 hours of development. The larva has characteristic external landmarks that are very useful for genetic analysis. Three thoracic (T1 to T3) and 8 abdominal (A1 to A8) denticle belts (rows of "hairs") provide major landmarks for each body segment (Fig. 16.13). Each belt is formed of 3–7 rows of denticles arranged in a characteristic manner. Other landmarks

include the prominent anterior mouth hooks and the posterior spiracles (part of the respiratory system).

The Molecular Genetics of Drosophila Embryonic Development

The combination of genetic and molecular approaches has led to a fairly sophisticated understanding of the processes governing embryonic development of *Drosophila*. The fact that over 40 articles have been published in the past 6 years illustrates the progress tha has been made (2 excellent recent texts are Lawrence 1992 and St. Johnston and Nusslein-Volhard 1992). This section provides a selected and simplified overview of some early events in the establishment of the embryonic body plan (Fig. 16.14).

A great deal of the information required for the establishment of the *Drosophila* embryonic body plan is synthesized maternally (in the ovary) and stored in the unfertilized egg. After fertilization, these maternal gene products act on the genome of the zygote (developing embryo) to initiate a cascade of gene expression that culminates in the development of a fully differentiated larva. Thus, many of the maternal genes directly or indirectly activate transcription of the zygotic genes. The maternal genes establish the major embryonic axes by selectively activating zygotic genes (such regulated genes will be referred to as "downstream" genes). This initiates a cascade of events that sequentially establishes more and more detailed pattern elements. Consequently, embryos mutant in maternal genes have the broadest impact on the development of the embryo whereas embryos mutant in zygotic genes are defective in more restricted portions of the embryonic body plan (Fig. 16.14). Figure 16.14 lists the different classes of zygotic genes in the approximate temporal order of their action. The gap genes are the first zygotic genes to be activated (by the maternal genes), followed by the pair rule and segment polarity genes.

The homeotic genes are activated relatively late. This class of genes is special in that they do not affect the establishment of the segments per se but only the character assumed by each segment. For instance, an embryo homozygous for a deletion of the *Bithorax* complex has the correct number of segments, but segments T3 to A8 all develop with a T2 character. We

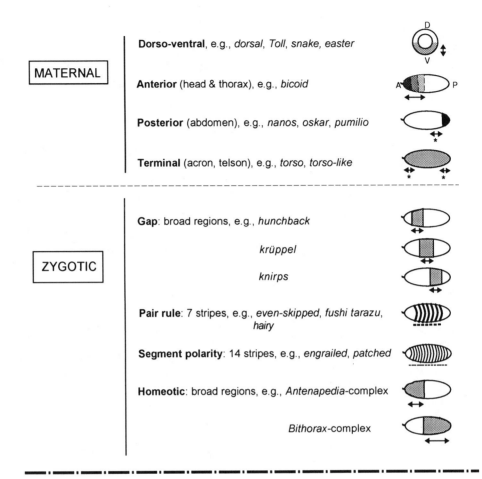

MATERNAL

Dorso-ventral, e.g., *dorsal, Toll, snake, easter*

Anterior (head & thorax), e.g., *bicoid*

Posterior (abdomen), e.g., *nanos, oskar, pumilio*

Terminal (acron, telson), e.g., *torso, torso-like*

ZYGOTIC

Gap: broad regions, e.g., *hunchback*

krüppel

knirps

Pair rule: 7 stripes, e.g., *even-skipped, fushi tarazu, hairy*

Segment polarity: 14 stripes, e.g., *engrailed, patched*

Homeotic: broad regions, e.g., *Antenapedia*-complex

Bithorax-complex

Homeobox: *bicoid, fushi tarazu*

Zn-finger: *hunchback, krüppel, knirps*

helix-loop-helix: *hairy*

tyrosine kinase: *torso*

Serine protease (secreted): *snake, easter*

Transmembrane (large extracellular domain): *Toll*

Extracellular: *patched*

16.14 Summary of genes involved in embryonic pattern formation. Two general classes of genes are required for establishment of the proper embryonic body plan: (1) maternal genes, which are expressed in the ovary but act in the early embryo; and (2) zygotic genes, which are expressed in the embryo and act immediately. All genes act in restricted regions of the embryo, as shown on the right. A cross-section of an embryo is shown on the top (dorsal is up) and longitudinal sections (anterior is to the left) for the embryos below. Shaded portions indicate regions where gene products are located. Arrows (or dashes for the pair rule and segment polarity genes) mark where the gene products are active, as indicated by the phenotype of mutants for those genes. In most cases the sites of gene product and gene action coincide. Exceptions to this rule are indicated by asterisks below the arrows. Many of the genes have been cloned. As shown at the bottom of the figure, the genes fall into a variety of functional classes.

will summarize a few well-characterized cases to illustrate different molecular "strategies" used by *Drosophila* for the establishment of the embryonic body plan.

The dorsal Gene and the Establishment of the Dorso-Ventral Pattern

Establishment of the dorso-ventral pattern depends on a different type of regulatory cascade involving 11 maternal genes. *dorsal*, which encodes a transcription factor, is at the bottom of this cascade and is the "effector" that ultimately regulates the transcription of a number of zygotic "downstream" genes. Interestingly, 3 of these genes (*pipe*, *nudel*, and *windbeutel*) are expressed during oogenesis not in the nurse cells but in the follicle cells. Their products are presumed to be incorporated into the vitelline membrane (Fig. 16.16). *snake*, *easter*, *spätzle*, and *gastrulation defective* are expressed in the nurse cells. These genes share the unique property of being secreted into the perivitelline space (Fig. 16.16). *Toll* is a transmembrane protein that receives the signal generated by *pipe–nudel–windbeutel* and transmitted by *snake–easter–gastrulation defective–spätzle*. *Toll* relays this signal to *pelle-tube*, which activates the release of *dorsal* from the cytoplasmic protein *cactus*. Upon release, *dorsal* migrates to the embryonic nuclei, where it regulates the transcription of downstream zygotic genes. The key to this regulatory cascade is that *dorsal* release does not occur uniformly around the circumference of the embryo but only along the ventral side (Fig. 16.14, top right). The mechanism of this localized activation is not understood, but the asymmetry of the signal is likely to result from differential gene expression in the ventral follicle cells of the egg chamber (Fig. 16.16).

In summary, the following strategies are used in the establishment of the dorso-ventral differentiation pattern of *Drosophila*.

1. Differential signaling originates from gene products expressed during oogenesis in the follicle cells that surround the oocyte. Only in the ventral portions of the developing embryo does this signal cross the perivitelline space. The signal is received by the transmembrane *Toll* protein and transmitted to *cactus,* causing the release of *dorsal* in the ventral portions of the embryo. Thus, ultimate regulation is at the level of cytoplasm-to-nucleus translocation of a transcription factor.

2. Because some of the perivitelline gene products encode serine proteases (e.g., *snake*, *easter*), it is likely that signal transduction across this space occurs by a proteolytic cascade, not unlike the mammalian clotting cascade.

3. The key gene in the dorso-ventral cascade encodes a transcription factor *(dorsal).*

The *bicoid* Gene and the Establishment of the Anterior Pattern

bicoid is a maternal gene that contains a homeobox.[2] In the ovary, *bicoid* mRNA is synthesized in the nurse cells and transported to the oocyte, where it accumulates exclusively at the anterior end. The products of the maternal genes *exuperantia*, *swallow*, and *staufen* are required for anterior localization because flies mutant in these genes yield embryos defective in *bicoid* mRNA localization. After fertilization, *bicoid* mRNA translation is activated and the protein diffuses from its anterior source, creating a decreasing antero-posterior concentration gradient (Fig. 16.14, Fig. 16.15, column 1). Through its homeobox, the *bicoid* protein binds to the promoter of zygotic genes such as *hunchback* (a zinc finger–containing transcriptional regulator), activating their transcription. *hunchback* acts in turn on a number of other downstream genes. Fig. 16.15 illustrates how the spatial distribution of *hunchback* transcription depends on the affinity of the *bicoid* protein to its promoter. If affinity is low, expression decreases fast along the anterior-posterior axis; if affinity is high, *hunchback* expression will extend further posteriorly because even small amounts of *bicoid* will be sufficient to bind to the *hunchback* promoter and activate its expression.

The importance of the shape of the *bicoid* concentration gradient is illustrated by the fact that an increase of *bicoid* gene dosage (and therefore *bicoid* mRNA concentration) will move the site of head formation more posteriorly. Embryos from mothers with 8 copies of the *bicoid* gene die, presumably because the changes in the spatial pattern of gene expression are so

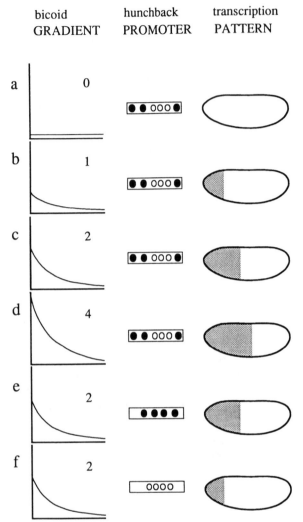

bicoid
GRADIENT

hunchback
PROMOTER

transcription
PATTERN

16.15 Spatial transcriptional regulation of the zygotic gap gene *hunchback* by the *bicoid* protein gradient. The left column shows the shape of the *bicoid* protein gradient as the maternal gene dosage (0, 1, 2, or 4) of *bicoid* is varied. The horizontal axis represents distance along the anterior-posterior axis, and the vertical axis shows the concentration of *bicoid* protein. The middle column shows the *bicoid*-binding sites in the regulatory region of *hunchback* (a-d) or two reporter (e-f) gene constructs. The closed circles indicate high affinity; the open, low-affinity binding sites. The right column shows the size of the anterior expression domain of a reporter gene containing the *bicoid*-binding sites shown in the middle column in the presence of the gradient shown in the left column. (a) No maternal copies of *bicoid*, wild-type *hunchback*. (b) One maternal copy of *bicoid*, wild-type *hunchback*. (c) Two maternal copies of *bicoid* (normal), wild-type *hunchback*. (d) Four maternal copies of *bicoid*, wild-type *hunchback*. (e) Two maternal copies of *bicoid*, reporter gene construct containing 4 high-affinity *bicoid*-binding sites. (f) Two maternal copies of *bicoid*, reporter gene construct containing 4 low-affinity *bicoid*-binding sites. Reproduced from St. Johnston and Nusslein-Volhard. 1992. "The Origin of Pattern and Polarity in the Orosophila Embryo," *Cell* 68:201–219. © Cell Press.

great that the embryo can no longer compensate for them. Thus, the spatial distribution and the quantity of a single gene product such as *bicoid* can have profound effects on embryonic development.

In summary, the pattern of *bicoid* gene expression illustrates some fundamental principles of the establishment of the *Drosophila* anterior body plan: First, spatial restriction of gene expression is achieved by mRNA localization. Second, a concentration gradient of a key transcriptional regulatory protein *(bicoid)* is achieved by synthesis from a localized source (the mRNA) at the anterior end and diffusion away from it toward the posterior end. Finally, differentiation along the anterior-posterior axis will be altered either if *bicoid* gene copy number is altered or if affinity of *bicoid* to the promoter of its target gene (e.g., *hunchback*) is altered.

Expression of Pair Rule Genes in Stripes

Some of the earliest genes to be expressed after fertilization are the gap genes (Fig. 16.15). They are expressed in unique territories of the embryo, sometimes overlapping slightly, sometimes separated by

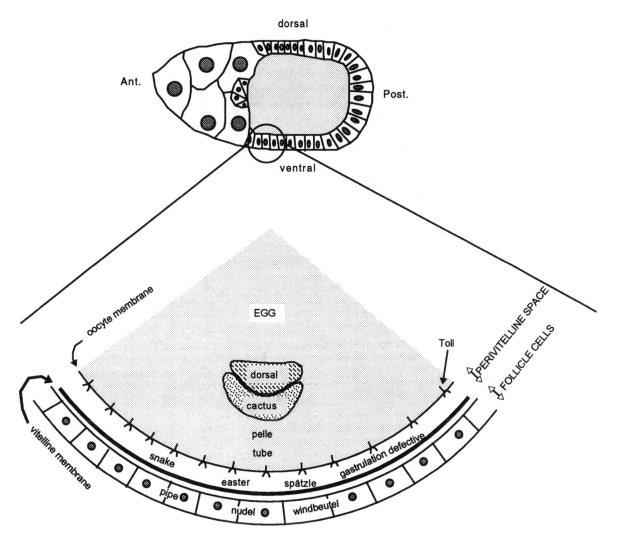

16.16 The dorso-ventral genes. The top of the figure shows a developing ovarian egg chamber. Fifteen interconnected nurse cells (5 are shown at the left) communicate with the oocyte (stippled at the right) to which they transfer their synthetic materials. Follicle cells surrounding the oocyte synthesize the protective layers of the oocyte (such as the vitelline membrane) and molecules such as *pipe*, *nudel*, and *windbeutel*, which participate in the dorso-ventral differentiation of the embryo (see bottom of the figure). The fluid-filled space between the vitelline membrane and the oocyte membrane define the perivitelline space. The *snake*, *easter*, *spätzle*, and *gastrulation defective* proteins are synthesized by the oocyte and secreted into the perivitelline space. *Toll* is a transmembrane receptor protein. The *pelle*, *tube*, *cactus*, and *dorsal* proteins are found in the egg (and embryo) cytoplasm.

small gaps. Thus, unique combinations of transcription factors are established along the anterior-posterior axis of the embryo. The striped pattern of pair rule gene expression takes advantage of this regionalization of transcription factors along the length of the embryo (Fig. 16.17). Interestingly, separate promoter elements "read" the unique transcription factor combination in each region of the embryo. This was shown by placing individual promoter elements next to a reporter gene such as beta-galactosidase. When transformed into the organism by *P* element–mediated transformation, these genes direct beta-galactosidase expression only in their corresponding domain (Fig. 16.18). In all likelihood, genes that are expressed later (e.g., segment polarity genes, homeotic genes) are similarly regulated by the different combinations of localized transcriptional activators and repressors.

In summary, segmentation of the embryo depends in part on the expression of pair rule genes in stripes. Pair rule gene expression in stripes is achieved: (1) by the distribution of transcriptional activators and repressors (maternal gene products, zygotic gap genes) in spatially restricted patterns, and (2) by the presence of separate promoter elements that can read the unique combination of transcriptional regulators in a given region of the embryo.

CONCLUSIONS

A wealth of information about *Drosophila* embryonic development has been assembled. This knowledge will be a great asset for the study of arthropod vectors, a

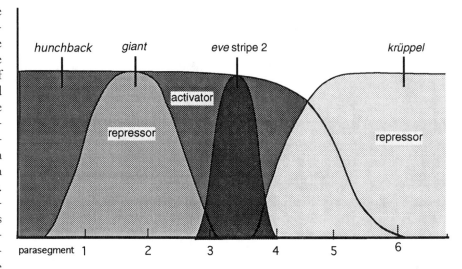

16.17   The spatial distribution of transcriptional activators and repressors determine the expression of the pair rule gene *even-skipped* (*eve*) as a stripe. The horizontal axis represents distance along the anterior-posterior axis (anterior is to the left), and the vertical axis shows the concentration of the transcriptional activators and repressors (these are all gap class genes). Repression is dominant over activation. What would happen to *eve* stripe 2 in an embryo that does not have functional *krüppel* gene product? Reprinted from Peter Lawrence, *The Making of a Fly,* © 1992, by permission of Blackwell Scientific Publications Ltd.

field that is still in its infancy. For instance, even though there is not yet a convenient method of reintroducing cloned genes into vectors, cloned vector genes can be transformed into *Drosophila*, thus providing an in vivo heterologous insect system. Knowledge acquired from *Drosophila* genes potentially important for vector biology could be extended to the study of the corresponding genes in vectors. For instance, a dorsal-related gene that probably regulates the *Drosophila* immune response was recently isolated (Ip et al. 1993). The isolation of the corresponding gene from insect vectors could be of importance for the study of the interaction of pathogens with their insect hosts.

NOTES

1. Balancer chromosomes are multiply inverted chromosomes that suppress recombination with their homologue. They are marked with dominant morphological markers that allow immediate

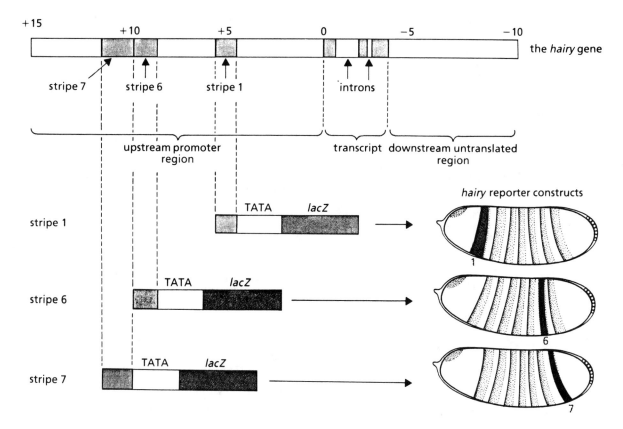

16.18   Each promoter element directs the expression of the pair rule *hairy* gene in a different stripe. The top of the figure is a schematic diagram of the *hairy* gene. The origin of the scale (in kilobases) is at the transcription initiation site. When the indicated DNA fragments were used to drive the expression of the beta-galactosidase (lacZ) reporter gene, expression occurred only in stripes 1, 6, or 7, as indicated in the diagrams at the right. Reprinted from Peter Lawrence, *The Making of a Fly*, © 1992, by permission of Blackwell Scientific Publications Ltd.

identification of the flies carrying them. Balancers are usually, but not always, lethal when homozygous and are useful for keeping mutant stocks of recessive lethal mutations.

2.   The homeobox is a DNA sequence motif that encodes a stretch of 60 amino acids called homeodomain. The homeodomain is involved in DNA sequence recognition. Homeobox genes encode DNA-binding proteins that bind to promoter regions of the genes that they regulate.

REFERENCES

Aeschlimann, A. 1958. Développement embryonnaire d'*Ornithodorus moubata* (Murray) et transmission transovarienne de *Borrelia duttoni*. *Acta Trop*. 15:15–64.

Aeschlimann, A., and E. Hess. 1984. What is our current knowledge of acarine embryology? In: D.A. Griffiths and C.E. Bowman, editors, *Acarology VI*, Vol.1. Chichester: Ellis Horwood. pp. 90–99.

Anderson, D.T. 1972. The development of hemimetabolous insects. In: S.J. Counce and C.H. Waddington, editors, *Developmental systems: Insects*, Vol. 1. New York: Academic Press. pp. 95–163.

―――. 1972a. The development of holometabolous insects. The development of hemimetabolous insects. In: S.J. Counce, and C.H. Waddington, editors, *Developmental systems: Insects,* Vol. 1. New York: Academic Press. pp. 165–242.

―――. 1979. Embryos, fate maps, and the phylogeny of arthropods. In: A.P. Gupta, editor, *Arthropod phylogeny.* New York: Van Nostrand Reinhold. pp. 59–105.

Clements, A.N. 1992. *The biology of mosquitoes,* Vol. 1. Development, Nutrition and Reproduction. London: Chapman and Hall. 509 p.

Crampton, J., A. Morris, G. Lycett, A. Warren, and P. Eggleston. 1990. Transgenic mosquitoes: A future vector control strategy. *Parasit. Today* 6:31–36.

Gambrell, F.L. 1933. The embryology of the black fly, *Simulium pictipes* Hagen. *Ann. Entomol. Soc. Am.* 26:641–671.

Hafen, E., A. Kuroiwa, and W.J. Gehring. 1984. Spatial distribution of transcripts from the segmentation gene *fushi tarazu* during *Drosophila* embryonic development. *Cell* 37:833–841.

Hagan, H.R. 1951. *Embryology of the viviparous insects.* New York: Ronald Press. 472 p.

Ip, Y.T., M. Reach, Y. Engstrom, L. Kadalayil, H. Cai, S. Gonzalez-Crespo, K. Tatei, and M. Levine. 1993. Dif, a *dorsal*-related gene that mediates an immune response in *Drosophila. Cell* 75:753–763.

Lawrence, P.A. 1992. *The making of a fly.* New York: Blackwell Scientific Publications. This is an excellent book that reviews *Drosophila* development in an accessible form.

Mahowald, A.P. 1992. Germ plasm revisited and illuminated. *Science* 255:1216–1217.

Mazur, P., K.W. Cole, J.W. Hall, P.D. Schreuders, and A.P. Mahowald. 1992. Cryobiological preservation of *Drosophila* embryos. *Science* 258:1932–1935.

Mellanby, H. 1936. The early embryonic development of *Rhodnius prolixus* (Hemiptera, Heteroptera). *Q. J. Microsc. Sci.* 78:71–91.

―――. 1937. The later embryology of *Rhodnius prolixus. Q. J. Microsc. Sci.* 79:1–42.

Munstermann, L.E. 1990. Linkage map of the yellow fever mosquito, *Aedes aegypti.* In: S.J. O'Brien, editor, *Genetic maps,* Vol. 3, 5th ed. Cold Spring Harbor, NY: Cold Spring Harbor Press. pp 179–183.

Nusslein-Volhard, C., and E. Wieschaus. 1980. Mutations affecting segment number and polarity in *Drosophila. Nature* 287:795–801.

Raminani, L.N. and E.W. Cupp. 1978. Embryology of *Aedes aegypti* (L.): Organogenesis. *Int. J. Ins. Morph. Embryol.* 7:273–296.

Rubin, G.M., and A.C. Spradling. 1982. Genetic transformation of *Drosophila* with transposable element vectors. *Science* 218:348–353.

Sander, K., H.O. Gutzeit, and H. Jäckle. 1985. Insect embryogenesis: Morphology, physiology, genetical and molecular aspects. In: G.A. Kerkut and L.I. Gilbert, editors, *Comprehensive insect physiology, biochemistry and pharmacology,* Vol. 1. New York: Pergamon Press. pp. 319–385.

St. Johnston, D., and C. Nusslein-Volhard. 1992. The origin of pattern and polarity in the *Drosophila* embryo. *Cell* 68:201–219.

17. PHYSIOLOGY OF MOSQUITOES

Henry H. Hagedorn

INTRODUCTION

In most respects, the physiology of vectors, including mosquitoes, is much like that of other insects and is covered in basic physiology textbooks. However, studies of the physiology of vectors are incomplete; much must be inferred from studies on model insects such as the moth *Manduca sexta*. Such inferences must be made with care, as it has become evident that there is considerable diversity in physiological systems among the insects and that model insects are unique to some degree. This is true even of comparisons within the Diptera. The cyclorraphan Diptera, which include *Drosophila melanogaster*, are highly specialized insects, making comparisons with mosquitoes less obvious than their taxonomy would suggest.

THE LARVAL MOSQUITO

Fortunately, the larval mosquito has been the object of much research regarding the salt and water balance in insects, which is the subject of this section. Why should this be of interest to the vector biologist? The distribution of mosquitoes is largely based on the availability of suitable sites for larval growth. Because larval mosquitoes are aquatic, water is essential. However, water sources vary considerably in composition, from the nearly distilled water resulting from rain to salt marshes and alkaline lakes. Although 95% of mosquito species live in fresh water, the distribution of some important vector and pest mosquitoes depends on their ability to cope with extreme situations, which has

been the subject of many investigations. Mosquito larvae have developed physiological mechanisms that allow them to invade niches that are extreme in terms of salt composition. *Aedes campestris* larvae have been collected from a lake in Canada in which sodium was 0.48 molar, bicarbonate was 0.38 molar, and the pH was 10.2! Some species can live equally well in fresh water and seawater (e.g., *Aedes campestris* and *Aedes dorsalis*) or in acid and alkaline lakes (e.g. *Aedes taeniorhynchus*). Rock pool mosquitoes such as *Opifex fuscus* from New Zealand are regularly exposed to either very high saline concentrations as water evaporates from the pool or to nearly fresh water as rain dilutes the pool. Brackish-water species live in areas such as salt marshes where fresh water mixes with seawater.

The ability of mosquito larvae to survive under varying conditions can be measured by examining hemolymph osmolarity in waters with different salt compositions. Like most other animals, insects must be able to regulate the composition of the hemolymph bathing their internal organs because cells are usually tolerant of only a narrow range of ionic and osmotic conditions. In mosquitoes that are able to live in diverse conditions, the composition of the hemolymph changes very little as the concentration of the external medium increases. An extreme example of this ability is *O. fuscus*, which lives in salty rock pools that vary widely in salt composition. Figure 17.1 describes the change in larval hemolymph osmolality as the concentration of the seawater in which the larvae were growing was

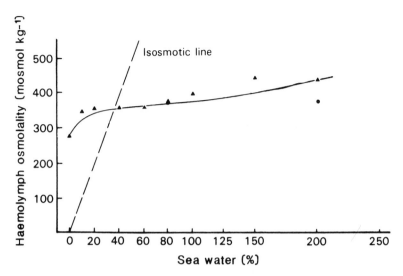

17.1 The mean osmolality of *Opifex fuscus* hemolymph taken from larvae reared in different concentrations of seawater. The isosmotic line indicates what the hemolymph osmolality would be if it were allowed to rise with the change in external seawater. Modified from S.W. Nicolson 1972, "Osmoregulation in larvae of the New Zealand saltwater mosquito *Opifex fuscus*," J. Entomol. (A) 47:101–108, with permission of The Company of Biologists Ltd.

high saline concentration, the opposite is true, and the internal salt concentration rises. Basically, the mosquito meets these challenges in two ways: it eliminates excess salts via the Malpighian tubules and rectum, and it takes on needed salts via the rectal papillae.

The Freshwater Mosquito

Aedes aegypti larvae are restricted to freshwater habitats. The larvae osmoregulate in dilute media, but osmoregulation breaks down if the osmolarity of the water nears that of the hemolymph. Figure 17.2 provides data for larvae of *Ae. aegypti* reared in dilute seawater. The curve in the graph is very different from the curve in Figure 17.1. As the concentration of seawater increased from distilled to 20%, the osmolality of the hemolymph remained near 250 mOsmoles. But as the osmality of the water rose to 250 mOsmoles (25% seawater), regulation failed and the hemolymph and water osmolalites rose together. The larvae died when the seawater concentration reached 50%.

In a freshwater species such as *Ae. aegypti*, the larvae drink about 300 nl of water each hour. Water movement into the animal across the cuticle is greatest via the anal papillae and can represent up to 33% of the insect's body weight per day, or about 40 nl/hr, assuming a body weight of 3 mg. Thus, the larvae in fresh water are stressed by water overload and scarcity of salts. They compensate by taking up salts via the anal papillae. Ninety percent of the active exchange of sodium and chloride occurs across the anal papillae, whereas uptake of potassium is passive. Loss of sodium from the hemolymph to the water by osmosis across the cuticle is less because the sodium binds to larger molecules such as proteins. This is also known to occur in terrestrial insects exposed to dehydration. Excess water is eliminated by the Malpighian tubules and rectum.

increased from 10% (essentially fresh water) to 200% (1.12 molar NaCl). The dashed line shows what the concentration would have been if hemolymph osmolality matched the concentration of the water. The graph demonstrates that in 10–20% seawater, the concentration of the hemolymph was maintained above that of the water. As the percentage of the seawater was increased from 40–200%, the osmolality of the hemolymph was kept nearly constant and much lower than the water. Over the entire range, the osmolality of the hemolymph was maintained between 300–400 mOsmoles. The obvious question raised by this display of physiological athletics is how do they do it?

The problem for larval mosquitoes is that while feeding they drink the solution in which they live. Salts and water also pass through the cuticle, which acts as a semipermeable membrane so that the water flows toward the region with the highest salt concentration. In fresh water, feeding and the flow of water into the animal across the cuticle results in excess water that the larva must eliminate. In water with a

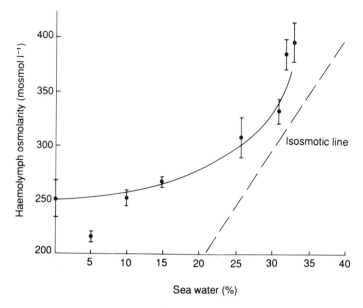

17.2 Osmolarity of larval *Aedes aegypti* hemolymph reared in different concentrations of seawater. Isosmotic line as in Fig. 17.1. Adapted from H.A. Edwards 1982, "Ion concentration and activity in the hemolymph of *Aedes aegypti*," *J. Exp. Biol.* 101:143–157, with permission of The Company of Biologists Ltd.

Whatever the route of entry, excess water ends up in the hemolymph. From there, active uptake of potassium by the Malpighian tubules results in the passive flow of water and other solutes into the lumen. The osmotic concentration of the primary urine secreted by the Malpighian tubules is identical to that of the hemolymph, but the concentration of potassium is naturally much higher and the sodium lower in compensation. In the rectum needed salts are actively pumped back into the hemolymph. The recovery of potassium is especially

important because it drives the activity of the tubules. Thus the animal produces a dilute urine, thereby eliminating the excess water load. *Ae. aegypti* fails to regulate when the salt concentration of the water rises above the normal hemolymph osmolarity (Fig. 17.2) because it cannot produce a urine that is more concentrated than the hemolymph. It apparently lacks the ability to reverse the direction of transport and move ions into the rectum from the hemolymph.

The Saline-Water Mosquito

The saline-water species *Aedes detritus* placed in distilled water produces a urine that is more dilute than the hemolymph (Fig. 17.3); in seawater, its urine is much more concentrated than the hemolymph. Thus, mosquitoes that can live in both dilute or saline waters, such as *Ae. detritus*, can turn on and off various mechanisms for salt uptake and elimination. In *Ae. aegypti*, the major route of salt uptake by

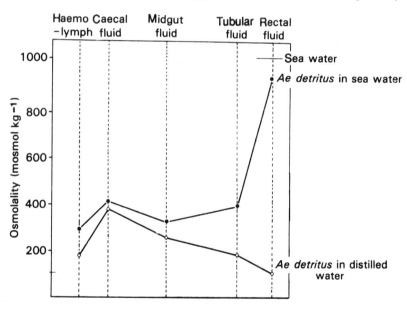

17.3 Osmolality of hemolymph and gut fluids from *Aedes detritus* reared in seawater or distilled water. Also indicated is the osmolality of seawater. Modified from J.A. Ramsay 1950, "Osmotic regulation in mosquito larvae," *J. Exp. Biol.* 27:145–157, with permission of The Company of Biologists Ltd.

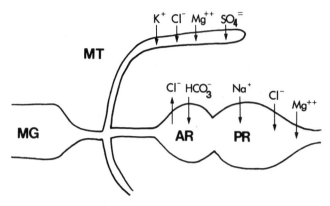

17.4 A diagram of the excretory system of *Aedes taeniorhynchus*. Demonstrated pathways of ion transport and their probable locations are shown. AR = anterior rectum, MG = midgut, MT = Malpighian tubule, PR = posterior rectum. Courtesy T.J. Bradley 1954.

and Cl⁻) into the lumen, corresponding to the concentration of the ions in the water. Figure 17.5 illustrates that the ability of the rectum to secrete a particular ion is inducible and that the degree of activation is a function of the amount of salt in the water. Thus, the presence of a distinct posterior rectum is unique to saline-water species, and the activity of the posterior part of the rectum permits the excretion of a concentrated urine (Fig. 17.3).

Mosquitoes that live in waters with high concentrations of sulfate, such as *Ae. campestris*, actively transport sulfate into the Malpighian tubules. This is unusual because most ions move into the tubule lumen following a concentration gradient set up by the large-scale transport of

larvae is the anal papillae. In saline-water species the uptake of ions via the papillae can be regulated. Thus, in *Ae. campestris*, ion uptake by the papillae is negligible in seawater but is high in fresh water. When larvae are transferred from seawater to fresh water, the change in ion uptake by the papillae takes several days to develop.

Saline-water species regulate their water deficit by drinking the water in which they live. Some species, such as *Ae. campestris,* increase their drinking rate 3-fold when transferred from fresh to seawater. Although drinking the saline solution supplies necessary water to balance that lost in the urine and by osmosis across the cuticle, it also adds to the salt load. Most of the salt is eliminated via the excretory system.

The Malpighian tubules of saline-water species produce a primary urine that is similar in osmotic pressure to that of the hemolymph; however, it is high in potassium just as is true of freshwater mosquitoes. The difference between saline-water and freshwater species is evident in the rectum. Morphologically, the rectum in some species is divided into anterior and posterior regions. As the primary urine enters the anterior rectum of *Ae. taeniorhynchus*, ions in short supply, such as potassium, are recovered. As shown in Figure 17.4 the posterior region of the rectum secretes all of the major ions commonly found in saline waters (Na⁺, K⁺, Mg2⁺,

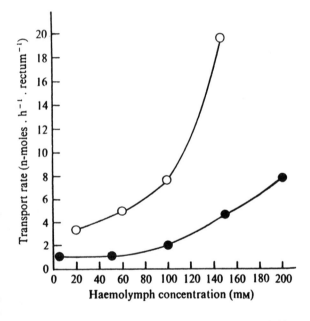

17.5 The relationship between the concentration of chloride (open circles) or sodium (closed circles) in artificial hemolymph bathing ligated recta of *Aedes taeniorhynchus* and the rate of transport of that ion. Adapted from T. J. Bradley and J. E. Phillips 1977, "The effect of external salinity on drinking rate and rectal secretion in the larvae of the saline-water mosquito *Aedes taeniorhynchus*," *J. Exp. Biol.* 66:87–100, with permission of The Company of Biologists Ltd.

potassium chloride. As shown in Figure 17.6, the level of sulfate transport is directly related to the concentration of sulfate in the water in which the mosquitoes live; sulfate transport can develop within a few hours after exposure, suggesting that sulfate transport proteins are synthesized and inserted into the tubule membrane in response to the presence of sulfate in the hemolymph. For some reason sulfate is not transported into the urine by the rectum as is the case for the other ions. Thus, sulfate is not concentrated and is present in the urine in concentrations equivalent to those in the hemolymph.

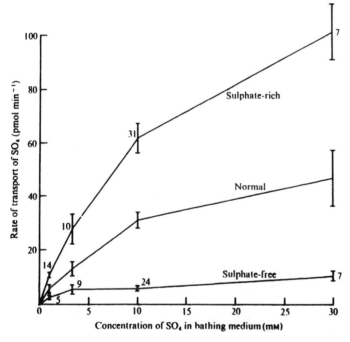

17.6   Change in sulfate uptake by Malpighian tubules of larval *Aedes taeniorhynchus* reared in seawater plus 89 mM sulfate, normal seawater, and sulfate-free seawater. At the 4th larval instar the Malpighian tubules were removed and incubated in a medium containing the indicated concentration of SO_4. Adapted from S.H.P. Maddrell and J. E. Phillips 1978, "Active transport of sulphate ions by the Malpighian tubules of larvae of the mosquito *Aedes campestris*," *J. Exp. Biol.* 72:181–202, with permission of The Company of Biologists Ltd.

The Brackish-Water Mosquito

Culiseta inornata and *Culex tarsalis* are found in salt marshes where fresh and saltwater mix. *Cs. inornata* cannot live in water with seawater concentrations of greater than 80%. This species seems to have adapted to the medium range of salt concentration and can regulate osmotic composition in waters ranging from 40–80% seawater (Fig. 17.7).

The recta of *Cs. inornata* and *Cx. tarsalis* are simple and do not have the divided regions found in certain other saline-water species. The urine in the rectum is neither concentrated nor diluted relative to the hemolymph, suggesting that these species are unable to alter the composition of the primary urine as it passes through the rectum beyond the recovery of needed ions such as potassium. However, the hemolymph of *Cx. tarsalis* contains variable levels of proline and serine, which increase as the animal is exposed to higher levels of salt in the water. Thus it appears that this species has a different mechanism for dealing with salt load. By increasing amino acid concentrations, the osmotic pressure of the hemolymph increases, which prevents the movement of salts into the hemolymph across the cuticle and from the gut. Thus, these insects have no need for specialized ion transport mechanisms in the rectum.

In Figures 17.1, 17.2, and 17.7 the relative abilities of fresh-, saline-, and brackish-water mosquitoes to regulate can be compared. Another measure of this ability can be obtained by comparing the maximum salt tolerance for *Ae. aegypti* (500 mOsm), *Cs. inornata* (800 mOsm), and *Ae. taeniorhynchus* (3000 mOsm).

Ultrastructure Recapitulates Physiology

How do the Malpighian tubules and rectum transport water and ions? There has been a considerable amount of work done on how the structure of these tissues correlates with their function. The tubules produce the primary urine by actively pumping potassium across the

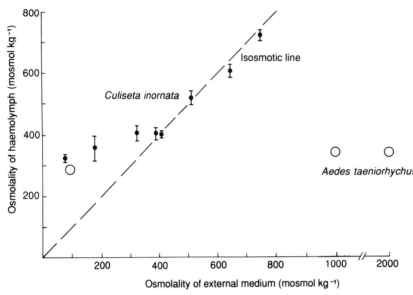

cell. On the lumenal side of the cell, the membrane has many microvilli (Figure 17.8) that often contain mitochondria. This membrane contains the potassium pumps, and the mitochondria provide the ATP to energize these pumps. Between the cells are smooth septate junctions that form a belt around the lumen side of the cells. These septate junctions form a barrier to molecules that move into the lumen between the cells. It has been demonstrated that they do act as a filter restricting the entry of larger molecules. Most hemolymph proteins are large enough to be excluded from this pathway.

17.7 Osmolality of hemolymph of *Culiseta inornata* reared in different salt concentrations in water. 1000 mOsmol/kg is equivalent to 100% seawater. Isosmotic line as in Fig. 17.1. Also shown are 3 points (0) for *Aedes taeniorhynchus* reared under similar conditions. Adapted from M. Garrett and T. J. Bradley 1984, "The pattern of osmotic regulation in larvae of the mosquito *Culiseta inornata*," *J. Exp. Biol.* 113:133–141, with permission of The Company of Biologists Ltd.

apical cell membrane into the tubule lumen from the cytoplasm of the cell. Channels exist on the basal membrane (hemolymph side) that allow potassium, water, and small ions to follow the resulting osmotic gradient. Larger organic molecules are not transported across the cell membrane but instead travel between the cells following the same gradient. Each mosquito tubule contains 2 cell types, the principal cell and the stellate cell (Figure 17.8). All of the physiological functions of the tubule have been attributed to the principal cell; the role of the stellate cells is not known. The basal cell membrane is exposed to the hemolymph and is highly folded. This membrane contains the potassium channels and anion channels that allow ions to move from the hemolymph into the cell. The many folds in the basal membrane increase the cell's surface, which therefore increases the filtering efficiency of the

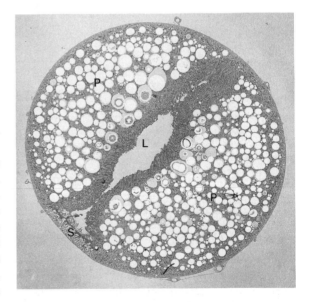

17.8 Structure of Malpighian tubules of larval *Aedes taeniorhynchus*. The tubule is composed of 2 cell types: the principal cell (P) and the stellate cell (S). The brush border around the lumen (L) is formed by microvilli of the principal cell. Figure courtesy of T.J. Bradley.

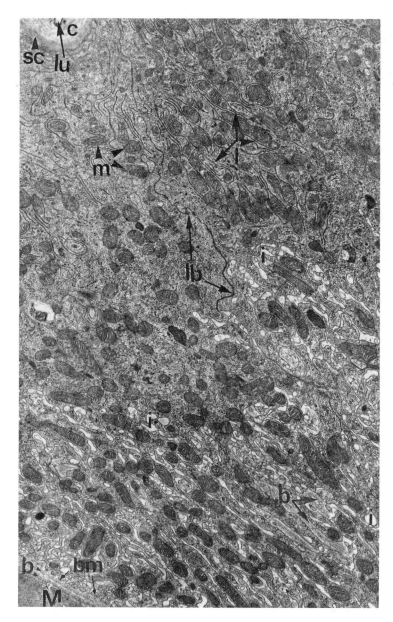

17.9 Ultrastructure of anterior rectum of *Aedes campestris* maintained in hyperosmotic medium. The lateral border is relatively straight and unspecialized whereas the apical and basal membranes are infolded. Mitochondria are evenly distributed. b = basement membrane, bm = basal plasma membrane, c = cuticle, i = basal infolding, l = apical lamellae, lb = lateral border, lu = lumen, M = muscle, m = mitochondria, sc = subcuticular layer. x = 12,900. Adapted from Meredith and Phillips; figure courtesy of J. Meredith 1973.

It is especially interesting to compare the ultrastructure of the rectum of fresh- and saltwater mosquito larvae (Fig. 17.11). As mentioned earlier, the rectum of the saltwater species, *Ae. campestris*, is divided into 2 sections, the anterior and posterior rectum. The anterior region is similar in structure and function to the rectum of the freshwater mosquito *Ae. aegypti*. Figure 17.9 illustrates the anterior rectum of *Ae campestris*. Both the apical and basal membranes are infolded to form microvillar-like structures. The apical membrane infolding extends to about 20% of the total cell depth. The basal infolding forms a canalicular system that extends throughout the cell. Mitochondria are randomly distributed throughout the cell. The contrast with the posterior rectum of *Ae. campestris* is striking (Figs. 17.10a,b). Here the apical membrane is much more highly infolded (Fig. 17.10a), extending to 60% of the total cell depth. The lamellae are thicker and more tightly packed. About 90% of the mitochondria are found in the apical region associated with the lamellae. The basal membrane is infolded to form canals as in the anterior rectum. The most remarkable aspect of this region is that the cell membranes are thrown up into folds or ridges with the opposing cells forming a complex channel with treelike branches that penetrate deeply into the cytoplasm (Fig. 17.10b).

The structure of the cells of the posterior rectum suggest that the most metabolically active region is the apical portion of the cell with its highly infolded lamellae and numerous mitochondria. This hypothesis has been confirmed by studies of the movement of ions across the rectal epithelium.

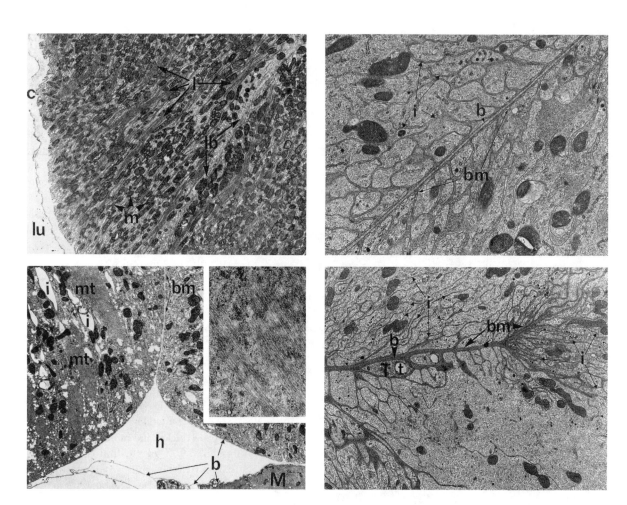

17.10a Ultrastructure of posterior rectum of *Aedes campestris*. Above is shown the apical border of the posterior rectal epithelium at x = 5000. Below is shown the basal border of the posterior rectal epithelium at x = 6000. The inset shows a magnified view of the microtubules at x = 24,000. h = hemocoel, mt = microtubular bundle, b = basement membrane, bm = basal plasma membrane, c = cuticle, i = basal infolding, l = apical lamellae, lb = lateral border, lu = lumen, M = muscle, m = mitochondria, sc = subcuticular layer. x = 12,900.

17.10b Ultrastructure of the posterior rectum of *Aedes campestris* showing views of the basal borders between 2 posterior rectal cells. Above x = 11,000. Below x = 7000. T = tracheal cell, t = trachea. Other abbreviations as in Figure 17.10a. Figures courtesy of J. Meredith.

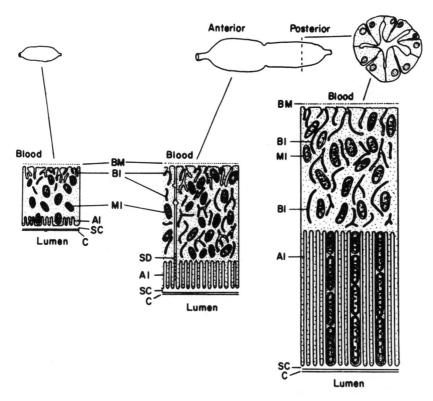

17.11 Morphology of the rectum of the freshwater mosquito *Aedes aegypti* (left) and the saltwater mosquito *Aedes campestris* (right). Drawn approximately to scale. The differences between the rectum of *A. aegypti* and *A. campestris* are evident, as are the differences between the anterior and posterior regions of the rectum of *A. campestris*. Note increase in basal infolding (BI) and the length of microvilli (apical infolds, AI) in the 3 regions. BM (basement membrane), MI (mitochondria), SD (septate junction), SC (subcuticular space), C (cuticle). Courtesy T.J. Bradley.

As shown in Figure 17.12, cation pumps (Na⁺, K⁺, and Mg2⁺) are hypothesized to exist in the apical membrane. These pumps require the ATP produced by the mitochondria to move ions into the lumen of the rectum so that a concentrated urine can be produced. The function of the complicated, treelike structure of the basal membrane, although not known, possibly provides the surface area needed to allow the ions in the hemolymph to penetrate deeply into the cell, where they would flow rapidly into the cytoplasm to replace the ions being pumped into the lumen.

Conclusions

Several conclusions are evident from this brief discussion of mosquito larvae survival in waters of diverse osmotic and ionic composition. First, the physiological mechanisms used vary considerably. Examples include the use of amino acids to adjust osmotic pressure of the hemolymph in brackish-water species and the development of the unique posterior rectum in saline-water species. Second, inducible pumps are found in both the rectum and Malpighian tubules in several saltwater species. Third, in laboratory experiments using *Ae. taeniorhynchus,* it has been possible to

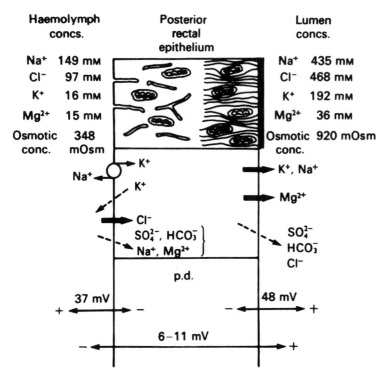

Haemolymph concs.

Na⁺	149 mM
Cl⁻	97 mM
K⁺	16 mM
Mg²⁺	15 mM
Osmotic conc.	348 mOsm

Na^+ 149 mM
Cl^- 97 mM
K^+ 16 mM
Mg^{2+} 15 mM
Osmotic conc. 348 mOsm

Posterior rectal epithelium

Lumen concs.

Na^+ 435 mM
Cl^- 468 mM
K^+ 192 mM
Mg^{2+} 36 mM
Osmotic conc. 920 mOsm

K^+
Na^+
K^+

K^+, Na^+
Mg^{2+}

Cl^-
SO_4^{2-}, HCO_3^-
Na^+, Mg^{2+}

SO_4^{2-}
HCO_3^-
Cl^-

p.d.

37 mV
48 mV

6–11 mV

17.12 A model for the transport of ions in the posterior rectum of *Aedes taeniorhynchus*. *top:* a diagrammatic representation of the ultrastructure of the cells in the posterior rectum. *middle:* The proposed sites of ion transport during fluid secretion. Solid arrows represent active transport, broken arrows represent passive movements. *bottom:* Average potential difference measurements across each plasma membrane and across the entire posterior rectal epithelium when recta are bathed in artificial hemolymph. Courtesy T.J. Bradley.

select for populations of mosquitoes with increased ability to cope with high saline conditions. Thus, selective pressure in the field is likely to lead to the development of populations of mosquitoes with differing abilities to adapt to local conditions.

THE ADULT MOSQUITO

The vector biologist is concerned with adult mosquito reproduction because the mosquito's requirement for blood makes mosquitoes capable of transmitting disease-causing pathogens. As a result, a considerable amount of work has been done on diverse aspects of adult reproduction. Other chapters in this text cover the physiology behind behaviors such as mating, host location, biting, digestion of the meal, and energy metabolism. This section covers the regulation of egg development.

The mosquito oocyte development has been well studied because the development of the oocyte is particularly easy to measure. Mosquitoes are also a good subject for biochemical and molecular work because large amounts of yolk proteins are produced in a short period of time. Early experiments demonstrated the importance of hormones in regulating egg development. For example, decapitation after a blood meal was shown to prevent egg development unless the operation was delayed for several hours. Transplantation experiments traced the effect to a group of cells in the brain. Before discussing the regulation of egg development in the mosquito, it is important to introduce the hormones involved and their role in the endocrinology of insects in general

The so-called classic scheme that was developed on the basis of experiments on large holometabolous insects such as *Hyalophora cecropia* and *Manduca sexta* demonstrated the influence of 3 hormonal factors on molting in insects: 20 hydroxyecdysone, juvenile hormone (JH), and an ill-defined factor called the brain hormone (Fig. 17.13). Each of these factors was thought to play a specific role—the brain hormone stimulated ecdysone production, ecdysone stimulated production of a new cuticle, and juvenile hormone determined whether the new cuticle was larval, pupal, or adult. A better understanding of the endocrinology of these factors resulted when their chemistry became known. Ecdysone was isolated in the 1950s, juvenile hormone in the 1960s, and the peptide brain hormones that regulate the production of ecdysone and juvenile hormone have only recently been sequenced and studied in

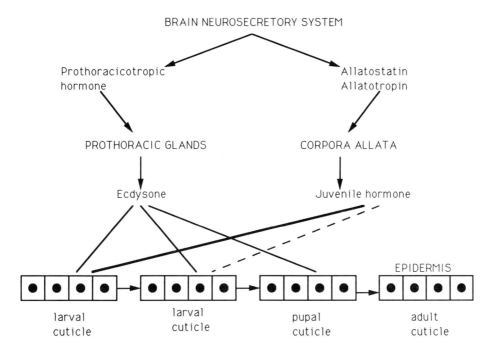

BRAIN NEUROSECRETORY SYSTEM

Prothoracicotropic
hormone

Allatostatin
Allatotropin

PROTHORACIC GLANDS

CORPORA ALLATA

Ecdysone

Juvenile hormone

EPIDERMIS

larval
cuticle

larval
cuticle

pupal
cuticle

adult
cuticle

17.13 The "classic scheme" for the endocrine control of molting and metamorphosis of holometabolous insects suggested that whether the epidermis produced larval, pupal, or adult cuticle depended on the hormones to which it was exposed. 20-hydroxyecdysone (ecdysone) stimulated the production of the cuticle in each case, but if the juvenile hormone titer was high, a larval cuticle was produced. If the titer was low, a pupal cuticle was produced; if it was absent, an adult cuticle was produced. Also evident in this figure is the hierarchical control over cuticle production via neurosecretory peptides such as prothoracicotropic hormone and allatotropin/allatostatin that regulate the production of ecdysone and juvenile hormones that affect the activities of target tissues.

detail. As more became known, it became clear that the endocrinology of insects is considerably more complex than the classic scheme suggested.

Ecdysone

The "molting hormones" consist of a small group of ecdysteroids characterized by a steroid nucleus having numerous hydroxyl groups that render the ecdysteroids water soluble, an unusual characteristic for a steroid hormone (e.g., estrogen). The structure of these molecules is shown in Fig. 17.14. The sources of ecdysone are the prothoracic gland in immature insects and the ovary (and perhaps the testis [Loeb 1984]) in the adult. In some insects, including the larval mosquito (Jenkins et al. 1992), other tissues, particularly the epidermis,

have been implicated in the synthesis of ecdy-sone. The active molecule in most insects is 20-hydro-xyecdysone. The hormone is produced as the relatively inactive ecdysone, which is enzymatically activated to 20-hydroxyecdysone in a number of tissues, especially in the fat body. In a few insects (some Hemiptera and Hymenoptera), the active hormone is makisterone A, which has an extra carbon atom on the side chain.

The ecdysteroids control a number of aspects of insect life, including molting, wandering behavior, the development of the nervous system, reproduction, and the production of sex pheromones. In some cases, the mode of action of the ecdysteroids involves the expression of genes that code for transcription factors

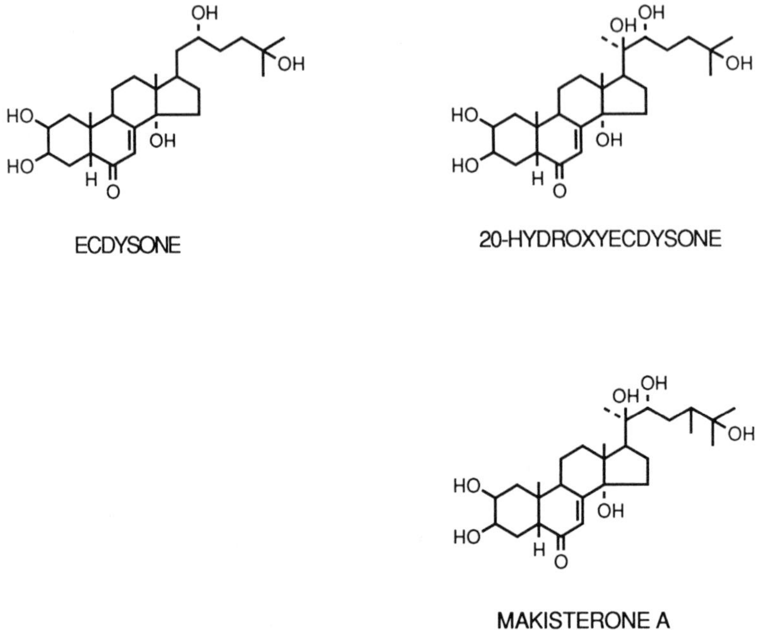

ECDYSONE

20-HYDROXYECDYSONE

MAKISTERONE A

17.14 The structural formulae for the ecdysteroids important in insect physiology. Ecdysone is the product of the prothoracic glands and is converted by several tissues to 20-hydroxyecdysone, which is considered to be the active form of the hormone. Makisterone A is the active hormone in some Hemiptera and Hymenoptera.

necessary to activate a 2nd set of genes. Transcription factors that bind ecdysone have been isolated from several insectes, including the mosquito (Chen et al. 1994), In the case of wandering behavior, the hormone has a direct effect on the nervous system: A new pattern of nerve impulses is produced that results in wandering of the insect. In the adult, the follicle cells of the ovary produce ecdysteroids that enter the developing oocyte as inactive conjugates, which later regulate the molting of the embryo. In the mosquito, the ecdysone from the ovary enters the hemolymph and has important effects on egg development.

Juvenile Hormone

In contrast to the relatively few members of the ecdysteroid family of hormones, the juvenile hormones found in insects are much more varied. Figure 17.15 lists the 9 forms of the JH molecule that are candidates

for hormonal status: JH I, II, and III; JH 0; 4-methyl JH; JHB3; MF; FA; and the acid of JH I. Of these, juvenile hormone III is the major form found in most insects, including mosquitoes. Juvenile hormones I and II are found only in Lepidoptera. JH 0 has been extracted from *Manduca* embryos. The evidence for a biological role for JH I and III is solid. What the other molecules do is less well understood. The source of juvenile hormone is the corpora allata. The mode of action of juvenile hormone is not well understood and probably varies.

An exciting development in the field of JH research has been the discovery that a number of insects, and their relatives, seem to use as hormones molecules that were previously thought to be precursors and breakdown products to JH (Fig. 17.16). The corpora allata of wandering stage *M. sexta* produce juvenile hormone acid, which is a normal breakdown product of juvenile

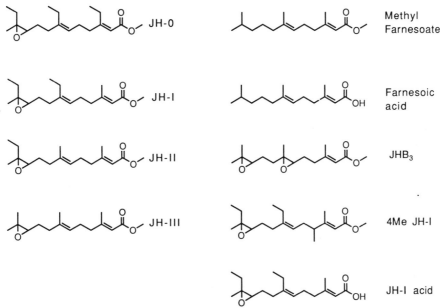

17.15 Nine forms of juvenile hormone have been found in insects. JH-I was the first to be isolated. JH-I, JH-II, and JH-III are all present during various stages of Lepidoptera. JH-III is the form found in most insects, including the mosquito *Aedes aegypti*. JH-O has been isolated from eggs of *Manduca sexta*. JHB3 is the bisepoxide form of JH found in some cyclorraphan Diptera, particularly *Drosophila melanogaster*.

hormone. There is evidence that the target tissues have the enzymatic capacity to convert the acid back to juvenile hormone. During the wandering stage the general presence of JH would disrupt normal development. Thus, the whole animal is not exposed to juvenile hormone—only the tissue that contains the enzymes capable of converting the acid to the active hormone. In 4th instar larvae of the cockroach *Diploptera punctata*, the corpora allata produce farnesoic acid (Yagi et al. 1990). The production of farnesoic acid seems to result from the loss of enzymes that convert farnesoic acid to juvenile hormone. In some crustaceans the mandibular organ produces methyl farnesoate, which may function as a hormone in these animals. Finally, the corpora allata of *Drosophila* and *Calliphora* have been found to produce JH bisepoxide, which has 2 epoxy groups instead of 1 (Richard et al. 1989). This molecule is biologically active in these insects.

Peptides

Many peptides that are hormones are products of specialized nerve cells called neurosecretory cells. These peptides travel down the axon to a site of release in the hemolymph called the neurohemal organ. It has become clear that in many cases these same peptides may also be produced by normal nerve cells and function as neurotransmitters or neuromodulators within the nervous system. The mode of action of most peptide hormones involves the stimulation of secondary messenger systems, such as cAMP, in target cells.

Our understanding and appreciation for the role of peptide hormones in insects has undergone a veritable renaissance. Many new peptides have been identified by their biological activity, some have been isolated and sequenced, and we have only scratched the surface in this dynamic area. The genes that code for these peptides can be isolated and studied for clues to their relationships and function. It is also possible that methods of control could be based on a thorough

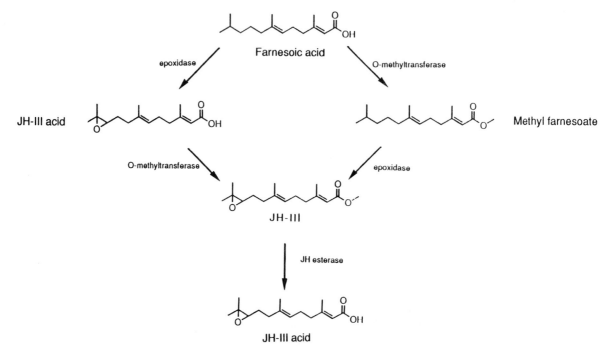

17.16 The final steps in the synthesis of juvenile hormone can occur via 2 alternative pathways. One involves the conversion of farnesoic acid to JH-III acid by the addition of an epoxy group. This is then formed into JH-III by the modification of the acid group to an ester. The alternative pathway involves the conversion of farnesoic acid to methyl farnesoate, which is then epoxidized to JH-III. The major degradation pathway for JH is the conversion of the ester group to an acid by the action of juvenile hormone esterase. Thus, JH-III acid can be either a precursor or a breakdown product.

knowledge of these hormones. For example, peptide hormone genes have been cloned into viruses that can then be used to infect insects.

Research over many years on the peptide hormone called the prothoracicotropic hormone (PTTH) in several Japanese laboratories finally resulted in the description of the sequences for 2 different peptides that appear to be able to activate ecdysone production by prothoracic glands. The 1st of these is considered to be the true PTTH of *Bombyx mori* (Kawakami et al. 1990). It is a dimer composed of 2 identical chains of 109 amino acids each. There is a single copy of this gene in the haploid genome. There is no homology of this peptide to any other peptide hormone yet sequenced. Hybridization of PTTH DNA to tissue sections shows reaction with only a single pair of dorsolateral neurosecretory cells in the brain that are identical to those identified by bioassay and antibodies against PTTH.

The 2nd peptide isolated by the Japanese group was found to be a member of a family of peptides called bombyxins. The bombyxins have a high degree of similarity to insulin (Kawakami et al. 1989). They are also dimers, but the A and B chains are different and are linked by disulfide bonds at exactly the same locations as those in insulin. There appear to be about 20 copies of the bombyxin genes in the diploid genome. Bombyxin DNA hybridizes to 8 (4 pairs) of middorsal cells of the brain. The function of bombyxin is unknown, but it is clear that molecules similar to insulin exist in many insects and other invertebrates.

One of the 1st peptide hormones to be isolated in insects was the adipokinetic hormone, AKH. This peptide is produced by the intrinsic cells of the corpora cardiaca. AKH has been isolated from a number of insects, forming a family of peptides, 8–10 amino acids long, that are related to the red-pigment concentrating hormone of crustacea. In some insects, AKH regulates lipid metabolism; in others it regulates carbohydrate metabolism. In many insects AKH is released during flight and regulates the mobilization of lipid or carbohydrate needed as fuel for flight (Keely et al. 1991).

Several peptides have been isolated and sequenced that affect juvenile hormone production by the corpora allata. An allatotropin, which stimulates juvenile hormone synthesis, was isolated from *M. sexta* (Kataoka et al. 1989). A group of peptides called allatostatins that inhibit the corpora allata were isolated from the cockroach *Diploptera punctata* (Pratt et al. 1991). Thus, peptides control the activity of the corpora allata.

Another class of peptide hormones that cause diuresis (production of urine) have been isolated from insects (Nicolson 1993). These include the diuretic hormones, or diuresins, that were first isolated from *Manduca sexta* and have since been found in several other insects. These are 30–45 amino acids long and cause fluid secretion by isolated Malpighian tubules via an effect of cAMP. A 2nd group of smaller peptides (8–10 amino acids) with diuretic effects are related to the leucokinins. These peptides were 1st isolated from *Leucophaea maderae* on the basis of their effects on contraction of the gut and were subsequently found to cause fluid secretion by mosquito Malpighian tubules. They appear to be widespread, having been isolated from the locust, cricket, and mosquito (Fig. 17.17). The N-terminal end, which is conserved in these species, appears to be essential for activity.

Leucokinin-like peptides

Leucophaea 1	Asp-Pro-Ala-Phe-Asn-Ser-Trp-Gly-NH2
Acheta 1	Ser-Gly-Ala-Asp-Phe-Tyr-Pro-Trp-Gly-NH2
Culex 2	Ser-Lys-Tyr-Val-Ser-Lys-Gln-Lys-Phe-Phe-Ser-Trp-Gly-NH2
Aedes 1	Asn-Ser-Lys-Tyr-Val-Ser-Lys-Gln-Lys-Phe-Tyr-Ser-Trp-Gly-NH2

Diuresin-like peptides

Manduca 1 Arg-Met-Pro-Ser-Leu-Ser-Ile-Asp-Leu-Pro-Met-Ser-Val-
Acheta   Thr-Gly-Ala-Gln-Ser-Leu-Ser-Ile-Val-Ala-Pro-Leu-Asp-Val-
Locusta Met-Gly-Met-Gly-Pro-Ser-Leu-Ser-Ile-Val-Asn-Pro-Met-Asp-Val-

Leu-Arg-Gln-Lys-Leu-Ser-Leu-Glu-Lys-Glu-Arg-Lys-Val-His-Ala-Leu-Arg-
Leu-Arg-Gln-Arg-Leu-Met-Asn-Glu-Leu-Asn-Arg-Arg-Arg-Met-Arg-Glu-Leu-
Leu-Arg-Gln-Arg-Leu-Leu-Leu-Glu-Ile-Ala-Arg-Arg-Arg-Leu-Arg-

Ala-Ala-   -Ala-Asn-Arg-Asn-Phe-Leu-Asn-Asp-Ile-NH2
Gln-Gly-Ser-Arg-   -Ile-Gln-Gln-Asn-Arg-Gln-Leu-Leu-Thr-Ser-Ile-NH2
Asp-Ala-Glu-Glu-Gln-Ile-Lys-Ala-Asn-Lys-Asp-Phe-Leu-Gln-Gln-Ile-NH2

17.17 Sequences of some peptides causing diuresis in insects. The leucokinins were originally isolated from *Leucophaea maderae*. Eight related peptides were isolated. Shown is the first of these, leucokinin I. Achetakinin I is 1 of 2 peptides in this family isolated from the cricket *Acheta domesticus*. Two members of the leucokinin family (culekinin I and II) have been isolated from the mosquito *Culex salinarius*. T.K. Hayes, personal communication. The diuresins, or diuretic hormones, are much longer peptides and have been isolated from *Manduca sexta, Acheta domesticus,* and *Locusta migratoria*. Similar peptides are likely to be present in the mosquito also. See Nicolson 1993 for a recent review.

Hormones and Molting

Figure 17.13 provides a simple view of the interactions among the hormones discussed. Our understanding of the molecular mechanisms behind these processes has become much more detailed as a result of recent experiments. Several of these findings are relevant here. First, it is clear that peptides have 2 general roles. They regulate the activity of glands producing other hormones (e.g., ecdysone and JH), and they also directly affect physiological processes, (e.g., diuresis, lipid and carbohydrate levels, heart rate, etc.). It has also become increasingly evident that a given peptide can have multiple roles. For example, allatotropin, initially isolated on the basis of its effects on JH production by the corpora allata, has also been found in the accessory glands of male locusts and has been shown to cause contraction of the oviducts in the female. Although the leucokinins were initially found to cause contraction of the gut, they are now known to be active in diuresis. These multiple physiological roles are likely related. For example, it has been suggested that the effect of leucokinins on diuresis is enhanced by the stirring of the hemolymph caused by contraction of the gut. The pace of discovery of new roles for peptide hormones suggests that we have discovered only the tip of an iceberg. Thus, it is likely that the future roles of peptides in insect physiology will be very complex. Because the genes that code for these peptides can be studied and manipulated, these molecules could provide new approaches to insect control using molecular biology.

These peptide hormones are produced by cells in, or associated with, the nervous system. This is significant because the release of at least some of these peptides is photo-periodically regulated; others are under different kinds of nervous control. An excellent example is the work of Truman (1971). His studies on Saturniid moths demonstrated a gated release of eclosion hormone, a 62–amino acid peptide eclosion hormone, from neurosecretory cells of the brain. A gated release means that once each day a "gate" opens during which time the hormone could be released. In the silkmoth *Antheraea pernyi* this gate appears several hours before dusk. However, although the gate appears daily, the hormone is not released until the process of pharate adult development is complete. Thus, many days go by without release of eclosion hormone. When the hormone is finally released it causes a programmed response in nerve cells regulating eclosion behavior, a stereotyped series of movements that results in the shedding of the pupal cuticle and escape of the adult moth from the cocoon. Studies in this area provide a mechanistic explanation for the observation that insects tend to pupate and/or eclose at certain times of the day, which is a common observation in various mosquito species. In this context it is relevant that eclosion hormone has been found to regulate larval as well as adult eclosion in many different insects. In connection to the discussion of multiple roles of hormones, eclosion hormone also causes the cuticle to become stretchable so that after the insect ecloses, the new cuticle can be expanded before it hardens. The process of hardening is controlled by another peptide hormone called bursicon.

Experiments on insect eclosion have also revealed that the hormone is not the only player in this physiological drama. It is evident that the release of the hormone determines when eclosion will occur, but in fact the target cells become capable of responding to the hormone before it appears. Thus, for example, in *A. pernyi*, the nervous system becomes sensitive to eclosion hormone about 4 hours before the hormone is actually released. This is believed to be caused by the programmed appearance of receptors in the target cells. The key point is that each cell of the body has its own physiological rhythms; the integration of the whole is not a function of the hormone by itself. Equally important is the state of target cells, which have mechanisms capable of measuring time and regulating the appearance of biologically important molecules accordingly. Studies on the periodic, or *per*, mutants of *Drosophila* are beginning to unravel the details of these cellular mechanisms.

MOSQUITO ENDOCRINOLOGY

We will now examine hormones in mosquitoes. Actually, despite its small size, the adult female mosquito is one of the better known insects in this respect. Shown in Figure 17.18 are the titer changes for ecdysteroids and juvenile hormone III from eclosion through the 1st blood meal. As will be discussed later,

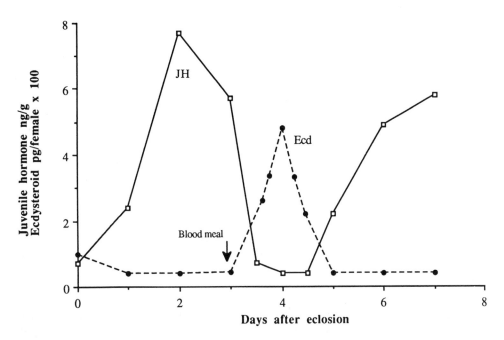

17.18   Changes in juvenile hormone and 20-hydroxyecdysone titers in the female *Aedes aegypti* from eclosion of the adult through a blood meal and the production of the 1st batch of eggs. The rise in juvenile hormone titers after eclosion of the adult stimulates previtellogenic development of the follicles, maturation of the fat body, and behavioral changes. By day 2 these physiological changes are complete. When the 1st blood meal is taken, juvenile hormone titers drop and 20-hydroxyecdysone titers rise. Not shown is the release of the egg development neurosecretory hormone (EDNH). The titer changes of this hormone are unknown. EDNH stimulates the ovaries to produce ecdysone, which is enzymatically converted to 20-hydroxyecdysone by the fat body. The 20-hydroxyecdysone stimulates vitellogenic growth of the oocytes. Growth of the oocytes is complete, and the eggs are laid 3 days after a blood meal. Juvenile hormone titers begin to rise again by the 2nd day after a blood meal, preparing the animal for the 2nd blood meal. Juvenile hormone titer changes are from Shapiro et al. 1986. 20-hydroxyecdysone titer changes are from Greenplate et al. 1985.

these hormones have multiple effects on the reproductive life of the female.

Hormones regulate physiological processes. A hormone regulates a process not only by turning it on but by ending it as well; in addition, the hormone must be able to adjust the level of the response. The presence, absence, and amount of a hormone can regulate a process in this way. Thus, it is not enough to know the structure of a putative hormone; one must also know where it is made, when it is present in the hemolymph, its titer changes, and its target tissues. We can examine

most of these questions by considering the juvenile hormones in the mosquito. The juvenile hormone titer changes shown in Figure 17.18 reflect the synthetic activity of the corpora allata (Fig. 17.19) and the activity of the most important catabolic enzyme, juvenile hormone esterase (Fig. 17.20). It is clear that the activity of the corpora allata and the rise in the JH titer after eclosion are coincident. After a blood meal the titer falls, the corpora allata stop making JH, and the levels of the esterase, which is produced in the fat body, rise. Thus, the process of regulating the titers of

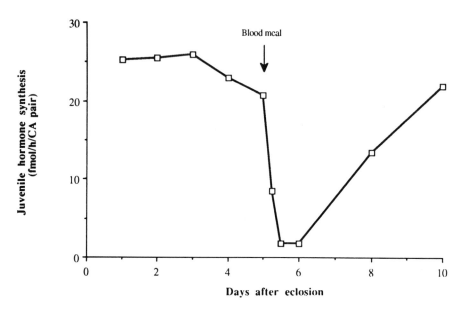

17.19 The changing juvenile hormone synthetic activity of the corpora allata was measured by incubating corpora allata of female *Culex pipiens* in a medium containing [3H]-methionine to label newly synthesized juvenile hormone. Synthesis of juvenile was found to be high in the newly eclosed female, to decline after a blood meal, and then increase again by the 3rd day after a blood meal. These data support those shown in Fig. 17.17 even though different mosquitoes were used. Modified from Readio et al. 1988.

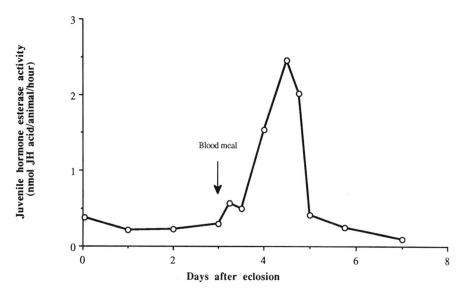

17.20 The activity of juvenile hormone esterase was determined by 1st incubating hemolymph taken from adult female *Aedes aegypti* with [3H]-juvenile hormone III and then measuring the amount of juvenile hormone acid produced. The activity of the enzyme was found to be low when juvenile hormone titers were high after eclosion but higher after a blood meal when juvenile hormone titers dropped. Comparing these data to those shown in Fig. 17.17, it is evident that the esterase activity was highest from 24–36 hr after a blood meal when the juvenile hormone titers were lowest. Data are from Shapiro et al. 1986.

JH involves the coordinated activity of several tissues. We know less about the regulation of 20-hydroxyecdysone titers in the female mosquito, but a similar hierarchy of controls must exist. It has recently been suggested that tissues other than the corpora allata may produce JH in mosquitoes (Borovsky et al. 1994a, b).

Egg Development in the Mosquito

What are the target tissues of JH and 20-hydroxyecdysone in the adult female? When the female ecloses, the follicles of the ovary contain 8 germ cells surrounded by a layer of follicle cells. Over the next 2–3 days, a single germ cell differentiates to become the oocyte, and the rest become nurse cells, or trophocytes (Fig. 17.21). During this period the follicles double in size, and the follicle cells multiply to keep up with the growing follicle. Changes are also occurring in the fat body as the amount of DNA doubles per cell, and a modest amount of ribosomal RNA is made. At eclosion, the female does not mate and shows no interest in obtaining a blood meal, but by 2 days after eclosion, her behavior changes and mating and host seeking begin. All of these events have been shown to be under the control of JH in several species of mosquito, so the target tissues of juvenile hormone in the newly eclosed female include the fat body, several cell types in the ovary, and the nervous system. Evidence is accumulating that the gut may be another target of JH, as mRNA coding for trypsin also accumulates after eclosion.

Once these tissues have responded to juvenile hormone, the female is ready to take a blood meal, and when this occurs, a series of extensive physiological changes take place. Immediately after a blood meal the JH titers drop, and the levels of 20-hydroxyecdysone rise (Fig. 17.18). The ovary, which is the source of the ecdysone, responds to the release of a peptide hormone from the medial neurosecretory cells of the brain that has been historically known either as the egg development neurosecretory hormone (EDNH) or the ovarian ecdysteroidogenic hormone. This peptide was recently sequenced and found to be related to neuroparsin. Although it has been established that EDNH causes the ovary to produce ecdysone, exactly how the blood meal causes the brain to release EDNH is not clear. There is some evidence that a rise in amino acids or the release of small peptides from the digestion of the meal trigger the gut and/or the ovary to produce a factor that causes the release of EDNH. The midgut of the mosquito contains about 500 cells that appear to produce peptide hormones (Brown and Lea 1989; Veenstra et al. 1995). By way of comparison, the nervous system is thought to have about 200 neurosecretory cells. Little is known about the peptides produced by the gut and their possible physiological roles.

The rise in 20-hydroxyecdysone titers has a multitude of effects on the vitellogenic phase of egg development, as the oocyte develops the yolk needed by the developing embryo. Under the regulation of this hormone, the fat body produces large amounts of the major yolk protein, vitellogenin, which travels through the hemolymph to the oocyte, where it is taken up by receptor-mediated endocytosis. The fat body also produces a serine carboxypeptidase, also taken up by the oocyte, that is important in degradation of the vitellogenin during embryogenesis. In the ovary, the vitelline envelope, which lies under the chorion, and an enzyme, dopa decarboxylase, which is

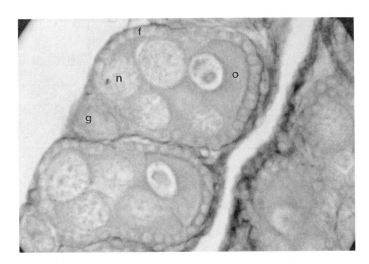

17.21   Ovarian follicles of *Aedes aegypti* 3 days after eclosion (non–blood-fed). Germarium (g), oocyte (o), follicle cells (f), nurse cell (n).

needed to harden and darken the chorion after oviposition, are produced. These are only a few of the many events in the fat body and ovary that are known to be regulated by 20-hydroxyecdysone. There are many other events that are not as well understood, such as an increase in the ploidy level of the fat body, the huge increase in fat body ribosomal RNA needed to produce the yolk proteins, and the production of the chorion.

There may also be effects of 20-hydroxyecdysone on behavior, although these have been harder to demonstrate experimentally. In particular, Bowen and Loess-Perez (1989) have shown that ecdysteroids are involved in the inhibition of host-seeking behavior that occurs after a blood meal in *Ae. aegypti*. A factor present in the male accessory glands is transferred to the female during mating and causes a change in female behavior such that she refuses to mate with other males. There is some evidence that in *Cx. tarsalis* this peptide is related to similar factors in *D. melanogaster* (Young and Downe 1987). Its effects appear to wear off after a batch of eggs is produced (Young and

Downe 1982). Other unidentified factors involved in regulating behavior are discussed in Chapter 3.

The Second Blood Meal

Egg production is cyclic in mosquitoes; after the 1st batch of eggs is laid the female may take a 2nd blood meal and begin the process of egg development again (Fig. 17.22). The morphological basis for Fig. 17.22 is the clear separation of the previtellogenic and vitellogenic stages of follicle growth by the blood meal. The physiological basis for this diagram is the fact that JH regulates previtellogenic growth of the follicle and 20-hydroxyecdysone regulates vitellogenic growth. At a deeper level the tissues involved, i.e., the fat body and ovary, lose their competence to respond to hormones that appear after a blood meal and must be exposed to juvenile hormone to regain competency. Thus, each blood meal results in the release of hormones that not only ensure the vitellogenic growth of the 1st follicle but also ensure the previtellogenic growth of the next. The role of juvenile hormone can therefore be seen to

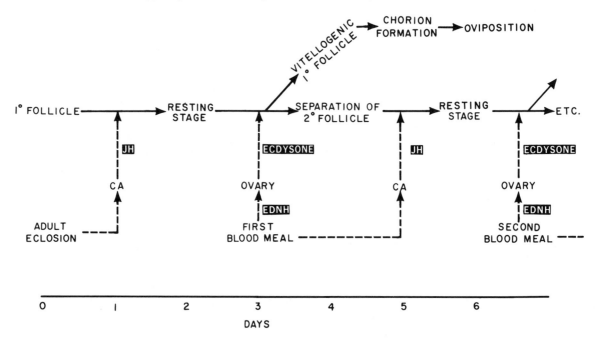

17.22 Mosquitoes can take several blood meals, each of which produce a batch of eggs. The endocrine basis for cyclic egg development is shown here. Each blood meal results in the release of hormones that not only ensure the vitellogenic growth of a follicle but also ensure the previtellogenic growth of the next.

reset the system for the next blood meal. Logically, one might expect the fat body to retain the large number of ribosomes and endoplasmic reticulum made in response to the blood meal for reuse during the 2nd cycle of egg development. Instead, all of these organelles are destroyed and recreated anew after the 2nd blood meal. The recovery of fat body responsiveness requires JH. As shown in Fig. 17.17, titers of JH do rise 36–48 hours after a blood meal, and it is during this period that responsiveness to 20-hydroxyecdysone returns. This issue of tissue competence to respond to hormones is important because it indicates that the state of the target tissue is just as important as the presence of the hormone. Competence in molecular terms probably means the presence of appropriate hormone receptors and may also mean that the structure of the DNA in the appropriate genes changes to allow an interaction with hormone receptor complexes. One of these hormone receptors, the ecdysone receptor gene, was cloned from a mosquito (Chen et al. 1994).

Studies on autogenous mosquitoes, which develop a batch of eggs without a blood meal, have shown that all of the major hormonal events that occur in anautogenous mosquitoes also take place. It seems that the major difference is that eclosion, rather than the blood meal, replaces the stimulus for the release of EDNH.

Some mosquitoes may require several blood meals to initiate full development of the oocytes (Gillies 1955). Such behavior has important implications for vector biologists because it increases the chances for transmission of pathogens.

Hormones and Metabolism

The diet of the adult mosquito consists of nectar and blood, meals that have entirely different compositions. Newly eclosed adults usually take a sugar meal, which is required for normal previtellogenic development of the oocytes, perhaps because it stimulates juvenile hormone production by the corpora allata. In the wild, mosquito larvae are often starved. Oocyte development in adults from such larvae is delayed, and the first blood meal taken by these animals stimulates previtellogenic oocyte development rather than deposition of yolk. There is growing evidence that JH stimulates the utilization of carbohydrate reserves, which may be an important function of the rising titers of JH after eclosion. In the normal female, the stored carbohydrate may come from the larval stage, whereas in the nutritionally deprived female, the reserves may come from sugar or blood meals. It is not known if mosquitoes have an AKH-like hormone that regulates lipid metabolism, although the involvement of a neurosecretory hormone in the deposition of fat has been demonstrated (Van Handel and Lea 1970).

Diuresis in the Adult

Those who have avoided the instinct to squash a feeding mosquito may have noticed that it produces a clear urine, sometimes while still feeding. *Ae. aegypti* typically takes a blood meal of 3.5 μl, 1.9 μl of which is plasma. Within the first 30 minutes after a blood meal, about 35% of the water in the plasma is excreted. The predominant cation in this urine is sodium, reflecting the composition of the plasma. The rate of urine production then slows dramatically, and potassium becomes the dominant cation as the red blood cells leak their contents. The production of this urine is controlled by peptides released from brain and/or nerve cord. Decapitation immediately after feeding reduces the flow of urine (Fig. 17.23). Extracts of the head cause urine production when injected into a decapitated female (Fig. 17.24b). Isolated Malpighian tubules also secrete fluid when incubated with a crude extract of heads (Fig. 17.24a). Peptides in these head extracts were separated by high performance liquid chromatography, and 3 fractions were found to have diuretic effects (Fig. 17.24). Fraction III affects fluid secretion by causing an increase in cAMP levels in the Malpighian tubules. Peptides related to the leucokinins have been isolated from several mosquitoes (Fig. 17.17) and have been found to cause cAMP and inositol triphosphate changes in the Malpighian tubules (C. Cady and H. Hagedorn, unpublished).

HORMONES AND MOSQUITO CONTROL

When larval mosquitoes are reared in water containing juvenile hormone they do not develop normally during the pupal period, resulting in the failure of adult emergence (Spielman and Williams 1966). This observation is consistent with the role of JH during metamorphosis in Lepidoptera in which JH must be absent during the pupal stage for normal metamorphosis to occur. Methoprene, an analog, of juvenile hormone, was the first insect growth regulator to be approved for use in insect, specifically mosquito, control. Control is most effective when larvae are exposed in the later instars. Thus, methoprene is most effective for use in flooded ponds, such as rice fields, where the development of larvae is somewhat synchronous. Formulations of methoprene that ensure slow release improve the level of control.

PARASITES OF THE MOSQUITO

Parasites of insects, including mosquitoes, have been shown to use, or manipulate, the hormones of the host to their own advantage. Two cases are known in which parasites use the ecdysone that appears after a blood meal to regulate the production of reproductive spores. One of these is a microsporan, *Amblyospora* sp., that has a life cycle that alternates between copepods and mosquito larvae. In the male adult mosquito the parasite sporulates, killing the host. In females, the parasite does not sporulate until after the blood meal, when the rise in 20-hydroxyecdysone titers stimulate sporulation. These spores enter the developing oocytes, resulting in vertical transmission to the next generation of mosquitoes (Lord and Hall 1983).

The second case involves a fungus, *Coelomomyces stegomyiae*, that also alternates between mosquito larvae and copepods. Mosquitoes that survive the fungal infection and become adults have hyphae throughout their bodies. Spores do not develop until after a blood meal, and again it is ecdysone that stimulates sporulation. In this case, however, the spores fill the developing follicles and the female exhibits normal oviposition behavior, but instead of depositing eggs, she deposits spores. Thus, the fungus uses the female mosquito as a mechanism for dissemination (Lucarotti 1992).

There is no evidence that a mosquito parasite that is a human pathogen interacts with host endocrinology in this way. However, the research is dated, and this question should be reinvestigated in light of our current understanding of mosquito physiology.

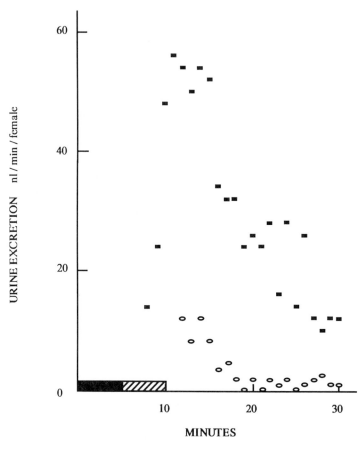

17.23 Decapitation of a mosquito shortly after a blood meal reduces the amount of urine secreted in the first 30 minutes after a blood meal. Filled squares are urine production in normal females. Open circles are urine production in decapitated females. Black bar represents feeding time. Hatched bar is time required for decapitation and waxing the wound. Drops of urine were counted and converted to nl using the relationship 1 drop = 16.6 nl. Adapted from Wheelock et al. 1988.

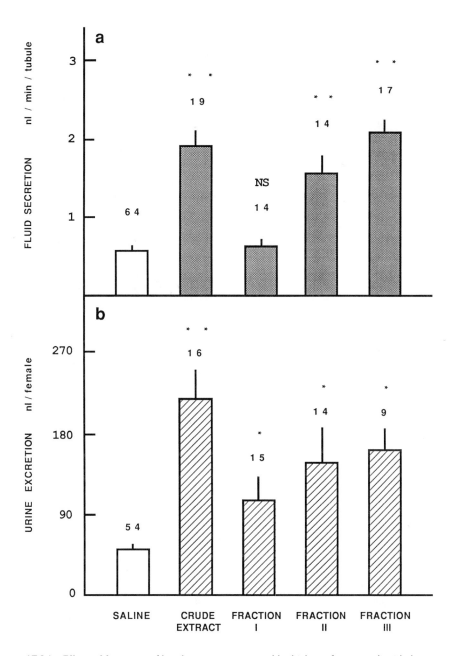

17.24   Effect of fractions of head extracts separated by high performance liquid chromatography on (a) fluid secretion by Malpighian tubules incubated with fraction being tested or (b) urine production by blood-fed decapitated females injected with fraction being tested. In (b) the females were also injected with ^{3}H-water, and the amount of urine produced was estimated by measuring the amount of ^{3}H-water excreted in vials. Adapted from Wheelock et al. 1988.

CONCLUSIONS

It should be clear from this chapter that the endocrinology of mosquitoes is important to vector biologists. Endocrines affect feeding behavior, nutrition, water balance, egg development, and parasite development. Note that the hierarchy of controls from neurosecretory peptide hormones to steroid (or terpenoid) hormones to 2nd messengers and receptor molecules in the target tissues are common features of endocrine systems in all animals. Despite its small size, the mosquito is no exception to this rule. As the possibility of the genetic engineering of mosquitoes nears reality, many more aspects of mosquito physiology will become important to the vector biologist.

ACKNOWLEDGMENT

Thanks are due to Dr. T. J. Bradley for reviewing the 1st section of this chapter and providing several figures and to Dr. J. Meredith for Figures 17.9 and 17.10.

REFERENCES

Bradley, T.J. 1985. The excretory system: Structure and function. In: G.A. Kerkut and L. I. Gilbert, editors, *Comprehensive insect physiology, biochemistry and pharmacology.* London/New York: Pergamon.

Bradley, T.J. 1987. Physiology of osmoregulation in mosquitoes. *Ann. Rev. Entomol.* 32:439–462.

Brown, M.R., and A.O. Lea. 1989. Neuroendocrine and midgut endocrine systems in the adult mosquito. *Adv. Disease Vector Res.* 6:29–58.

Clements, A.N. 1992. *The biology of mosquitoes,* Vol. 1, Chap. 6. London: Chapman and Hall.

Hagedorn, H.H. 1985. The role of ecysteroids in reproduction. In: G.A. Kurkut and L.I. Gilbert, editors, *Comprehensive insect physiology, biochemistry, and pharmacology,* Vol. 8, Endocrinology. Oxford, New York, Sydney, Paris, and Frankfurt: Pergamon Press. pp. 205–262.

Hagedorn, H.H. 1994. The endocrinology of the adult female mosquito. *Adv. Disease Vector Res.* 10:109–148.

Nicolson, S.W. 1993. The ionic basis of fluid secretion in the insect Malpighian tubule: Advances in the last ten years. *J. Insect Physiol.* 39:451–458.

Raikhel, A.S. 1992. Vitellogenesis in mosquitoes. *Adv. Disease Vector Res.* 9:1–39.

CITED REFERENCES

Borovsky, D., D.A. Carlson, R.G. Hancock, H. Rembold, and E. Van Handel. 1994. De novo biosynthesis of juvenile hormone III and I by the accessory glands of the male mosquito. *Insect Mol. Biol.* 24:437–444.

Borovsky, D., D.A. Carlson, I. Ujvary, and G.D. Prestwich. 1994. Biosynthesis of (10R)-juvenile hormone III from farnesoic acid by I *Aedes aegypti* ovary. *Arch. Insect Biochem. Physiol.* 27:11–25.

Bowen, M.F., and S. Loess-Perez. 1989. A re-examination of the role of ecdysteroids in the development of host-seeking inhibition in blood-fed *Aedes aegypti* mosquitoes. In: D. Borovsky and A. Spielman, editors, *Host regulated developmental mechanisms in vector arthropods.* Vero Beach: University of Florida. pp. 286–291.

Bradley, T.J., and J.E. Phillips. 1977. The effect of external salinity on drinking rate and rectal secretion in the larvae of the saline-water mosquito *Aedes taeniorhynchus. J. Exp. Biol.* 66:97–110.

Chen, J-S., W-L Cho, and A.S. Raikhel. 1994. Analysis of mosquito vitellogenin cDNA, similarity with vertebrate phosvitins and arthropod serum proteins. *J. Mol. Biol.* 237:641–647.

Edwards, H.A. 1982. Ion concentration and activity in the haemolymph of *Aedes aegypti* larvae. *J. Exp. Biol.* 101:143–151.

Garrett, M., and T.J. Bradley. 1984. The pattern of osmotic regulation in larvae of the mosquito *Culiseta inornata. J. Exp. Biol.* 113:133–141.

Gillies, M.T. 1955. The pre-gravid phase of ovarian development in *Anopheles funestus. Ann. Trop. Med. Parasitol.* 49:320–325.

Greenplate, J.T., R.L. Glaser, and H.H. Hagedorn. 1985. The role of factors from the head in the regulation of egg development in the mosquito *Aedes aegypti. J. Insect Physiol.* 31:328–329.

Jenkins, S.P., M.R. Brown, and A.O. Lea. 1992. Inactive prothoracic glands in larvae and pupae of *Aedes aegypti:* Ecdysteroid release by tissues in the thorax and abdomen. *Insect Biochem. Molec. Biol.* 22:553–559.

Kataoka, H., A. Toschi, J.P. Li, R.L. Carney, D.A. Schooley, and S.J. Kramer. 1989. Identification of an allatotropin from adult *Manduca sexta. Science* 243:1481–1483.

Kawakami, A., M. Iwami, H. Nagasawa, A. Suzuki, and H. Ishizaki. 1989. Structure and organization of four clustered genes that encode bombyxin, an insulin-related brain secretory peptide of the silkmoth *Bombyx mori. Proc. Natl. Acad. Sci. USA* 86:6843–6847.

Kawakami, A., H. Kataoka, T. Oka, A. Mizoguchi, M. Kimura-Kawakami, T. Adachi, M. Iwami, H. Nagasawa, A. Suzuki, and H. Ishizaki.1990. Molecular cloning of the *Bombyx mori* prothoraciotropic hormone. *Science* 247:1333–1335.

Keeley, L.L., T.K. Hayes, J.Y. Bradfield, and Y.-H Lee. 1991. Metabolic neuropeptides. In: J.J. Menn, T.J. Kelly, and E.P. Masler, editors, *Insect Neuropeptides*, American Chemical Society Symposium Series #453. Columbus, OH: ACS.

Loeb, M.J., E.P. Brandt, and M.J. Birnbaum. 1984. Ecdysteroid production by testis of the tobacco budworm, *Heliothis virescens*, from last larval instar to adult. *J. Insect Physiol.* 30:375–381.

Lord, J.C., and D.W. Hall. 1983. Sporulation of *Amblyospora* (Microspora) in female *Culex salinarius:* Induction by 20-hydroxyecdysone. *Parasitol.* 87:377–383.

Lucarotti, C.J. 1992. Invasion of *Aedes aegypti* ovaries by *Coelomomyces stegomyiae. J. Invert. Pathol.* 690:176–184.

Maddrell, S.H.P., and J.E. Phillips. 1978. Active transport of sulphate ions by the Malpighian tubules of larvae of the mosquito *Aedes campestris. J. Exp. Biol.* 72:181–202.

Meredith, J., and J.E. Phillips. 1973. Rectal ultrastructure in salt- and freshwater mosquito larvae in relation to physiological state. *Z. Zellforschung Mikr. Anat* 138:1–22.

Nicolson, S.W. 1972. Osmoregulation in larvae of the New Zealand saltwater mosquito *Opifex fuscus. J. Entomol.* (A) 47:101–108.

Pratt, G.E., D.E. Farnsworth, D.F. Fok, N.R. Siegel, A.L. McCormack, J. Shabanowitz, D.F. Hunt, and R. Feyereisen. 1991. Identity of a second type of allatostatin from cockroach brains: An octadecapeptide amide with a tyrosine-rich address sequence. *Proc. Natl. Acad. Sci. USA* 88:2412–2416.

Ramsay, J.A. 1950. Osmotic regulation in mosquito larvae. *J. Exp. Biol.* 27:145–157.

Readio, J., K. Peck, R. Meola, and K.H. Dahm. 1988. Corpus allatum activity (*in vitro*) in female *Culex pipiens. J. Insect Physiol.* 34:131–135.

Richard, D.S., S.W. Applebaum, T.J. Sliter, F.C. Baker, D.A. Schooley, C.C. Reuter, V.C. Henrich, and L.I. Gilbert. 1989. Juvenile hormone bisepoxide biosynthesis in vitro by the ring gland of *Drosophila melanogaster*. A putative juvenile hormone in the higher Diptera. *Proc. Natl. Acad. Sci. USA* 86:1421–1425.

Shapiro, A.B., G.D. Wheelock, H.H. Hagedorn, F.C. Baker, L.W. Tsai, and D.A. Schooley. 1986. Juvenile hormone and juvenile hormone esterase in adult females of the mosquito *Aedes aegypti. J. Insect Physiol.* 32:867–877.

Truman, J.W. 1971 Hourglass behavior of the circadian clock controlling eclosion of the silkmoth *Antheraea pernyi. Proc. Nat. Acad. Sci. USA* 68:595–599.

Van Handel, E., and A.O. Lea. 1970. Control of glycogen and fat metabolism in the mosquito. *Gen. Comp. Endocrinol.* 14:381–384.

Wheelock, G.H., D.H. Petzel, J.D. Gillett, K.W. Beyenbach, and H.H. Hagedorn. 1988. Evidence for hormonal control of diuresis after a blood meal in the mosquito *Aedes aegypti. Arch. Insect Biochem. Physiol.* 7:75–89.

Yagi, K. J., K.G. Konz, B. Stay, and S.S. Tobe. 1990. Production and utilization of farnesoic acid in the juvenile hormone biosynthetic pathway by corpora allata of larval *Diploptera punctata. Gen. Comp. Endocrinol.* 81:284–294.

Young, A.D.M., and A.E.R. Downe. 1983. Influence of mating on sexual receptivity and oviposition in the mosquito, *Culex tarsalis. Physiol. Entomol.* 8:213–217.

Young, A.D.M., and A.E.R. Downe. 1987. Male accessory gland substances and the control of sexual receptivity in female *Culex tarsalis. Physiol. Entomol.* 12:233–239.

18. THE VECTOR ALIMENTARY SYSTEM

William S. Romoser

INTRODUCTION

This chapter focuses on the adaptations by which blood-feeding arthropods acquire and process matter/energy in the form of vertebrate blood and how these activities bring them into contact with human and other vertebrate pathogens. Specifically covered are the structure and function of a generalized insect alimentary system, the structure and function of alimentary systems in insects and ticks specialized for blood-feeding, and the alimentary canal as a habitat for blood-borne vertebrate microorganisms. Understanding the structure and function of arthropod alimentary systems forms the basis for developing an understanding of the activities of microorganisms within these systems. Because the pathogenic microorganisms vectored by arthropods spend a significant part of their lives in the alimentary canal, interactions between these microbes and the arthropod gut epithelium are key elements in determining vector competence and host specificity.

Given the vast amount of information available, this chapter is of necessity somewhat general, although specific cases are cited when appropriate. General accounts of the structure and function of the insect alimentary system can be found in Applebaum (1985), Chapman (1982; 1985a; 1985b), Dow (1986), King and Akai (1984), Phillips et al. (1988), Romoser and Stoffolano (1994), Snodgrass (1935), Turunen (1985), and Wigglesworth (1972).

STRUCTURE AND FUNCTION OF THE INSECT ALIMENTARY CANAL

The alimentary canal in insects is a tube (commonly coiled) that extends from the anterior oral opening (true mouth) to the posterior anus. The mouthparts are considered to have been derived for the most part from primitive, bilateral appendages surrounding the mouth (Chap. 1). Discussion of arthropod mouthparts is beyond the scope of this chapter, but useful recent discussions may be found in Smith (1985) (insects in general) and Lehane (1991) (blood-feeding insects).

The insect alimentary canal (Fig.18.1a) is formed by a layer of epithelium 1 cell thick that has a noncellular basal lamina or basement membrane present on the hemocoel side. Three major regions of the canal are the foregut, midgut, and hindgut. In the embryo, the foregut and hindgut arise as ectodermal invaginations, and like the ectodermal cells that form the arthropod integument, these cells retain the capacity to secrete a noncellular, chitinous layer continuous with the integumentary cuticle. Both the foregut and hindgut are lined with this noncellular intima and, as with the integument, the specific composition and nature of this lining is differentiated spatially in structure and function. The midgut is generally viewed as being of endodermal origin. Distally closed evaginations, the Malpighian tubules, open into the lumen of the alimentary canal at the junction between the midgut and hindgut.

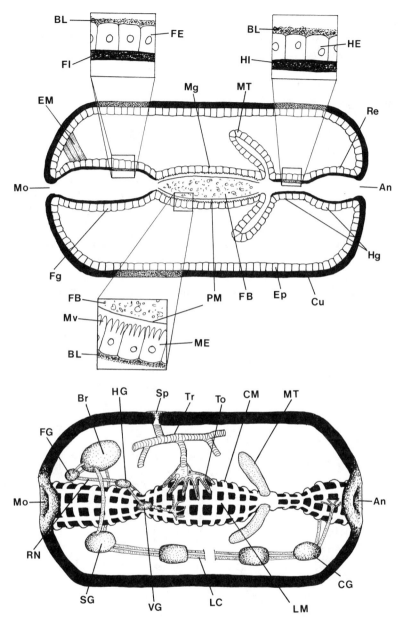

18.1   Diagram of the key elements of the insect alimentary canal. (A) sagittal section; (B) Relationship between the alimentary canal and other systems. Drawing by Aaron Power. An = anus, BL = basal lamina, Br = brain, Cu = cuticule, CG = caudal ganglion, CM = circular muscle, EM = extrinsic muscle, Ep = epidermis, Fg = foregut, FB = food bolus, FE = foregut epithelium, FG = frontal ganglion, FI = foregut intima, Hg = hindgut, HE = hindgut epithelium, HG = hypocerebral ganglion, HI = hindgut intima, LC = longitudinal connective, LM = longitudinal muscle, Mg = Midgut, Mo = mouth, Mv = microvillus, ME = midgut epithelium, MT = Malpighian tubule, PM = peritrophic membrane, Re = rectum, RN = recurrent nerve, SG = subesophageal ganglion, Sp = spiracle, Tr = trachea, To = tracheole, VG = ventricular ganglion.

The musculature of the arthropod alimentary canal consists of both intrinsic and extrinsic fibers (Figs. 18.1a, b). The intrinsic muscles form circular, longitudinal, and/or irregular networks around the gut and provide the alternate waves of contraction and relaxation (peristalsis) that propel food along its length. The rectum is particularly rich in muscle fibers. Whereas intrinsic visceral muscles such as those associated with the alimentary canal connect with one another, the extrinsic muscles of the alimentary canal attach at one end to the gut and the other end to the cuticle. Contraction of these muscles causes luminal expansion and is typically associated with various pumping actions. Action antagonistic to the extrinsic muscles is provided by intrinsic muscles or by the elasticity inherent in specialized regions of the intima such as in the pharyngeal pump of mosquitoes. Extrinsic muscles also play a suspensory role. As with all arthropod muscles, visceral muscle fibers are striated.

A well-developed tracheal/tracheolar network (Fig. 18.1b) facilitates the movement of oxygen to the alimentary epithelium and associated muscles and helps hold structures in place in a fashion similar to vertebrate mesentery. The muscles of the foregut are typically innervated by fibers associated with the so-called stomatogastric nervous system and the ventricular ganglia (Fig. 18.1b) are located on either side of the gut in the region of the foregut/midgut junction. In some cases, neurosecretory cells have been found in the ventricular ganglia. Although there is considerable variation among the different insect groups, the ventricular ganglia have neural connections with the hypocerebral ganglion, which lies on the dorsum of the esophagus just behind the brain. The recurrent nerve connects the hypocerebral ganglion, and hence the ventricular ganglia, to the frontal ganglion, which in turn has neural connections with the brain. The hindgut muscles receive fibers from the caudal ganglion of the ventral chain. Some gut muscles appear not to receive any innervation.

Each major gut region is specialized for particular functions. The foregut is involved primarily with the ingestion, conduction, and storage of food; the midgut with the digestion and absorption of food; and the hindgut with excretion and egestion of waste materials from the midgut and Malpighian tubules and with regulation of hemolymph composition. Structural characteristics associated with the various specialized functions are often evident.

In generalized forms (Fig. 18.2), the mouthparts surround the true mouth. The cavity formed by the various appendicular mouthparts is subdivided into the cibarial (preoral) cavity, into which the true mouth opens, and the salivarium, into which the common salivary duct opens. The foregut intima is impermeable and varies along its length in thickness and degree of sclerotization. In the pharynx, into which the true

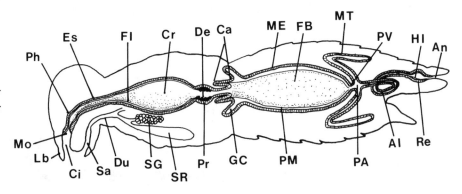

18.2 Generalized insect alimentary canal. An = anus, Al = anterior intentine, Ca = cardia, Ci = cibarium, Cr = crop, De = denticle, Du = duct, Es = esophagus, FB = food bolus, Fl = foregut intima, GC = gastric caeca, Hl = hindgut intima, Lb = labrum, ME = midgut epithelium, Mo = mouth, MT = Malpighian tubule, Ph = pharynx, PA = pyloric ampulla, PM = peritrophic membrane, Pr = proventriculus, PV = pyloric valve, Re = rectum, Sa = salivarium, SG = salivary gland, SR = salivary reservoir. From William S. Romoser and John G. Stoffolano, Jr., *The Science of Entomology*, 3rd edition. Copyright © 1994 Wm. C. Brown Communications, Inc., Dubuque, Iowa. All rights reserved. Reprinted with permission.

mouth opens, the intima is typically somewhat thickened and elastic in association with the pumping function of this structure. The esophagus is a conducting tube between the pharynx and the crop, which is a variously modified food storage structure. The intima lining the esophagus and crop is comparatively thin. In insects that ingest solid food, e.g., grasshoppers and cockroaches, there is typically a secondary triturating (chewing) structure, the proventriculus or gastric mill, in which the intima may be formed into sclerotized denticles (teeth).

The junction between the foregut and midgut is located in a rather complex structure called the cardia. Among morphologists who study the Diptera (true flies) and Siphonaptera (fleas), the cardia is often called the proventriculus, but this is a very different structure from the proventriculus of the more generalized insects like the Orthoptera (grasshoppers, crickets, etc.) and Blattaria (cockroaches). The cardia forms as an intussusception composed of both fore- and midgut epithelia. Muscles within the folds of the cardia act as sphincters whereas the inner and reflected layers of foregut epithelium produce a valve effect. In fact, the term "stomodael valve" is sometimes used for the cardia. The outer layer of the cardia is the cardial epithelium, and the foregut-midgut junction is located at the point where the cardial epithelium and reflected wall of the esophagus join. In histological sections this junction is evident as the point where the foregut intima ends.

The midgut is composed of epithelial cells that secrete the digestive enzymes, absorb water, and absorb the products of digestion. A typical midgut epithelial cell is illustrated in Figure 18.3, and an electron photomicrograph of a representative midgut epithelial cell is shown in Figure 18.4. In histological form, midgut epithelial cells vary from columnar to squamous depending upon the degree of distension by food. Typically the apical (luminal) side of the cell is

microvillate, and a mucopolysaccharide coating is attached to the surface of the plasma membrane, forming the glycocalyx. The glycocalyx ranges from about 20–200 nm depending on the species (Chapman 1985a). The microvilli provide an enormous surface area for the absorption of materials from the lumen. On the hemocoel side, the plasma membrane is formed into a complex network of invaginations, the basal labyrinth. Mitochondria are found among many of the regions of cytoplasm associated with the basal labyrinth. As with the microvilli, the basal labyrinth provides a large surface area through which materials

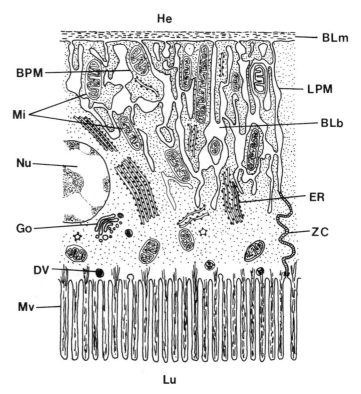

18.3 Ultrastructure of a generalized insect midgut epithelial cell. BLm = basal lamina, He = hemocoel, LPM = lateral plasma membrane, BLb = basal labyrinth, BPM = basal plasma membrane, DV = dense vesicle, ER = endoplasmic reticulum, Go = Golgi, Lu = lumen, Mi = mitochondria, Mv = microvillus, Nu = nucleus, ZC = zonula continua. Adapted from Berridge 1970. *A structural analysis of intestinal absorption.* In: A.C. Neville, ed., *Insect ultrastructures*, Symposia of the Royal Society of London, No. 5.

may be transported. A basal lamina (or basement membrane) separates the basal plasma membrane, including openings from the basal labyrinth from the hemocoel and hemolymph. The basal lamina may be granular in appearance or may have a distinct lattice-like structure. Laterally, the midgut epithelial cells are joined apically for about half of their length by intercellular junctions called zonula continua. More basally distinct intercellular spaces are evident and are bounded by unjoined lateral plasma membrane. Within the cytoplasm there is usually an abundance of rough endoplasmic reticulum (as would be expected in cells that synthesize materials extensively for export). Regenerative or replacement cells (Fig. 18.4) can be found at the bases of the actively secreting and absorbing epithelial cells. When the active cells die, the regenerative cells differentiate into active midgut epithelial cells.

A noncellular, chitinous peritrophic matrix is usually formed around the food bolus (Fig. 18.2). Depending on the insect species and stage, this membrane. forms

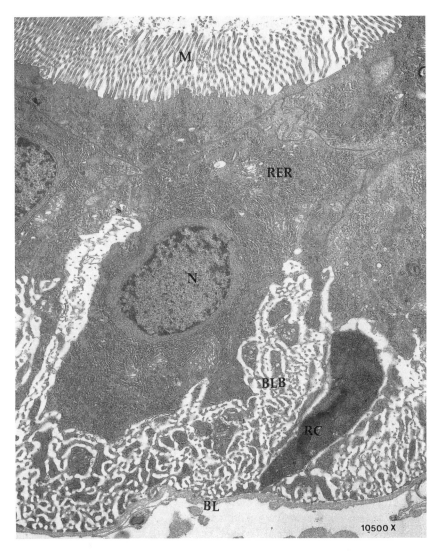

18.4 Ultrathin section of mosquito midgut epithelial cell and regenerative cell. BL = basal lamina, BLB = basal labyrinth, M = microvilli, N = nucleus, RC = regenerative cell, RER = rough endoplasmic reticulum (10,500 X). Courtesy of Dr. K. Lerdthusnee.

from a secretion produced by most or all of the midgut epithelial cells (Chap. 19). This matrix delaminates from the midgut epithelium and basically conforms to the shape and size of the food bolus. Or the peritrophic matrix forms a more or less cylindrical tube secreted by specialized cells in the cardial epithelium.

Because the peritrophic matrix is located between the food bolus and the midgut epithelium, it may play a significant role in the interactions between microbes and the midgut epithelium (see Chap. 19).

The midgut and hindgut (Fig. 18.2) are typically separated by a sphincter/valve arrangement called the pyloric valve. Distally closed Malpighian tubules open into an expanded region posterior to the pyloric valve called the pyloric ampulla. As mentioned earlier, the hindgut, like the foregut, is lined with a chitinous intima; however, the intima is permeable to water and various solute molecules. Two regions of the hindgut are readily recognizable: the anterior intestine and the rectum. Subdivision of the anterior intestine into an anterior ileum and posterior colon is sometimes evident. The anterior intestine, rectum, and Malpighian tubules function as the major excretory system of insects. Nitrogenous and other wastes, ions, and so on are secreted into the lumen of the Malpighian tubules and pass to the lumen of the hindgut where they join undigested waste from the midgut. Water, ions, and other small molecules that are needed by the insect are reabsorbed in the hindgut, particularly in the rectum. Rectal absorption is commonly facilitated by the presence of several lobelike or leaflike projections into the lumen, the rectal papillae, which are highly specialized absorptive structures. A recent discussion of excretory function in insects can be found in Bradley (1985).

For insects that undergo complete metamorphosis (holometabolous forms), the larval and adult stages usually live in different environmental circumstances and have different feeding habits. Correlated with this is a dramatic rebuilding of the alimentary canal during metamorphosis. In contrast, insects that undergo simple metamorphosis (hemimetabolous forms) (Chap. 1) usually live in the same environment and display the same feeding habits throughout the life cycle. In these insects, the alimentary system remains basically the same for the life of the insect.

THE ALIMENTARY SYSTEM IN HEMATOPHAGOUS INSECTS

The use of vertebrate blood as a source of nutriment has evolved independently several times in the class Insecta, and many convergent similarities in the alimentation process are evident in diverse taxa. This section focuses on the principal groups of blood-feeding arthropods: (1) order Phthiraptera, suborder Anoplura, the sucking lice (Ferris 1951; Marshal 1981); (2) order Hemiptera, family Reduviidae, subfamily Triatominae, the kissing bugs, and family Cimicidae, the bed, bird, and bat bugs (Usinger 1966); (3) order Siphonaptera, fleas (Rothschild et al. 1986); (4) order Diptera, the bloodsucking Diptera, including mosquitoes (Snodgrass 1959), black flies, sand flies, biting midges, tabanids (horse and deer flies), and the biting muscoids *(Stomoxys)*, and the tsetse fly, *Glossina*. The ticks (class Arachnida, order Acari) are examined in a later section.

Blood-feeding forms are found among insects that undergo simple metamorphosis as well as those that undergo complete metamorphosis (Table 18.1). Among blood-feeding insects that undergo simple metamorphosis (bed bugs, kissing bugs, and sucking lice), both nymphal and adult males and females ingest blood; therefore alimentary structure and function remain essentially the same throughout the life cycle. In contrast, among insects that undergo complete metamorphosis (with the exception of certain blood-feeding dipteran larvae in the family Calliphoridae, e.g., *Auchmeromyia* spp., the Congo floor maggot, and others), only adults ingest blood; larvae display altogether different feeding habits that are reflected in very different alimentary structure and function. In these insects, the alimentary canal undergoes a dramatic reconstruction (metamorphosis) during the pupal stage.

Blood-feeding insects that undergo complete metamorphosis may be further subdivided on the basis of whether both sexes or only females take blood meals (Table 18.1). For example, among the nematocerous Diptera (mosquitoes and relatives) only females ingest blood, whereas both males and females take nectar (sugar) meals. However, among the biting muscoid flies, both sexes are blood-feeders. The use of the nutrients derived from a blood meal varies considerably among the different blood-feeding groups. Basically a blood meal may be utilized in one or more of the following ways: (1) for the synthesis of yolk material in eggs, i.e., the process of vitellogenesis; (2) in growth and development during the larval or nymphal stage; and (3) as a source of energy for mobility and body maintenance.

In Table 18.1, it is evident that different groups feed on blood during different stages of the life cycle, and that some depend solely on blood whereas others ingest nectar in addition to blood. Those insects that rely

TABLE 18.1 Feeding patterns and symbionts in blood-feeding insects

Metamorphosis	Taxon[a]	Common name	Larval feeding	Adult food male	Adult food female	Use of blood[b]	Symbionts	Location of symbionts
Simple	**O. Pthiraptera** So. Anoplura	sucking lice	blood	blood	blood	1, 2, 3	+	ventral wall of midgut; ovaries
	O. Hemiptera F. Cimicidae	bird, bat, and bed bugs	blood	blood	blood	1, 2, 3	+	fat body
	F. Reduviidae Sf. Triatominae	kissing bugs	blood	blood	blood	1, 2, 3	some +	blood storage region of midgut lumen
Complete	**O. Siphonaptera**	fleas	miscellaneous organic debris; blood drops from adults	blood	blood	1, 2, 3	some +	lumen of midgut
	O. Diptera	true flies						
	F. Psychodidae (Sf. Phlebotominae)	sand flies	miscellaneous organic debris	nectar	blood and nectar	3	–	–
	F. Culicidae	mosquitoes	microplankton	nectar	blood and nectar	3	–	–
	F. Simuliidae	black flies	microplankton and decaying organic matter	nectar	blood and nectar	3	–	–
	F. Ceratopogonidae	biting midges	microbial growth, some scavengers and predators	nectar	blood and nectar	3	–	–
	F. Tabanidae	horse and deer flies	predators; some possibly predators	nectar and pollen	blood and nectar	2, 3	–	–
	F. Muscidae (*G. Stomoxys*)	stable flies	decaying plant matter	blood and nectar	blood and nectar	2, 3	–	–
	(*G. Glossina*)	tsetse flies	secretions from uterine glands	blood	blood	1, 2, 3	+	midgut wall

[a] O. = order, So. = suborder, F. = family, Sf. = subfamily, G. = genus
[b] 1 = growth and development, 2 = maintenance, 3 = egg development

solely on blood throughout the life cycle, for example the blood-feeding Hemiptera, utilize the blood nutrients in all 3 of the ways mentioned. Tsetse flies, *Glossina* spp., also depend solely on blood for the entire life cycle, but the larvae obtain nutrients indirectly from adult blood meals. A single larva develops within the well-developed "uterus" of the adult female and is nourished by secretions from special uterine glands. Some species of fleas also obtain blood nutrients indirectly during the larval stage. In this case the adults that are feeding on a host literally squirt droplets of blood out of the anus that are then ingested by the larvae. Insects such as the stable fly *Stomoxys calcitrans*, which feeds solely on blood (but only in the adult stage), utilizes other sources of nutrients for growth, development, and so on during the larval stage. The same is true for the nematocerous Diptera (Yuval 1992) and Tabanids, except that the blood nutrients are used for vitellogenesis, and energy for flight and long-term survival is derived mainly from the sugar in nectar meals.

Vertebrate blood lacks certain vital nutrients, particularly vitamins in the B group (Chap. 2), and there is a correlation between the sole reliance on blood throughout the life cycle and the presence of symbiotic microorganisms (Table 18.1). Thus the sucking lice, the bloodsucking Hemiptera, the fleas, and the tsetse flies all harbor symbionts that probably provide the nutrients missing from the diet of vertebrate blood. Experimental deprivation of these insects of their symbionts causes the inhibition of growth and development in general and of reproductive development in females. The symbionts can be free-living in the gut lumen or harbored in specialized cells called mycetocytes, which are sometimes organized into a specialized structure referred to as a mycetome. Mycetocytes and mycetomes are variously located, depending on the species of insect. In nymphs and adult male sucking lice a single mycetome is located in the ventral midgut wall; in adult females the symbionts are associated with the ovaries. Likewise, symbionts are located in the midgut wall of tsetse flies. In the kissing bugs and fleas, symbionts live freely in the midgut lumen. In the bed, bat, and bird bugs, symbionts are widely distributed throughout the body as well as in specialized mycetomes associated with the abdominal fat

body in females and the vasa deferentia in the males. Information on symbionts may be found in Buchner (1965) and Marshal (1981).

The following discussion is based on comparison of the alimentary systems in the major hematophagous insect groups, with mosquitoes representing the nematocerous Diptera (Table 18.2; Figs. 18.5–9). Movement of blood into the foregut of blood-feeding forms is achieved by means of 1 or 2 pumping structures. In the bloodsucking Hemiptera and the tsetse fly (Figs. 18.6, 18.9) the cibarium is the only pumping organ, whereas in the remaining hematophagous groups both the cibarium and pharynx act as pumping organs. The foregut intima that lines pumping structures is typically thickened and elastic, and the extrinsic muscles that dilate the pump lumen are opposed by the elasticity of the modified intima that closes the lumen (see Fig. 18.8b). A 1-way valve effect sustains a directional flow of blood toward the midgut. Pappas (1988) measured the activity of the cibarial and pharyngeal pumps

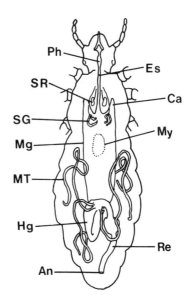

18.5   Sucking louse alimentary canal. An = anus, Ca = caeca, Es = esophagus, Hg = hindgut, Mg = midgut, My = mycetome, MT = Malpighian tubule, Ph = pharynx, Re = rectum, SG = salivary gland, SR = salivary reservoir. Redrawn from A.G. Marshal 1981, *The ecology of ectoparasitic insects*, Academic Press, San Diego.

TABLE 18.2 Comparative alimentary structure and function of representative hematophagous insects

Common name	Cibarial pump	Pharyngeal pump	Nature of crop	Crop function	Nature of midgut	Blood storage	Blood digestion	Site of digestion/ absorption	Peritrophic membrane
sucking lice (Fig. 18.5)	+	+	–	–	comparatively large and saclike; gastric caeca in some	midgut	batch	midgut/ midgut	–[a]
kissing bugs (Fig. 18.6)	+	–	–	–	two major regions: saclike anterior and tubular posterior[b]	anterior midgut	continuous	posterior midgut/ posterior midgut	+ –[c]
fleas[d] (Fig. 18.7)	+	+	–	–	barrel shaped	midgut	batch	midgut/ midgut	–
mosquitoes (Fig. 18.8)	+	+	two dorsal and one ventral diverticulum	nectar and storage[e]	tubular anterior and saclike posterior	posterior midgut	batch	posterior midgut/ posterior midgut	+ (secreted by midgut epithelium)
tsetse flies (Fig. 18.9)	+	–	ventral diverticulum	blood storage	longitudinally divided into four regions[f]	anterior midgut and crop	continuous	secretory midgut/ posterior midgut	+ (secreted by proventriculus)

[a] Peritrophic matrix "seems to be absent" (Peters 1992).
[b] Posterior midgut can be further divided into two regions. Anterior midgut is also the site of diuresis, ion regulation, carbohydrate digestion, hemolysis, and lipid processing (Billingsley 1990).
[c] Extracellular membranes somewhat different from those found in other insects; they appear to lack chitin (Peters 1992)
[d] Well-developed proventricular spines disrupt blood cells.
[e] Nectar can be absorbed in the anterior midgut.
[f] Midgut divided into (1) anterior, (2) mycetome, (3) secretory, and (4) posterior regions

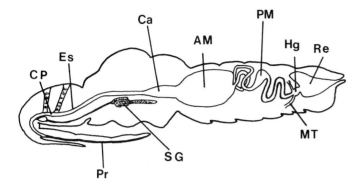

18.6   Triatomid (kissing) bug alimentary canal. Based on Harwood and James 1979, after Miall. AM = anterior midgut, Ca = cardia, CP = cibarial pump, Es = esophagus, Hg = hindgut, Pr = proboscis, PM = posterior midgut, Re = rectum, SG = salivary gland.

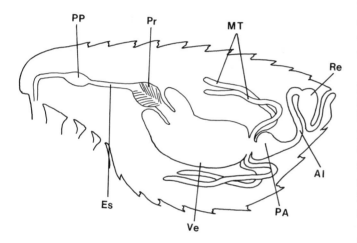

18.7   Flea alimentary canal. Based on Harwood and James 1979, after Faarch. AI = anterior intestine, Es = esophagus, PP = pharyngeal pump, MT = Malpighian tubules, PA = pyloric ampulla, Pr = proventriculus, Re = rectum, Ve = ventriculus.

electromyographically in several mosquito species and provided a detailed account of the pumping sequence in which the cibarial pump works in alternation with the pharyngeal pump.

As with generalized forms, the esophagus serves as a conducting tube, connecting the pharynx directly with the cardia (proventriculus) in the sucking lice (Fig. 18.5), bloodsucking true bugs (Fig. 18.6), and

fleas (Fig. 18.7). The esophagus can also connect the pharynx and the crop, as in the bloodsucking Diptera (Fig. 18.8).

The crop in the bloodsucking Diptera (e.g., Fig. 18.8) is typically a blind sac or diverticulum that opens into the esophagus and extends back into the abdomen, where it is free to expand due to the flexibility of the telescoping abdominal segments. As with the crop in other kinds of insects, the diverticulum is an impermeable storage organ. The nature of the intimal lining of the foregut determines the impermeability of both the diverticulum and the rest of the foregut. Anastomosing networks of muscle fibers propel the diverticular contents. In mosquitoes (Fig. 18.8), in addition to a large ventral diverticulum, 2 smaller dorsal diverticula open into the esophagus and expand into bilateral anterior cavities between the 2 sets of indirect flight muscles.

The cardia (e.g., Fig. 18.8) regulates the passage of materials from the foregut to the midgut and prevents reflux of materials back into the foregut from the midgut. For example, the regulation of the passage of sugar solutions (nectar) from the diverticulum of nematocerous Diptera into the midgut is mediated via the cardia. In some bloodsucking insects, such as tsetse flies, the cardia secretes and forms the peritrophic membrane.

The midgut in hematophagous insects varies from the more or less saclike structures found in the sucking lice and fleas to midguts, which display distinct anterior to posterior structural-functional differentiation. For example, at least 2 major regions are evident in the bloodsucking Hemiptera (Fig. 18.6), the saclike anterior midgut and the tubular posterior midgut, both of which may be further subdivided histologically and functionally (Billingsley 1990). Likewise in the tsetse flies (Fig. 18.9) and other biting muscoids, the midgut is differentiated longitudinally. At least 4 regions have been described (Billingsley 1990): the anterior midgut, the mycetome, the secretory midgut, and the posterior midgut. In the mosquito (Fig. 18.8)

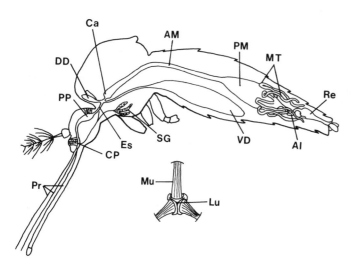

18.8 Mosquito alimentary canal. Below, cross-section of pharyngeal pump. AI = anterior intestine, AM = anterior midgut, Ca = cardia, CP = cibarial pump, DD = dorsal diverticulum, Es = esophagus, MT = Malpighian tubule, PM = posterior midgut, PP = pharyngeal pump, PR = proboscis, Re = rectum, SG = salivary gland, VD = ventral diverticulum (crop) Mu = muscle, Lu = lumen. Modified from R.E. Snodgrass, 1959, *The anatomical life of the mosquito*. Smithsonian Misc. Coll., Vol. 139, No. 8, Washington, D. C.

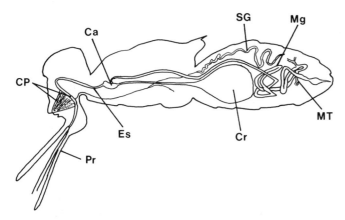

18.9 Tsetse fly alimentary canal. Modified from Glasgow 1963. Ca = cardia, Cr = crop, CP = cibarial pump, Es = esophagus, Pr = proboscis, SG = salivary gland, Mg = midgut, MT = Malpighian

and other nematocerous Diptera, the midgut is longitudinally divided into a tubular anterior and saclike posterior midgut. The midgut, or specialized portions of it, is highly expandable, a process facilitated by the telescoping abdominal segments. Histological and ultrastructural studies of midgut cells have revealed various specializations that have formed the basis for functional interpretations. An excellent discussion of such interpretations appears in Billingsley (1990). The electron photomicrograph of a midgut epithelial and associated regenerative cell (Fig. 18.4) illustrates some of the ultrastructural characteristics.

The destination and storage of blood varies among the different blood-feeding forms (Table 18.2). For the most part, it is initially directed to the midgut, but in the case of the tsetse flies, the crop receives overflow blood from the midgut. The destination and storage of blood in the midgut of insects (which show longitudinal specialization of the midgut) also vary. In the bloodsucking Hemiptera (Fig. 18.6), and in tsetse flies (Fig. 18.9), it is stored in the saclike anterior midgut. In mosquitoes and other bloodsucking Nematocera, blood is directed through the tubular anterior midgut and into the posterior midgut.

As mentioned earlier, only female nematocerous Diptera ingest blood, whereas both males and females ingest flower nectar. These sugar meals are directed to and stored in the impermeable diverticula and are subsequently released into the midgut, where absorption occurs. Both sexes of the stable fly, *Stomoxys calcitrans*, ingest nectar that is likewise directed to the diverticulum. The process of sugar meal movement from the crop into the midgut is probably closely regulated in relation to the physiological needs within the hemolymph (Gelperin 1971). Ingested nectar has an osmotic concentration of solutes well above the osmotic concentration in the hemolymph. Thus, storing nectar in the impermeable diverticulum, or diverticula in the case of mosquitoes, and then slowly releasing it for absorption probably protects the insect from osmotic shock and enables it to ingest a concentrated source of energy. The "switch mechanism," whereby blood is directed to the posterior midgut and nectar (sugar solutions) to the diverticula, has not been elucidated, but sensilla associated with the mouthparts and in the cibarial cavity, as well as the stomatogastric nervous system, are probably involved.

Hematophagous insects commonly ingest several times their weight in blood, and blood meal size varies with several factors, including temperature, stage, feeding history, etc. Representative estimates of blood meal size appear in Figure 18.10. Regulation of blood meal size is generally mediated by stretch receptors that respond to distention. These receptors are associated with the muscles along the alimentary canal itself and/or the expandable body wall of the abdomen. For example, multipolar neurons, suggestive of stretch receptor function, have been described in various parts of the foregut in adult tsetse flies (Chapman 1985b). Further, cutting the ventral nerve cord in female *Aedes aegypti* mosquitoes results in the ingestion of much larger than normal blood meals (Gwadz 1969).

The time it takes for a given arthropod to digest a blood meal is influenced by the volume ingested, ambient temperature, age, and blood meal source as well as other factors. Estimates of average time for blood meal digestion are provided in Lehane (1991). Time required for digestion varies. It takes 4 hours for *Pediculus humanus* (the human body louse), 60–130 hours for various mosquito species, 168 hours for the bed bug *Cimex lectularius*, and 376 hours for the kissing bug *Triatoma infestans*.

The sustained presence of blood in the midgut and subsequent release of the undigested remains are mediated through the operation of the pyloric valve. The control of this valve has not been thoroughly studied;

however, in mosquitoes the passage of the undigested remains of a blood meal appears to be under hormonal control, release of blood from the midgut into the hindgut apparently being induced by the ecdysone secreted by the ovaries (Rosenberg 1980).

Blood digestion and absorption occur in the midgut (Table 18.2). Lehane (1991) describes 2 basic strategies in this respect, batch and continuous digestion. Batch digestion occurs in the sucking lice, fleas, and nematocerous Diptera. The blood bolus is digested

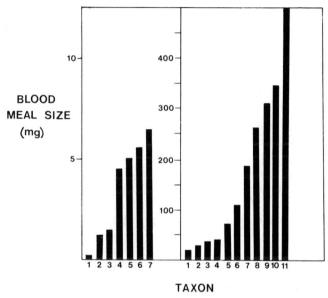

TAXON

18.10 Estimated amounts of blood ingested by various arthropods. Data from Balashov (1972) and Gooding (1972). 0–10 mg scale: 1 = *Leptoconops kertezi* (Diptera, Ceratopogonidae), 2 = *Pediculus humanus* (Phthiraptera, Pediculidae), 3 = *Simulium rugglesi* (Diptera, Simuliidae), 4 = *Aedes aegypti* (Diptera, Culicidae), 5 = *Culex pipiens* (Diptera, Culicidae), 6 = *Anopheles quadrimaculatus* (Diptera, Culicidae), 7 = *Cimex lectularius* (Hemiptera, Cimicidae). 0–500 mg scale: 1 = *Stomoxys calcitrans* (Diptera, Muscidae), 2 = *Psorophora ciliata* (Diptera, Culicidae), 3 = *Glossina morsitans* (Diptera, Muscidae), 4 = *Chrysops silacea* (Diptera, Tabanidae), 5 = *Tabanus quinquerittatus* (Diptera, Tabanidae), 6 = *Glossina brevipalpus* (Diptera, Muscidae), 7 = *Rhodnius prolixus* (Hemiptera, Reduviidae), 8 = *Ixodes persulcatus* (Acari, Ixodidae), 9 = *Triatoma infestans* (Hemiptera, Reduviidae), 10 = *Tabanus sulcifrons* (Diptera, Tabanidae), 11 = *Dermacentor pictus* (Acari, Ixodidae).

over its entire surface, and apparently the same cells are involved in the synthesis and secretion of digestive enzymes as well as the absorption of the products of digestion. In continuous digestion, found in the blood-sucking Hemiptera and tsetse flies, blood is passed gradually from the storage portion of the midgut into the more specialized posterior regions where digestion and absorption occur.

Peritrophic matrices are formed in some bloodsucking insects and presumably not in others. Peritrophic matrices are apparently absent in the sucking lice and fleas but present in the bloodsucking Diptera. Extra-cellular membranes occur around the blood bolus in the kissing bugs but probably do not contain chitin and are different in other ways from typical peritrophic matrices (Peters 1992). The 2 basic patterns of peritrophic matrix formation described earlier are illustrated by the bloodsucking Diptera. In mosquitoes, the midgut epithelium secretes the peritrophic matrix around the blood bolus, and a plug of peritrophic matrix material forms, separating the lumen of the tubular anterior midgut from the posterior midgut, which contains the blood meal. The suggestion has been made that this plug of material separates the blood-digesting/absorbing posterior midgut from the tubular anterior midgut into which slugs of nectar (sugar solution) stored in the diverticula could be released from the diverticula and digested and absorbed in the anterior midgut at the same time blood is being digested in the posterior midgut (Richardson and Romoser 1972). In tsetse flies, the peritrophic matrix is secreted and formed by the cardia and runs posteriorly throughout the midgut as a blood-containing tube.

Earlier interpretations portrayed the peritrophic matrix as a structure that prevents the gut epithelial cells from the abrasive action of food particles. Although this may be true in some insects that ingest particulate food, the presence of a peritrophic matrix in many fluid-feeding insects, including those that ingest blood, has resulted in other hypotheses regarding such parameters as permeability, involvement in the process of digestion, interaction with or protection from parasites in the blood, and so on. The position of this noncellular matrix in the midgut between the food bolus, in which ingested parasites and microbes may reside, and the midgut epithelium (the "gateway to the hemocoel"), makes this structure of great interest in vector biology (see Chap. 19).

As explained earlier, the foregut, cardia, and probably the midgut are innervated by the stomatogastric nervous system. The detailed functioning of the stomatogastric system has not been described, but involvement in monitoring diverticular distention and the operation of valves or sphincters associated with the crop and cardia seems likely.

In addition to digestion and absorption of food and excretory functions, the alimentary canal is also involved in the process of ecdysis. It provides the expansion needed to direct hemostatic pressure against the preformed ecdysial cleavage lines in the undigested old cuticle, causing the exuvia to split and allowing the next instar to emerge. Some insects gulp air to aid in the expansion process; others gulp water.

PROCESSING THE BLOOD MEAL

The acquisition of a meal usually involves finding a host that, like the insects themselves, moves about. Hematophagous insects are of necessity periodic feeders. When a blood-feeding insect does successfully ingest a blood meal, a cascade of events is set into motion that culminates in both the extraction of nutrients from the meal and disposal of the undigested waste. This section presents an overview of the processes by which the components of vertebrate blood are converted to raw materials used by the blood-feeding insect. More comprehensive discussions of this topic may be found in Gooding (1972) and Lehane (1991). Clements (1992) also contains very useful discussions of blood meal digestion, focusing on mosquitoes.

Blood processing by a hematophagous insect involves several major steps: (1) the removal of excess water from the blood meal, (2) the breakdown of vertebrate blood cells (hemolysis), (3) the hydrolytic degradation of macromolecules in the blood meal (digestion), and (4) the absorption of small molecules produced by digestion into the midgut epithelial cells and subsequently into the hemocoel.

As with cells and biological fluids in general, blood is approximately 80% water. By volume, vertebrate blood is approximately 55% plasma (the fluid fraction) and 45% cells (Dow 1986). The weight of excess water is no doubt a liability to an insect, a liability that is addressed almost immediately after blood is ingested. Water is removed from a blood meal by an osmotic gradient between the midgut lumen, the midgut epithelial cells, and the hemolymph. This gradient is probably produced by the active transport of ions, such as sodium and potassium, and facilitates the passive diffusion of water from the midgut lumen (Chap. 17). Correlated with the absorption of water from the blood meal, for example in bloodsucking bugs and mosquitoes, is an increase in volume of the extracellular spaces of the basal labyrinth. At the same time, the urine flow in the Malpighian tubules (diuresis) increases significantly, promoting completion of the water removal process by rapidly shunting it to the hindgut for egestion. Diuresis is probably under hormonal control in all hemotophagous insects. For example, in response to a blood meal, a diuretic hormone is detectable in the hemolymph of the bloodsucking bug *Rhodnius prolixus* (Maddrell and Gardiner 1976). In the mosquito *Aedes aegypti*, peptides stored in the head are thought to control diuresis (Wheelock et al. 1988). Removal of water not only allows an insect to resume mobility as quickly as possible following a blood meal but also aids in the clumping and congealing of the blood bolus, an effect that probably aids the digestive process.

Most of the protein and other nutrients in vertebrate blood are locked up in the cells; the breakdown of these cells (hemolysis) releases the cellular macromolecules, making them accessible to the digestive enzymes. Hemolysis may be achieved mechanically or biochemically. For example, in mosquitoes, there is a correlation between the presence and extent of development of the cibarial armature (Coluzzi et al. 1982) and the degree of red blood cell breakdown. The proteolytic enzyme trypsin probably also functions as a major hemolytic factor in mosquitoes. Other hemolytic factors, small peptides and free fatty acids, have been recognized in hematophagous insects.

Blood-feeding insects have full complements of hydrolytic enzymes, including proteases, carbohydrases, and esterases that are used to split macromolecules in blood into absorbable units. Because vertebrate blood is mostly protein, proteases play a prominent role in blood digestion (Fig. 18.11). The strategy in protein digestion in hematophagous insects is similar to that in other animals. Protein molecules are degraded into large polypeptides by endopeptidases (for example, trypsin and chymotrypsin), and then single amino acids or dipeptides are cleaved from both ends of the large peptides by endopeptidases (for example, aminopeptidases and carboxypeptidases, which act respectively at the N-terminal and C-terminal ends of a polypeptide chain). For example, analyses of enzyme activity in mosquito midguts have revealed the presence and activity of trypsin (Fig. 18.12) and chymotrypsin as well as aminopeptidase (Fig. 18.12) and carboxypeptidase activity (Clements 1992). Likewise, glycosidase (Fig. 18.12) and esterase activity has been detected in the midguts of various mosquitoes.

The synthesis of enzymes occurs in the midgut epithelium, and it appears to be initiated in response to a blood meal in the midgut. Several kinds of stimuli

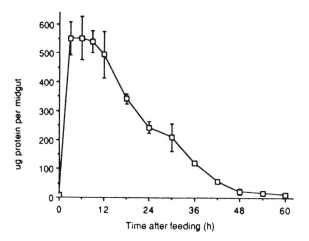

18.11 Protein digestion following blood meal in the mosquito *Anopheles stephensi*. Adapted from P.F. Billingsley and H. Hecker 1991, *Blood digestion in the mosquito* Anopheles stephensi *Liston (Diptera: Culicidae): Activity and distribution of trypsin, aminopeptidase and x-glucosidase in the midgut. J. Med. Entom.* 28:865–867. Used with permission.

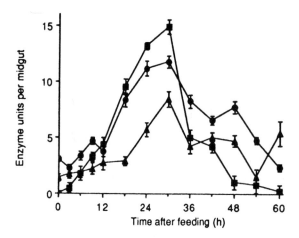

18.12 Enzyme activity following a blood meal in the mosquito *Anopheles stephensi*; squares = trypsin, circles = aminopeptidase, triangles = alpha-glucosidase. Adapted from P.F. Billingsley and H. Hecker 1991. *Blood digestion in the mosquito* Anopheles stephensi *Liston (Diptera: Culicidae): Activity and distribution of trypsin, aminopeptidase and x-glucosidase in the midgut. J. Med. Entom.* 28:865–867. Used with permission.

can be involved in inducing the synthesis and secretion of enzymes: neural, secretogogue, osmotic, and mechanical. Even in mosquitoes, the picture is incomplete, but evidence points to the action of a secretogogue (a chemical in the blood meal) as the most important stimulus involved in the induction of trypsin synthesis (Briegel and Lea 1975), although mechanical and osmotic factors may also be involved (Graf and Briegel 1989). Studies involving the experimental removal of known hormone-secreting tissues have provided evidence of endocrine involvement in the control of enzyme synthesis (Clements 1992). The amino acid sequence of one of the midgut trypsins has recently been elucidated (Barillas-Mury et al. 1992). This group's studies of midgut enzyme synthesis and regulation at the molecular level have revealed the presence of early and late trypsins that function in regulation of enzyme synthesis and digestion of blood meals (Chap. 2).

Structural changes in the midgut epithelium in association with blood-feeding have been described for a number of hematophagous insects (Billingsley 1990).

A particularly rigorous and quantitative series of studies (Hecker et al. 1974; Hecker and Rudin 1981) have been carried out with mosquitoes. A major structural change associated with the presence of a blood meal in the midgut is, of course, the profound stretching of the posterior midgut epithelium. This stretching results in the stretching of the basal lamina, which nearly doubles the pore size of the basal lamina (Reinhardt and Hecker 1973). Other changes include an increase in the cytoplasmic volume of the midgut epithelial cells, increases in the surface area of both rough and smooth endoplasmic reticulum, and the appearance of secretory vesicles that, on the basis of immunocytochemical labeling, contain trypsin (Rudin and Hecker 1979). These changes are directly associated with the extensive protein (enzyme) synthesis in response to the presence of a blood meal.

The absorption process occurs differently in insects that carry out continuous digestion versus those that digest by the batch method. In insects that continuously digest, for example, tsetse flies (Table 18.2), absorption occurs in a specialized gut region posterior to the region where digestion occurs; in those with batch digestion, e.g., mosquitoes (Table 18.2), the same cells that synthesize and secrete digestive enzymes apparently also carry out absorption.

Although no specific structural changes have been observed in association with absorption, the transitory appearance of various substances in the gut epithelial cells, e.g., lipid granules, is taken as an indication of absorptive activity. Structural adaptations that clearly facilitate the movement of molecules across cell membranes are evident in the enormous surface area afforded by the microvilli on the luminal (apical) side of the midgut and by the extensive basal labyrinth on the hemocoel side (basal).

Processes involved in absorption of nutrients range from simple diffusion to various energy-using mechanisms (active transport). For example, the absorption of sugar into the hemolymph from the the lumen of the anterior midgut is by simple diffusion. The glucose concentration gradient between the midgut lumen and the hemolymph is maintained by the synthesis of the disaccharide trehalose (linkage of 2 glucose molecules) in the hemolymph. The absorption of amino acids has not been described in hematophagous insects, but given the high concentration of amino acids characteristic of insect hemolymph, luminal amino acids are probably transported to the hemolymph by active transport. Likewise, little is known about lipid absorption or the absorption of various other molecules, such as vitamins and minerals, in hematophagous insects.

In addition to the midgut epithelial cells that carry out digestion and absorption and the regenerative cells, scattered endocrine-like cells have been identified in several hematophagous insect species, including several mosquitoes, sand flies, adult fleas, and the triatomine bug *Rhodnius prolixus* (a bloodsucking hemipteran) (Brown and Lea 1989). In the mosquito *Aedes aegypti*, the cytoplasm of these cells is less electron dense than that of the other midgut cells. Some of these cells reach the lumen and have microvilli; others do not. It is possible that these cells are involved with the coordination of alimentary and excretory processes with feeding behavior.

ALIMENTARY STRUCTURE AND FUNCTION IN TICKS

Compared to that of hematophagous insects, the tick alimentary system has received much less attention. In Coons et al. (1986) adult *Dermacentor variabilis* (the American dog tick) is used as a representative hard tick (family Ixodidae) and *Ornithodorus moubata* as a representative soft tick (family Argasidae). Coons et al. contains detailed descriptions of our current knowledge of the tick alimentary system. Other texts that include information on the alimentary process in ticks are Balashov (1968; 1983), Woolley (1988), and Evans (1992).

Ticks, like insects, possess 3 general regions (Fig. 18.13) in the alimentary canal, the foregut, midgut, and hindgut. And like insects, the foregut and hindgut are lined with a chitinous intima that is continuous with the integumentary cuticle. Peritrophic matrix has been found in the midguts of at least some species of Ixodidae and Argasidae (Peters 1992). Also, circular and longitudinal visceral muscles propel blood and undigested wastes along the length of the alimentary canal.

The foregut is composed of a sucking pharynx and food-conducting esophagus. Posterior movement of ingested blood is presumably maintained by valves in the foregut. A valvular structure separates the foregut and midgut. The midgut is composed of the anterior ventriculus and posterior rectal tube. The ventriculus is greatly expandable, a process facilitated by the presence of multiple blind sacs or diverticula. The undifferentiated midgut epithelial cells in unfed adult ticks have few microvilli, lack a glycocalyx, and have relatively few cytoplasmic organelles. Lipid inclusions, glycogen granules, and residual bodies remaining from the nymphal stage can be present. The rectal tube connects the diverticulate ventriculus to the hindgut, which consists of an anterior, well-musculated small intestine (rectal bulb) and posterior rectal sac (rectum or anal canal). One or 2 pairs of Malpighian tubules open into the small intestine.

The foregut functions in the acquisition of blood and its movement into the midgut. Digestion of the blood meal takes place in the ventriculus and, in contrast to

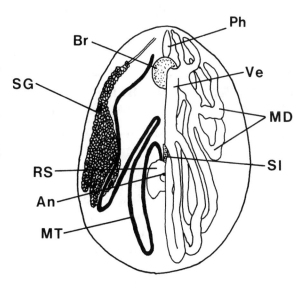

18.13 Ixodid tick alimentary canal. (An) anus, (Br) brain, (Ph) pharynx, (MD) middle diverticulum, (MT) Malpighian tubule, (RS) rectal sac, (SG) salivary gland, (SI) small intestine, (Ve) ventriculus. Adapted from Balashov 1972. *Bloodsucking ticks (Ixodoidea): Vectors of diseases of man and animals.* Trans. (T500) Medical Zoology Dept. U.S. Naval Medical Research Unit No. 3, Cairo, Egypt. Misc. Publications of the Entomol. Soc. America, Vol. 8.

insects, is an intracellular, endocytotic process occurring in the midgut epithelial cells. Undigested wastes remain in the cells as residual bodies, which form from secondary lysosomes (the products of fusion of lysosomes and endosomes). Midgut epithelial cells filled with residual bodies slough into the lumen and are replaced by replacement cells. In addition to digestive and replacement cells, female ixodid ticks also have vitellogenic cells which, along with the fat body, produce vitellogenin, the precursor molecule that is converted to the yolk protein vitellin in the ovaries. Digestive, replacement, and vitellogenic cells differentiate from unspecialized midgut epithelial cells. Apparently, argasid ticks lack well-defined vitellogenic cells, and the midgut does not produce large quantities of vitellogen. Although the basic process of blood meal digestion appears to be similar in hard and soft ticks, the timing in each is correlated with reproductive differences between the 2 families. The Malpighian tubules are involved in the excretion of nitrogenous wastes. The occurrence of water reabsorption in the hindgut has not been clearly established.

THE ARTHROPOD GUT AS A GATEWAY AND HABITAT FOR VECTOR-BORNE PATHOGENS

This chapter is not intended to describe the detailed mechanisms of arthropod host/microbe interactions in the alimentary canal; however, a few general comments in this regard seem appropriate. Both intrinsic and extrinsic factors are involved in determining the competence of a given individual arthropod to support the life activities of pathogenic microorganisms long enough to be transmitted to a vertebrate host. The alimentary canal is often the only arthropod "internal" habitat to which many vertebrate blood-borne pathogens are exposed. Hence a significant number of the intrinsic factors that influence vector competence no doubt act within the alimentary canal. In an evolutionary context, it is in the alimentary canal that microbial and arthropodan genomic expressions first come into contact and have the potential to act as agents of natural selection on one another. What, then, do microbes

do in the arthropod alimentary canal, and how might they be influenced by alimentary processes?

Upon ingestion, blood typically goes to the midgut. Pathogenic microorganisms contained therein, depending on the species involved, follow 1 of 3 patterns: (1) Some use the midgut as a gateway to the hemocoel, infect the midgut epithelial cells soon after ingestion, and then escape into the hemocoel; (2) some use the midgut as a gateway to the hemocoel, but only after they undergo cyclic and/or multiplicative changes in the lumen; and finally, (3) some remain in the alimentary canal, later to be shed from the arthropod via the mouthparts or the rectum.

An example of the 1st pattern is the attachment to, and subsequent infection of, midgut epithelial cells by arboviruses (Chap. 4). Arboviruses attach to receptor molecules associated with the epithelial cell membranes and enter the host cells soon after contact. Within the midgut cells they replicate and are eventually released into the hemocoel, where they can infect other tissues, including the salivary glands and ovaries (Hardy 1988; Leake 1992). A good example of the 2nd pattern is the malaria parasites that carry out fertilization within the midgut lumen, forming the ookinetes that then penetrate the midgut epithelium and lodge between the epithelial cells and the basal lamina, where they undergo further differentiation before invading the hemocoel. Plague bacilli in fleas and the trypanosomes, which cause Chagas' disease, are examples of the 3rd pattern. Plague bacilli multiply in the midgut, often reaching a point where they block the lumen and prevent the movement of blood (taken during subsequent feeding attempts) into the midgut (Lehane 1991). When a blocked flea attempts to feed, plague bacilli are regurgitated into the feeding puncture. In the case of the triatomine bugs and the trypanosomes that cause Chagas' disease, the trypanosomes eventually invade the lumen of the rectum and are released in the droplets of fluid that pass from the anus during blood meal ingestion (Chap. 10).

Within the arthropod alimentary canal, a microorganism ingested with a blood meal encounters a multitude of structural and physiological/biochemical characteristics that can influence its survival. For example, the noncellular peritrophic matrix can be an effective physical barrier, preventing the midgut epithelium from infection or penetration. Ponnudurai et al. (1981) suggest that in the case of human malarial plasmodia, vector specificity among anopheline mosquitoes is determined by the rate of peritrophic matrix formation versus the rate of ookinete production. Other factors in the alimentary canal that can interfere with a microbe's success include various sorts of cuticular structures such as the cibarial armature or spines protruding into the lumen; sudden rushes of fluid that occur with the ingestion of blood or sugar meals, with the voiding of the rectum associated with defecation or with the flow of fluid from the lumens of the Malpighian tubules; batteries of hydrolytic enzymes secreted in response to a blood meal; changes in the osmolarity of the contents of the midgut and rectum when small molecules, ions, and water are absorbed into the hemocoel or when waste materials are flushed into the hindgut lumen from the Malpighian tubules; and variations in the hydrogen ion concentration of the luminal contents.

In a more passive way, the alimentary environment may fail to provide for some particular need or needs of a given pathogen. For example, specific cell surface receptor molecules necessary for the successful attachment of an arbovirus may be lacking, in very low density, or be occluded in some way, thus preventing cell entry and subsequent replication of the virus. Or the alimentary canal may fail to provide some critical nutrient or nutrients, or a microhabitat suitable for pathogen development. Further, a specific chemical signal (or signals) required to stimulate multiplication and/or cyclic changes may be absent.

Although many aspects of the biology of vector arthropods and pathogens have been extensively studied, our understanding of the molecular dynamics of arthropod host/microbe interactions, including those that determine vector competence and host specificity, is very limited. However, the potential for great strides in this area has increased dramatically in recent years with impressive developments in molecular biology and the advent of sophisticated molecular and immunocytochemical tools for in situ labeling studies in association with light and electron microscopy

(Howard 1993; Beltz and Burd 1989). For a recent example of current approaches and thinking, Miller and Lehane (1993) provide a thought-provoking overview of the interactions between parasitic protozoa, the peritrophic matrix, and cell surface molecules in their host arthropods.

REFERENCES AND FURTHER READING

Applebaum, S.W. 1985. Biochemistry of digestion. In: G.A. Kerkut and L.I. Gilbert, editors, *Comprehensive insect physiology, biochemistry, and pharmacology*, Vol. 4. Oxford and New York: Pergamon Press. pp. 279–311.

Balashov, Y.S. 1972. *Blood-sucking ticks (Ixodoidea)—Vectors of Diseases of Man and Animals.* (A translation.) *Misc. Publ. Entomol. Soc. Amer.* 8(5):161–376.

Balashov, Y.U., ed. 1983. *An atlas of tick ultrastructure.* A.S. Raikel, translator; A.S. Raikel and H. Hoogstraal, editors. College Park, MD: Entomol. Soc. Amer. Special Publication.

Barillas-Mury, C., R. Graf, H.H. Hagedorn, and M.A. Wells. 1991. cDNA and deduced amino acid sequence of a blood meal-induced trypsin from the mosquito *Aedes aegypti. Insect Biochem.* 21:825–831.

Beltz, B.S., and G.D. Burd. 1988. *Immunocytochemical techniques: Principles and practice.* Cambridge, MA: Blackwell Scientific Publications.

Berridge, M.J. 1970. A structural analysis of intestinal absorption. In: A.C. Neville, editor, *Insect ultrastructure.* Oxford: Blackwell Scientific Publications. pp. 135–151.

Billingsley, P.F. 1990. The midgut ultrastructure of hematophagous insects. *Ann. Rev. Entomol.* 35:219–248.

Billingsley, P.F., and H.H. Hecker. 1991. Blood digestion in the mosquito, *Anopheles stephensi* Liston (Diptera: Culicidae): Activity and distribution of trypsin, aminopeptidase, and a-glucosidase in the midgut. *J. Med. Entomol.* 26(6):865–871.

Bradley, T.J. 1985. The excretory system: Structure and physiology. In: G.A. Kerkut and L.I. Gilbert, editors, *Comprehensive insect physiology, biochemistry, and pharmacology*, Vol. 4. Oxford and New York: Pergamon Press. pp. 421–465

Briegel, H., and A.O. Lea. 1975. Relationship between protein and proteolytic activity in the midgut of mosquitoes. *J. Insect Physiol.* 21:1597–1604.

Brown, M.R., and A.O. Lea. 1989. Neuroendocrine and midgut endocrine systems in the adult mosquito. In: *Advances in disease vector research*, Vol. 6. New York: Springer-Verlag. pp. 29–58

Buchner, P. 1965. *Endosymbiosis of animals with plant microorganisms*. New York: Wiley-Interscience.

Burgess, L., and J.G. Rempel. 1966. The stomodael nervous system, the neurosecretory system, and the gland complex in *Aedes aegypti* (L.). *Can. J. Zool.* 44:731–765.

Chapman, R.F. 1982. *The Insects—Structure and function*, 3rd ed. Cambridge, MA: Harvard University Press.

Chapman, R.F. 1985a. Structure of the Digestive System. In: G.A. Kerkut and L.I. Gilbert, editors, *Comprehensive insect physiology, biochemistry, and pharmacology*, Vol. 4. Oxford and New York: Pergamon Press. pp. 165–211.

Chapman, R.F. 1985b. Coordination of Digestion. In: G.A. Kerkut and L.I. Gilbert, editors, *Comprehensive insect physiology, biochemistry, and pharmacology*, Vol. 4. Oxford and New York: Pergamon Press. pp. 213–240.

Clements, A.N. 1992. *The biology of mosquitoes*, Vol.1. Development, nutrition, and reproduction. New York and London: Chapman and Hall.

Coluzzi, M., A. Concretti, and F. Ascoli. 1982. Effect of cibarial armature of mosquitoes (Diptera, Culicidae) on blood-meal haemolysis. *J. Insect Physiol.* 28:885–888.

Coons, L.B., R. Rosell-Davis, and B.I. Tarnoski. 1986. Bloodmeal digestion in ticks. In: J.R. Sauer and J.A. Hair, editors, *Morphology, physiology, and behavioral biology of ticks*. New York: John Wiley & Sons. pp. 248–279.

Dow, J.A.T. 1986. Insect midgut function. *Adv. Insect Physiol.* 19:187–303.

Evans, G.O. 1992. *Principles of acarology*. Oxon, UK: C*A*B International.

Farmer, J., S.H.P. Maddrell, and J.H. Spring. 1981. Absorption of fluid by the midgut of *Rhodnius*. *J. Exp. Biol.* 94:301–316.

Ferris, G.F. 1951. The sucking lice. *Mem. Pacific Coast Entomol. Soc.* 1:1–320.

Gelperin, A. 1971. Regulation of feeding. *Ann. Rev. Entomol.* 16:365–372.

Glasgow, J.P. 1963. *The distribution and abundance of tsetse*. New York: Macmillan Co.

Gooding, R.H. 1972. Digestive processes of haematophagous insects. *Quaest. Entomol.* 8:5–60.

Graf, R., and H. Briegel. 1989. The synthetic pathway of trypsin in the mosquito *Aedes aegypti* L. (Diptera: Culicidae) and in vitro stimulation in isolated midguts. *Insect Biochem.* 19:129–137.

Gwadz, R.W. 1969. Regulation of blood meal size in the mosquito. *J. Insect Physiol.* 15:2039–2044.

Hardy, J.L. 1988. Susceptibility and resistance of vector mosquitoes. In: T.P. Monath, editor, *The arboviruses: Epidemiology and ecology*, Vol. 1. Boca Raton, FL: CRC Press. pp. 87–126.

Harwood, R.F., and M.T. James. 1979. *Entomology in human and animal health*, 7th ed. New York: Macmillan Publishing Co.

Hecker, H., R. Brun, and C. Reinhardt. 1974. Morphometric analysis of the midgut of female *Aedes aegypti* (L.) (Insecta, Diptera) under various physiological conditions. *Cell Tissue Res.* 152:31–49.

Hecker, H., and W. Rudin. 1981. Morphometric parameters of the midgut cells of *Aedes aegypti* (L.) (Insecta, Diptera) under various conditions. *Cell Tissue Res.* 219:619–627.

Howard, G.C., editor. 1993. *Methods in nonradioactive detection*. Norwalk, CT: Appleton and Lange.

King, R.C., and H. Akai. 1984. *Insect ultrastructure*, Vol. 2. New York: Plenum Press.

Leake, C.J. 1992. Arbovirus-mosquito interactions and vector specificity. *Parasit. Today* 8(4):123–128.

Lehane, M.J. 1991. *Biology of blood-sucking insects*. London: Harper Collins Academic.

Maddrell, S.H.P., and B.O.C. Gardiner. 1976. Diuretic hormone in adult *Rhodnius prolixus*: Total store and speed of release. *Physiol. Entomol.* 1:265–269.

Marshall, A.G. 1981. *The ecology of ectoparasitic insects*. New York: Academic Press.

Miller, N., and M.J. Lehane. 1993. Peritrophic membranes, cell surface molecules and parasite tropisms within arthropod vectors. *Parasit. Today* 9(2):45–50.

Peters, W. 1992. *Peritrophic membranes*. New York: Springer-Verlag.

Phillips, J.E., N. Audsley, R. Lechleitner, B. Thomson, J. Meredith, and M. Chamberlin. 1988. Some major transport mechanisms of insect absorptive epithelia. *Comp. Biochem. Physiol.* 90A(4):643–650.

Ponnudurai, T., P.F. Billingsley, and W. Rudin. 1988. Differential infectivity of Plasmodium for mosquitoes. *Parasit. Today* 4(11):319–321.

Reinhardt, C., and H. Hecker. 1973. Structure and function of the basal lamina and of the cell junctions in the midgut epithelium (stomach) of female *Aedes aegypti* L. (Insecta, Diptera). *Acta Tropica* 30:213–236.

Richards, A.G., and P. Richards. 1971. Origin and composition of the peritrophic membrane of the mosquito, *Aedes aegypti. J. Insect Physiol.* 17:2253–2275.

Richardson, M.W., and W.S. Romoser. 1972. The formation of the peritrophic membrane in adult *Aedes triseriatus* (Say) (Diptera: Culicidae). *J. Med. Entomol.* 9(6):495–500.

Romoser, W.S., and J.G. Stoffolano Jr. 1994. *The science of entomology*, 3rd ed. Dubuque, IA: Wm. C. Brown Publishers.

Rosenberg, R. 1980. Ovarian control of blood meal retention in the mosquito *Anopheles freeborni. J. Insect Physiol.* 26:477–480.

Rothschild, M., Y. Schlein, and S. Ito. 1986. *A Colour Atlas of Insect Tissues—Via the Flea.* London: Wolfe Publishing.

Rudin, W., and H. Hecker. 1979. Functional morphology of the midgut of *Aedes aegypti* L. (Insecta, Diptera) during blood digestion. *Cell Tissue Res.* 200:193–203.

Smith, J.J.B. 1985. Feeding mechanisms. In: A. Kerkut and L.I. Gilbert, editors, *Comprehensive insect physiology, biochemistry, and pharmacology*, Vol. 4. Oxford and New York: Pergamon Press. pp. 33–86.

Snodgrass, R.E. 1935. *Principles of insect morphology.* New York: McGraw-Hill Book Co.

Snodgrass, R.E. 1959. *The anatomical life of the mosquito.* Smithsonian Misc. Collections, Vol. 139, Number 8. Washington, DC: Smithsonian Institution.

Turunen, S. 1985. Absorption. In: G.A. Kerkut and L.I. Gilbert, editors, *Comprehensive insect physiology, biochemistry, and pharmacology*, Vol. 4. Oxford and New York: Pergamon Press. pp. 241–277.

Usinger, R.L. 1966. *Monograph of cimicidae* (Hemiptera-Heteroptera). Thomas Say Foundation, Vol. 7. College Park, MD: Entomological Society of America, 595 p.

Wheelock, G.D., D.H. Petzel, J.D. Gillett, K.W. Beyenback, and H.H. Hagedorn. 1988. Evidence for hormonal control of diuresis after a blood meal in the mosquito *Aedes aegypti. Arch. Insect Biochem. and Physiol.* 7:75–89.

Wigglesworth, V.B. 1972. *The principles of insect physiology*, 7th ed. London: Chapman and Hall.

Woolley, T.A. 1988. *Acarology.* New York: John Wiley & Sons.

Yuval, B. 1992. The other habit: Sugar feeding by mosquitoes. *Bull. Soc. Vector Ecol.* 17(2):150–156.

19. THE PERITROPHIC MATRIX OF INSECTS

Marcelo Jacobs-Lorena and Maung Maung Oo

INTRODUCTION

The gastrointestinal tract of most insects possesses a layer of acellular material separating ingested food from the gut epithelial cells. This layer is called peritrophic membrane or matrix (PM). Our knowledge about this structure is incomplete; however, there has been a recent surge of interest in PM because of its possible significance as a barrier to various pathogens.

READING SOURCES

The literature on the peritrophic matrix is vast. Three general sources of review articles are Peters (1992), by far the most complete and recent source; Richards and Richards (1977), which although dated, remains one of the most useful introductory texts on the subject; and Peters (1976), another well-written review.

INITIAL REMARKS

Name

This chapter differs from the usual treatment of the subject in 2 respects: the name and the emphasis on PM types. The "peri" in "peritrophic" comes from the Greek word for around; "trophic" is from the Greek word for food. Thus the name fits because the PM invariably surrounds the food bolus. However, the concept of membrane has evolved significantly since the term "peritrophic membrane" was first coined over 100 years ago. Today "membrane" signifies a lipid bilayer, which the PM is certainly not. Moreover, the PM of certain insects is not a firm membrane but a sheath of friable cheesy material of amorphous appearance covering the food bolus. The word "matrix" appropriately describes this structure. Accordingly, the term "peritrophic matrix" is used throughout this chapter.

Types of PM

As will be described later, there are 2 classes of PM, type 1 and type 2, that are now universally accepted. This chapter is unusual because it emphasizes the distinct biology of these 2 types. Thus, the abbreviations PM1 and PM2 will be used often and when appropriate.

Even though the PM is found in an extremely broad array of animal phyla (Peters 1992), this chapter focuses only on insects of medical importance. Thus, statements made in this text might not apply to PMs in every organism.

PERITROPHIC MATRIX

What Is the Peritrophic Matrix?

The PM is an extracellular matrix containing chitin that lines the gut epithelium of most insects. It was first described in 1762 by Lyonet in a caterpillar (Peters 1976). The name "peritrophic membrane" was first proposed by Balbiani (1890), who referred to this structure as a "membranous sac that directly encloses

TABLE 19.1 Comparison properties of PM1 and PM2

	PM1	**PM2**
Secretory cells	most cells in the expandable part of the midgut	specialized cells of the cardia at the foregut and midgut junction
Secretory stimulus	expansion of midgut epithelium	none; secreted constitutively
Rate of secretion	highly variable among species and also among individuals. Range 6 to 48 hr	1 to 10 mm/hr, 2 to 5 mm/hr most common
Thickness	2 to 20 μm is common	usually less than 1 μm
Chitin	present in most PMs	present in most PMs

the food bolus inside the gut." This definition remains valid, even though various other definitions have also been proposed. For practical purposes the PM can be thought of as a structure that functions strictly in the gut. However, there are some odd exceptions such as the case of some beetles that use the PM for building cocoons.

PM1 AND PM2

PM1 and PM2 are 2 types of peritrophic matrix that have different properties (Fig. 19.1 and Table 19.1). Each insect species and each developmental stage (larva versus adult) produces either PM1 or PM2 but not both.

PM1

The PM1 is a thick extracellular matrix secreted around a blood meal by midgut epithelial cells. The thickness of PM1 is typically ranges from 2–20 μm. PM1 is the most common type of PM in bloodsucking insects, such as mosquitoes, black flies, and sand flies. Notable exceptions are the tsetse fly (*Glossina* spp.) and the stable fly *Stomoxys calcitrans*, which secrete PM2 (Lehane 1976).

Secretion

In insects that secrete PM1, no PM is present in the gut prior to the blood meal. Accordingly, no PM can be detected in insects kept in the laboratory on a sucrose diet. The secretion of the PM1 is triggered by the dramatic distention of the midgut epithelium during ingestion of the blood meal. Most epithelial cells surrounding the blood mass are believed to contribute to the formation of the PM1. Even while the insect is feeding, a large amount of liquid is removed by diuresis from the blood meal through the gut wall. Thus, hematophagous insects can ingest blood meals that are often equal or even twice their own body weight. The Malpighian tubules then capture the excess liquid and eliminate it through the hindgut. After liquid removal, a large mass of compacted erythrocytes remain, in the lumen of the expandable midgut. Electron microscopy reveals a clear cell-free zone between the blood mass and the distended epithelium as early as 2 minutes after the blood meal (abm) (Reid and Lehane 1984). It is from this clear zone that the PM is formed. By feeding mosquitoes with a blood-ferritin mixture, Perrone and Spielman (1988) showed that ferritin was present in the clear zone at 2 hr abm. Based on this result, the authors concluded that the clear zone represents extruded plasma and not PM material. Although demonstrating that plasma components might be incorporated into the PM, these experiments do not rule out the likely possibility that PM components secreted by epithelial cells make up at least part of the material in the clear zone.

Maturation

The PM1 is initially soft and fragile and cannot be physically isolated by dissection. Its presence can only be demonstrated microscopically after sectioning fixed guts. As the PM matures, it gradually thickens and solidifies and is consequently easier to dissect. When viewed by electron microscopy, the PM progressively acquires structure, frequently (but not always) in the form of 1 or more layers. The thickness of the mature PM1 varies from 1 individual to another, but its structure (i.e., layering) is characteristic for each species (Table 19.1). The time required for PM1 maturation is also species-specific (Table 19.2).

Induction

Several lines of evidence strongly suggest that the signal that activates PM secretion is the physical distention of the midgut epithelium. For instance, ingestion of a partial blood meal by *Anopheles* and *Simulium* does not trigger the secretion of a PM, although in *Aedes* a correlation appears to exist between the volume of blood ingested and the thickness of the PM1 formed (Freyvogel and Jaquet 1965; Reid and Lehane 1984). These results suggest that the chemical composition of the food cannot be the sole trigger for PM secretion and the *volume* of food ingested is a major determinant of PM1 secretion. Thus, in *Anopheles* and *Simulium*, PM secretion obeys the "all or none" rule, whereas in *Aedes* the degree of distention correlates with the amount of PM secreted. The strongest support for the hypothesis that distention is the major signal for PM secretion comes from the experiments of Freyvogel and Jaquet (1965), who used enemas (rectal injections) to show that saline, water, and even *air* can trigger the formation of the PM. Nothing is known about the mechanism by which the induction actually occurs. Since dramatic changes in cell shape take place, it is possible that certain cytoskeletal components could be involved in the induction pathway. The cloning of genes encoding PM components likely will provide additional tools to investigate this interesting question. It is also possible that stretch receptors on the gut wall elicit signals that activate certain neurological

TABLE 19.2   Time of PM1 formation in some medically important blood-feeding insects

First detected	Mature	First detected	Reference
Aedes aegypti	5 hr	12–17 hr	Stohler 1957
	4–8 hr	5–8 hr	Freyvogel and Stäubli 1965
		12 hr	Perrone and Spielman 1988
Anopheles gambiae		13 hr	Freyvogel and Stäubli 1965
Anopheles stephensi		32 hr	Freyvogel and Stäubli 1965
	12 hr	48 hr	Berner et al. 1983
Simulium ornatum	2–10 min	12–24 hr	Reid and Lehane 1984
Simulium equinum			
Simulium lineatum			
Simulium vitattum	20 min	6 hr	Ramos et al. 1993 (in prep.)
Phlebotomus longipes	< 24 hr	48 hr	Gemetchu 1974
Phlebotomus perniciosus	30 min	36 hr	Walters et al. 1993

Note: The times of peritrophic matrix type 1 formation in mosquitoes (*Aedes*, *Anopheles*), black flies (*Simulium*), and sand flies (*Phlebotomus*) are listed. It should be emphasized that "first detection" and "maturation" are based on highly subjective criteria and that in most cases an exhaustive time course of PM formation has not been attempted. Moreover, in any given experiment the parameters measured vary largely from individual to individual. Thus, the listed values serve only as guidelines.

pathways and ultimately produce the transcription of particular genes through chemical mediators. A way to test this possibility would be to observe PM formation after disruption of neuronal pathways.

PM2

Adults of many higher Diptera, the majority of which are non–blood-feeding, secrete PM2. The PM2 is a thin tubular sleeve, usually less than 1 µm thick, that lines the entire intestine. As noted earlier, the tsetse fly is an example of hematophagous insect that secretes PM2. Although most hematophagous insects secrete PM1 as adults, the larvae always secrete PM2. Thus, mosquitoes, black flies, and sand flies secrete PM2 during larval life and PM1 during adult life. Nothing is known about the relationship at the molecular level between the PM2 and PM1 of the same organism.

The Cardia

The PM2 is produced by a group of specialized cells called "cardia," situated at the junction of the foregut and the midgut. (In the literature this organ is often incorrectly referred to as the "proventriculus.") The cells of the cardia are continuous with the single-layer gut epithelium. In the region of the cardia, the epithelium folds twice upon itself, creating a protected pocket from which the PM2 is secreted (Fig. 19.2). The structure of the cardia is variable and is characteristic of each species. Different cell types can be identified microscopically within the cardia (King 1988). This differentiation is especially pronounced in the more evolutionary advanced species. When viewed with the electron microscope, the PM2 frequently has a layered appearance. Interestingly, the different layers seem to originate from different regions of the cardia, and each group of cells appears to be the origin of a specific PM2 component (Fig. 19.2b). This suggests that different cell types are specialized in the synthesis of different PM2 components. When genes encoding PM components are cloned, it will be possible to test this hypothesis by in situ hybridization techniques.

Secretion

The PM2 is secreted continuously, independent of food ingestion. Thus, the PM2 is a long and thin tube that originates in the cardia (foregut-midgut junction),

lines the entire midgut and hindgut, and is excreted with the feces through the anus. The rate of formation of the PM2 can be measured by various methods. The most direct is to physically measure the PM length that is extruded from the anus during a given time interval. The 2nd method takes advantage of 2 properties of some PM2s:

1. When appropriately stained (e.g., with the dichroitic dye Congo Red) and viewed with polarized light, the PM2 shows a regular pattern of cross striations.

2. When the organism is given a "cold pulse" by being momentarily placed at 5°C, the cross-banding pattern is disturbed. To measure the rate of PM2 formation, 2 "cold pulses" are given, separated by a defined time interval at the rearing

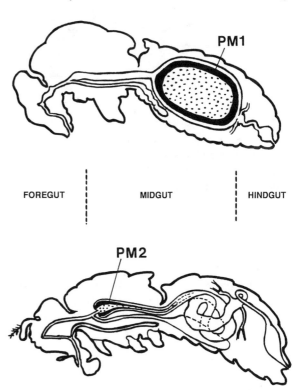

19.1 Schematic diagrams of PM1 and PM2 in *Aedes aegypti* and *Drosophila melanogaster*, respectively. The regions of the foregut, midgut, and hindgut are compared in 2 insects.

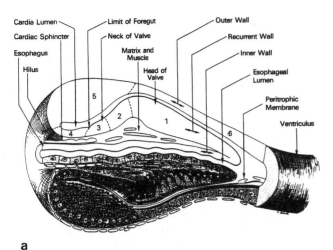

a

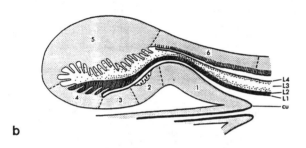

b

19.2 Schematic diagram of the cardia and its PM2 formation zone in *Drosophila melanogaster.* (a) Basic morphology of the cardia as seen in saggital section. Anterior is to the left. The epithelium has been numbered 1–6 according to the morphology of the cells in that zone. (b) Stylized diagram of peritrophic matrix formation, showing the association of the 4 layers of the peritrophic matrix with specific regions of cardia epithelium (not drawn to scale). L1, the innermost layer of the peritrophic matrix, forms adjacent to the foregut cuticle (cu); L2 forms over zone 4; L3, over zone 5; and L4, over zone 6. Reproduced from King, "Cellular organization and peritrophic membrane formation in the cardia (proventriculus) of *Drosophila melanogaster*," *Journal of Morphology,* by permission of Wiley-Liss, a division of John Wiley and Sons, Inc., copyright © 1988.

temperature. The distance between cross-banding pattern disturbances is then measured. When this distance is divided by the time between the cold pulses, the rate of PM2 formation can be obtained (Becker 1978).

A 3rd method is to give 2 separate pulses of a radioactive precursor (e.g., ^{14}C-glucose) and then subject the dissected PM2 to autoradioagraphy. The rate of formation can be calculated by dividing the distance between the labeled zones by the time interval between the 2 radioactive precursor injections (Peters 1992). Rates of PM2 formation for both larvae and adults is usually in the 1–10 mm/hr interval but most commonly fall in the 2–5 mm/hr range. In adult tsetse flies the rate is approximately 1 mm/hr (Harmsen 1973). Considering that an adult fly is somewhere between 6–14 mm long, this is an impressive rate of PM2 secretion. Unlike PM1, PM2 secretion occurs in the absence of food intake. However, the rate of PM2 formation tends to be lower in starving animals.

Ultrastructure of Peritrophic Matrix and PM-Secreting Cells

The PM of both types appears as homogeneous or laminated structures when ultrathin sections are viewed by electron microscopy. Microvilli of PM-secreting cells are usually embedded in the PM material or its precursor. In some insects, when the whole mount preparation is visualized with the electron microscope after negative staining or shadow casting, a highly regular arrangement of microfibrils is revealed. These can have random orientation or be disposed in a honeycomb or hexagonal pattern. Some of these patterns could be cast by the regular arrangement of microvilli of the epithelial cells (Richards and Richards 1977). The ultrastructural appearance of PM1 or PM2 and of their secreting cells depends on the individual species and on the time in relation to the blood meal.

PM1

The PM1 is secreted by the majority of the epithelial cells of the posterior midgut. This is in contrast to the PM2, which is secreted by the specialized cardia cells. Unlike the invariant morphology of the cardia cells, which constitutively secrete PM2, the PM1-secreting midgut cells display marked changes in

(A) Before blood meal.

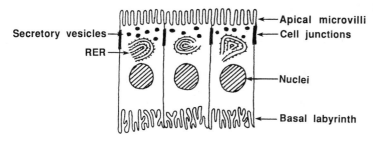

Secretory vesicles → ← Apical microvilli
← Cell junctions
RER →
← Nuclei
← Basal labyrinth

(B) After blood meal.

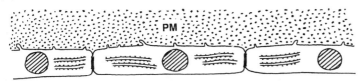

PM

19.3   Schematic diagram of ultrastructural changes in PMI secreting cells after blood-feeding. Apical microvilli and basal labyrinth largely disappear to accommodate the flattening of the epithelial cells that accompanies the dramatic distention of the midgut. As the PMI forms, secretory vesicles disappear and the RER whorls unfold. Not all of these changes occur in all insects.

morphology after ingestion of a blood meal. Upon blood-feeding, the high cuboidal to columnar lining cells are stretched out like a balloon to become flattened (Fig 19.3). Extensive infoldings, called labyrinths, exist on basal surface to accommodate stretching. Microvilli arranged in close array on the apical surface are separated after blood-feeding, probably because microvilli stretch to provide increased surface area (Ramos, Mahowald, and Jacobs-Lorena 1994). Cells are securely connected to each other at their lateral surfaces by cell junctions such as septate junctions, gap junctions, and hemidesmosomes.

Organelles for protein synthesis and secretion, such as RER and Golgi apparatus, are abundant in the epithelial cells. However, the gut epithelial cells of *Aedes* and *Anopheles* are morphologically different. In *Aedes aegypti*, the RER cisternae are in parallel arrays or grouped into whorls resembling fingerprints. After a blood meal, the whorls unfold and cytoplasmic volume is expanded. Secretory granules are absent in unfed gut but a small number of vesicles appear after blood-feeding (Hecker 1977; Perrone and Spielman 1988). By contrast, *Anopheles gambiae* contains a large number of apical granules before the blood meal. RER of unfed cells consists of vesicles and of short and long cisternae, parallel oriented cisternae, and occasionally whorls. After blood-feeding, the apical granules disappear, the RER markedly proliferates, and the whorls are replaced by parallel cisternae (Berner et al. 1983).

The sand fly, *Phlebotomus longipes*, which is the vector for human leishmaniasis, exhibits similar ultrastructural changes upon blood-feeding. Conspicuous whorls or large linear formations of RER are found in starved sand flies. After blood-feeding, dome-shaped apical surfaces of the epithelial cells disappear, presumably by stretching, and RER whorls unwind to become parallel to the flat apical surface. The cytoplasm is rich in ribosomes. Clear vesicles and lipoid spheres appear after blood-feeding, but their relationship to PM secretion is unknown. The PM forms as an irregular lattice of electron-dense and -lucent areas rather than a laminated structure (Gemetchu 1974).

In black flies, which are the vectors for onchocerciasis, lamination of PM into distinct layers occurs. After blood-feeding, microvilli significantly decrease in number and become disorganized, probably because of stretching (Ramos, Mahowald, and Jacobs-Lorena 1994). Precursor materials can be found between the individual villi at an early stage. With time, the microvilli reorganize, and the lamination of PM becomes more obvious (Reid and Lehane 1984). The epithelial cells are rich in RER and contain electron-dense apical vesicles that disappear after blood-feeding (Ramos, Mahowald, and Jacobs-Lorena 1994).

In summary, the secretory activity after blood ingestion results from secretion of preformed products in *Anopheles* and mainly from stimulating the synthetic activity in *Aedes*. Varying participation of both components, namely the exocytosis of secretory vesicles and the activation of protein synthesis, is evident in other hematophagous insects. No information is available on whether vesicle content or changes in RER organization are related to the production and secretion of PM precursors, digestive enzymes, or both.

PM2

The morphology of the PM2-secreting cells was studied in detail in the fruit fly, *Drosophila melanogaster*, by King (1988). The epithelial cells in the cardia can be divided into 6 zones according to their morphology (Fig. 19.1). PM2 appears to have distinct layers, and each layer is secreted by distinct formation zones, each composed of morphologically different cells. The major portion of the PM2 is secreted by zones 4 and 5, which form 2 main layers of the PM2.

Zone 4 cells produce a Periodic Acid-Shiff (PAS) positive mass of amorphous or finely filamentous material that forms a thick inner layer of the PM2 (Fig. 19.2b). This layer is lined internally by a thin electron-dense layer, which is a continuation of the cuticular lining of the foregut. The PAS stain, which is specific for certain carbohydrates, suggests that the secreted proteins might be glycosylated. Zone 4 cells are cuboidal to short, columnar, and are characterized by abundant rough endoplasmic reticulum (RER), which suggests active protein synthesis interspersed with conspicuous Golgi bodies. A few pale vesicles, which are considered to be secretory granules, are found at the apical region.

The outer finely granular layer is secreted by the epithelial cells of zone 5 and covered externally by a delicate layer that begins as a thin coating over the flat apical ends of the microvilli of the zone 6 cells. Zone 5 cells are much taller than those of zone 4 and display similar abundance of RER and Golgi bodies. The apical ends form dome-shaped cytoplasmic "pegs" that project into the lumen. The pegs contain numerous large indistinct vesicles filled with poorly stained flocculent material that is different from the vesicle content

of zone 4 cells. Long apical microvilli are embedded in extracellular secretion containing fine granules.

Epithelial cells in both zones are bound to each other by septate junctions near apical surfaces where lateral membranes are somewhat folded together. Below the apical region, cells are separated by a narrow intercellular space that is interrupted by frequent desmosomes and gap junctions. In summary, one of the major conclusions from these studies is that at least in *Drosophila*, components of different PM2 layers seem to be secreted by distinct groups of cardia cells.

Dissection of the Peritrophic Matrix

The PM1 is formed only after a blood meal and has a definite sequence of formation and degradation. The time frame of these events is unique for each blood-sucking insect. A significant proportion of liquid is removed from the blood meal by diuresis even while the insect feeds. By the time the PM matures, it surrounds a compact mass of blood cells.

To induce PM1 formation under experimental conditions, insects are usually fed with blood on an anesthetized animal. Alternatively, blood can be fed by use of a special feeding apparatus covered with Parafilm or an animal skin. Artificial membrane feeding is extremely useful to test the effect of a specific substance mixed into the blood meal, such as an antibody, an inhibitor, or another chemical. The PM1 is dissected at a time when it is fully mature and easy to handle (Table 19.2). Cold-immobilized insects are dissected using thin watchmaker's forceps by first removing the abdominal exoskeleton to expose the blood-filled midgut. Next, the midgut epithelial wall is peeled away to release the round mass of blood, or "ball," contained by the thick PM1. The PM can be separated from the blood by sectioning the ball and washing the blood away from the PM (Fig 19.4). Billingsley and Rudin (1992) recently described a method to induce PM formation in the absence of blood or of any exogenous proteins.

Because the PM2 is secreted continuously, no special treatment of the insect is necessary for dissection of the PM2. After the gut is removed from the abdomen, tearing and peeling off the midgut epithelium will expose the PM2 (Fig 19.5).

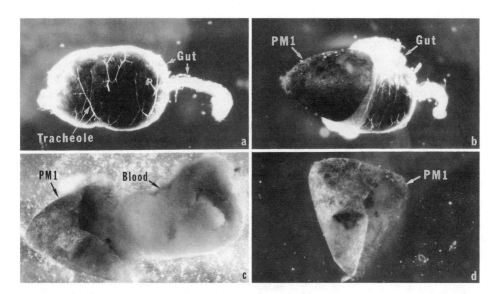

19.4 Dissection of the midgut and of the PM1 from an adult *Aedes aegypti* mosquito. (a) The distended midgut surrounds the PM1. (b) The partially "peeled" gut epithelium exposes the underlying PM1. The PM1 contains the blood meal. (c) Breaking of the PM1 releases the inner blood mass. (d) The same PM1 fragment as in (c) after removal of the blood.

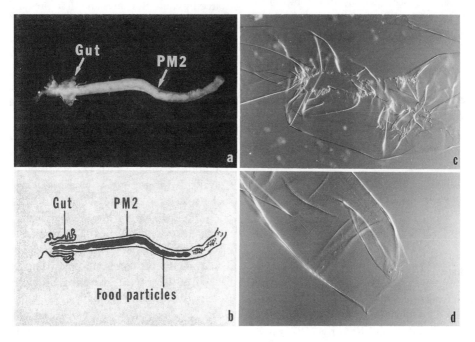

19.5 Dissection of the PM2 from an *Aedes aegypti* mosquito larva. (a) A PM2 tube filled with food particles, as seen under the dissecting microscope. The retracted gut wall covers the left end of the tube. (b) Schematic representation of the image in panel (a), (c), and (d) are microphotographs of a PM2 after removal of the food contents, observed by differential interference contrast (Nomarski) optics. (c) A wrinkled portion of the PM2. (d) An open end of the PM2.

Peritrophic Matrix Components

Chitin is almost always present in the PM. Chitin serves as a scaffold to which proteins and other components attach, thus giving it structural strength. The determination of the composition of the PM is not as straightforward as it may at first appear. One of the problems is contamination by ingested food. This is especially true for PM1, because its formation is usually induced by a blood meal that is rich in proteins and other components from the mammalian host. Thus, most of the available data are for PM2s. However, contamination by food remnants as well as by bacteria and other organisms that populate the gut is also a concern for PM2. Another concern is that the PM is located at the site where high concentrations of hydrolytic (digestive) enzymes are present. Thus, the recovered components may not be those originally present in the PM. For instance, in the case of PM1, the blood meal triggers the secretion not only of PM components but also of digestive enzymes. Thus, it is not unreasonable to expect that the PM composition might change as a function of time after the blood meal due to breakdown of its components. The amount of available material is another limiting factor in the determination of PM composition. The thin PMs must be individually dissected to accumulate enough material for analysis. The work of Ono and Kato (1968, cited in Peters 1976) illustrates this point. To determine the composition of the silkworm PM2, they had to dissect about 30,000 PMs to obtain 18 g of starting material for their analysis.

Chitin, protein, and carbohydrates have been reported to make up the following proportions of the PM.

Chitin 4	~ 13%
Protein 21%	~ 51%
Carbohydrates	~ 15%

As stated earlier, most of the measurements were made for PM2. These determinations do not seem to be all that rigorous. As Richards and Richards (1977) point out, the sum of all the components is never above 75% and is commonly less than 50%. No explanation for these discrepancies has been offered.

Molecular Characterization of Peritrophic Matrix Proteins

Although protein constitutes a substantial proportion of PM material, molecular characterization is hindered by the contaminating food proteins, digestive enzymes, and bacteria. Only a few studies have dealt with the identification of PM proteins.

Stamm et al. (1978) separated the PM2 proteins of blow flies and flesh flies by SDS electrophoresis. Several bands ranging from 10–200 kDa were identified by Coomassie blue and PAS stains. In the blow fly *Calliphora erythrocephala*, several protein bands were identified, and some of them were found in both larvae and adults. Larger proteins were PAS positive, suggesting glycosylation. Comparable results were obtained in the case of the flesh fly *Sarcophaga barbata*. Interestingly, a 17 kDa protein appears to be common between blow flies and flesh flies in both larval and adult stages. A high molecular weight band of about 200 kDa, which was positive only with PAS, was shared by adult blow flies and flesh flies and by blow fly larvae. Both species have similar living habits. Similar results were obtained for the tsetse fly *Glossina morsitans* (Stamm et al. 1978). Dorners and Peters (1988) analyzed by SDS-PAGE the larval PM2 protein of the black fly *Odagmia ornata*. Ten bands were identified ranging from 10–140 kDa. Among them, only 1 band of 54 kDa was found to be glycosylated.

The composition of PM1 proteins from any organism has not been reported so far. Similarly, no high resolution, 2-dimensional gel electrophoretic analysis is available for any PM. Our laboratory has initiated such analysis, seeking the identification of genes encoding PM components. A 2-dimensional gel electrophoresis study of the PM1 protein of the adult black fly, *Simulium vitattum*, revealed that this PM has a relatively simple composition. Two major proteins of 61 and 66 kDa were identified (Ramos and Jacobs-Lorena 1994). Similar studies on *Aedes aegypti* and *Anopheles gambiae* mosquitoes revealed a more complex protein composition with approximately 40 major protein spots. Of these, about 15 appear to be common between *Aedes* and *Anopheles* (Oo and Jacobs-Lorena, unpublished). An artificial meal consisting of latex particles suspended in saline solution can induce PM1 in both organisms. At least 15–20 of the major latex meal-induced PM proteins migrated identical to the blood-induced PM proteins on 2-dimensional gels, indicating that the protein-free meal induces many of the same blood-induced mosquito PM1 genes (Moskalyk, Oo, and Jacobs-Lorena, submitted for publication).

In summary, both PM1 and PM2 contain an array of proteins of varying complexity and sizes. A few protein bands with similar sizes appear to be shared between species or between different developmental stages. It is not clear whether the proteins that are similar in size are actually the same; the significance of this finding remains to be determined. Some of the PM2 proteins are glycosylated, and the extent of glycosylation varies widely. The cloning of genes encoding these proteins will provide additional tools to explore PM structure and function.

Permeability of Peritrophic Matrix

The question of PM permeability is important because digestive enzymes must cross the PM to reach their target (the food bolus) and digestion products must traverse the PM to reach the absorptive epithelium.

Much more is known about the permeability of PM2 than of PM1. For instance, to determine whether the PM2 from mosquito larvae is permeable to ferritin, one can incorporate this marker into the food and determine microscopically whether ferritin has traversed the PM2. A similar experimental approach is not possible for the adult mosquito, because at the time of food ingestion the PM1 does not exist. In fact, this type of experiment (incorporation of ferritin into the food) was used by Perrone and Spielman (1988) to suggest that components of blood plasma proteins may be incorporated into the PM1 when it forms. Thus, one of the problems of determining the permeability of PM1 resides in the difficulty of introducing the test substance into this thick, closed sac.

Other technical constraints must be considered. For instance, many marker molecules, including dyes, colloidal gold, and proteins, tend to aggregate under certain conditions; thus, PM porosity may not correspond to the nominal particle size of the test substance. Degradation of the test substance (e.g., a protein) in the harsh environment of the midgut must also be considered. Although dextrans appear to be good markers, the possibility that they could be adsorbed onto other proteins (e.g., onto the blood albumin) should be evaluated.

The permeability of PM2 to different substances varies somewhat from organism to organism and from larva to adult. In every case, the PM was found to be impermeable to ferritin (450 kDa) but usually permeable to molecules around 30–40 kDa (e.g., horseradish peroxidase, 40 kDa). One surprising discrepancy was noted when the permeability of the PM of mosquito larvae was measured (Peters and Wiese 1986). Although the permeability of the PM2 of *An. stephensi* larvae to fluorescence-labeled dextran was in the "normal range," parallel measurements determined that *Ae. aegypti* larval PM2 was impermeable even to the smallest dextran fraction and only barely permeable to Evans Blue (981 daltons). The significance of this observation is unclear. In adult tsetse flies, myoglobin (17 kDa) and horseradish peroxidase (40 kDa) penetrate the PM2 whereas hemoglobin (68 kDa) may or may not penetrate (Wigglesworth 1929; Peters 1992). The shape of the molecule and other physical properties (charge, hydrophobicity, etc.) can substantially affect permeability. Thus, one should be careful when extrapolating the results with test substances to "real life" situations.

Intriguing results were reported by Zhuzhikov (1964) on permeability measurements of PM2 of the house fly. The dissected PM2 was tied at both ends with a silk thread to form a "sausage" containing a sealed internal compartment. A solution of starch and iodine was placed on one side (inside) of the PM and human salivary amylase on the other side. When the amylase traverses the PM2, it digests the starch, and the solution turns blue. Zhuzhikov reported that amylase was able to traverse the PM2 from the outside in but not in the reverse direction and concluded that the PM2 is unidirectionally permeable to the enzyme. These properties correspond to what one would expect in vivo because digestive enzymes secreted by the midgut epithelium do traverse the PM2 from the outside in. Unfortunately, these interesting results have not since been repeated.

Borovsky (1986) conducted experiments to estimate the permeability of PM1 from *Culex nigripalpus*. Adult mosquitoes were fed on blood and dissected 24 hr later, after the PM1 had formed. The fluid in the ecto-peritrophic space (the space between the PM1 and the midgut epithelium) was then sampled and analyzed for the size of the peptides. Proteins with sizes up to 23 kDa were found. Thus, Borovsky estimated that proteins up to this size can penetrate the PM1 presumably from inside out. These results should be considered to be preliminary because some experimental problems remain to be solved and the origin (from the food bolus or from the epithelium) of the larger proteins in the ectoperitrophic space has not been demonstrated.

The Peritrophic Matrix as a Barrier to Pathogen Invasion

Pathogens transmitted by bloodsucking insects nearly always enter the insect via the blood meal. The pathogen must then reach the gut epithelium. In the majority of the cases, the pathogen traverses the epithelium and continues to develop in the insect body cavity. Because the PM completely surrounds the blood meal and separates the ingested parasite from the epithelium, the PM constitutes a potential barrier for pathogen invasion. Obviously, this is not an absolute barrier; otherwise the insect would not be able to support development of the pathogen and would not be a disease vector in the first place. When considering the possible role of the PM as a barrier for pathogen invasion, it is critical to consider the time required for PM formation and relate it to pathogen development. Three possible scenarios are possible: (1) the pathogen attaches and/or traverses the gut as soon as it is ingested and before the PM

has formed, (2) the pathogen first develops in the gut lumen and then traverses a mature PM to reach the epithelium, and (3) the pathogen moves toward the gut epithelium after the PM breaks down.

In the 1st case (pathogen attaches/traverses gut soon after ingestion) the PM probably does not constitute a significant barrier. Viruses and most microfilariae belong to this category. For instance, *Onchocerca volvulus*, the causative agent of river blindness, is transmitted by the black fly, whose PM1 matures relatively fast (Table 19.2). Lewis (1953) states that microfilariae remain alive in the gut of black flies for up to 24 hours after an infectious blood meal. However, Laurence (1966) demonstrated that most of the ingested microfilariae that traverse the gut do so within 30 minutes of ingestion and then only slowly until 2–4 hr after the blood meal (Fig. 19.6). In this experiment approximately 25% of the ingested microfilariae remain trapped within the PM and die. In other experiments the proportion of trapped microfilariae tended to be higher. Perrone and Spielman (1986) also showed that microfilariae of *Brugia*

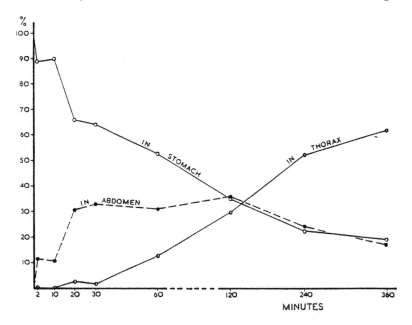

19.6   Percentages (geometric means) of the microfilariae of *Onchocerca volvulus* found in the stomach, abdomen, and thorax of *Simulium damnosum* 2–360 min after an infective blood meal. Reproduced with permission from B. R. Laurence 1966.

malayi penetrate the mosquito gut soon after ingestion with the blood meal and before PM1 formation.

The malarial parasite *Plasmodium* belongs to the 2nd category. After ingestion, the gametocytes go through a complete sexual cycle in the midgut lumen and develop into motile ookinetes, a process that takes 16–24 hr depending on the species. Major invasion of the epithelial cells occurs about 30 hr after the blood meal, at a time when the PM1 is fully formed and mature (Table 19.2). Thus, the PM1 does constitute a barrier. Elegant work by Huber et al. (1991) suggests that *P. gallinaceum* secretes a chitinase in order to penetrate the PM1 of *Ae. aegypti*. Huber et al. also report that pure chitinase (devoid of contaminating proteases) is sufficient to physically disrupt the PM1. Subsequently, Shahabuddin et al. (1993) demonstrated that inhibition of chitinase activity by allosamidin completely blocks transmission of the parasite. Moreover, these authors demonstrate that the chitinase secreted by the parasite is activated by the mosquito-secreted trypsin. These findings reveal sophisticated mechanisms of adaptation of the parasite to the PM1 and digestive enzymes secreted by its host. The PM1 of *An. stephensi* was reported not to contain chitin (Berner et al. 1983). The means by which the malaria parasite penetrates the PM1 of this mosquito and whether additional enzymes are required for PM penetration in general are issues that remain to be resolved. Interestingly, the protozoan *Babesia microti* apparently uses the contents of a specialized organelle to traverse the solid PM1 of the tick *Ixodes scapularis* (Rudzinska et al. 1982).

The development of *Leishmania* in sand flies is an example of the 3rd category, in which the pathogen moves to the gut after PM breaks down. Recently Shahabuddin et al. (submitted for publication) showed that anti-trypsin antibodies ingested with the blood meal can block malaria transmission. The initial steps of the *Leishmania* life cycle include the transformation of amastigotes into promastigotes, which divide rapidly within the blood meal. PM breakdown after several days was once believed to trigger the next phase of parasite development, attachment to the gut epithelium and anterior migration. Schlein et al. (1991) have shown that *Leishmania* may actually rely on chitinase

to penetrate the PM, in a similar way as the malarial parasite. Moreover, chitinase activity has also been demonstrated in several trypanosomatids. This suggests that *Trypanosoma brucei*, the causative agent for African sleeping sickness, may use the same mechanism to escape the preformed PM2 of the tsetse fly. More recently Schlein et al. (1992) presented evidence that damage of the chitin-containing cuticular lining of the cardiac valve could enhance transmission of *Leishmania* by stimulating regurgitation of the parasites and deposition in the host tissue. Thus, the 3rd mode of transmission (escape after PM breakdown) may not occur.

Other Roles Played by the Peritrophic Matrix

Several other functions have been attributed to the PM, but none has ever been demonstrated conclusively. The almost ubiquitous occurrence of the peritrophic matrix among arthropods is a strong, albeit indirect, argument that it must play some essential role. If it had no role, why would the PM be preserved in evolution? In the previous section, evidence was presented that the PM directly interacts with at least some parasites (e.g., malaria and *Leishmania*). However, this interaction does not warrant the conclusion that protection of the insect from parasites is one of the functions of the PM. In fact, the opposite might be true. The PM may be a structure that serves other functions and evolutionarily predates vector-parasite interactions. The argument can thus be made that the parasites evolved means to traverse the PM as opposed to insects evolving a PM to protect themselves from parasites.

PM can also serve some role in digestion. It has been argued that the PM completely separates the food bolus from the intestinal epithelium. Here again, it is useful to discuss PM1 and PM2 separately. The role of the PM1 in digestion of a blood meal has been tested experimentally in mosquitoes. Mosquitoes were fed (or force-fed) a saline solution, followed 24 hr later by a blood meal. Different results were observed for 2 mosquito species: *Ae. aegypti* formed a PM1 thicker than normal after this regimen, whereas *An. stephensi* formed no detectable PM (Berner et al. 1983; Billingsley and Rudin 1992). The reasons for a thicker PM in

Ae. aegypti are not clear, but it might be attributed to "superinduction" of the PM genes caused by the 1st stimulus (the saline meal). *An. stephensi* apparently stores PM components in cytoplasmic vesicles that are secreted by the stimulus of saline feeding. The relatively short time between the saline feeding and the blood feeding might not be sufficient to renew the stored PM components, explaining the absence of new PM formation. In any event, the significant result was that blood digestion was not altered by the presence of a thicker PM in *Aedes aegypti* or by the absence of a PM in *Anopheles stephensi*. Taken at face value, these results contradict the supposed role of PM1 in blood digestion. However, these experiments were performed in laboratory conditions and did not measure the *efficiency* of digestion. In other words, the results only showed that the blood disappeared from the lumen of the gut (presumably because of digestion) and that the flies did not die. It is still possible that in nature flies that form a PM digest blood more efficiently and produce eggs faster and in larger numbers, conferring to PM-secreting flies a selective advantage. The experiments of Billingsley and Rudin (1992) also addressed the effect of the PM1 on infectivity of the fly by *Plasmodium*. Infection of *An. stephensi* was unaffected by the absence of the PM, whereas infection of *Ae. aegypti* was partially inhibited by the presence of a thickened PM. The latter result supports the model that the PM constitutes a partial barrier to parasite transmission.

No experiments are available that directly test the role of PM2 in food digestion; however, a number of published reports point to the interesting possibility that the PM2 serves as a solid support to digestive enzymes. For instance, Walker et al. (1980) localized leucine amino peptidase to the *Drosophila* PM2. Peters and Kalnis (1985) found that aminopeptidases are strongly attached to the PM2 of 8 different insects. By immunological methods, Patel, Mahowald, and Jacobs-Lorena (manuscript in preparation) have observed that a trypsinlike enzyme is found almost exclusively attached to the PM2 of *Drosophila melanogaster*. These findings suggest a model whereby the PM2 serves as an attachment site to digestive enzymes. As food moves along the PM2, it is digested

by these immobilized enzymes. In fact, Waterhouse (1954) determined that in drone fly and blow fly larvae, the food moves along the gut about 10 times faster than the rate of PM secretion (food motion is probably aided by peristaltic movements). Conceivably, attachment of enzymes to the PM2 might confer selective advantage because much more food can be digested per molecule of enzyme than if it were secreted into the lumen of the gut and rapidly excreted with the food bolus. Moreover, by attaching to the PM2, digestion would take place at the interface between the food bolus and ectoperitrophic space (the space between the PM2 and the epithelium), facilitating the diffusion of the proteolytic products toward the absorptive epithelium.

Extensive investigations of the distributions of many digestive enzymes in larvae of several insects have led Terra (1990) to propose an interesting model for the role of the PM2 in compartmentalizing digestion. The PM2 defines 2 compartments within the gut lumen: the endoperitrophic space, which is the space within the PM2 tube; and ectoperitrophic space, which is the space defined by the gut epithelium on the outside and the PM2 on the inside. It is usually difficult to sample the fluid in the ectoperitrophic space. Terra and colleagues took advantage of the fact that in certain insect larvae the cecum (Fig 19.7) is unusually large, allowing sampling of ectoperitrophic fluid from the lumen of the cecum. Analysis of a number of different digestive enzymes showed that they tend to be unevenly distributed within these compartments: enzymes that digest large molecules tend to be enriched within the endoperitrophic space whereas enzymes that digest smaller molecules tend to be enriched in the ectoperitrophic space. As expected, the enzymes that are found predominantly in the endoperitrophic space are smaller than those that do not cross the PM2. The model proposes that large food molecules are degraded within the endoperitrophic space to generate small oligomers that diffuse into the ectoperitrophic space. In this compartment the oligomers are digested by enzymes specialized in the digestion of such small molecules. The final degradation of the smallest oligomers (dimers) takes place by membrane-bound and intracellular enzymes. In addition, the

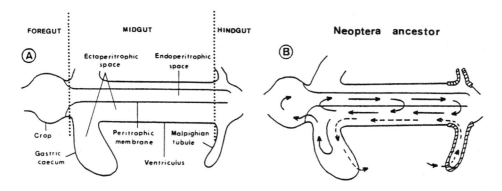

FOREGUT | MIDGUT | HINDGUT | Neoptera ancestor

Ectoperitrophic space | Endoperitrophic space

Crop

Gastric caecum

Peritrophic membrane

Malpighian tubule

Ventriculus

19.7   Generalized diagram of the insect gut (A) and representation (B) of fluid fluxes (dotted arrows). Reproduced with permission from Terra 1990, *Annual Review of Entomology*, vol. 35, © 1990 by Annual Reviews Inc.

model theorizes, by a flow of liquid moving from the Malpighian tubules toward the cecum, the concentration of the small molecules in the ectoperitrophic space (Fig 19.7). Experimental evidence for such flow has been previously obtained by the use of dyes incorporated into the food. The model is attractive; additional experimental evidence that these compartments are in fact physiologically important will greatly strengthen its significance. A number of other functions have been attributed to the PM. Among them is the protection of the gut epithelium from abrasion or damage by food particles. There is little experimental evidence to either support or rule out such functions.

SUMMARY AND PROSPECTS

The PM is an acellular structure that lies between the food and the gut epithelium and is found in the great majority of arthropods. Despite the large body of information available on the PM, it is surprising how little is known about its function. Its interaction with certain parasites (e.g., malaria and *leishmania*) is one of the most significant properties that have been revealed so far. In contrast to the vast amount of information on PM morphology and physiology, little experimentation has been done at the molecular level. This line of investigation is promising. The molecular characterization of genes that participate in PM formation should advance our understanding of this structure significantly, and with some luck, it may even lead to some fundamental discovery relating to disease control.

REFERENCES

Balbiani, E.-G. 1890. Etudes anatomiques et histologiques sur le tube digestif des cryptops. *Arch. Zool. Exp. Gen.* Ser. 2, 8:1–82.

Becker, B. 1978. Determination of the formation rate of peritrophic membranes in some Diptera. *J. Insect Physiol.* 24:529–533.

Berner, R., W. Rudin, and H. Hecker. 1983. Peritrophic membranes and protease activity in the midgut of the malaria mosquito, *Anopheles stephensi (Liston)* (Insecta: Diptera) under normal and experimental conditions. *J. Ultrastr. Res.* 83:195–204.

Billingsley, P.F., and W. Rudin. 1992. The role of the mosquito peritrophic membrane in bloodmeal digestion and infectivity of *Plasmodium* species. *J. Parasitol.* 78:430–440.

Borovsky, D. 1986. Proteolytic enzymes and blood digestion in the mosquito, *Culex nigripalpus. Insect Biochem. Physiol.* 3:147–160.

Dorner, R., and W. Peters. 1988. Localization of sugar components of glycoproteins in peritrophic membranes of larvae of Diptera (Culicidae, Simuliidae). *Entomol. Gen.* 14:11–24.

Freyvogel, T.A., and C. Jaquet. 1965. The prerequisites for the formation of a peritrophic membrane in culicidae females. *Acta Trop.* 22:148–154.

Freyvogel, T.A., and W. Stäubli. 1965. The formation of the peritrophic membrane in culicidae. *Acta Trop.* 22:118–147.

Gemetchu, T. 1974. The morphology and fine structure of the midgut and peritrophic membrane of the adult female, *Phlebotomus longipes* Parrot and Martin (Diptera: Psychodidae). *Ann. Trop. Med. Parasit.* 68:111–124.

Harmsen, R. 1973. The nature of the establishment barrier for *Trypanosoma brucei* in the gut of *Glossina pallidipes*. *Trans. R. Soc. Trop. Med. Hyg.* 67:364–373.

Hecker, H. 1977. Structure and function of midgut epithelial cells in culicidae mosquitoes (Insecta, Diptera). *Cell Tissue Res.* 184:321–341.

Huber, M., E. Cabib, and L.H. Miller. 1991. Malaria parasite chitinase and penetration of the mosquito peritrophic membrane. *Proc. Nat. Acad. Sci. USA* 88:2807–2810.

King, D.G. 1988. Cellular organization and peritrophic membrane formation in the cardia (proventriculus) of *Drosophila melanogaster*. *J. Morphol.* 196:253–282.

Laurence, B.R. 1966. Intake and migration of the microfilariae of *Onchocerca volvulus* (*Leuckart*) in *Similium damnosum* Theobald. *J. Helm.* 40:337–342.

Lehane, M.J. 1976. Formation and histochemical structure of the peritrophic membrane in the stablefly, *Stomoxys calcitrans*. *J. Insect Physiol.* 22:1551–1557.

Lewis, D.J. 1953. *Simulium damnosum* and its relation to onchocerciasis in Anglo-Egyptian Sudan. *Bull. Entomol. Res.* 43:597–644.

Perrone, J.B., and A. Spielman. 1986. Microfilarial perforation of the midgut of a mosquito. *J. Parasit.* 72:723–727.

Perrone, J.B., and A. Spielman. 1988. Time and site of assembly of the peritrophic membrane of the mosquito *Aedes aegypti*. *Cell Tissue Res.* 252:473–478.

Peters, W. 1976. Investigations on the peritrophic membranes of Diptera. In: H.R. Hepburn, editor, *The insect integument*. New York: Elsevier Scientific Publishing Co. pp. 515–543.

Peters, W. 1992. *Peritrophic membranes*. New York: Springer-Verlag.

Peters, W., and M. Kalnins. 1985. Aminopeptidases as immobilized enzymes on the peritrophic membranes of insects. *Entomol. Gener.* 11:025–032.

Peters, W., and B. Wiese. 1986. Permeability of the peritropic membranes of some diptera to labelled dextrans. *J. Insect Physiol.* 32:43–49.

Ramos, A., A. Mahowald, and M. Jacobs-Lorena. 1994. Peritrophic matrix of the black fly *Simulium vittatum*: Formation, structure, and analysis of its protein components. *J. Exp. Zool.* 268:269–281.

Reid, G.D., and M.J. Lehane. 1984. Peritrophic membrane formation in three temperate simuliids, *Simulium ornatum*, *S. equinum* and *S. lineatum*, with respect to the migration of onchocercal microfilariae. *Ann. Trop. Med. Parasit.* 78:527–539.

Richards, A.G., and P.A. Richards. 1977. The peritrophic membranes of insects. *Ann. Rev. Entomol.* 22:219–240.

Rudzinska, M.A., A. Spielman, S. Lewengrub, J. Piesman, and S. Karakashian. 1982. Penetration of the peritrophic membrane of the tick by *Babesia microti*. *Cell Tissue Res.* 221:471–481.

Schlein, Y., R.L. Jacobson, and J. Shlomai. 1991. Chitinase secreted by *Leishmania* functions in the sand fly vector. *Proc. R. Soc. Lond.* (B)245:121–126.

Schlein, Y., R. L. Jacobson, and G. Messor. 1992. *Leishmania* infections damage the feeding mechanism of the sand fly vector and implement parasite transmission by bite. *Proc. Natl. Acad. Sci. USA* 89:9944–9948.

Shahabuddin, M., T. Toyoshima, M. Aikawa, and D.C. Kaslow. 1993. Transmission-blocking activity of a chitinase inhibitor and activation of malarial parasite chitinase by mosquito protease. *Proc. Natl. Acad. Sci. USA* 90:4266–4270.

Stamm, B., J. D'Haese, and W. Peters. 1978. SDS gel electrophoresis of proteins and glycoproteins from peritrophic membranes of some Diptera. *J. Insect Physiol.* 24:1–8.

Stohler, H. 1957. Analyse des infektionsverlaufes von *Plasmodium gallinaceum* im Darme von *Aedes agypti*. *Acta Trop.* 14:302–352.

Terra, W.R. 1990. Evolution of digestive systems of insects. *Ann. Rev. Entomol.* 35:181–200.

Walker, V.K., B.W. Geer, and J.H. Williamson. 1980. Dietary modulation and histochemical localization of leucine aminopeptidase activity in *Drosophila melanogaster* larvae. *Insect Biochem.* 10:543–548.

Walters, L.L., K.P. Irons, H. Guzman, and R.B. Tesh. 1993. Formation and composition of the peritrophic membrane in the sand fly, *Phlebotomus perniciosus* (Diptera: Psychodidae). *J. Med. Entomol.* 30:179–198.

Waterhouse, D.F. 1954. The rate of production of the peritrophic membrane in some insects. *Aust. J. Biol. Sci.* 7:59–72.

Wigglesworth, V.B. 1929. Digestion in the tsetse-fly: A study of structure and function. *Parasit.* 21:288–321.

Zhuzhikov, D.P. 1964. Function of the peritrophic membrane in *Musca domestica* L. and *Calliphora erythrocephala* Meig. *J. Insect Physiol.* 10:273–278.

20. THE SALIVARY GLANDS OF DISEASE VECTORS

Kenneth R. Stark and Anthony A. James

INTRODUCTION

The salivary glands of hematophagous arthropods play an important role in blood-feeding and the transmission of diseases. The glands produce a saliva that not only facilitates rapid and efficient feeding but also may be involved with the initial metabolism of the blood meal. In addition, many pathogens are transmitted to vertebrate hosts through the secretion of saliva. In this chapter the development and physiology of vector salivary glands are reviewed in general terms, and the role of saliva in blood-feeding and its involvement in enhancing parasite transmission are described.

DEVELOPMENTAL AND MORPHOLOGICAL ASPECTS OF VECTOR SALIVARY GLANDS

In the majority of vector species, it is the adults that feed on blood and therefore transmit diseases. However, in the triatomine bugs and ticks all stages feed on blood, and immature ticks are important vectors in many instances (e.g., Lyme disease). Nevertheless, the focus of most studies, and hence this chapter, has been on the salivary glands of adult vectors.

The development of adult salivary glands is as varied as the phyla that feed on blood. In related nonvector arthropod species, the glands appear to be of ectodermal origin and are formed from discrete embryonic epithelial primordial cells, and this generalization may apply to vector species as well. In the holometabolous Insecta such as the Diptera (including mosquitoes, sand flies, black flies, and tsetse), the adult glands are distinct from the larval glands. For these insects, different groups of cells form the larval and adult glands during embryogenesis. In the subadult stages, the glands remain relatively undifferentiated, often as rings or small placodes of cells located near the larval glands. These cells have the characteristics of imaginal discs because they are arranged in a single layer, are mitotically active, and are presumably diploid. During metamorphosis, these cells divide further and undergo significant changes in shape to achieve the final form of the adult glands. Following adult eclosion in holometabolous insects, particularly mosquitoes, the glands undergo a period of rapid synthesis of proteins before the adults are ready to feed on blood. In the hemimetabolous insects (e.g., triatomine bugs), salivary gland development is less well characterized, but the glands appear to be the same in both subadult and adult stages. The glands enlarge at every molt, presumably as a result of cell division and cell growth.

The development of tick salivary glands in the subadult stage is also not well characterized. After the final molt, the glands in the adult hard tick are relatively inactive. After the tick attaches to a host, however, the glands initiate a sequential series of protein syntheses that reflect the stages of the feeding process. For example, there is an initial and rapid synthesis of a cement protein that attaches the tick firmly to the host and seals the area around the proboscis to the wound site, possibly preventing fluid leakage. Cells in the tick salivary gland can take up to 2–3 days to reach their maximum size and production capability.

The structure of adult salivary glands varies among the phyla. In general, the glands consist of 1 or a few lobe- or saclike structures composed of a single layer of cells with distinct apical and basal regions. The layer is organized as an epithelium and has a basement membrane that surrounds the outside of the glands. There are 3 basic types of gland structure: alveolar, reservoir, and tubular. The gland structure in ticks is alveolar, composed of individual cells attached to a branching duct. The reservoir gland structure consists of an epithelium with cells surrounding a large extracellular space. The cells secrete material into this space, and the material then flows through a duct during feeding. Mosquitoes and some flies have tubular glands, which consist of a single layer of cells surrounding a duct. The duct can be completely or partially chitinized. Each cell has a large extracellular acinus in which the products of secretion are stored. Categorization of glands in this manner is not exclusive because variations and combinations of these 3 basic types exist.

The cells within a salivary gland vary in their structure and function. Mosquito salivary glands are a good example of this variability (Fig. 20.1). In the mosquito a structural and functional dimorphism exists between the sexes, reflecting the fact that only the females feed on blood. The salivary glands of both sexes are paired organs located in the thorax, and each gland consists of 3 lobes connected to a main salivary duct. Some morphological differences exist between the salivary glands of anopheline and *Aedes* species. The salivary ducts are lined with chitin and extend the full length of the glands in *Aedes* and *Culex* species but only into the proximal regions in *Anopheles*. These tubular glands consist of a single-layered epithelium of predominantly secretory cells surrounding the salivary duct. The common salivary duct leads anteriorly to a salivary pump located at the base of the salivary stylet.

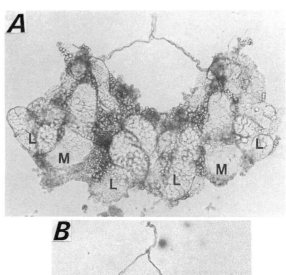

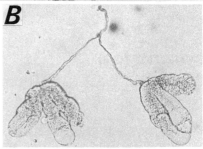

20.1 Adult salivary glands from the mosquito *Aedes aegypti*. (A) A pair of glands dissected from a 5-day, postemergence female. Note the common salivary duct and association with the fat body. (B) A pair of glands dissected from an adult male. These glands are approximately one-fifth of protein mass of the female glands. L = lateral lobe, M = medial lobe.

The lobes of the male mosquito appear morphologically and histochemically homogeneous, and the glands are approximately one-fifth the size of the female glands, possibly because males feed on only sugars. Male salivary products include a-glucosidase, a-amylase, a bacteriolytic factor, and a nonspecific esterase. These products are present in similar quantities in both sexes.

The female salivary glands (Fig. 20.1A) in mosquitoes are morphologically different from those of the male (Fig. 20.1B); female glands also show differentiation between and within the lobes. The female gland has 2 identical lateral lobes and a shorter and wider median lobe. The lateral lobes can be divided into proximal (male-like) and distal regions. A narrow area of small cells separates the 2 regions, probably representing a transition zone. The median lobe consists of a region of large secretory cells separated from the rest of the gland by a separate "neck" that contains nonsecretory cells implicated morphologically in fluid transport. Thus, the glands are organized into regions of at least 3 cell types. Histochemical and molecular analyses of female *Aedes aegypti* salivary glands have demonstrated that different regions of the glands secrete different proteins. The proximal lateral lobes produce enzymes involved in sugar feeding and are functionally and morphologically similar to the adult male salivary glands. Other secretory cell types, located in the median lobe and distal lateral lobes, appear to be female-specific. The neck region appears structurally to be female-specific; however, the male must have some analogous mechanism of fluid transport. Furthermore, the adult female appears to have some control over the release of salivary products depending on whether she is feeding on sugar or blood. When feeding on sugar, only proteins associated with sugar-feeding are secreted. When feeding on blood, the female salivates both sugar- and blood-feeding components.

The median and distal lateral lobes of female glands bind lectins not found on other regions of the glands, indicating that there are different carbohydrate moieties from those in the proximal lobes associated with the basement membrane. In addition, the distal lateral and medial lobes produce apyrase and in *Aedes aegypti* express a female-enriched gene, *D7*, which is the major protein synthesized in female glands. Interestingly, these lobes are invaded preferentially by sporozoites during the mosquito cycle of malaria parasites. The median lobe can be distinguished histochemically from the distal lateral lobes and differs in the binding of some lectins. In *Ae. aegypti*, the median lobes accumulate tachykinin-like proteins, sialokinins, that have a dilative effect on vertebrate vasculature.

The regulation of salivary gland secretion can be hormonal, neuronal, or both. Application of serotonin and dopamine to fly and tick salivary glands, respectively, causes an increased flow of saliva from dissected glands maintained in culture. Substances such as pilocarpine (a cholinergic agonist), which acts on the ganglia, also stimulates salivation when applied topically to ticks, thus indicating a nervous system component. In general, the mechanisms by which salivation is initiated in vector arthropods are poorly characterized and are a potentially fruitful area of investigation.

The flow of saliva through the mouthparts is facilitated by a salivary pump. This structure is located at the base of the mouthparts and produces sufficient pressure to force the liquid saliva through the narrow channels of the salivary ducts.

FUNCTIONS OF THE SALIVARY GLANDS

Non–Blood-Feeding Roles of Salivary Glands

Although the principal focus of attention on vector salivary glands is their role in blood-feeding and the transmission of disease agents, they have a number of other important roles. In arthropods in general, saliva is a medium for dissolving and solubilizing food and providing enzymes that initiate digestion. This function is clearly evident in vectors, especially in those that feed on both sugar and blood. In mosquitoes saliva contains α-amylases and α-glucosidases that digest sugars, and saliva is likely to be the primary source of enzymes for this digestion.

Salivary gland secretions can also play a role in the maintenance of the feeding mouthparts. The proboscis of a probing vector is a complex structure composed of long stylets originating from different segments in the head. These stylets fit together to form a strong but flexible structure capable of penetrating the skin of vertebrate hosts. Researchers have proposed that saliva acts as a lubricant for the mouthparts and as a medium for keeping the structural elements together. Saliva may also lubricate the chitinous structures of those vectors with chewing or biting mouthparts.

The salivary glands in certain vectors play a role in processes such as water secretion during feeding. During a feeding regime that often lasts several days, hard ticks take in a large amount of fluid. The water in the ingested blood is cycled back through the salivary glands where it is returned to the host. The tick uses this method to regulate the amount of fluid in its body as well as to deliver salivary activities important in feeding. There are other examples in insects in which the production of a hygroscopic saliva is used to maintain fluid levels within the insect. Thus, salivary glands are complex organs involved in several physiological functions of the vectors in addition to their role in blood-feeding.

Hematophagy and the Host Response

Blood-feeding presents significant challenges to the vector arthropod. There are the general problems of host location, digestion of blood, diuresis, and in those vectors that feed on blood for solely reproductive purposes, the coordination of blood-feeding and vitellogenesis. One of the significant challenges is the act of feeding itself. After finding a host, the arthropod must locate vascular tissue. Since vertebrate skin is not completely vascularized, it is quite possible that an arthropod probing with small mouthparts will fail to locate vascular tissue.

The various orders of hematophagous arthropods have evolved different mouthpart structures to assist in this difficult task of locating blood. Mosquitoes and triatomine bugs have long, flexible feeding stylets that enable them to feed either directly from cannulated arterioles and venules or to feed from a laceration-induced hematoma (Chap. 1). Phlebotomine sand flies (Chap. 9) have a much shorter proboscis and thus must feed on the superficial capillary beds. The biting flies (for example, black flies and tsetse flies) have only chewing and biting mouthparts, which restrict their feeding to superficial hematomas that form in the lacerated tissue. These flies rely heavily on the pharmacological properties of their saliva to find blood. Ticks (Chaps. 1 and 12) often feed for several days on a single host and literally can burrow into the skin to feed from a hematoma that forms around their mouthparts.

The ultimate effect of hematophagy on the vertebrate host is tissue and vascular laceration. Normally, the host responds to the damage by a complicated, interconnected cycle of hemostasis and inflammation. Tissue damage causes the activation of platelets and coagulation factors leading to platelet degranulation that in turn induces vascular changes via inflammatory reactions producing erythema, edema, and pain. Depending on the extent of the damage, the coagulation pathway is activated to cleave fibrinogen to form a fibrin clot and thereby stop the flow of blood through the wound. However, in damage to small vessels, platelet aggregation and vasoconstriction are usually sufficient to close the wound. This reaction is quite efficient and can occur in less than 30 seconds. The analogy of a pinprick works well to describe the physical damage that occurs when an arthropod first begins to feed. When a finger is pricked by a sharp needle of small diameter, the 1st drop of blood is easily obtained; however, the second drop can only be obtained by forcefully squeezing the fingertip. This rapid cessation of bleeding is due principally to vasoconstriction and platelet aggregation. If such a response were to occur unchecked, the arthropod would not achieve a successful blood meal.

In addition to hemostasis, vertebrate blood represents a potential challenge in itself (Chap. 2). Blood transports nutrients and defends against foreign invasion. Thus, blood contains an array of molecules that are potentially toxic to an unsuspecting hematophagous arthropod, such as complement proteins, macrophages, neutrophils, tumor necrosis factor (TNF), and antibodies. An arthropod that has successfully located and withdrawn blood is now faced with the prospect of having ingested a potentially hazardous meal. There are a number of specific and nonspecific defense mechanisms that pose a threat to the integrity of the insect midgut. These mechanisms include the cytolytic and cytotoxic components of the complement system. Complement particles (e.g., C3b) ingested during the blood meal could become activated inside the vector by interacting with the midgut surface and thereby induce lysis of midgut epithelial cells. Similarly, macrophages, neutrophils, and/or TNF could also participate in cytolytic reactions against the vector midgut. In the laboratory, after a vector has fed repetitively on a host, antibodies against vector salivary proteins are produced. In principal, antigen-antibody complexes formed during subsequent feeding cycles could also pose a cytotoxic threat to the vector midgut epithelium.

The pain response also potentially threatens the feeding vector. The act of probing itself is painful. In addition, hemostasis and inflammation induced by blood-feeding causes the release of bradykinin, which contributes significantly to the pain response of classical inflammation. Pain perceived by the vertebrate could then lead to either increased grooming or a violent response that could terminate vector feeding.

In summary, hematophagous vectors must somehow obtain blood from a potentially physiologically and physically hostile vertebrate host. The host response to blood-feeding centers on hemostasis because all hematophagous arthropods (and blood-feeding ectoparasites in general) cause localized blood vascular lacerations in the area they probe. Hemostasis can also be initiated by inflammation and humoral and cellular immune responses directed against vector salivary compounds that are released during blood-feeding. The actions of hemostasis, inflammation, and the physical act of blood-feeding potentially cause host pain, which could lead to the physical removal of the vector. Thus, to achieve successful hematophagy arthropods must effectively combat the host response. Antihemostatic, antiinflammatory, and immunosuppressive activities that contribute to a successful blood meal have been described and characterized in the saliva and/or salivary gland extracts for several species of blood-feeding insects and other arthropods, as well as for hematophagous leeches.

Pharmacological Properties of Arthropod Saliva

The first clues that saliva plays an important role in blood-feeding came from salivary duct transection experiments using mosquitoes, triatomine bugs, and tsetse flies. These experiments showed that although salivating and nonsalivating animals fed equally well from blood through a latex membrane, the nonsalivating animals tended to probe longer on living hosts. Experiments with tsetse flies that had their salivary glands removed showed that many flies did not survive extended engorgement, indicating that salivary gland secretions may play a role in maintaining the flow of blood through the mouthparts. Since these initial experiments, researchers have been able to identify and

characterize a variety of biochemical activities from both salivary gland homogenates and salivary secretions from oil- and pilocarpine-induced salivation. In the wild, salivation is probably critical for the rapid location of blood vessels or the formation of hematomas for successful blood-feeding. The evasion of a host immune response is probably more important for extended blood-feeders such as ticks.

Table 20.1 shows a compilation of the salivary activities that have been characterized in hematophagous vectors and are thought to be involved with blood-feeding. The pharmacological effects of saliva result in a decreased time required to feed on blood and an increase in the probability of locating blood in the surface epithelium and deeper tissues. The common denominator of vector salivary products was shown initially to be the platelet aggregation inhibitor, apyrase. Research in the last few years has shown that in addition to platelet inhibitors, vasodilatory agents and anticoagulants are common among all blood-feeding vectors. Vectors ingest a mixture of blood and saliva while feeding, and the saliva could play a role in neutralizing bioactive molecules present in blood, as well as assist in blood-finding.

Platelet Inhibitors

An important component of hemostasis that determines the success of blood-feeding is platelet aggregation. All hematophagous arthropods, and ectoparasites in general, have been shown to contain an antiplatelet activity attributable to apyrase (Table 20.2). Considering the evidence that platelet aggregation is central to host hemostasis and the importance of platelet aggregation in response to minor blood vessel damage, this common mechanism is not surprising. Apyrase is believed to be important for blood-finding because apyrase activity is inversely proportional to probing time in mosquitoes. Probing time is defined as the time spent locating vasculature before beginning engorgement. Apyrase from *Aedes aegypti* belongs to the gene family that includes 5'-nucleotidases. Apyrases are enzymes that catalyze the degradation of ADP and ATP to AMP and inorganic phosphates. They do not hydrolyze AMP, which distinguishes apyrase activity from general 5'-nucleotidases. ADP, a

TABLE 20.1   Reported arthropod salivary gland activities with proposed roles in blood-feeding

Reported activity	Product (if known)
Sand flies	
Antiplatelet	Apyrase
Vasodilator (Erythema inducing factor)	Maxadilan
Macrophage-activation inhibitor	Maxadilan (not proven)
Mosquitoes	
Hemagglutinin	
Anticoagulant	Anti-fXa, antithrombin
Antitumor necrosis factor	
Antiplatelet activity	Apyrase
Unknown	D7 (female-specific protein)
Vasodilators	(a) tachykinin-like (b) catechol oxidase
Hard ticks	
Antihistamine	
Antiplatelet	Apyrase
Anticoagulants	(a) Anti-fVIIa, anti-fVa (b) Antiprothrombinase
Kininase (Antibradykinin)	Carboxypeptidase N-like
Antianaphylatoxin	Carboxypeptidase N-like
Vasodilator	Prostaglandin E2 (PGE2)
Anti-PAF (platelet activating factor)	PGE2
Immunosuppression	
Neutrophil-activation inhibitor	

TABLE 20.1 (Continued)   Reported arthropod salivary gland activities with proposed roles in blood-feeding

Reported activity	Product (if known)
T-cell activation inhibitor	
Anticomplement (alternate pathway)	
Soft ticks	
Anticoagulant	TAP (Tick anticoagulant peptide)
Antiplatelet	Apyrase
Triatomine bugs	
Antiplatelet	Apyrase
Anticoagulants	(a) Anti-fVIII (b) Anti-thrombin (rhodniin)
Tsetse flies	
Antiplatelet	Apyrase
Anticoagulant	Antithrombin
Black flies	
Anticoagulants	(a) Antithrombin (b) Anti-fXa

component of the granules in platelets, is also released by damaged cells and is one of the important signal molecules that lead to platelet recruitment and platelet aggregation. Other molecules that can activate platelets are thrombin, collagen, prostaglandin H_2, thromboxane A_2, and platelet activating factor (PAF). Vector salivary compounds directed against collagen and prostaglandin H_2 have not been described. However, antithrombins are often present in vector saliva. These antithrombins are usually thought to be involved in anticoagulation but could also conceivably be involved in inhibiting platelet aggregation. Antithromboxane activities are also known to exist that could contribute to platelet inhibition as well as providing an

TABLE 20.2 Salivary apyrases of vector arthropods[a]

Species	Cation cofactors	pH optimum[b]
Mosquitoes		
Aedes aegypti	Ca++, Mg++, Sr++	9.0
Anopheles stephensi	Ca++, Mg++	9.0
An. freeborni	Ca++, Mg++	9.0
Sand flies		
Lutzomyia longipalpus	Ca++	8.0
Phlebotomus argentipes	Ca++	8.0
P. papatasi	Ca++	8.0
P. perniciosus	Ca++	8.0
Triatomine bugs		
Rhodnius prolixus	Ca++	7.5
Fleas		
Oropsylla bacchi	Ca++, Mg++	7.5
Orchopea howardii	Ca++, Mg++	7.5
Xenopsylla cheopsis	Ca++, Mg++	
Ticks		
Ornithodorus moubata	Ca++, Mg++	7.5
Ixodes dammini/scapularis	Ca++, Mg++	7.5

[a] after Ribeiro et al. 1991, *Comp. Biochem. and Physiol.* 100.
[b] averaged optima for ADP and ATP

antiinflammatory response. Anti-PAF activity attributable to the prostaglandin E_2–like molecule has been described in ticks.

Vasodilators

Another apparently universal challenge to hematophagy is presented by vasoconstriction. As described earlier, in addition to platelet aggregation vasoconstriction is an important hemostatic response, particularly in small wounds. Every hematophagous arthropod examined secretes a vasodilator. These substances most likely counteract vasoconstriction that occurs during hemostasis following injury and bring the vessels closer to the surface, enabling the insect direct access to the vasculature. The vasodilators in vector saliva are generally thought to cause the erythema observed following the bite of an arthropod, which reflects increased capillary permeability. This increased permeability contributes to a surface hematoma on which the vectors can feed. Vasodilation is most significant in vectors that have short feeding stylets (e.g., phlebotomine sand flies) or chewing mouthparts (biting flies). Indeed, maxadilan, the most potent vasodilator described to date, was isolated from a sand fly.

Vasodilatory substances appear to be unique for each group of hematophagous arthropods (Table 20.3). For example, the bloodsucking bug *Rhodnius prolixus* induces vasodilation through a secreted nitric oxide (NO) binding protein, whereas sand flies secrete maxadilan, a peptide that induces vasodilation similar to mammalian vasoactive peptide, CGRP (calcitonin gene-related peptide). Ticks secrete a prostaglandin E_2–like molecule. Interestingly, the vasodilators in mosquitoes vary in members of the subfamilies. *Ae. aegypti* and *Ae. triseriatus* secrete a tachykinin-like molecule, and *Anopheles albimanus* secretes a catechol-oxidase. Thus, during evolution, vasodilatory substances probably had not been optimized before the ancestral separation of these 2 major mosquito groups.

Anticoagulation Factors

As discussed earlier, coagulation and the formation of a fibrin clot are essential for stopping major bleeding and providing long-term support to platelet plugs. Except for ticks, the kinetics of coagulation are longer than the time required for a vector to obtain blood. Hence coagulation probably does not determine the ability of an arthropod to locate blood; however, anticoagulants have been discovered in most of the salivary glands of the hematophagous vectors examined. The presence of anticoagulants in mosquitoes, tsetse flies, black flies, and triatomine bugs as well as ticks suggests that coagulation affects the success of blood-feeding by arthropods. Because anticoagulant-negative genetic mutants are currently unavailable, researchers can only speculate on the physiological role of the anticoagulant

TABLE 20.3 Vasodilatory activities in vector saliva

Species	Activity
Mosquitoes	
Aedes aegypti	tachykinin-like
Aedes triseriatus	tachykinin-like
Anopheles albimanus	catechol oxidase/ peroxidase
Other flies	
Lutzomyia longipalpus	maxadilan
Simulium vittatum	unknown
Ticks	
Ixodes dammini/scapularis	prostaglandin E2-like
Amblyomma americanum	prostaglandin E2-like
Boophilus microplus	prostaglandin E2-like
Triatomine bugs	
Rhodnius prolixus	nitric oxide binding protein

TABLE 20.4 Anticoagulant activities found in vector saliva

Species	Activity
Triatomine bugs	
Rhodnius prolixus	(a) anti-fVIIIa
	(b) rhodniin, antithrombin (Kazal-type inhibitor)
Ticks	
Ornithodorus moubata	TAP, anti-fXa (Kunitz-type inhibitor)
Dermacentor andersoni	anti-fVa, Anti-fVIIa
Ixodes scapularis	not identified
Rhipicephalus appendiculatus	antiprothrombinase (not against fXa)
Mosquitoes	
Anopheles rossi, An. jamesi	not identified
An. freeborni, An. stephensi	not identified
Ae. aegypti	anti-fXa
An. gambiae	antithrombin
Tsetse flies	
Glossina morsitans	antithrombin (not proteinaceous)
G. austeni	antithrombin
Black flies	
Simulium vittatum	(a) anti-fXa (b) Anti-thrombin

found in these arthropods. Anticoagulants are possibly necessary to maintain the flow of blood through the mouthparts during feeding. In addition, anticoagulants could prevent a clot from forming within a vector-induced hematoma. As mentioned previously, antithrombins could affect both anticoagulation and platelet inhibition.

Anticoagulants vary in their specific activity according to the hematophagous species (Table 20.4). They often attack the common pathway in the coagulation cascade, specifically targeting factor Xa (fXa) and thrombin (Fig. 20.2). However, inhibitors against other factors have also been characterized. Except for *Glossina morsitans*, the anticoagulants characterized are all proteins. The best-characterized anticoagulants are the antithrombin rhodniin from *R. prolixus* and the anti-factor Xa TAP (tick anticoagulant peptide) from *Ornithodorus moubata*. Although both of these factors act as serine protease inhibitors, TAP is related to the Kunitz class of serine protease inhibitors

whereas rhodniin is related to Kazal-type protease inhibitors. In addition, TAP appears to be a protease that produces its inhibition through the proteolytic cleavage of fXa whereas rhodniin seems to act as a competitive inhibitor of thrombin. Unfortunately, because rhodniin was purified from whole animal extracts (and an earlier report described an antithrombin present in the midgut of *R. prolixus*) this anticoagulant may not be

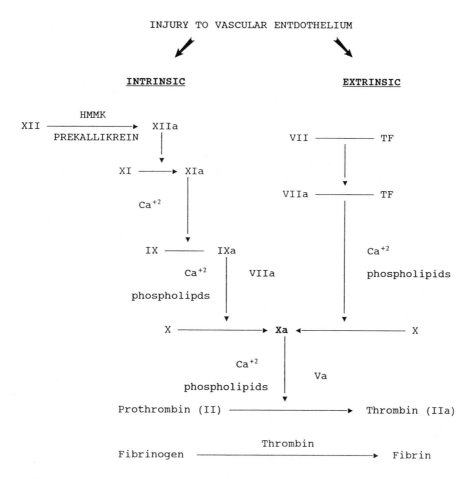

INJURY TO VASCULAR ENTDOTHELIUM

INTRINSIC   EXTRINSIC

XII ——HMMK——▶ XIIa   VII ————— TF
    PREKALLIKREIN

        XI ——▶ XIa   VIIa ————— TF

    Ca^{+2}

        IX ——— IXa   Ca^{+2}
            Ca^{+2} │ VIIa   phospholipids
        phospholipds

        X ————————▶ Xa ◀———————— X

                Ca^{+2}
                            Va
            phospholipids │

Prothrombin (II) ————————————▶ Thrombin (IIa)

                        Thrombin
Fibrinogen ————————————————▶ Fibrin

20.2   A schematic representation of the coagulation cascades leading to the activation of factor Xa to form the active prothrombinase (a complex of factors Xa and Va, calcium, and phospholipids). The extrinsic pathway is activated by clear-cut damage to the vascular wall and release of tissue factor from endothelial cells that causes the release of tissue cell. The intrinsic pathway occurs when internal structural defects exist on the vascular lining or when coagulation factors come in contact with other activating surfaces (e.g., glass). The prothrombinase complex cleaves prothrombin to release the active serine protease, thrombin. Thrombin then acts on fibrinogen to release active fibrin for formation of the hemostatic plug. Calcium and phospholipids are required cofactors for many steps of the coagulation cascade. *HMMK* = high molecular mass kallikrein; *TF* = tissue factor; roman numerals indicate coagulation factors, "*a*" indicates active coagulation factors.

of salivary gland origin. Thus, its role in blood-feeding remains obscure. The mechanisms of action and

inhibitor types of the other anticoagulants have not been elucidated.

Other Factors

In addition to the properties described, many other activities occur in arthropod saliva. Some of these activities may play an important role in neutralizing biochemically active components of blood. For example, a recently described tumor necrosis factor identified in female mosquitoes and the macrophage-activation inhibitor in sand flies have been proposed to play protective roles during ingestion of blood. The anticomplement activity of ticks could be responsible for preventing damage to the midgut. In addition an anticomplement activity could reduce the production of the anaphalotoxins, C5a and C3a, thus limiting the inflammatory response to blood-feeding; however, this activity was originally described as an adjunct to preventing host rejection of ticks by the alternate complement pathway. Ticks have a full array of pharmacological activities that could play an immunosuppressive role. These activities are important because ticks feed for extended periods and risk host rejection by the immune system much like a skin graft. A hemagglutinin has also been described in anopheline mosquitoes that could play a role in digestion by clumping the erythrocytes in the midgut during digestion. Although the pain response seems to be an important host response for the blood-feeding vector to evade, only one antibradykinin has been described, and this was found in ticks.

Convergent Evolution

Hematophagy in the various arthropod phyla represents a remarkable example of convergent evolution. The ability to feed on blood has arisen independently in various groups that have been separated for hundreds of millions of years. The fact that so many of the species have salivary activities that act to mitigate specific aspects of vertebrate hemostasis, inflammation, and the immune system emphasizes the nontrivial aspect of blood-feeding. A comparative analysis of the salivary gland activities points to essential elements required for all blood-feeding vectors. The ability to synthesize and secrete platelet inhibitory factors, vasodilatory activities, and anticoagulants appears to be a prerequisite for survival. Thus, in the study of the salivary glands of an uncharacterized vector, the identification of analogous activities can be a starting point for the molecular analysis of that species.

Analysis of the origin and molecular evolution of activities with specific roles in blood-feeding is also intriguing. The majority of compounds are proteins and therefore products of genes. In many cases these genes have highly regulated temporal, spatial, and sex-specific expression. The salivary gland–specific gene expression in mosquitoes is a good example of this highly specialized expression pattern. The ancestral progenitor genes in mosquitoes are assumed not to have the same or similar expression patterns as the current genes, but this may not be true of all hematophagic species. The ancestral feeding habits may influence which genes are later adapted to blood-feeding roles.

In the mosquito *Aedes aegypti*, the salivary apyrase is a member of the 5'-nucleotidase family. Through evolution, perhaps via gene duplication and divergence of one of the duplicated copies, a gene that encoded a widespread and common cellular enzyme acquired the proper enhancer and control elements that now direct its expression in a highly specific manner. The fact that apyrases in all hematophagic arthropod taxa appear to be similar biochemically suggests that this conversion may be relatively straightforward. Perhaps a gene encoding a secreted form of apyrase exists and can be recruited easily to a blood-feeding role.

The origin of the vasodilatory agents appears to represent the other extreme of convergent evolution. All arthropods secrete a compound that has a vasodilatory effect on vertebrate vasculature but with a wide variety of biochemically different proteins and peptides serving as the source of this activity. It is highly unlikely that these originated in the same gene families. Interestingly, there are groups such as the ticks that appear to have similar types of activities (prostaglandin E_2-like); however, within the mosquitoes, the vasodilatory activities differ significantly in members of the major subfamilies, the Culicinae and Anophelinae. These differences may indicate the ancestral feeding habits of each group. Most of the Arachnida (the class that includes ticks) are predatory and insectivorous. Genes that encode products such as proteases that were useful in the tick ancestral feeding modes may have been converted easily to a role in blood-feeding as anticoagulants. However, in the mosquitoes it is generally believed that the ancestral insects fed on sugar, much as the males do now. The evolution of different efficient vasodilatory agents occurred because the anophelines and culicines adapted these activities to a new feeding behavior as they proceeded along their divergent evolutionary paths.

The study of the molecular evolution of the genes encoding the anticoagulant activities should be intriguing. Both ticks and the triatomine bug, *R. prolixus*, have anticoagulants that appear to be noncovalently acting serine protease inhibitors distinct from the "serpins," although as described previously there are significant differences between the 2 groups. These protease inhibitors may have evolved from other secreted salivary protease inhibitors that were used by the predatory ancestors of these groups. It should be pointed out that the origin of blood-feeding in the triatomines has not been resolved. There are arguments to propose that the ancestral insects were predatory; others suggest that they were herbivorous, feeding on the hard seeds of plants. Perhaps a molecular systematic analysis of some of the salivary proteins could contribute to the resolution of this matter.

Anticoagulants in other groups are only now being characterized. Mosquitoes appear to vary within groups in the type of anticoagulant activities, and preliminary work has shown that *Ae. aegypti* has an anti-FXa, but *An. gambiae* has an antithrombin. It will be interesting to examine systematic relationships among the subfamilies using these activities as markers.

In conclusion, the molecular and comparative analysis of activities in the salivary glands of vector arthropods has identified some necessary requirements for the evolution of hematophagy. In addition, the analysis of genes and the gene products has revealed some interesting relationships within major groups of vector insects, especially the mosquitoes. It remains to be seen whether the genes that encode some of these activities or the activities themselves could be targets for future vector control strategies.

PARASITE TRANSMISSION

The relationship between vector and pathogen and the role of arthropod saliva in the transmission of disease is fascinating. Because of the inter-relationship of hemostasis, inflammation, and the immune response, many of the properties that facilitate and contribute to the success of blood-feeding may also enhance parasite disease transmission. This clearly is the case for leishmaniases and may prove to be a general property for arthropod-borne diseases.

Parasites first enter a vector with the blood meal, and most are eventually ejected during salivation into the vertebrate host. Thus, most parasites have ample opportunity to interact with their vector's salivary glands and/or salivary products by entry at the feeding site. Furthermore, all arthropod-borne diseases have parasitemia. For example, malarial parasites invade erythrocytes, leishmanial parasites invade macrophages, and arboviruses can be free in the blood. The action of vector saliva on blood may facilitate these phases of the pathogen life cycle. Filarial worms and the causative agents for Chagas' disease, *Trypanosoma cruzi*, are exceptions to emission during salivation. The worms rupture and emerge from the vector mouthparts during blood-feeding; *T. cruzi* are excreted in the feces during feeding. Both parasites enter the host at the feeding site, the former by wriggling their way in, and the latter by the host rubbing feces into the wound.

Three types of vector-parasite interactions that enhance transmission can be predicted from experimental findings and theoretical modeling: (1) parasites can increase the probability of their transmission by modifying arthropod salivary activities, (2) an infected host can be modified by a parasite such that the arthropod vector feeds more successfully on the infected host, and (3) specific pharmacological substances secreted by the arthropod during blood-feeding may enhance parasite transmission directly.

Modification of Salivary Activities

Infection of an arthropod by a parasite can alter the quality or quantity of specific components of the products in the salivary glands, resulting in enhanced transmission of the parasite. Malaria sporozoites infect the female-specific salivary gland lobes (distal-lateral and medial) of mosquitoes, the same lobes that are utilized only in blood-feeding. The parasite invasion causes cellular damage in the glands resulting in a 4–5-fold reduction in apyrase activity. Interestingly this does not affect salivation during probing. As mentioned earlier, studies have shown that probing time is inversely proportional to apyrase levels. Experiments have shown that sporozoite-infected mosquitoes take longer to probe when blood-feeding. This increased probing time possibly results in the release of more sporozoites; however, such a correlation has not been shown in experiments using an artificial feeding apparatus. Also, the infected mosquitoes demonstrate more interrupted feedings and therefore bite more frequently before achieving a successful blood meal. Therefore 1 infected mosquito can infect multiple individuals. In addition, sporozoites are ejected during the 1st phase of salivation. Thus, the act of probing could direct more sporozoites to the salivary glands and ducts and lead to a higher multiplicity of infection. In conclusion, parasite infection disrupts apyrase activity, interrupts mosquito feeding, and thus enhances disease transmission by infecting more individuals.

Many parasites and arboviruses must cross the vector midgut to the hemocoel as part of their development. In fact, vector competence often depends on whether a particular parasite or virus can cross the gut wall. Increased transmission of Rift Valley fever virus (RVFV) occurs when mosquitoes are coinfected with microfilaria. The microfilariae presumably rupture the midgut epithelium, thus increasing transmission by allowing a more efficient dissemination of the virus. Additionally, parasites cause cellular damage to the vector salivary glands; however, it is not clear yet if a decrease in any particular salivary activity leads to increased penetration across the gut wall. Decreased activity in either the anticomplement or anti-TNF activity in infected vectors could result in ingestion of complement factors and TNF, which could damage the midgut, Parasites or viruses could then penetrate the midgut more effectively, increasing the probability of and decreasing the time required for dissemination, thus enhancing infection and subsequent transmission.

Enhanced Feeding on the Infected Host

Many arthropod-borne infectious diseases cause erythema in the vertebrate host, indicating an increase in vascular permeability and vasodilation. Just as vasodilators in vector saliva enhance blood-finding, parasite-induced vasodilation in the vertebrate host would decrease the time required for a mosquito to blood-feed. Mathematical modeling has predicted that an arthropod will be able to feed more successfully on an infected host with parasite-induced erythema. In addition to erythema, many parasites disrupt host hemostasis mechanisms by virtue of their infectious cycle and therefore could enhance vector feeding efficiency on infected hosts. For example, malaria parasites replicate preferentially not only in erythrocytes but in a variety of hematopoietic stem cells and are known to cause thrombocytopenia (decreased platelet count). Likewise, RVFV causes hemorrhagic disorders by disrupting platelets. In both situations, feeding on an infected host with a low platelet count should be more efficient than feeding on a noninfected host with normal levels of functioning platelets. Experiments that compared the feeding rates on RVFV- or malaria-infected hosts with uninfected hosts showed that mosquitoes fed faster on the infected hosts. In addition, cutaneous leishmaniasis infection in a variety of rodents causes erythema as well as a loss of hair at the site of infection. Thus, sand flies can feed more readily at the wound site of infected hosts. Therefore, because more vectors are infected, disease transmission is enhanced.

Direct Transmission Enhancement

The best way to directly mediate parasite-vector interaction is via salivary biochemical activities. Several examples of this type of transmission enhancement exist. Ticks are the likely candidate for such a parasite-vector relationship because of the numerous activities present in tick saliva (see Table 20.1), and tick-infected hosts have been shown to be severely immunocompromised. The hard tick, *Ixodes scapularis* (formerly *I. dammini*), serves as a vector for *Borrelia burgdorferi*, the causative agent of Lyme disease. The transmission of infectious spirochetes by a tick bite is more efficient than by syringe injection of the parasites. Experiments have shown that immune serum effectively destroys *B. burgdorferi*, and that neutrophils alone phagocytose the parasites in vitro in the absence of immune serum. The neutrophil-inhibiting activity of *I. scapularis* saliva has been proposed to enhance Lyme disease transmission.

The infectivity of spirochetes injected into an animal model with and without tick saliva should be compared to determine if this is occurring. If tick saliva can be shown to enhance transmission, then the salivary fraction containing the neutrophil-inhibiting activity could be tested for Lyme disease transmission enhancement. *I. scapularis* saliva also contains a powerful anticomplement activity specific for the alternate pathway. Lysis of microorganisms, and parasites in particular, by the alternate complement pathway is well documented. The alternate complement pathway may also be important in the host defense against Lyme disease. Thus, tick saliva may enable *B. burgdorferi* to evade initial lysis by both phagocytic cells and the alternate complement pathway and therefore greatly enhance the infectivity of entering spirochetes. Other tick-borne infections may also be enhanced by tick saliva and should be investigated.

The best-characterized interaction between vector saliva and parasite transmission is the *Leishmania* spp. and phlebotomine sand fly interaction (Chap. 9). Leishmaniases are widespread diseases affecting the rural areas of most developing countries. Patients can die from the more severe mucocutaneous and visceral infection. However, the majority of leishmaniasis infections cause skin sores that can lead to physical disfigurement and immune suppression and therefore are predominantly a public health concern. The *Leishmania* life cycle involves obligate developmental stages within the sand fly vector. The parasite must replicate eventually within vertebrate macrophages or reticuloendothelial cells (see Fig. 20.3). During *Leishmania* metacyclogenesis, certain glycoproteins become expressed on their cell surfaces so that the infectious metacyclic promastigotes, when injected during the blood meal, are maximally opsonized by macrophages without activating the complement cascade. Normally foreign antigens are presented by macrophages to appropriate B- and T-lymphocytes, which causes the secretion of antibodies specific for the antigen, and/or secretion of lymphokines to cause leukocyte activation. The surface glycoproteins expressed on metacyclic promastigotes could then activate the alternate complement pathway. *Leishmania* do appear to cause the release of C3a, indicating the activation of complement; however, C3b becomes deposited on the cell

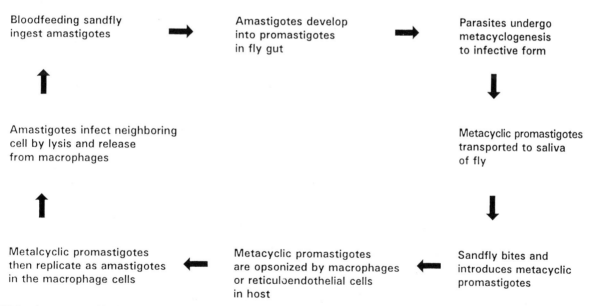

20.3 A summary of *Leishmania* life cycle in sand flies and transmission of vertebrate macrophages. Important sites of development and metamorphosis are indicated.

surface of the parasite and may facilitate its entry into macrophages. Thus, *Leishmania* seems to be well equipped to deal with the mammalian immune system. However, once phagocytosed the infected macrophage expresses *Leishmania* antigens on its cell surface with class II MHC (major histocompatibility). T-cells and B-cells recognize the expressed foreign antigen and secrete lymphokines such as IL–2 and INF-γ, causing the macrophage to become activated and lyse, thereby destroying the intracellular parasite. How *Leishmania* possibly avoids destruction by macrophage activation is currently being studied.

In studies utilizing experimental animal models, *Leishmania* injected by a syringe require several hundred times more parasites to cause disease than would be expected to occur in nature. However, when *Leishmania* was injected in the presence of sand fly saliva, as few as 10 parasites caused an infection; no infection was detected without saliva. The proposed *Leishmania* enhancing factor (LEF) present in sand fly saliva may be attributable to an antimacrophage activity. When macrophages are incubated with sand fly salivary gland extract, macrophages fail to present class I antigens and do not respond to IL–2 or INF-γ. Chromatographic studies of sand fly saliva initially indicated that the antimacrophage activity and the vasodilator, maxadilan, are similar to calcitonin gene-related peptide. CGRP is a neuropeptide hormone with known vasodilator activities which has recently been shown to inhibit macrophage function and exacerbate *L. major* infections in mice, albeit not as effectively as sand fly saliva. Also, the sand fly vasodilator activity has been shown to be 500 times that of CGRP, and its antimacrophage activity is about 10 times that of CGRP. Although it is possible that the sand fly recruited a gene encoding a neuropeptide for blood-feeding purposes, CGRP and LEF/maxadilan molecular weight differences are significant, and they do not share any antigenic determinant sites. Maxadilan-like molecules have been identified in a number of sand fly species, and cloned cDNAs are available for several of these. Experiments with better-characterized maxadilan-like peptides from a variety of sand flies are being performed to determine whether LEF, the antimacrophage activities, and the vasodilatory activity are properties of the same molecule.

An interesting corollary to the utilization of secreted salivary proteins to enhance transmission has been recently suggested for filarial worms and mosquitoes. Microfilariae are present in much lower levels than expected in the superficial blood vessels for a blood-feeding mosquito to maintain the infectious cycle. Thus, investigators have proposed that microfilariae respond to a component of mosquito saliva as a chemotaxin and therefore congregate in the superficial capillary bed at the feeding site to be maximally ingested during the blood meal.

Other Enhancements of Disease Transmission

Other vector-host and -parasite interactions exist that are important factors in the transmission of disease. Experiments have shown that more sporozoites are ejected from malaria-infected mosquitoes that were fed previously on hosts with antisporozoite antibody titers. Some researchers have proposed that because malaria sporozoites exist extracellularly in the mosquito, antisporozoite antibodies ingested in a blood meal from an immunized host interact with the sporozoite antigen. This antibody-sporozoite complex thus somehow facilitates parasite dissemination and therefore increases transmission efficiency. This could affect the efficacy of malaria vaccines directed against sporozoites. This mechanism of transmission enhancement presupposes that either the mosquito saliva does not have an anti-antibody activity or that the malaria sporozoites have decreased this speculative salivary property.

Thogoto viral transmission occurs at a much higher rate from an infected tick to an uninfected tick while feeding on the same nonpermissive host. Because of the immunosuppressive activities of tick saliva, virus could evade the immune system of the vertebrate host and infect the tick, where it can successfully replicate. This mode of vector-parasite interaction with a nonviremic host could be important in spreading disease among ticks and thereby increase the probability of transmission to permissive vertebrate hosts. Thus, such disease enhancement would be similar to those circumstances in which arthropod saliva directly causes transmission enhancement.

Coevolution of Vectors and Parasites

Arthropod-borne parasites have apparently coevolved with the evolution of blood-feeding to gain easier access to vertebrate hosts by evading immune surveillance systems. Whereas some parasites require both arthropod and vertebrate hosts for the support of their life cycle, the majority of arboviruses do not require both hosts for replication. Transovarial transmission may be sufficient to maintain the viruses in the mosquitoes. Thus, mammals and humans may be accidental hosts to these viruses. At some time during evolution, arboviruses gained access to the arthropod salivary glands, possibly during a coinfection with another parasite, and were ejected during blood-feeding. Those viruses that could replicate in their new vertebrate host became easily established in the immune-compromised environment created by the arthropod saliva, thus greatly expanding their host range.

CONCLUSION

Saliva secreted by a variety of arthropods has antihemostatic properties, particularly antiplatelet activity, which helps facilitate the location of blood. Apyrase is seemingly found in all arthropods, underlining the major importance of ATP and ADP in the recruitment of platelets and the central role of platelets in the initiation of hemostasis. Similarly, anticoagulants and vasodilators are present in the salivary glands of most hematophagus arthropods, indicating that vasoconstriction and coagulation present universal challenges to blood-feeding. Additional antihemostatic, antiinflammatory, and immunosuppressive activities are found in arthropod saliva, which increase the success of blood-feeding and therefore arthropod survival. Blood-feeding is not a trivial process, and hematophagous arthropods have responded with a complicated armament to combat the many problems associated with blood biochemistry. In addition, the arthropod-borne parasites, which must face many of the same vertebrate defense mechanisms in establishing an infection, have evolved several clever ways of manipulating and/or utilizing the salivary activities secreted during the blood meal to enhance their transmission. Such parasite-vector interactions may explain why attempts to vaccinate against vector-borne parasites have been unsuccessful.

Future studies with arthropod saliva and its role in both blood-feeding and parasite transmission should enable researchers to develop more effective measures to control vector-borne infectious diseases. For instance, in leishmaniasis, a vaccination for LEF could diminish the transmission enhancement by sand flies. If the LEF activity proves to be contained within the maxadilan protein, sand flies would have more difficulty feeding from vaccinated humans and therefore bite other mammals for their blood meal. Thus, the spread of leishmaniasis would be limited by the decreased efficiency of parasite transmission and the decreased biting rate of sand flies on humans. Also, studies of gene expression in arthropods could provide the means to genetically engineer vectors that would predominate in the wild but be refractory to pathogen infection. For example, the antisense messenger RNA or a ribozyme to dengue fever virus or other flaviviruses could be expressed in the salivary glands of adult female mosquitoes. Thus, when the virus infects the mosquito salivary glands, its RNA genome would not be translated. In addition, studies are currently under way to determine the genetic means of natural vector refractoriness to diseases such as malaria and filariases. As these genes are mapped and their mechanisms understood, new refractory vectors could be engineered and manipulated to ensure that these new strains replace the natural permissive strains. Although much work is still needed to attain these long-term goals, especially in the area of a reliable and efficient vector transformation system, much of the groundwork exists. Thus, the salivary glands and pharmacological properties of arthropod saliva present many academic and medical challenges. Future research on these organisms should not only provide insight into the interaction between vector, blood, and parasite but enable a better understanding of hemostasis, inflammation, and infectious disease transmission.

REFERENCES AND FURTHER READING

Davie, E.W., K. Fujikawa, and W. Kisiel. 1991. The coagulation cascade: Initiation, maintenance and regulation. *Biochemistry* 30:10363–10370.

Georgilis, K., A.C. Steere, and M.S. Klempnen. 1991. Infectivity of *Borrelia burgdorferi*: Correlates with resistance to elimination by phagocytic cells. *J. of Infectious Disease* 163:150–155.

James, A.A. 1994. Molecular and biochemical analyses of the salivary glands of vector mosquitoes. *Bulletin l'Institut Pasteur* 92:133–150.

James, A.A., and P.A. Rossignol. 1991. Mosquito salivary glands: Parasitological and molecular aspects. *Parasit. Today* 7:267–271.

Marinotti, O., A.A. James, and J.M.C. Ribeiro. 1990. Diet and salivation in female *Aedes aegypti* mosquitoes. *J. Insect Physiol.* 36:545–548.

Mustard, J.F., and M.A. Packham. 1977. Normal and abnormal haemostasis. *Brit. Med. Bull.* 33:187–191.

Ribeiro, J.M.C. 1987. Role of saliva in bloodfeeding and arthropods. *Ann. Rev. Entomol.* 32:463–478.

———. 1989. Role of saliva in tick/host interactions. *Exp. App. Acarol.* 7:15–20.

———. 1989. Vector saliva and its role in parasite transmission. *Exp. Parasitol.* 69:104–106.

Ribeiro, J.M.C., P.A. Rossignol, and A. Spielman. 1984. Role of mosquito saliva in blood vessel location. *J. Exp. Biol.* 108:1–7.

———. 1985. Mathematical model of parasite-vector interaction. *Exp. Parasitol.* 60:118–132.

Rossignol, P.A., and A.M. Rossignol. 1988. Models of parasite transmission enhancement by vector-parasite interactions. *Parasitol.* 97:363–372.

Rossignol, P.A., and A. Spielman. 1982. Fluid transport across the salivary glands of a mosquito. *J. Insect Physiol.* 28:579–583.

Titus, R.G., and J.M.C. Ribeiro. 1988. Salivary gland lysates from the sand fly *Lutzomyia longipalpis* enhance *Leishmania* infectivity. *Science* 239:1306–1308.

———. 1990. The role of vector saliva in transmission of arthropod-borne disease. *Parasitol. Today* 6:157–160.

Vargaftig, B.B., M. Chignard, and J. Benveniste. 1981. Present concepts on the mechanisms of platelet aggregation. *Biochem. Pharm.* 30:263–271.

Waxman, L., D.E. Smith, K.E. Arcuri, and G.P. Vlasuk. 1990. Tick anticoagulant peptide (TAP) is a novel inhibitor of blood coagulation factor FXa. *Science* 248:593–596.

21. FAT BODY AND HEMOLYMPH

Miranda C. van Heusden

INTRODUCTION

The insect fat body is the principal tissue for intermediary metabolism. It is functionally diverse and is instrumental in both biosynthesis and storage of lipids, carbohydrates, and proteins. Hence it performs the functions associated with mammalian liver and adipose tissue. Because the fat body produces many of the hemolymph metabolites, it strongly influences the overall physiology of the insect.

Hemolymph is the extracellular fluid that fills the hemocoel and surrounds all tissues. It has many functions, including transport of nutrients, waste products, and hormones. One important characteristic of insect hemolymph is its storage function, which results in high concentrations of organic molecules. This chapter provides an overview of the structure and physiology of the fat body and the circulatory system. Note that beyond the basic characteristics described here an enormous variability exists among species.

FAT BODY

Structure

Fat body is a diffuse tissue localized mainly in the abdomen. Smaller amounts also are present in the thorax and the head (Dean et al. 1985). It consists of sheets, pads, or ribbons 2–3 cell layers thick (Fig. 21.1). Fat body is often divided into 2 parts: the visceral fat body surrounding the midgut, instrumental in protein synthesis and storage, and the peripheral fat body adjacent to the integument, which stores lipids

and glycogen (although exceptions exist). The amorphic structure of the fat body is possibly an adaptation to the open circulatory system in which transport of metabolites occurs mainly by diffusion. Because the fat body is only a few cell layers thick and distributed throughout the body, a considerable amount of surface area is exposed to the hemolymph, reducing diffusion distance and resulting in efficient exchange of metabolites. The fat body is surrounded by a basal lamina that is permeable to metabolites, including proteins.

Trophocytes, also called adipocytes, are the main cell type of the fat body, and their functional diversity may be unequaled by any other metazoan cell type. Synthesis occurs in these cells, as well as storage of proteins, lipids, and glycogen. In some species other cell types are present: chromatocytes, which are filled with pigment and influence the insect color pattern; urocytes, which store urate that possibly originates from the catabolism of nucleic acids at the end of protein synthesis; mycetocytes, which contain symbiotic microorganisms; and oenocytes, which may function in the synthesis of lipids for the cuticle.

The ultrastructure of the fat body changes during development. During larval feeding periods the fat body cells actively synthesize protein, which is reflected in the abundant rough endoplasmatic reticulum and Golgi complexes. The so-called storage proteins make up the major portion of the synthesized protein. The larval stages are also characterized by the storage of lipids and glycogen in the fat body. At the

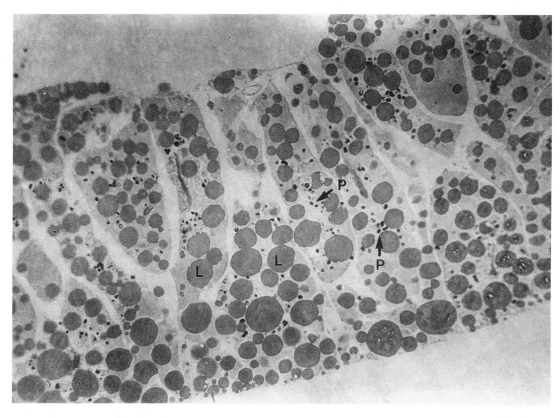

21.1   Toluidine blue stained section of a fat body ribbon from 5th instar larva of *Manduca sexta*. L = lipid droplet, P = protein granule. Magnification = 470x. Courtesy of E. Willot, R. Nagle, and L. Bew.

end of larval and the beginning of pupal development, proteins (mainly storage proteins) are resequestered from the hemolymph into the fat body and protein granules appear in the trophocytes. The larval fat body can also store tyrosine in vacuoles that contain phenolic precursors required by the epidermis for cuticular tanning. At the end of larval development, a change in cellular activity occurs: Peroxisomes, mitochondria, and endoplasmic reticulum are destroyed in autophagic vacuoles. In the adult insect, the fat body functions mainly as a site of storage and synthesis of metabolites necessary for reproduction and flight. The cells contain glycogen deposits and lipid droplets as well as many protein granules. There is a sexual dimorphism in adult fat body: Usually male fat body has larger lipid and carbohydrate stores whereas

female fat body has more endoplasmic reticulum, reflecting the role of trophocytes in mate-seeking flights and reproduction, respectively.

The change from larval to adult fat body occurs by different mechanisms. Adult adipocytes can be derived from larval adipocytes by reorganization of the cytoplasm (e.g., in Lepidoptera and mosquitoes) or by lysis of the larval cells and differentiation of imaginal cells in the pupa (e.g., in higher Diptera) or by a combination of both.

Protein Synthesis and Storage
The amount of fat body DNA varies during development. Polyploidy (a chromosome number that is a multiple of the normal diploid number) is a common phenomenon in insect cells, and Diptera are known for

their polyteny in many cell types (chromosomes consisting of many identical chromatids). Polyploidy has been described in the fat body of *Rhodnius prolixus* and *Aedes aegypti*, for example. Juvenile hormone (JH) and ecdysteroids appear to play a role in the regulation of ploidization. By providing multiple copies of the genome, polyploidy enhances selective transcription of a specific gene at a high rate. One example is the high level of synthesis of yolk protein precursors during oocyte development in *Locusta migratoria*, at which constitute time vitellogenic proteins comprise the major portion of the proteins synthesized by the fat body.

The fat body is the main source for synthesis of hemolymph proteins. In the larval stages, the storage proteins constitute most of the proteins synthesized by the fat body. Storage proteins are usually hexameric macromolecules that are high in aromatic amino acids. Their subunits have a molecular weight around 80 kDa. These proteins serve as storage reservoirs for amino acids necessary for the construction of adult tissues. They are secreted into the hemolymph during larval stages but are resequestered selectively into the fat body at the end of larval development (Kanost et al. 1990). The major protein synthesized by and secreted from the fat body in the adult stage is vitellogenin. It comprises 70–90% of the protein secreted by the adult female fat body. In flies and mosquitoes, protein-feeding activates the endocrine system, resulting in an accumulation of protein synthesis organelles in trophocytes. The role of JH and ecdysone in the stimulation of vitellogenin synthesis is described in Chapter 15.

Carbohydrate Synthesis and Storage

Carbohydrates are the major energy source in many insect species (Steele 1981); they also form a major component of the exoskeleton. Carbohydrates are stored in the fat body as glycogen. All enzymes for gluconeogenesis are present in the fat body (Chap. 22). Fat body glycogen is degraded by phosphorylase, which has to be activated by a kinase, which in turn is activated by ATP, Mg^{2+}, and Ca^{2+}. The resulting glucose–6-phosphate is conjugated to diphosphoglucoside to form trehalose–6-phosphate, which is subsequently dephosphorylated to trehalose. Trehalose is released into the hemolymph.

Lipid Synthesis and Storage

Lipids are often synthesized from carbohydrate precursors. Glycerolipids are synthesized de novo from glycerophosphate via phosphatidic acid. Phosphatidic acid then loses the phosphate, and the diacylglycerol (DG) formed is acetylated to triacylglycerol (TG) or converted to glycerophospholipids of choline and ethanolamine. TG is the main lipid storage form in the fat body. In general myristic, palmitic, and oleic acid are the main fatty acids synthesized and incorporated in glycerides and phospholipids. However, the presence of small amounts of long-chain polyunsaturated fatty acids in both phospholipids and prostaglandins has been demonstrated in many insect species (Stanley-Samuelson and Dadd 1983). The mobilization of lipids from the fat body is regulated by an adipokinetic hormone (AKH) released from the corpora cardiaca (Chap. 22). A lipase hydrolyses TG to DG, which is released into the hemolymph.

THE CIRCULATORY SYSTEM

Structure

Insects have an open circulatory system. The hemolymph flows through the entire body cavity, or hemocoel. A thin permeable membrane, the basal lamina, lines the hemocoel and separates the hemolymph from tissues. The flow of hemolymph is directed by body movements and a number of pulsatile organs, such as the dorsal vessel and the accessory pulsatile organs (Miller 1985). The dorsal vessel, which consists of a layer of striated muscle fibers, usually extends from the abdomen through the thorax to the head. It is composed of the heart (the abdominal portion), which shows segmental swellings with ostia, and the aorta (the thoracic and cephalic portion), which is a simple tube in front of the heart. Usually, the dorsal vessel pumps hemolymph from the posterior to the anterior end. However, reversal of blood flow has been observed in *Anopheles quadrimaculatus* (Clements 1992). Ostial valves are openings in the heart that either permit hemolymph to flow in the dorsal vessel and prevent backflow (incurrent ostia) or allow free flow of hemolymph out of the heart, usually without valves (excurrent ostia). Despite the extensive innervation of the heart in some species, the contractions of the dorsal vessel are myogenic. The heartbeat is under neurohormonal control. Besides being a contractile organ, it has also been suggested that the heart is a secretory organ. Protein release from heart tissue has been demonstrated in *L. migratoria* and in *Calpodes ethlius* (Fife et al. 1987).

The ventral diaphragm (also called alary muscle) plays an important role in hemolymph circulation. It is usually restricted to the abdomen, where it divides the hemocoel into the perineural sinus (around the ventral nerve cord) and the pericardial (or perivisceral) sinus. The structure of the diaphragm varies between species from a few vestigial remnants to a continuous layer covering the whole nerve cord. The extent to which the diaphragm develops also depends on the insect stage. For example, in larval *An. quadrimaculatus* no ventral diaphragm is present, but in the pupal and the adult stages a well-developed diaphragm forms between perineural and pericardial sinus (Jones 1954). In some mosquito species (e.g., *Ae. aegypti*), the diaphragm contracts in a peristaltic manner and thereby aids the general circulation of the hemolymph.

Hemolymph is circulated into the appendages by various accessory pulsatile organs located at the base of the legs, wings, and antennae. These organs are basically hemolymph-containing ampullae, surrounded by muscles that pump the hemolymph into the appendages (Miller 1985).

Hemolymph Composition

Hemolymph is the major water storage compartment of the insect. Hemolymph pH varies between species from slightly acidic to slightly alkaline (6.0–8.2). In general, the buffering capacity of hemolymph is low. Because respiration in insects occurs through the tracheolar system, hemolymph plays no role in the transport of CO_2 or O_2 Hemolymph contains several types of cells, the classification of which is still controversial. Lackie (1988) described 8 major types: prohemocytes, plasmatocytes, granular cells, coagulocytes, adipohemocytes, spherulocytes, oenocytoids, and crystal cells (Fig. 21.2). However, the number of hemocyte types varies among species. The main functions of hemocytes are phagocytosis and encapsulation of foreign materials,

coagulation, storage/distribution of nutrients, and protein synthesis. Because hemolymph plays an important role as storage compartment, it shows high levels of organic molecules, such as amino acids/peptides/proteins, carbohydrates, and lipids.

Transport and Storage Functions of Hemolymph

Hemolymph has many functions, foremost among which are those of transport and storage of nutrients and metabolic intermediates, such as proteins, carbohydrates, and lipids.

Insects typically have high levels of free amino acids in their hemolymph. Generally all amino acids are present, usually in the L-form (but D-alanine also occurs). Proline is present in high concentrations in insects that fuel flight with proline (*Glossina morsitans* and *Leptinotarsa decemlineata;* Bursell 1981). Levels of free amino acids in the hemolymph of *An. stephensi* increase 60–70% after a normal blood meal; however, when the blood meal is infected with a malaria parasite (*Plasmodium berghei*) the increase is less pronounced (~15–25%). This is in part caused by a nutritionally deficient blood meal of the infected host. It also results from the utilization of amino acids (especially methionine and histidine) by the developing malaria parasite.

Besides free amino acids, hemolymph contains peptides that function as hormones or play an important role in amino acid storage/transport; for example, Tyr- or Phe-rich peptides are required for cuticlular sclerotization (Bodnaryk 1978), and hemolymph of *G. austeni* contains several peptides of which the Tyr- and Phe-rich peptides are transferred at a high rate to the developing larvae.

Protein levels in hemolymph generally increase during each instar but decrease during molt. Some of the more important hemolymph proteins include storage proteins (in larvae), vitellogenin and microvitellogenin (in adults), lipophorin, lectins, antibacterial proteins, and clotting proteins (Chap. 15), enzymes (such as phenoloxidases and lysozymes), JH-binding proteins, and chromoproteins (such as insecticyanin and carotenoid-binding proteins). Although several of these proteins are described in more detail throughout this and other chapters in this volume,

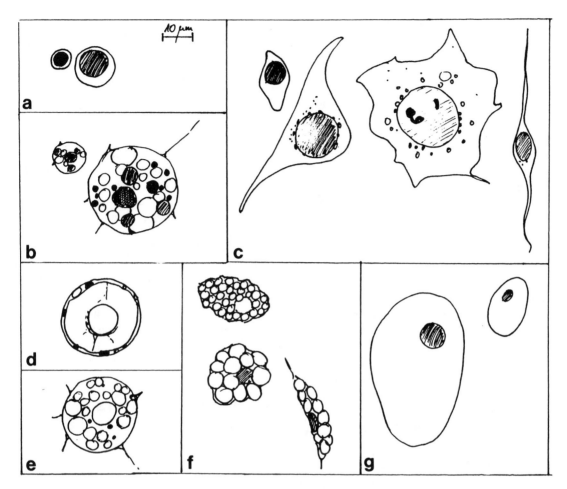

21.2 Schematic representation of lepidopteran hemocytes. (a) prohemocyte, (b) granular hemocyte, (c) plasmatocyte, (d) coagulocyte, (e) adipohemocyte, (f) spherulocyte, (g) oenocytoid. Courtesy of T. Trenczek.

Kanost et al. (1990) provide more detailed information on hemolymph proteins.

Insects store carbohydrate in hemolymph; therefore, the hemolymph carbohydrate content in insects is high compared to that in vertebrate blood. The major carbohydrate in insect hemolymph is trehalose, a nonreducing disaccharide that can be present at high concentrations without affecting the redox potential of the hemolymph. Generally lower levels of glucose occur and sometimes small amounts of glycogen are present. Carbohydrate levels are under hormonal control (Chap. 22).

Many different types of lipids can be found in hemolymph. Because lipids are insoluble in the aqueous environment of the hemolymph, they must be transported by lipoproteins. In general 1 lipoprotein occurs, called lipophorin (Lp), which falls in the high density class (1.063–1.210 g/ml) (Beenakkers et al. 1985). It is composed of apoproteins and a range of lipids. The main lipids are phospholipids and diacylglycerol. Smaller and varying amounts of other neutral lipids occur, including triacylglycerol, monoacylglycerol, sterolesters, fatty acids, carotenoids, and hydrocarbons. Recently the lipophorin of *Ae. aegypti* was found to contain mainly triacylglycerol as neutral lipid, in contrast to all other insect species studied so far.

An important feature of the insect lipophorin (in contrast to vertebrate lipoproteins) is that it functions as a reusable lipid shuttle: It continually transports lipids between tissues without being taken up and hydrolyzed intracellularly. Lipophorin can change in density and composition according to physiological or developmental circumstances. In larvae, lipophorin functions mainly in the transport of dietary lipid to the fat body, where lipids are stored for use in the adult. After adult emergence, lipophorin functions mainly in the redistribution of stored lipids to peripheral tissues. In insects that fly long distances (such as *Manduca sexta* and *L. migratoria*), sustained flight induces a change of lipophorin to a low density form, or LDLp (d ≈ 1.03–1.06 g/ml), as a result of diacylglycerol uptake from fat body. LDLp transports increased amounts of diacylglycerol to the active flight muscle. A lipid transfer particle was shown to play a role in diacylglycerol transfer from fat body to lipophorin. Lipophorin also plays an important role in the supply of lipids to the developing oocyte in *M. sexta* and in *R. prolixus*. In *G. morsitans*, lipophorin may play an important role in the transport of large amounts of diacylglycerol from fat body to the uterine gland during late pregnancy.

Other Functions of Hemolymph

Hemolymph plays an important role in thermoregulation. During flight, the circulation of the hemolymph controls the temperature of the thorax (Mullins 1985). Hemolymph volume fluctuates in response to changing physiological or developmental conditions and thereby affects the internal pressure of the insect. An increase in hemocoel pressure is of vital importance during ecdysis, oviposition, and expansion of the wings in the newly emerged adult. Hemolymph also plays an important role in osmoregulation, for example, in the adaptation of mosquito larvae to waters of different salinity. In more primitive insects inorganic ions (Na^+ and Cl^-) are the major osmoeffectors. In higher insects organic molecules are more important as osmoeffectors. Some larvae, for example *Culex tarsalis*, osmoconform in water of high salinity (> 400 milliosmol/liter) by accumulating proline, serine, and trehalose in the hemolymph. Another important function of hemolymph is the defense against foreign materials (Chaps. 23 and 31).

CONCLUSION

During the development of a parasite in its vector, the parasite often contacts (or passes through) the hemolymph of the vector. Therefore, the study of hemolymph and fat body of disease vectors is necessary to better understand parasite-vector interactions. Much of the present knowledge on fat body and hemolymph has been obtained from studies of nonvector species because they are larger and easier to rear. However, an important factor to consider is the enormous diversity among species. The tendency to project data obtained from a few species to all insects is dangerous and often wrong. For example, although for a long time it was assumed that diacylglycerol is the major neutral lipid in insect hemolymph, recently several mosquito species were shown to transport lipid in the form of triacylglycerol. The continuing development of sensitive molecular techniques will facilitate the physiological and biochemical study of vector species.

ACKNOWLEDGMENTS

The author wishes to thank Drs. A. Smith, F. Noriega, and R. Ziegler for their critical reading of the manuscript.

REFERENCES

Beenakkers, A.M. Th., D.J. Van der Horst, and W.J.A. Van Marrewijk. 1985. Insect lipids and lipoproteins and their role in physiological processes. *Prog. Lipid Res.* 24:19–67.

Bodnaryk, R.P. 1978. Structure and function of insect peptides. *Adv. Insect Physiol.* 13:69–132.

Bursell, E. 1981. The role of proline in energy metabolism. In: R.G.H. Downer, editor, *Energy metabolism in insects.* New York: Plenum Press. pp. 135–154.

Clements, A.N. 1992. *The biology of mosquitoes.* Vol. 1: Development, nutrition and reproduction. London: Chapman & Hall.

Dean, R.L., J.V. Collins, and M. Locke. 1985. Structure of the fat body. In: G.A. Kerkut and L.I. Gilbert, editors, *Comprehensive insect physiology, biochemistry, and pharmacology,* Vol. 3. Oxford: Pergamon Press. pp. 155–210.

Fife, H.G., S.R. Palli, and M. Locke. 1987. A function for pericardial cells in an insect. *Insect Biochem.* 17:829–840.

Gillett, J.D. 1982. Circulatory and ventilatory movements of the abdomen in mosquitoes. *Proc. Roy. Soc. Lond.* (B)215:127–134.

Jones, J.C. 1954. The heart and associated tissues of *Anopheles quadrimaculatus* Say (Diptera: Culicidae). *J. Morphol.* 94:71–124.

Kanost M.R., J. K. Kawooya, J.H. Law, R.O. Ryan, M.C. Van Heusden, and R. Ziegler. 1990. Insect Haemolymph Proteins. *Adv. Insect Physiol.* 22:299–396.

Lackie, A.M. 1988. Hemocyte Behaviour. *Adv. Insect Physiol.* 21:85–178.

Miller, T.A. 1985. Structure and physiology of the circulatory system. In: G.A. Kerkut and L.I. Gilbert, editors, *Comprehensive insect physiology, biochemistry, and pharmacology,* Vol. 3. Oxford: Pergamon Press. pp. 289–353.

Mullins, D.E. 1985. Chemistry and physiology of the hemolymph. In: G.A. Kerkut and L.I. Gilbert, editors, *Comprehensive insect physiology, biochemistry, and pharmacology,* Vol. 3. Oxford: Pergamon Press. pp. 355–400.

Stanley-Samuelson, D.W., and R.H. Dadd. 1983. Long-chain polyunsaturated fatty acids: Patterns of occurrence in insects. *Insect Biochem.* 13:549–558.

Steele, J.E. 1981. The role of carbohydrate metabolism in physiological functions. In: R.G.H. Downer, editor, *Energy metabolism in insects.* New York: Plenum Press. pp. 101–103.

22. ENERGY METABOLISM

Rolf Ziegler

INTRODUCTION

Insects, like all animals, must constantly expend energy for movement, transport, breathing, synthesis, reproduction, and growth. This life-sustaining energy is acquired from the environment by ingesting food. Although an insect has to expend energy constantly, it cannot feed constantly. Therefore, an insect will, when possible, ingest more food than it needs and use the excess to accumulate chemical energy stores. If the environment is less favorable (when the insect cannot feed) or if it needs a burst of energy, it will mobilize these energy stores to ensure survival.

Every insect faces situations in which it cannot feed, such as when it molts. Larvae of the Lepidoptera *Manduca sexta* feed more or less constantly except during molting, when they are unable to feed for 24 hours (Reinecke et al. 1980). During the feeding phase, an insect can also run out of food. Vectors are hematophagous (bloodsucking) and typically feed intermittently. They feed to repletion and then do not feed for extended periods ranging from several days to years, depending on the species and food supply. In addition, insects face situations when they need huge amounts of energy. During flight, an insect's energy consumption can increase by more than 100-fold (Sacktor 1975). In addition, during oogenesis an insect requires a great deal of energy, which comes mostly from food, but may also necessitate utilizing stored energy (e.g., autogenous mosquitoes, which tap into reserves accumulated as larvae). An insect, therefore, must be able to switch its energy metabolism quickly from accumulation of reserves to mobilization and back again. These switches must be well regulated to mobilize sufficient energy quickly and prevent waste.

In general, an insect's energy metabolism and major metabolic pathways are similar to those of other animals. Although I briefly review these pathways in this chapter, my main focus is the control of energy metabolism and areas in which the energy metabolism of insects, especially arthropod vectors, differs from mammals. The primary energy stores in insects, fat body and hemolymph are reviewed in Chapter 21.

REQUIREMENTS OF FOOD

Energy metabolism starts when an insect ingests food. Food supplies the fuel from which the chemical energy necessary to sustain life is liberated. Energy can be gained from lipids, carbohydrates, or proteins, but each one of these compounds cannot be used under every condition. For example, anaerobic conditions preclude the use of lipids for energy. Food also provides essential substances that an insect cannot synthesize by itself: some fatty acids, essential amino acids, vitamins, minerals, and cholesterol.

The basic nutritional needs of all animals are similar; differences occur mainly in how they acquire the nutrients necessary for a balanced diet. Some insects can live on a restricted diet, extracting the needed substances from a source containing only trace quantities of these substances (Dadd 1973; 1985). See Merritt et al. (1992)

for a review of the uptake of food by mosquito larvae. Vectors ingest blood, which is rich in proteins and lipids but low in carbohydrates; thus, some vectors require an additional carbohydrate source. B vitamins are found in low concentrations in blood; triatomines and blood-sucking hemiptera therefore have their diet supplemented by bacterial symbionts (Dadd 1985).

DIGESTION AND ABSORPTION OF FOOD

Food must be digested and then absorbed to be useful to an insect. In insects both digestion and absorption take place mainly in the midgut. The digestive enzymes of insects and their special adaptations to the needs of insects have attracted much attention in recent years (Chap. 18).

CONVERSION OF FOOD AND METABOLIC STORES TO ENERGY

Insects convert food into energy much like other animals. Food is broken down and oxidized to form energy; the end products are CO_2 and H_2O. The insect gains the energy as electrons are transported in several steps along a redox gradient to oxygen. The energy liberated during this process can be harnessed and used as ATP.

Carbohydrates

Complex carbohydrates are hydrolyzed to individual sugars, which are introduced into glycolysis. During glycolysis glucose is broken down into 2 molecules of pyruvate, which have 3 carbon atoms. This cleavage results in the formation of 2 molecules of ATP (adenosine triphosphate) per molecule of glucose. In addition, 2 reducing equivalents are gained as NADH (reduced form of NAD^+, nicotinamide adenine dinucleotide) (Fig. 22.1). ATP, upon hydrolysis, delivers the energy for life-sustaining and energy-demanding processes in an organism; reducing equivalents can be used to generate ATP.

Pyruvate enters the mitochondria, where 1 carbon atom is removed with the concomitant formation of another reducing equivalent of NADH (Fig. 22.1). The remaining 2 carbon atoms (an acetyl group) are introduced into the citric acid cycle (or tricarboxylic

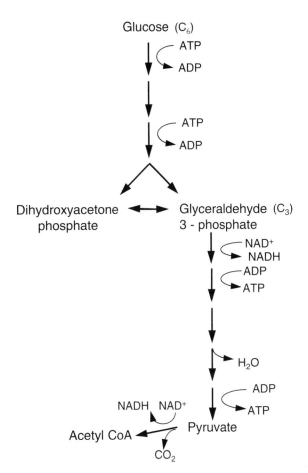

22.1   Glycolysis

acid or Krebs cycle) (Fig. 22.2) with the help of coenzyme A (CoA, a universal activator of acyl groups). In the citric acid cycle 1 guanosine triphosphate (GTP) molecule is formed, which is equivalent to 1 molecule of ATP. In addition, 3 NADH molecules and 1 $FADH_2$ molecule (reduced form of FAD, flavin adenine dinucleotide) are obtained.

Transport of Reducing Equivalents into Mitochondria

To gain energy from NADH formed during glycolysis, reducing equivalents must enter the mitochondria and be removed from NADH. (The citric acid cycle is located inside the mitochondria, so NADH formed in the citric acid cycle is not transported.) The removal of the reducing equivalent regenerates NAD⁺, and glycolysis can continue. The inner mitochondrial membrane, however, is impermeable to NADH and NAD⁺. To circumvent this problem, electrons are transported into the mitochondria and not NADH. In the mammalian heart and liver, this is achieved by the malate-aspartate shuttle, which transfers its electrons to NAD⁺ inside the mitochondria, forming intramitochondrial NADH. This results in the formation of 3 molecules of ATP from each NADH molecule. Insect flight muscle, however, uses the glycerol phosphate shuttle (Fig. 22.3). In this shuttle dihydroxyacetone phosphate, which is formed during glycolysis (Fig. 22.1), takes up the hydrogen from NADH, resulting in the formation of glycerol–3-phosphate and NAD⁺. Glycerol–3-phosphate delivers the reducing equivalents to an enzyme in the mitochondrial membrane. The electrons are transferred to FAD, generating $FADH_2$, which leads to the formation of only 2 ATP molecules. Dihydroxyacetone phosphate is regenerated and diffuses out of the mitochondria. In addition, for insect flight muscle a 1-pyrroline–5-carboxylate/proline shuttle has been proposed (Candy 1985) for the transport of reducing equivalents into mitochondria.

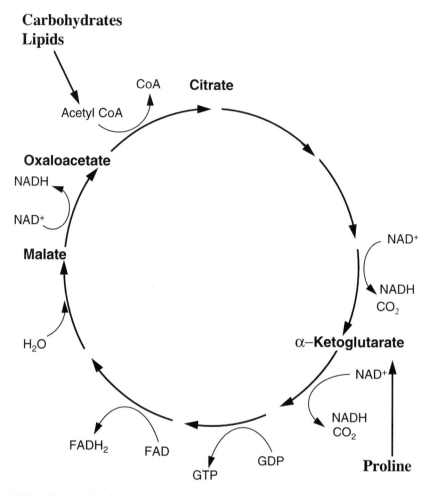

22.2   Citric acid cycle

Oxidative Phosphorylation

Inside the mitochondria, the difference in the electron-transfer potential of NADH or $FADH_2$ relative to that of O_2 is used to form ATP. The electrons are transferred from NADH or $FADH_2$, in a series of discrete steps, to oxygen. This process leads to the pumping of protons out of the mitochondrial matrix and the formation of a pH gradient and transmembrane electrical potential. When protons flow back to the mitochondrial matrix through an enzyme complex, ATP is synthesized, a process called oxidative phosphorylation.

During oxidative phosphorylation, NADH produces 3 ATP molecules whereas $FADH_2$ produces 2. In mammalian heart and liver, the total energy gained from 1 molecule of glucose is 38 ATP molecules. The insect flight muscle, which needs a tremendous amount of energy, for example, ATP, gains only 36

Cytosol

Mitochondrial Membrane

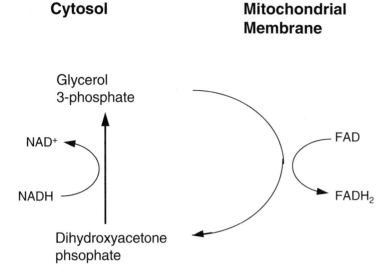

22.3   Glycerol phosphate shuttle

(Fig. 22.4). One $FADH_2$ and 1 NADH molecule are formed for every 2 carbon atoms removed. $FADH_2$ and NADH are used to produce ATP by oxidative phosphorylation. Acetyl CoA enters the citric acid cycle, and more energy is produced (see section on conversion of food). Lipids are rich in chemical energy; the oxidation of 1 palmitate (C_{16}) molecule forms 131 ATP molecules. Because the activation of palmitate to palmitoyl-CoA requires 2 molecules of ATP, the net gain is 129.

Lipids provide more energy than carbohydrates because they are in a more reduced form than carbohydrates, and the energy is produced by oxidation. In addition, carbohydrates are highly hydrated,

molecules of ATP per molecule of glucose because of the glycerol phosphate shuttle, which transfers electrons to $FADH_2$ and not to NADH. A possible explanation for this contradiction could be that at the beginning of flight, metabolism increases very quickly, using up the available NAD^+, which must be regenerated immediately. This is possible with the glycerol phosphate shuttle, because its components are synthesized at the same time as NADH. This shuttle also allows the transport of reducing equivalents into the mitochondria even when the NADH concentration in the cytoplasm is lower than inside the mitochondria.

Lipids

The lipids used to gain energy are mainly triacylglycerol, diacylglycerol, and free fatty acids. These lipids are hydrolyzed by lipases to free fatty acids and glycerol. Glycerol is used for synthesis of fats or is introduced into glycolysis. The fatty acids are mostly used for energy. They are transported as acyl-carnitine into the mitochondria, where they are transferred to CoA to form acyl CoA (Downer 1985). Carnitine then leaves the mitochondria and can be reused. Two-carbon units of the acyl CoA are sequentially transferred to CoA (forming acetyl CoA) in a process called (β-oxidation

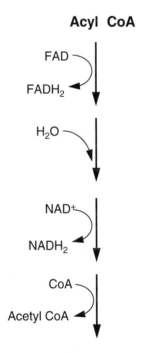

Acyl CoA

Acyl CoA shortened by two carbon atoms

22.4   β-Oxidation

making them even heavier, whereas the hydrophobic lipids are anhydrous. Thus, 1 g of mostly anhydrous lipid stores more than 6 times the energy of 1 g of hydrated glycogen. However, hydrophobic lipids are not soluble in hemolymph and need special transport proteins, lipoproteins (Chap. 21).

Proteins

To gain energy from proteins, they must first be digested by proteases to free amino acids. Amino acids can be deaminated and introduced into the citric acid cycle (see section on conversion of food). The introduction into the citric acid cycle occurs at different levels depending on the amino acid. The amount of energy recovered also varies for different amino acids. The contribution of proteins to total energy production is normally small. Some insects, such as tsetse flies and the Colorado potato beetle, use proline as a source of energy to power flight (see the section on use of proline to power flight).

During insect excretion, a primary urine is formed in the Malpighian tubules. Useful molecules are reabsorbed in the insect hindgut. The energy necessary for reabsorption appears to be obtained from the oxidation of proline (Phillips et al. 1986).

SYNTHESIS OF RESERVES

Stores of chemical energy are exceedingly important for all animals. In insects, the amount of food ingested determines the size of larvae. A large mosquito larva results in a large adult; a large adult female survives starvation longer, takes larger blood meals, and produces more offspring. Although the formation of reserves costs the insect a substantial amount of energy, the energy it recovers from mobilizing them is much greater.

Carbohydrates

Glucose is either ingested with food or synthesized from pyruvate or amino acids. Complex sugars in food are broken down, and nonglucose sugars are converted into glucose. Glucose is first phosphorylated to glucose–6-phosphate, which then can be used for the synthesis of the major carbohydrate reserves (trehalose and glycogen) as well as chitin. Chitin, a carbohydrate, is a polymer of N-acetylglucosamine (Kramer et al. 1985) and with proteins forms the cuticle or exoskeleton of insects. Even though the exoskeleton is shed at each molt, a large portion of it is reabsorbed and reused for the formation of the new cuticle.

Glycogen is a large molecule with molecular weights ranging from 10^6–10^8. It is formed by first converting glucose–6-phosphate into glucose–1-phosphate. Glucose–1-phosphate reacts with uridine triphosphate (UTP) to form uridine diphosphate glucose (UDP–glucose). With the help of glycogen synthase, UDP–glucose donates its glucose to a growing glycogen molecule by forming an $\alpha(1$–$4)$-glucosidic bond that creates long-chain molecules. Glycogen, however, is heavily branched. The "branching" enzyme breaks an $\alpha(1$–$4)$-link and creates an $\alpha(1$–$6)$-link. This increases the solubility of glycogen and its rate of synthesis and degradation. The cost for the addition of 1 glucose molecule to glycogen is 2 molecules of ATP.

Glucose–6-phosphate is also a substrate for the synthesis of trehalose. One glucose–6-phosphate can combine with UDP–glucose to form trehalose–6-phosphate. Trehalose–6-phosphate is dephosphorylated by trehalose phosphatase. The formation of 1 molecule of trehalose is made possible by the cleavage of 3 molecules of ATP (Chippendale 1978; Friedman 1985).

Control of the Synthesis of Complex Carbohydrates

Because the substrates for the synthesis of glycogen and trehalose are identical, the synthesis must be well regulated. Glucose–6-phosphate activates both trehalose synthase and glycogen synthase. Both enzymes need UDP–glucose, which is found in low concentration. Because the Km (Michaelis-Menten constant = substrate concentration at half maximal velocity) of trehalose synthase for UDP–glucose is much lower than the Km of glycogen synthase, trehalose is formed first. When the trehalose level increases, trehalose synthase is inhibited, and increasing levels of UDP–glucose promote glycogen synthesis (Murphy and Wyatt 1965). The synthesis of chitin, which also starts with glucose–6-phosphate, is controlled by 20-hydroxyecdysone (Kramer et al. 1985).

Whether carbohydrates are synthesized or metabolized appears to depend on hormones and the availability of substrates for synthesis. When insects feed and sufficient substrate is available, reserves are synthesized. The amount of reserves accumulated varies according to insect species. Normally larvae accumulate reserves and adults use them; however, adults can also accumulate reserves.

Lipids

Lipids are synthesized from absorbed fatty acids, carbohydrates, or proteins. Fatty acid synthesis starts with acetyl CoA, which is obtained from carbohydrates or proteins. Acetyl CoA is then carboxylated to malonyl CoA. This condenses with an acetyl group forming acetoacetyl through the loss of CO_2. The acetyl group and later the growing fatty acid is linked to the fatty acid synthase. Through successive additions of malonyl CoA, palmitate is synthesized. For the synthesis of 1 molecule of palmitate (C_{16}), 49 molecules of ATP are used. Complete oxidation of palmitate, however, will yield 129 ATP molecules (80 ATP molecules more than invested).

In summary, the synthesis of fatty acids resembles the reverse of the degradation; however, both pathways are well separated. Fatty acid synthesis takes place in the cytosol, whereas the degradation of fatty acids occurs in the mitochondrial matrix. The growing fatty acid is bound to a multienzyme complex and not released until the synthesis is complete. In addition, during degradation NADH is formed, whereas for synthesis NADPH (reduced form of nicotinamide adenine dinucleotide phosphate) is needed. The products of degradation are bound to CoA. The substrates for synthesis are derived from acetyl CoA, which is converted to malonyl CoA.

Fatty acids can be used for the synthesis of diacylglycerol, triacylglycerol, or phospholipids. For the synthesis of di- and triacylglycerol, glycerol is phosphorylated to form glycerol–3-phosphate, which is then acylated to form phosphatidic acid, phosphorylated diacylglycerol. If the phosphate group is replaced by another fatty acid, triacylglycerol is formed, which is the major storage form of lipids. Some phospholipids are synthesized partially by the same pathway.

Control of Lipid Synthesis

Adult mosquitoes feeding on sugar synthesize glycogen during the first 6–8 hours and then switch to lipid synthesis and accumulate much more lipid than glycogen (Van Handel 1984). The switch to lipid synthesis appears to be controlled by the median neurosecretory cells of the brain (MNC). If the MNC are removed, the mosquito continues to synthesize glycogen but not lipids; if the MNC are reimplanted, the mosquito switches glycogen synthesis off, but lipid synthesis is not switched on (Van Handel and Lea 1970). After a blood meal, a similar change in synthesis is found; however, the change in synthesis after a blood meal is not influenced by the removal of the MNC. The chemical identity of the active substance in the MNC is unknown.

Proteins

Nonessential amino acids can be synthesized from glucose or acetate (Candy 1985; Chen 1985). Protein synthesis from amino acids follows the general rules of protein synthesis.

The addition of 1 amino acid to a growing protein chain requires 3 ATP molecules. The folding of a protein into its final and active form can either be spontaneous or can require ATP. For example, the folding of rhodanese (an ubiquitous mitochondrial protein of unknown function) requires about 130 molecules of ATP.

STARVATION

Developmental and environmental factors preclude insects from feeding constantly. Therefore, insects encounter periods of starvation. Some vectors can survive extremely long periods without feeding; the kissing bug *Rhodnius* feeds only once per larval instar. Ticks are even more amazing; certain species survive for years without food. They digest a blood meal slowly and store part of it in the gut for later use (Sonenshine 1991). To survive several years without food, the metabolic rate of these ticks must slow tremendously, and the activity of reserve-degrading enzymes must fall to almost zero. Unfortunately, the effect of starvation on energy metabolism has not been examined in ticks.

Starvation in Larvae

In a starving insect, the respiratory rate decreases quickly, which means that its metabolism is reduced. The respiration rate of larvae of *Manduca sexta*, for example, drops 75% within 10–15 hr after feeding stops (Ziegler 1984). Despite the reduction of metabolism, reserves are mobilized; thus reserve-degrading enzymes are activated. Glycogen phosphorylase in starving larvae of *Manduca sexta* is activated maximally within 4 hours after the cessation of feeding.

In *Manduca* larvae, as in most insects, trehalose is the main sugar in the hemolymph and glucose a minor sugar. Hemolymph trehalose concentration in insects appears to be controlled; hemolymph glucose concentration does not appear to be controlled. Glucose is taken up by the gut, transported to the fat body, and converted quickly to trehalose; thus the level of hemolymph glucose seems to depend only on the speed of uptake and the speed of conversion to trehalose. If the larva stops feeding, glucose levels decrease by about 65% in half an hour. This decrease in hemolymph glucose appears to trigger the release of adipokinetic hormone (AKH) from the corpora cardiaca. AKH activates glycogen phosphorylase (GP), and therefore trehalose concentration remains high (Gies et al. 1988). If glucose is supplied to starving larvae, the activation of GP is prevented or reversed (Ziegler 1984). If starvation continues, GP is slowly inactivated. After about 48 hr the activity of GP is back to control levels even though only part of the glycogen reserves are used up. What controls the inactivation of GP is not known.

Starvation in Adults

In starving adult insects, carbohydrate and lipid reserves are mobilized in a manner similar to that in larvae. Hemolymph lipid concentration increases, whereas the level of trehalose in hemolymph decreases, despite the mobilization of glycogen. It is tempting to speculate that this mobilization of reserves is controlled by AKH. However, in adult *Locusta migratoria* (Goldsworthy 1984) and in adult *Manduca sexta* (Ziegler 1991), carbohydrate and lipid reserves are mobilized during starvation without any involvement of a hormone from the corpora cardiaca. In adult *Manduca*

sexta there are indications that a low level of hemolymph trehalose induces the mobilization of reserves. If trehalose is injected, lipid levels in the hemolymph decrease and GP is inactivated (Ziegler 1991). It would be interesting to examine enzyme activities during starvation of certain arthropod vectors, which can survive for weeks, months, or even years without food.

In adult female insects, starvation causes the resorption of developing eggs. In most insects, egg maturation is controlled by juvenile hormone (JH). The corpora allata, which produce JH, are inactivated by starvation. Tsetse flies are truly viviparous and give birth to fully grown larvae. The energy demand on the female during pregnancy is excessive, and starvation results in abortion of the developing larvae. The control of this process is not understood.

INSECT FLIGHT

Flight is an event that requires a tremendous increase in energy consumption and has a well-defined start and end. Consequently, the metabolism of the insect flight muscle has been more thoroughly examined than the metabolism of other parts of the insect. Flight muscles of insects are among the most metabolically active muscles. An adult human needs about 2000–3000 kcal per day. If the muscles of a 150-lb adult human were to consume as much energy as the flight muscles of a locust, 7500 kcal per hour would be required. To gain this much chemical energy (e.g., from potatoes), a human would have to eat 20–25 pounds of potatoes per hour.

Transport Systems

The activity of insect flight muscle is fully aerobic. Oxygen is transported in the trachea, largely by diffusion; however, in many insects gas exchange is facilitated by ventilation of air sacs, which, because of the small size of insects, is effective (Mill 1985). Fine ramifications of the tracheae, the tracheoles, penetrate the muscle and come into close proximity to the mitochondria, thereby minimizing the diffusion distance. In adaptation to the high metabolic rate, insect flight muscles have developed a high density of mitochondria:

30–40% of the fiber volume is occupied by mitochondria (Beenakkers et al. 1985).

With such high activity, stores of metabolic fuels in the muscle are insufficient for sustained flight. Triatomines, for example, *Rhodnius* and *Triatoma,* appear to be exceptions because they store huge amounts of lipids in their flight muscles (Candy 1985). In other insects fuels for the muscles come from fat body via the hemolymph. Insects have an open circulatory system (Chaps. 1 and 21). They do not have a capillary system like mammals, in which the diffusion distances are small. However, the plasma membrane of the insect muscle is deeply invaginated into the fiber by the transverse, or T-tubule system, which probably is also used for the transport of substrates. A possible compensation for the less efficient open circulatory system is the high concentration of sugars, lipids, and amino acids in the hemolymph (Beenakkers et al. 1985).

Estimates of Energy Expenditure During Flight

Because insect flight muscles are fully aerobic, their metabolic activity can be determined by measuring oxygen consumption. Respiratory measurements, taken during rest and during flight, show that oxygen consumption can increase by a factor of more than 100 (Sacktor 1975; Kammer and Heinrich 1978). In mammals and birds, increases of up to a factor of 10 have been observed. The energy expenditure of flying insects can also be determined by measuring the depletion of energy stores. In locusts and in *Manduca sexta,* values of energy used, which were determined by these different methods, agree reasonably well (Ziegler 1984). Increases as low as 4-fold in the metabolic rate of mosquitoes during flight have been reported; however, after a blood meal, mosquitoes can exhibit up to a 6-fold increase in oxygen consumption (Clements 1992). This would indicate that the energy expenditure per hour for the digestion of a blood meal is larger than for flight, which seems unlikely.

Fuels for Flight

Insects use different fuels to power flight. Insects that do not feed as adults (some Lepidoptera) or that fly long distances (locusts) primarily use lipids for flight (Beenakkers et al. 1981). Locusts also use some carbohydrates to power flight, especially at the onset. Insects such as flies, mosquitoes, hymenoptera, and some lepidoptera obtain the energy needed for flight from carbohydrates. Many insects use a mixture of carbohydrates and lipids. Insects that only use carbohydrates in flight tend to fly for shorter times. There are exceptions; mosquitoes, for example, which power flight with carbohydrates, can stay airborne for several hours even as young unfed adults. If they have been feeding, much of the flight energy comes from food in the crop (Clements 1992).

Lipids, which are mobilized to gain energy, are transported in mammals in the form of free fatty acids whereas most insects use diacylglycerol; mosquitoes use triacylglycerol hemolymph (Chap. 21). Lipid concentrations in insect hemolymph can be extremely high; in adult *Manduca sexta* concentrations of 150 mg/ml have been found (Ziegler 1991). Free fatty acids in such high concentration in hemolymph would harm the insect, whereas the neutral diacylglycerol can be tolerated. However, diacylglycerol is not soluble in aqueous media and has to be transported by a lipoprotein, lipophorin.

There is a high turnover of free fatty acids in the kissing bug *Triatoma infestans* (Soulages et al. 1988). The rate is so high during rest that despite the low concentration of free fatty acids, they may be more important as an energy source than diacylglycerol. However, the role of free fatty acids in flying *Triatoma infestans* has not been examined.

Control of Energy Metabolism During Flight

Energy metabolism in flight muscle is well controlled to ensure efficiency. Critical control points are at the start of flight (with the tremendous increase in the rate of energy production) and then at the switch from one fuel to another. In the locust flight muscle, stored ATP and phosphoarginine (which is a buffer for energy-rich phosphates) are used up within a second of flight. Therefore, energy must be released quickly from chemical stores. The 1st store to be used is muscle glycogen, followed by hemolymph trehalose and fat body glycogen, and finally fat body lipid. Muscle glycogen phosphorylase, which mobilizes glycogen, is activated by increasing levels of Ca^{2+} in the contracting muscle. Enzymes of the glycolytic pathway are also activated. Within the first 2 seconds of flight in locust flight muscle the level of free phosphate increases 3-fold, the level of ADP increases 5-fold, and the level of AMP 27-fold, as shown by NMR (nuclear magnetic resonance) spectroscopy. These changes activate glycogen phosphorylase, phosphofructokinase, hexokinase, and pyruvate kinase (Wegener et al. 1991). Hemolymph trehalose enters the cell and is cleaved by trehalase; the glucose released is phosphorylated by the activated hexokinase and can then be introduced into glycolysis. The activation of glycogen phosphorylase in the fat body is controlled by hormones in some insects.

Another important regulatory point in flight muscle metabolism is the change from carbohydrates to lipids before carbohydrates are used up completely. In mammalian heart muscle, the use of carbohydrate is inhibited by the effect of high citrate concentration on phosphofructokinase, an enzyme involved in glycolysis; however, phosphofructokinase from insect muscle is insensitive to citrate. Recently it was shown that fructose–2,6-bisphosphate, a potent activator of phosphofructokinase, decreases by 80% during the first 15 min of flight. A decrease of this magnitude reduces the activity of locust phosphofructokinase in vitro by 95%. Thus, fructose–2,6-bisphosphate could well be the regulator that accomplishes the switch from carbohydrate to lipid use (Wegener 1990).

Use of Proline to Power Flight

The proline concentration in the hemolymph of various insects decreases at the beginning of flight. In most insects proline appears to provide intermediates for the citric acid cycle (Beenakkers et al. 1985). In some insects, such as the tsetse fly, *Glossina morsitans*, and the Colorado potato beetle, *Leptinotarsa decemlineata*, proline is the main fuel used to power flight (Bursell 1981). In these insects proline can be completely oxidized but is mostly partially oxidized (Fig. 22.5). Proline is first converted to glutamate by 2 dehydrogenases, forming 1 $FADH_2$ molecule and 1 NADH molecule. Glutamate is deaminated to (α-ketoglutarate, which enters the citric acid cycle. (α-ketoglutarate goes through part of the

citric acid cycle to form malate. During this conversion 1 NADH, 1 $FADH_2$, and 1 GTP molecule are formed with the concomitant loss of 1 molecule of CO_2. The 4-carbon malate remains in the citric acid cycle or is decarboxylated to pyruvate. The decarboxylation is performed by an NAD-dependent malic enzyme, yielding 1 NADH molecule in the process. Thus the total yield is 14 ATP molecules for the partial oxidation of proline. Pyruvate either can be reintroduced into the citric acid cycle and completely oxidized or it can serve as an ammonia acceptor (from the deamination of glutamate) to form alanine. In the tsetse fly and the Colorado potato beetle, the oxidation of pyruvate is inhibited by proline. In other insects, which use proline to spark the citric acid cycle, a high percentage of the proline used is completely oxidized.

The resynthesis of 1 proline molecule from pyruvate and acetyl CoA costs 3 ATP molecules. Therefore, acetyl CoA converted to energy by partial oxidation of proline yields a net of 11 molecules of ATP, whereas the normal oxidation of acetyl CoA in the citric acid cycle produces 12. Proline has an advantage over lipids because it is water soluble and does not require lipoprotein for transport; however, probably all insects have hemolymph lipoproteins (Chap. 21), including the proline-dependent tsetse flies (Ochanda et al. 1992).

Proline Synthesis

Proline levels in insects are high; for example, in tsetse flies, proline concentrations in tissue fluid in excess of 200 mMoles have been reported (Bursell 1978). Even these concentrations, however, are too low for extended flight. Proline is synthesized in fat body from alanine (Fig. 22.5). Alanine enters the mitochondria, where it is transaminated with (α-ketoglutarate to pyruvate. Pyruvate is carboxylated at the expense of 1 ATP molecule and introduced into the citric acid cycle as oxaloacetate. Oxaloacetate takes up the acetyl group from 1 acetyl CoA (originating from the metabolism of fatty acids), forming (α-ketoglutarate and 1 NADH. (α-ketoglutarate is transaminated with alanine to glutamate, which at the expense of 1 $FADH_2$ molecule and 1 NADH molecule reforms proline (Bursell 1981; Beenakkers et al. 1985). The formation of proline from alanine and acetyl CoA has a net cost of 3 molecules of ATP.

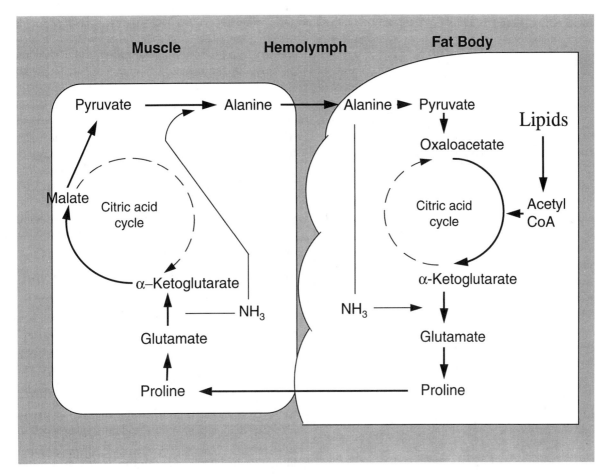

22.5 Proline metabolism

The rate of synthesis of proline is slow. In tsetse flies it is only 2.5–3.3% of the rate of usage during flight. Tsetse flies have long rests after short flights. Proline is the major fuel for flight in tsetse flies; however, other fuels may also be used. Hargrove (1976) calculated that the 1.3 µmoles of proline found in resting *Glossina pallidipes* would be enough for 2 min of flight; however, females were able to fly for 8 min and males for 14 min. Bursell (1978) pointed out that the proline content differs markedly in different animals. He found between 1.3 and 4.2 µmoles of proline per *Glossina morsitans*, which is nearly enough to support 8 min of flight. According to Bursell, the mature *Glossina morsitans* females that he used had better-developed flight muscles than the young females of *Glossina pallidipes* used by Hargrove (1976). Thus it is likely that they also used more proline. The possibility that a 2nd substrate is used to power flight should be reexamined.

Control of Proline Metabolism

The rate of proline oxidation increases strongly during the transition from rest to flight and is stimulated by the increase in ADP concentration. Different sites for the control by ADP have been discussed (Bursell 1981; Beenakkers et al. 1985). Proline is synthesized if the level of proline is low; proline synthesis is inhibited if proline concentration is high. Proline synthesis appears to be stimulated by an AKH.

REPRODUCTION

Reproduction is a major event in the life of an adult insect. The females invest huge amounts of energy and reserves, and in some cases, males may also make a substantial investment. The female tick *Hyalomma impletatum* can convert 55% of its body weight at repletion into more than 10,000 eggs (Sonenshine 1991).

Energy Costs of Reproduction

Obtaining quantitative data on the energy costs of reproduction is difficult. The process is of long duration and is not as well defined as flight. It is also difficult to identify good controls. In larvae and males other energy-consuming processes are going on that disqualify them for comparison. Virgins often do not produce eggs and thus could be considered good controls; however, they produce yolk proteins. In addition, most insects feed during or shortly before reproduction and consequently not only should changes in reserves be considered when the energy consumption is examined but also the amount of food taken up and the rate of assimilation.

Vitellogenin, the major yolk protein, can make up 15% of all the protein synthesized in fat body or 60% of the exported protein (Wyatt 1980). In addition to yolk proteins, eggs contain large amounts of lipids and carbohydrates. In *Manduca sexta* eggs, nearly 50% of the dry weight is lipid, and only about 30% is protein (Kawooya and Law 1988). The total caloric content of eggs from *Aedes* mosquitoes is constant, whereas the contribution by lipid can vary between 56% and 81% (Briegel 1990).

Tsetse flies have special reproductive adaptations because they are larviparous (Langley 1977). Tsetse flies do not produce large amounts of vitellogenin; however, an accessory gland is transformed into a uterine milk gland that supplies the developing larva with all its needed nutrients. Tsetse flies produce only 1 egg about every 9 days. At 25°C the larva hatches 4 days after ovulation and goes through 3 instars during the next 5 days. The larva is deposited fully grown and ready to pupate. The female takes several blood meals, feeding on 2 consecutive days after larviposition and once or twice more during pregnancy. The last meal is taken on the 6th or 7th day of pregnancy. Later, the developing larva is so large that the female can no longer ingest a blood meal. The energy needed to support the growth of the larva comes mostly from the blood meals. The uterine milk that feeds the larva contains about equal amounts of lipid and protein throughout development. The early blood meals appear to be used for the synthesis of most of the lipid, which is synthesized by the fat body and then transferred to the uterine gland later during pregnancy. The protein in uterine milk seems to be synthesized in part by the fat body and in part by the uterine gland from amino acids derived from the last blood meal during pregnancy (Langley and Bursell 1980; Langley et al. 1981). The main uptake of nutrients by the larva occurs in the 3rd instar.

Hormonal Control of Energy Metabolism During Reproduction

Vitellogenin synthesis, which requires a great deal of energy, is controlled in most insects by juvenile hormone. In mosquitoes ecdysone has this function (see Chap. 17). The effect of these hormones on energy metabolism in vitellogenesis, however, is an indirect one.

Pimley (1983) reports that extracts of the brains of tsetse flies stimulate protein synthesis by the uterine gland. In these experiments the gland was incubated in a salt solution and not in a full medium; therefore, it is likely that free amino acids in the brain extract stimulated protein synthesis.

AKH, which mobilizes energy stores, is not involved in mobilizing reserves for egg maturation. The amount of energy needed is large, but the demands are spread out over a comparatively long time, whereas the actions of AKH are comparatively short.

HORMONES CONTROLLING ENERGY METABOLISM

Although several hormones indirectly affect the energy metabolism (for example, JH and ecdysone), only a very few have a direct effect. Two hormones, an unnamed factor from the median neurosecretory cells (MNC) of the mosquito brain and adipokinetic hormone (AKH) are discussed here. The MNC of mosquitoes control whether glycogen or lipid is synthesized (Van Handel and Lea 1970). The chemical identity of this substance is unknown.

AKH is the only known insect hormone that directly influences the mobilization of energy stores. It is a peptide that is synthesized and stored in the corpora cardiaca. Peptides of the AKH family probably are present in all insects. Apparently, AKH mobilizes reserves only in situations when a large amount of energy is needed quickly (as in insect flight) or, in some cases, during starvation. AKH mobilizes lipid reserves for flight in locusts and *Manduca sexta*. This mobilization of lipids by AKH most likely is found in other insects in which flight is fueled by lipids. In locusts, AKH also controls the mobilization of carbohydrates for flight (Van Marrewijk et al. 1986), and there is evidence that this occurs in Diptera as well (Vejbjerg and Normann 1974). In the larvae of *Manduca sexta*, AKH mobilizes carbohydrate stores during starvation by activating glycogen phosphorylase. Other functions have been suggested for AKH, for example, the inhibition of lipid and protein synthesis (Kanost et al. 1990), and the stimulation of heme biosynthesis in a cockroach, *Blaberus discoridalis* (Keeley et al. 1995). Octopamine is possibly a 3rd hormone that directly controls the energy metabolism. It can mobilize lipids in insects, although to a lesser degree than the adipokinetic hormone.

Tsetse flies and the Colorado potato beetle power flight mostly with proline. There are reports that corpora cardiaca extracts can stimulate proline synthesis by the fat body in both insects. Thus, AKH is possibly involved in the control of proline metabolism. The following effects were observed in vitro upon the addition of aqueous extracts of corpora cardiaca to fat body from tsetse flies: inhibition of lipid synthesis (Pimley and Langley 1981), stimulation of the release of free fatty acids, and stimulation of proline synthesis (Pimley and Langley 1982). AKH mobilizes the major fuel for flight in some insects; in tsetse flies proline is the primary fuel. The ability to mobilize lipids gave AKH its name, and inhibition of lipid synthesis also has been proposed as an action of AKH (Kanost et al. 1990). Therefore, all these effects in tsetse flies are likely controlled by AKH; however, some questions remain. The responses are seen at concentrations of corpora cardiaca extracts orders of magnitudes lower than what is needed in other insects. Surprisingly, all these effects are seen only in vitro—no response has been seen in vivo. The experiments showing release of free fatty acids should be repeated with lipophorin in the incubation medium. It is more likely that under physiological conditions, when lipophorin is present, diacylglycerol is released instead of free fatty acids.

In vivo, the injection of corpora cardiaca extracts increased the concentration of total hemolymph carbohydrates in tsetse flies. This extract is also hypertrehalosemic in cockroaches and lipid-mobilizing in locusts (Mwangi and Awiti 1989). An increase in hemolymph sugar levels after 1 hour of flight has been reported in tsetse flies; however, these results are deceptive, because tsetse flies cannot fly for an hour. In this experiment the insects were actually in a rotating cage and were thus agitated, not flying, for an hour. Nevertheless, this study indicates that tsetse flies likely have an AKH that can control the mobilization of carbohydrate stores, possibly during flight. Further experiments are necessary to clarify the possible role of carbohydrates and how carbohydrate levels are controlled during the flight of tsetse flies.

Little is known about the control of AKH secretion from the corpora cardiaca. Flight causes the release of AKH, but it is unknown which flight-induced change is the signal. The brain controls the secretion of AKH by the nervi corporis cardiaci II, which originate in the protocerebrum and innervate the corpora cardiaca. Octopamine has been reported to be involved in the control of AKH release in locusts (Orchard 1987). However, no octopamine was found in axons innervating the glandular lobes of the corpora cardiaca, which synthesize and store AKH, nor were octopamine receptors found on the corpora cardiaca (Konings et al. 1989).

SUMMARY

The energy metabolism of insects is similar to that of other animals; however, there are also some important differences. The transport forms of carbohydrate and lipid are trehalose and diacylglycerol, respectively, and not glucose and free fatty acids as in mammals. Diacylglycerol is transported by a lipoprotein, lipophorin, which is specific for insects. The regulation of energy metabolism is also clearly different in that some of the key enzymes respond to different activators and inhibitors. The hormones involved in the control are unique to insects.

Most of our knowledge of the energy metabolism of insects has been accumulated in nonvector insects because they are easier to study; however, special methods have been developed and used to examine carbohydrate and lipid metabolism in mosquitoes. In general, a great deal of work remains to be done on the energy metabolism of arthropod vectors. Arthropod vectors do have special adaptations, which are potentially useful as targets for control measures. For example, some vectors can survive long bouts of starvation, and others can process large quantities of blood. Flight metabolism also has unique aspects in some insect vectors.

The knowledge acquired about other insects will facilitate the design of experiments that can also be applied to arthropod vectors. With the advanced purification and sequencing methods developed in recent years, it is possible to isolate peptide hormones from arthropod vectors. These hormones can be sequenced and synthesized. Synthetic hormones will make it easier to examine the role of hormones in the control of energy metabolism by in vivo and in vitro experiments. Other questions concerning energy metabolism are still better tackled first in model insects such as *Manduca sexta* rather than in arthropod vectors.

ACKNOWLEDGMENTS

The author is grateful to Mrs. D. Engler, Mr. F. Bartnek and Drs. J. R. Gasdaska, J. H. Law, and R. Van Antwerpen for critically reading the manuscript and for many helpful comments. Thanks are due to Mr. G.M. Grace for help with the computer graphics program.

REFERENCES

Beenakkers, A.M.Th., D.J. Van der Horst, and W.J.A. Van Marrewijk. 1981. Role of lipids in energy metabolism. In: R.G.H. Downer, ed., *Energy metabolism in insects.* New York: Plenum Press. pp. 53–100.

Beenakkers, A.M.Th., D.J. Van der Horst, and W.J.A. Van Marrewijk 1985. Biochemical processes directed to flight muscle metabolism. In G.A. Kerkut and L.I. Gilbert, editors, *Comprehensive insect physiology, biochemistry and pharmacology,* Vol. 10. Oxford: Pergamon Press. pp. 451–486.

Briegel, H. 1990. Metabolic relationship between female body size, reserves, and fecundity of *Aedes aegypti. J. Insect Physiol.* 36:165–172.

Bursell, E. 1978. Quantitative aspects of proline utilization during flight in tsetse flies. *Physiol. Entomol.* 3:265–272.

Bursell, E. 1981. The role of proline in energy metabolism. In: R.G.H. Downer, editor, *Energy metabolism in insects.* New York: Plenum Press. pp. 135–154.

Candy, D.J. 1985. Intermediary metabolism. In: G.A. Kerkut and L.I. Gilbert, editors, *Comprehensive insect physiology, biochemistry and pharmacology,* Vol. 10. Oxford: Pergamon Press. pp. 1–41.

Chen, P.S. 1985. Amino acid and protein metabolism. In: G.A. Kerkut and L.I. Gilbert, editors, *Comprehensive insect physiology, biochemistry and pharmacology,* Vol. 10. Oxford: Pergamon Press. pp. 177–217.

Chippendale, G.M. 1978. The functions of carbohydrates in insect life processes. In: M. Rockstein, editor, *Biochemistry of insects.* New York: Academic Press. pp. 1–55.

Clements, A.N. 1992. *The biology of mosquitoes.* Vol. 1: Development, nutrition and reproduction. London: Chapman and Hall.

Dadd, R.H. 1973. Insect nutrition: Current developments and metabolic implications. *Ann. Rev. Entomol.* 187:381–420.

Dadd, R.H. 1985. Nutrition: Organisms. In: G.A. Kerkut and L.I. Gilbert, editors, *Comprehensive insect physiology, biochemistry and pharmacology,* Vol. 10. Oxford: Pergamon Press. pp. 313–390.

Downer, R.G.H. 1985. Lipid metabolism. In: G.A. Kerkut and L.I. Gilbert, editors, *Comprehensive insect physiology, biochemistry and pharmacology,* Vol. 10. Oxford: Pergamon Press. pp. 77–113.

Friedman, S. 1985. Carbohydrate metabolism. In: G.A. Kerkut and L.I. Gilbert, editors, *Comprehensive insect physiology, biochemistry and pharmacology,* Vol. 10. Oxford: Pergamon Press. pp. 43–76.

Gies, A., T. Fromm, and R. Ziegler 1988. Energy metabolism in starving larvae of *Manduca sexta. Comp. Biochem. Physiol.* 91A:549–555.

Goldsworthy, G.J. 1984. The endocrine control of flight metabolism in locusts. *Adv. Insect Physiol.* 17:149–204.

Hargrove, J.W. 1976. Amino acid metabolism during flight in tsetse flies. *J. Insect Physiol.* 22:309–311.

Kammer, A.E., and B. Heinrich. 1978. Insect flight metabolism. *Adv. Insect Physiol.* 13:133–228.

Kanost, M. R., J.K. Kawooya, J.H. Law, R.O. Ryan, M.C. Van Heusden, and R. Ziegler. 1990. Insect haemolymph proteins. *Adv. Insect Physiol.* 22:299–396.

Kawooya, J.K., and J.H. Law. 1988. Role of lipophorin in lipid transport to the insect egg. *J. Biol. Chem.* 263:8748–8753.

Keeley, L.I., J.Y. Bradfield, S.M. Sowa, Y.-H. Lee, and K.-H. Lu. 1994. Physiological actions of hypertrechalosemic hormones in cockroaches. In: *Perspectives in comparative endocrinology*. Canada: National Research Council of Canada. pp. 475–485.

Konings, P.N.M., H.G.B. Vullings, W.M.J.B. Van Gemert, R. De Leeuw, J.H.B. Diederen, and W.F. Jansen. 1989. Octopamine-binding sites in the brain of *Locusta migratoria*. *J. Insect Physiol.* 35:519–524.

Kramer, K.J., C. Dziadik-Turner, and K. Daizo. 1985. Chitin metabolism in insects. In: G.A. Kerkut and L.I. Gilbert, editors, *Comprehensive insect physiology, biochemistry and pharmacology*, Vol. 3. Oxford: Pergamon Press. pp 75–115.

Langley, P.A. 1977. Physiology of tsetse flies (*Glossina* spp.) (Diptera: Glossinidae). *Bull. Ent. Res.* 67:523–574.

Langley, P.A., and E. Bursell. 1980. Role of fat body and uterine gland in milk synthesis by adult female *Glossina morsitans*. *Insect Biochem.* 10:11–17.

Langley, P.A., E. Bursell, J. Kabayo, R.W. Pimley, M.A. Trewern, and J. Marshall. 1981. Haemolymph lipid transport from fat body to uterine gland in pregnant females of *Glossina morsitans*. *Insect Biochem.* 11:225–231.

Merritt, R.W., R.H. Dadd, and E.D. Walker. 1992. Feeding behavior, natural food, and nutritional relationships of larval mosquitoes. *Ann. Rev. Entomol.* 37:349–376.

Mill, P.J. 1985. Structure and physiology of the respiratory system. In: G.A. Kerkut and L.I. Gilbert, editors, *Comprehensive insect physiology, biochemistry and pharmacology*, Vol. 3. Oxford: Pergamon Press. pp. 517–593.

Murphy, T.A., and G.R. Wyatt. 1965. The enzymes of glycogen and trehalose synthesis in silk moth fat body. *J. Biol. Chem.* 240:1500–1508.

Mwangi, R.W., and L.R.S. Awiti. 1989. Hypertrehalosaemic activity in corpus cardiacum-corpus allatum-aorta complex and adipokinetic response of *Glossina morsitans*. *Physiol. Entomol.* 14:61–66.

Ochanda, J.O., E.O. Osir, E.K. Nguu, and N.K. Olembo. 1992. Isolation and properties of 600-kDa and 23-kDa haemolymph proteins from the tsetse fly, *Glossina morsitans*: Their possible role as biological insecticides. *Scand. J. Immunol.* Suppl. 11. 67:41–47.

Orchard, I. 1987. Adipokinetic hormone—an update. *J. Insect Physiol.* 33:451–463.

Phillips, J.E., J. Hanrahan, M. Chamberlin, and B. Thomson. 1986. Mechanisms and control of reabsorption in insect hindgut. *Adv. Insect Physiol.* 19:329–422.

Pimley, R.W. 1983. Neuroendocrine stimulation of uterine gland synthesis in the tsetse fly, *Glossina morsitans*. *Physiol. Entomol.* 8:429–437.

Pimley, R.W., and P.A. Langley. 1981. Hormonal control of lipid synthesis in the fat body of the adult female tsetse fly, *Glossina morsitans*. *J. Insect Physiol.* 27:839–847.

Pimley, R.W., and P.A. Langley. 1982. Hormone stimulated lipolysis and proline synthesis in the fat body of the adult tsetse fly, *Glossina morsitans*. *J. Insect Physiol.* 28:781–789.

Reinecke, P., J.S. Buckner, and S.R. Grugel. 1980. Life cycle of laboratory-reared tobacco hornworms, *Manduca sexta*, a study of development and behavior, using time lapse cinematography. *Biol. Bull.* 158:129–140.

Sacktor, B. 1975. Biochemistry of insect flight. Part I—Utilization of fuel by muscle. In: D.H. Candy and B.A. Kilby, editors, *Insect biochemistry and function*. London: Chapman and Hall. pp. 1–88.

Sonenshine, D.E. 1991. *Biology of ticks*, Vol. 1. New York: Oxford University Press.

Soulages, J. L., O.J. Rimoldi, O.R. Peluffo, and R.R. Brenner. 1988. Transport and utilization of free fatty acids in *Triatoma infestans*. *Biochem. Biophys. Res. Commun.* 157:465–4

Van Handel, E. 1984. Metabolism of nutrients in the adult mosquito. *Mosq. News* 44:573–579.

Van Marrewijk, W.J.A., A.Th.M. Van den Broek, and A.M.Th. Beenakkers. 1986. Hormonal control of fat-body glycogen mobilization for locust flight. *Gen. Comp. Endocrinol.* 64:136–142.

Van Handel, E., and A.O. Lea. 1970. Control of glycogen and fat metabolism in the mosquito. *Gen. Comp. Endocrinol.* 14:381–384.

Vejbjerg, K., and T.C. Normann. 1974. Secretion of hyperglycaemic hormone from the corpus cardiacum of flying blowflies, *Calliphora erythrocephala. J. Insect Physiol.* 20:1189–1192

Wegener, G. 1990. Elite invertebrate athletes: Flight in insects, its metabolic requirements and regulation and its effects on life span. In: K. Nazar, R.L. Terjung, H. Kaciuba-Uscilko, and L. Budohoski, editors, *International perspectives in exercise physiology.* Champaign, IL: Human Kinetics Books. pp. 83–87.

Wegener, G., N.M. Bolas, and A.A.G. Thomas. 1991. Locust flight metabolism studied *in vivo* by 31P NMR spectroscopy. *J. Comp. Physiol. B.* 161:247–256.

Wyatt, G.R. 1980. The fat body as a protein factory. In: M. Locke and D.S. Smith, editors, *Insect biology in the future.* New York: Academic Press. pp. 201–225.

Ziegler, R. 1984. Metabolic energy expenditure and its hormonal regulation. In K.H. Hoffmann, editor, *Environmental physiology and biochemistry of insects.* Berlin: Springer-Verlag. pp. 95–118.

Ziegler, R. 1991. Changes in lipid and carbohydrate metabolism during starvation in adult *Manduca sexta. J. Comp. Physiol. B.* 161:12.

23. IMMUNE RESPONSES OF VECTORS

Susan M. Paskewitz and Bruce M. Christensen

INTRODUCTION

The ability to differentiate between self and nonself is a necessary adaptation in a world of pathogens and parasites. When recognition of nonself occurs, an organism mounts a defensive, or "immune," response in an effort to destroy or expel the foreign invader. The nature of these defenses is diverse, ranging from phagocytosis in many organisms to antibody production and complement cascades in mammals. Because insects are economically important as agricultural pests and disease vectors, there is much interest in describing the mechanisms operating in insect immunity. Understanding immune responses of vectors is important in 2 contexts. First, we need to assess the ways vectors might avoid destruction by biological control agents. Second, immune responses play a critical but underestimated role in the complex relationships that exist between arthropod vectors and the human and animal pathogens they transmit. Just as strong immune responses can reduce or restrict the vectorial capacity of some hosts, weakened responses can enhance the ability to transmit disease agents. An understanding of the methods by which parasites avoid these responses can suggest mechanisms that might be exploited for parasite control.

Although the arthropod immune response lacks the specificity of antigen-antibody complementarity, they do possess internal defense mechanisms that are surprisingly specific and effective in destroying pathogens and parasites. Because much of the information available on insect immunity has been derived from studies of nonvector species, this chapter is not limited to information obtained specifically from vector biology studies. However, the class Insecta is massive in size and wonderfully diverse, and undoubtedly this diversity also applies to the mechanisms operating in immune responses. How accurately can we apply data derived from immune studies with lepidopteran larvae or pupae to adult hematophagous dipterans, or from holometabolous to hemimetabolous insects? These are serious questions that have not yet been adequately answered. Further, many vectors are unique in having physiological processes associated with blood-feeding for egg production that can interact with the immune system. Thus, although the primary model systems for studying insect immune responses have been Lepidoptera, vectors are now being studied because new tools are available to overcome some of the limitations of working with small organisms. Some of the information that follows, therefore, is likely to change or be modified as additional species and groups of insects are subjected to critical studies.

There are 3 possible outcomes following exposure of an arthropod to a parasite via an infective meal: (1) In a susceptible arthropod, the parasite receives the appropriate stimuli from a compatible biochemical environment and develops and/or reproduces successfully in the vector; (2) in a resistant arthropod, some or all of the parasites are recognized as foreign by the cellular/humoral components in the hemolymph, and the arthropod initiates an immune response that can effectively sequester and destroy the parasite; or (3) in a refractory arthropod, the parasites do not elicit an immune response and although they can be successful in their migration to and invasion of the appropriate tissue, they fail to develop due to a physiological or biochemical incompatibility. Obviously, the genetic makeup of both the arthropod and the parasite influences the outcome of the relationship, and the manner by which the parasite responds to the host environment plays a role equal to that of the host's response to the parasite. This chapter focuses on resistance mechanisms, that is, the cellular and biochemical aspects of immune responses in insect vectors of disease agents.

CELLS AND TISSUES INVOLVED IN ARTHROPOD IMMUNE RESPONSES

The Cuticular and Gut Barriers

Arthropods possess a rigid cuticle that functions as an excellent barrier to potential pathogens. Entry of microorganisms through this exoskeleton usually requires a wound or some form of specialized entry mechanism on the part of the microbe. The most common route of entry for a pathogen or parasite is to be ingested by the arthropod. Many types of pathogens proceed no farther, undergoing complete development within the gut, and are passed on through the feces or through regurgitation. Most arthropods produce some form of a chitinous peritrophic matrix (previously referred to as a peritrophic "membrane") that can also act as a physical barrier (Chap. 19). How effective the peritrophic matrix is in limiting infection is debatable. Parasites that successfully penetrate the gut and gain access to the hemocoel then face an environment that is compatible or incompatible depending on the cellular, biochemical, and molecular interactions that occur between the parasite and the arthropod.

The Hemolymph

The functional tissue responsible for many of the immune responses is the insect blood, or hemolymph, which consists of hemocytes and plasma. However, the ability to respond to invading organisms is not restricted to this specific effector system, and other tissues can have immunologic capability as well.

The cellular portion of the hemolymph is composed of circulating hemocytes that function as the 1st line of defense against invading pathogens (Fig. 23.1). Categories of hemocyte types based on ultrastructural morphology and function vary depending on the organism examined, the experimental techniques employed, and the individual scientists conducting the studies. As a result, different classifications have been reported for the same genus and even the same species of vector. A good generalized classification for the insects is summarized in Table 23.1. Additional useful methods for classification rely on identifying hemocyte populations by means of fractionating them on density gradients and then producing monoclonal antibodies to cell surface determinants.

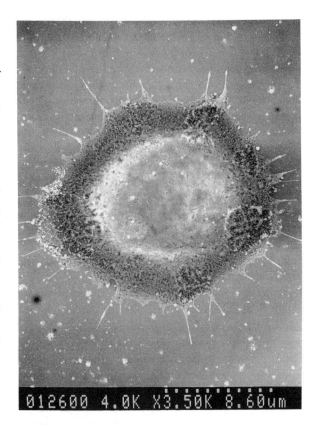

23.1   Scanning electron micrograph of spreading plasmatocyte from *Aedes aegypti*

TABLE 23.1 General overview of insect hemocyte classification and characteristics

Hemocyte type	Size (μm)	Inclusions (granules)	Stability (in vitro)	Other characteristics
Prohemocytes	6–13	none	very stable	high nuclear: cytoplasmic ratio Precursor cell?
Plasmatocytes	10–15	occasional small when present	stable	produce numerous cytoplasmic extensions capable of ameboid movement
Granular cells	8–20	numerous	unstable	some cytoplasmic extensions, usually lyse rapidly in vitro
Spherule cells	3–16	large spherular inclusions	very stable	membrane-bound inclusions cause irregular "morula" appearance
Oenocytoids	12–39	none	very stable to labile	eccentric nucleus and large nucleolus, few organelles

Modified from Rowley and Ratcliffe 1981; Gupta 1986; Drif and Brehelin 1993

Most researchers today recognize prohemocytes, the presumed stem cells from which other hemocyte types differentiate, plasmatocytes, and granulocytes, although some researchers suggest that all hemocytes represent developmental phases of a single cell type. Prohemocytes are small round cells with a high nuclear to cytoplasmic ratio, and they constitute a small percentage of the total hemocyte population. Plasmatocytes are the "macrophages" of insects. This is the most abundant hemocyte type, generally comprising over 60% of the population. Plasmatocytes are ameboid cells that readily attach and spread on surfaces (Fig. 23.1). These cells are extremely important in insect immunity and are actively involved in phagocytosis, nodule formation, encapsulation reactions, and wound healing. Granulocytes are rounded cells that are packed with granules. These cells degranulate rapidly in vitro and during a variety of immune responses including phagocytosis, nodule formation, and encapsulation (Fig. 23.2). Other cells, including coagulocytes (cystocytes), spherulocytes, and oenocytoids occur less often, and their functions are unclear. The podocytes, vermiform cells, and thrombocytoids sometimes mentioned in the literature are probably not distinct cell populations because ultrastructurally they appear to be similar to plasmatocytes. A number of

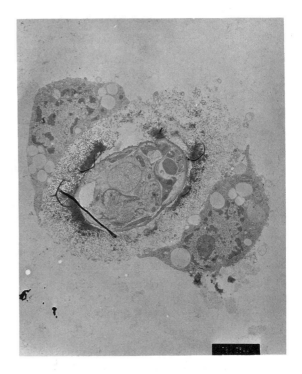

23.2 Plasmatocytes in proximity to microfilaria undergoing melanotic encapsulation in *Aedes trivitattus*.

studies categorizing hemocyte types have been conducted for vector species (Table 23.2). In Diptera, in vitro studies using hemocytes have been hampered by the extreme lability of some hemocyte types, which lyse as soon as they are exposed to air.

TABLE 23.2 Vector species and studies on hemocytes

Species	Study
Panstrongylus megistus	Barracco and Loch 1989
Dermacentor variabilis	Sonenshine 1991
Anopheles stephensi	Foley 1978
Glossina austeni	Kaaya and Ratcliffe 1982
Glossina morsitans	Kaaya and Ratcliffe 1982
Culex quinquefasciatus	Kaaya and Ratcliffe 1982
Culex pipiens	Drif and Brehelin 1983
Aedes aegypti	Drif and Brehelin 1983
Aedes albopictus	Bhat and Singh 1975
Simulium vittatum	Luckhart, Cupp, and Cupp 1992
Rhodnius prolixus	Jones 1967a,b

Hemocytes can be free, sessile, or arranged into aggregates termed hemopoietic or phagocytic organs and pericardial cells. The majority of the hemocyte studies have been carried out on free hemocyte populations, but there is evidence that phagocytic organs can also contribute to immune responses. Furthermore, in mammals certain lymphocytes are capable of invading tissues. Infiltrating, or invasive, hemocytes also have been reported for insects in response to cuticular grafts and could be important for response to parasites that are not free in the hemocoel.

In addition to hemocytes, other tissues can be involved in the production of immune system components. For example, the fat body plays a major role in the synthesis and release of many of the antibacterial proteins involved in humoral responses. The integument also secretes these compounds. For example,

when the cuticule of *Bombyx mori* is abraded, the underlying epidermal cells produce the antibacterial peptide cecropin. The midgut also produces important immune response components. For example, in the tobacco hornworm, *Manduca sexta,* an antibacterial protein is produced by regenerative cells of the midgut epithelium at the time of metamorphosis from 5th instar to pupae. During metamorphosis, the gut undergoes dissolution by histolytic enzymes, and the antibacterial substance probably helps to destroy gut bacteria and prevent contamination of the nutrient-rich hemolymph. In another example, the midgut cells of cockroaches infected with larval acanthocephala have been shown to produce the enzyme phenoloxidase (PO), which is important in melanotic encapsulation of parasites. Filarial worms have been found melanized within muscles and Malpighian tubule cells, although a breakdown of the Malpighian tubule syncytium can allow the inward passage of hemolymph components in this instance. Finally, antibacterial activity occurs in the salivary glands, crop, and components of the reproductive systems of various insects. Thus, in insects a widespread ability of various tissues to respond to invasive threats exists.

METHODS OF ACTION

Humoral Immunity in Insects

Insect immune responses are often separated into cellular and cell-free, or humoral, responses, although humoral responses can be cell-mediated events. Humoral immune component production can be induced in many insects by an injection of nonpathogenic bacteria, heat-killed pathogens, or fungal or bacterial cell wall products as well as by sterile wounds. Originally, the antibacterial response noted after induction was attributed mainly to insect proteins that are closely related to the chicken-type lysozymes. However, work using the pupae of the cecropia moth, *Hyalophora cecropia,* resulted in the description of 2 new classes of antibacterial proteins, the cecropins and attacins. This model insect is advantageous because immune protein synthesis can be induced during diapause when few other proteins are being produced and it also has a large quantity of hemolymph accessible for analysis. This work has inspired a number of scientists to investigate similar phenomena in other groups; the growing list of antibacterial peptides identified from insects is summarized in Table 23.3. In general, induced antibacterial factors are not specific for the bacterial species used for induction but instead are active against many bacterial targets. No group of insects has been identified that produces representatives of all groups of insect antibacterials identified.

TABLE 23.3   List of antibacterial peptides isolated or cloned from insects

Diptericin superfamily	Cecropins	Lysozyme	Defensins	Other
Diptericins	Cecropins	Lysozyme	Defensin	Coleoptericin
Attacins	Bactericidin		Sapecins	Drosocin
Sarcotoxin II	Sarcotoxin I		Sarcotoxin III	Pyrrhocoricin
Abaecin	Ceratotoxin		Phormicins	Andropin
Apidaecin			Royalisin	
Hymenoptaecin				

Diptericins

The diptericin superfamily includes attacins, sarcotoxin II, diptericins, abaecin, and apidaecin. Attacins are large (20 kDa) and occur in both basic and acidic forms. Putative attacins have been identified in *Sarcophaga, Glossina, Drosophila,* and *Aedes aegypti.* Attacins act at the level of gene transcription and prevent production of the major outer membrane proteins in *Escherichia coli,* thereby causing membrane breakdown. The action of attacin on the outer wall possibly permits cecropins and lysozyme to penetrate. Sarcotoxin II (from *Sarcophaga*) is closely related to the attacins. Diptericins are smaller (9kDa) and have a proline-rich domain (P) and a glycine-rich domain (G). Attacins have a repeated sequence similar to the G domain, and sarcotoxin II has both G repeats and a portion of a P repeat. Two other types of hymenopteran proteins, the apidaecins and abaecins, are much smaller (2–4 kDa). Apidaecin contains only a P domain, whereas abaecin has both a P and part of a G domain. Coleoptericin, found in a tenebrionid beetle, has no homology to known peptides, but the peptide is glycine rich and active against gram-negative bacteria, characteristics that are similar to diptericins. Hymenoptaecin, from *Apis mellifera,* is 93 amino acids long and glycine rich. This antibacterial also is somewhat similar in sequence to diptericins.

Cecropins

Cecropins are small (4 kDa), basic, devoid of cysteines, and form 2 amphipathic alpha helices; these molecules act on both gram-negative and gram-positive bacteria. In *Hyalophora* there are 3 families of related cecropin peptides. Although first described in insects, recent studies have shown that these peptides also occur in vertebrates (pigs) and thus may be widespread phylogenetically. Among insects, homologues have been identified in many lepidopterans and in several dipterans, including *Drosophila, Ae. aegypti, Simuliium, Anopheles, Sarcophaga,* and *Glossina* spp. The DNA sequence is highly conserved between *Drosophila* and *Sarcophaga,* with 73% nucleotide similarity. The mechanism of cecropin action has been intensively studied. Apparently, pores are formed in the bacterial cell inner membranes with consequent cell lysis. The presence of cholesterol in the membrane reduces the effectiveness of cecropins to form pores, which is consistent with the evidence that eukaryotes are resistant to these molecules. Andropin, an antibacterial protein that is confined to the ejaculatory duct of adult male fruit flies, has no sequence homology with cecropins, but the 2 peptides may have similar secondary structures.

Lysozymes

Since its discovery in 1922, lysozyme has been used as a model for investigating the 3-dimensional structure of proteins and the mechanism of enzyme action. This enzyme must have appeared early in evolutionary history because it has been found in bacteriophages, plants, invertebrates, and vertebrates. Lysozyme was the first antibacterial factor identified in insect hemolymph. It has been purified or cloned from a number of insects, including *Hyalophora, Galleria, Manduca, Locusta, Spodoptera, Calliphora, and Drosophila*. Lysozymes are generally 14–17 kDa proteins that are bactericidal to some gram-positive bacteria such as *Bacillus megaterium* and *Micrococcus lysodeikticus* (*M. luteus*). This enzyme breaks down the amino acid–sugar polymer (peptidoglycan) that forms the cell wall of many bacteria. In *Hyalophora*, it has been hypothesized that lysozyme serves mainly to remove the cell wall sacculus that is left after the action of cecropins and attacins. In Lepidoptera, synthesis of this enzyme is induced upon bacterial injection, but in *D. melanogaster* synthesis is suppressed under these conditions. In *Drosophila*, lysozymes form a multigene family with at least 7 members. Different genes are expressed in the midgut and in the salivary glands. Some forms of this enzyme have digestive rather than immune functions in several insects, including *Musca* and *Drosophila*, as well as in mammalian foregut fermenters. In general, midgut lysozymes have neutral or acidic pI's, not the strongly basic lysozymes involved in immune responses. Finally, it should be noted that additional "duck-type" lysozymes have been isolated from several birds and bear no DNA or amino acid sequence level resemblance to chicken-type lysozymes, a group that contains all known insect lysozymes. Nothing is known about the presence of these alternative lysozymes in invertebrates.

Defensins

Defensins are 4 kDa cationic peptides that contain 6 cysteine residues forming 3 disulfide bonds. They are structurally well defined, and are all characterized by an alpha helix, containing both hydrophobic and hydrophilic groups, joined by 2 disulfide bridges to an antiparallel beta sheet. Insect defensins have been reported from Diptera (sapecins, phormicins), Hymenoptera, Coleoptera, and Odonata. These molecules were originally considered homologous to defensins that occur in mammals, where they are found in neutrophils and macrophages and contribute to the destruction of bacteria and viruses. However, the 3-dimensional structures of the proteins and the disulfide bond formations are entirely different and are more closely related to charybdotoxins, scorpion-derived toxins that function as potassium–channel blockers. In insects, defensins are most potent against gram-positive bacteria, although some activity against gram-negative strains has been noted. In *Sarcophaga*, defensins are expressed in hemocytes in response to body injury and during pupal and embryonic development. This group is related to a peptide found in royal jelly of honeybees (royalisin).

Gene Regulation of Antibacterial Proteins

Regulation of gene expression of some of these antibacterial factors has been examined. In all cases studied so far, the increase in antibacterial proteins results from elevated levels of the mRNAs, usually in the fat body (Chap. 15). Comparisons of the promoter regions of 2 attacin genes, cecropins and lysozyme, in *H. cecropia* revealed a common sequence. A further search revealed that this sequence was similar to a binding site for transcription factor NF-k (kappa) B found in mammals. This binding site was first identified in the enhancer of the immunoglobulin light chain gene. Since then, NF-kB has been found to regulate a number of genes involved in mammalian immune, inflammatory, and acute phase responses through its interaction with the NF-kB binding sites. NF-kB occurs in the cytoplasm, where it is bound to an inhibitor protein. The release of NF-kB from the inhibitor is mediated by protein phosphorylation by either protein kinase C or cAMP-dependent protein kinase. Interestingly, the binding factor cecropia immunoresponsive factor (CIF) from *H. cecropia* has been identified and shares a number of features with NF-kB. CIF may be regulated in a manner similar to NF-kB because the inducers lipopolysaccharide (LPS) and phorbol 12-myristate 13-acetate (PMA) stimulate quick responses in both systems. Similar NF-kB related binding motifs have been identified in *D. melanogaster* in cecropins A2 and B and diptericin and in *Sarcophaga peregrina*. Putative-binding proteins from both species also have been identified; thus the molecular basis for this type of response to bacteria is probably widespread among organisms. Understanding the mechanisms for induction of the genes can suggest mechanisms by which pathogens manage to avoid these defense systems.

Antibacterial Proteins in Vectors

Information is scarce about antibacterial proteins in vectors, even in those vectors that transmit bacterial diseases. Many bacterial diseases, including anthrax, bacillary dysentery, typhoid, and cholera, can be mechanically transmitted by insects and do not interact with the immune system. Most of the biologically transmitted bacterial or rickettsial diseases are vectored by ticks or lice. In these arthropods, the bacteria are usually confined to the gut, and transmission is via the feces or regurgitation. However, the spirochetes *Borrelia duttoni* or *B. hermsii* (tick-borne relapsing fever) and *B. recurrentis* (louse-borne relapsing fever) multiply within the hemocoel of their vectors and are well exposed to the immune system. *B. burgdorferi* spirochetes (Lyme disease) and *Rickettsia tsutsugamuchi* rickettsias (scrub typhus) must also travel through the hemocoel to reach the salivary glands in *Ixodes* ticks and trombiculid mites, respectively. These pathogens are able to avoid or suppress the host response. Another possibility is that the vector organisms cannot mount an antibacterial defense; however, antibacterials have been demonstrated in other evolutionarily ancient groups, including the Odonata, the horseshoe crab, and the millipede (although mollusks seem to have little antibacterial synthetic capacity). It is unlikely that ticks and mites, which spend considerable time off-host moving through leaf litter rich in fungi and bacteria, have no internal defenses against these organisms. Nonetheless, all tick and sucking louse stages are obligate blood-feeders (and blood is a relatively sterile food source); thus internal exposure to bacteria is rare and the need for a humoral defense low. However, reduviid vectors of Chagas' disease are also obligate blood-feeders in all stages, and in *Rhodnius prolixus*

both lysozyme and other antibacterial activity (perhaps cecropin-like) is induced on inoculation with bacteria.

In other vectors, lysozyme activity has been identified in the salivary glands of mosquitoes, and bacterial inhibitors have been found in the crop of the sand fly *Phlebotomus papatasi*, in which sugar meals are stored. However, nectars are notoriously devoid of bacterial contamination due to the extremely high osmotic pressure, so the function of bacterial inhibitors in the crop is not clear. A bacteria-inducible lysozyme has not been identified in dipteran vectors.

Cecropin and attacin-like factors have been induced in the hemolymph of the tsetse fly *Glossina morsitans morsitans*, and a probable cecropin has been induced in a cell line of the mosquito *Aedes albopictus*. Southern blot analysis of *Ae. aegypti* and *Simulium* probed with heterologous cecropin clones suggests that these molecules occur in these species as well. Antiattacin antibodies also appear to recognize polypeptides present in hemolymph from *Aedes* and *Simulium*. Apart from these few examples, little information about antibacterials in dipteran vectors is available, in part because a direct relevance to disease transmission was not evident earlier and because obtaining adequate hemolymph samples is difficult in many of the Diptera. However, recent studies have shown that antibacterials can in fact have a broader target range. The demonstrated effect of cecropins and/or the magainin peptides from frogs on filarial worms, malaria organisms, trypanosomes, and leishmanial parasites has provoked more interest in this overlooked area. Finally, to some extent the difficulties of obtaining adequate samples can be overcome with tools for directly identifying genes for some of the more evolutionarily conserved antibacterial peptides and for microanalysis of protein sequences.

Other Bacteria-Inducible Proteins

In addition to those proteins with bactericidal activity, other proteins also are induced following bacterial injection into some Lepidoptera. These proteins include hemolin (P4), the major inducible protein in *H. cecropia* and *M. sexta*, as well as scolexin (M13), identified from *M. sexta*. Scolexin is produced by the epidermis and midgut in *M. sexta* after bacterial injection and can agglutinate sheep red blood cells and trigger hemocyte coagulation in vitro. Hemolin is a member of the immunoglobulin (Ig) superfamily and is discussed later.

Antifungal Proteins in Insects

An antifungal protein (AFP) has been purified from the hemolymph of larval *S. peregrina*. This protein is expressed constitutively; its action against fungi is enhanced in the presence of one of the inducible antibacterial proteins, sarcotoxin IA. AFP is a histidine-rich peptide that consists of 67 amino acids.

Hemolysins

In many invertebrates, hemolysins have been identified that rupture red blood cells in vitro, but their role in vivo is unknown. It has been suggested that hemolysins could be evolutionarily related to the vertebrate complement system components perforin and C9. In insects, these molecules have been little studied, but a midgut trypanolysin that acts against *Trypanosoma brucei brucei* and *T. congolense* has been identified in *G. palpalis*.

Antiviral Mechanisms in Arthropods

Little is known about the effectiveness of insect defense reactions against viruses, but many viruses attack insects. The gut can form a primary barrier to invasion of viral particles into the hemocoel; it has been estimated that there is a 50–60% reduction in infectivity of some viruses that have passed through the midgut. Hemocytic immune responses in cultured *Ae. aegypti* and *Bombyx mori* larvae were not found. Baculovirus infections in *Trichoplusia ni* larvae apparently do not stimulate immune responses; however, antiviral activity in the hemolymph and gut of *B. mori* has been reported, and viral particles can sometimes be phagocytosed. Susceptibility to flavivirus infection in *Ae. aegypti* is apparently under genetic control, although whether this represents resistance or refractoriness is unknown.

Cellular Immunity in Insects

Phagocytosis

Phagocytosis was the first of the cellular defense reactions of animals to be studied by Elie Metchnikoff in the mid-1800s. This Russian scientist observed the phenomenon in several invertebrates, including the starfish and the copepod *Daphnia*. Phagocytosis is a primary defense against bacteria and other particles, such as various protozoan spores, small enough to be engulfed. The process requires first that contact between the invader and the phagocyte take place. Contact in vertebrates can be facilitated by chemotactic factors, but in insects it has been difficult to prove that such factors are necessary. Certainly, chemotaxis would not be operative during phagocytosis of inert objects such as glass or fibers. Instead, there is ample opportunity for random contact between cells and foreign materials because of the free movement of hemocytes in an open body cavity.

Once contact is made, attachment occurs, which can be mediated by serum factors or opsonins. Opsonins are molecules that promote phagocytosis (or encapsulation) by attaching to the target and then interacting with the phagocyte. Vertebrate examples of opsonins are plasma antibodies and components of the complement system. In mollusks and crustaceans, the opsonizing ability of hemagglutinins (which cause red blood cells to clump) and lectins is well documented; however, the presence of opsonins has been a controversial area in insect immunity. Although hemagglutinin activity has been identified in many insects, opsonic functions have only rarely been attributed to these molecules (see the section on recognition molecules), and several studies have shown reduced phagocytosis after preincubation of particles in agglutinins. One alternative is that attachment proceeds directly through receptors found on the hemocyte membranes.

Once the invader or particle attaches to the phagocyte, uptake proceeds by surrounding the invader with filopodia or by ingestion in coated vesicles. After uptake, the invader must be killed. In vertebrates, a number of antimicrobial systems have been identified, including superoxide anion, acid pH, lysozyme, lactoferrin, cationic proteins, and myeloperoxidase-H_2O_2 halide systems. In insects little is known about the specific killing mechanisms, but evidence suggests that a peroxidase/superoxide killing system such as that found in snails and vertebrates is lacking.

Phagocytosis in Diptera occurs less often for those species with low numbers of hemocytes. For example, it has been reported that in *Chironomus* larvae, phagocytosis occurs rarely and late in the response to injected bacteria, with the primary response being humoral melanotic encapsulation.

Nodule Formation

Although small infections with bacteria are dealt with through phagocytosis, the response to more overwhelming infections is nodule formation. Nodules are composed of a loose association of hemocytes, and the foreign particles sometimes become melanized. Hemolin, the major induced protein after bacterial injection in several Lepidoptera, possibly functions as a hemocyte modulator either to prevent excessive aggregation in nodules or to cause the release of sessile hemocytes for nodule formation.

Encapsulation

The main defense mechanism of insects against invaders that are too large to be phagocytosed is encapsulation. Encapsulation usually involves the hemocytes in the formation of a layered, multicellular sheath that sometimes becomes melanized. Some dipteran vectors have low numbers of hemocytes; in these species melanization can occur without the formation of the cellular sheath. This is often termed humoral melanotic encapsulation, but hemocytes can be involved in the initial stages during the formation of this type of capsule. The type of capsule formed can also depend on the type or species of parasite invading the hemocoel.

Encapsulation responses have been described for a variety of parasite infections, including microsporans in grasshoppers and mosquitoes. Since these parasites are protozoa, related to malaria and leishmanial parasites as well as trypanosomes, and because they are often used for biological control, the humoral and cellular factors that limit their development are of special interest. In general, these parasites sometimes elicit strong hemocyte encapsulation reactions as well as melanization, but the responses are often insufficient to constrain microsporan development. Such responses usually do not occur in normal hosts.

Phenol Oxidase

The formation of melanin has been studied in detail (Fig. 23.3). A careful study of the cuticular sclerotization and melanization pathways, which are closely related to the immune melanization response biochemistry, yields much useful information. Of primary importance in melanin formation are the phenol oxidase enzymes (PO). Phenol oxidases are copper binding enzymes that occur in most organisms, including fungi, plants, and animals. In insects, 2 types of PO have been recorded: the laccase-type and the tyrosinase-type. The laccase-type enzymes are involved in cuticular sclerotization and can act on some of the same substrates (p- and o-diphenols but not monophenols) as the tyrosinase-type PO (o-diphenols and monophenols). The known tyrosinase-type enzymes are evolutionarily related to the hemocyanins, the oxygen-carrying pigments found in many lower arthropods, but they have different functions.

The terminology associated with these enzymes can be confusing. Phenol oxidases that catalyze the hydroxylation of tyrosine, a monophenol, to DOPA are called monophenol oxidases. The diphenol oxidases act on o-diphenols, including catecholamines such as DOPA and dopamine, to produce reactive quinones. Diphenol oxidases also oxidize 5,6-dihydroxyindole to indolequinone forms that can polymerize with or without additional proteins to form various types of melanin. Diphenol and monophenol oxidase activities can occur within the same enzyme, which may be called a "tyrosinase."

The PO enzymes are important in many aspects of insect biology and have been purified from a number of species. POs are involved in melanization and sclerotization of the cuticle and of eggs or egg cases in some insects. POs also are involved in wound healing as well as in the immune system. Thus, it is not surprising that in some insects there can be multiple PO genes. In mammals, a single enzyme, tyrosinase, has diphenol oxidase, monophenol oxidase, and indole dehydrogenase activities. But in extracts from *D. melanogaster*, at least 4 DOPA-staining bands can be resolved using native polyacrylamide gel electrophoresis. Two of these bands have only diphenol oxidase activity whereas the other 2 have both diphenol and

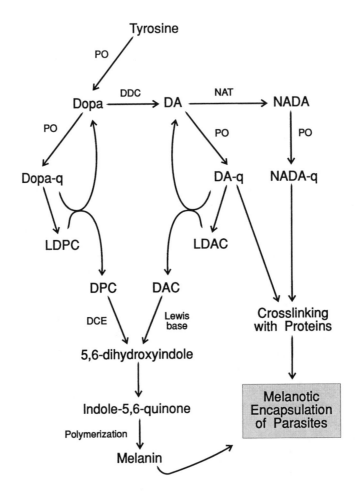

23.3   Biochemical pathways for formation of melanotic materials during encapsulation of parasites. The biochemistry of mel-anotic encapsulation is likely initiated by the hydroxylation of tyrosine by phenol oxidase (PO) to L-dopa (Dopa). This can result in the decarboxylation of L-dopa by the action of dopadecarboxylase (DDC) to form dopamine (DA), and DA can be acetylated through the enzymatic activity of N-acetyltransferase (NAT) to form N-acetyldopamine (NADA).   All of these compounds (dopa, DA, and NADA) can be oxidized by PO to their respective quinones, dopaquinone (Dopa-q), dopamine-quinone (DA-q), and acetyldopamine-quinone (NADA-q). Intramolecular cyclization of Dopa-q and DA-q results in the for-mation of leukodopachrome (LDPC) and leukodopaminechrome (LDAC), respectively. LDPC and LDAC react with Dopa-q and DA-q to form dopachrome (DPC) and dopaminechrome (DAC), and during these reactions Dopa-q and DA-q are reduced back to Dopa and DA, respectively. DPC undergoes a decarboxylative structural rearrangement by the action of dopachrome conversion enzyme (DCE) to form 5,6-dihydroxyindole. 5,6-dihydroxyindole also is formed by the isomeriza-tion of DAC by a general base catalyzed reaction. The oxidation of 5,6-dihydroxyindole to indole–5,6-quinone and the poly-merization of indole–5,6-quinone result in the formation of melanin. DA-q, NADA-q, and to a certain extent Dopa-q can react with nucleophilic groups of protein molecules, together with hemocytes and melanin polymers, to form melanotic cap-sules that can effectively sequester parasites.

monophenol oxidase activity. The 2 diphenol oxidase bands are affected by 2 genes (Dox A–2 and Dox A–3) that are separately mutable and probably encode protein components of a PO. It is possible that a combination of gene products associate as subunits to form the complete PO. The Dox-A2 gene has been cloned from *Drosophila*, but the deduced protein encoded bears no resemblance to that deduced from sequences of tyrosinases cloned from human, mouse, and *Neurospora* or to hemocyanins cloned from mollusks or arthropods. Mutations of the Dox-A2 gene severely affect cuticular sclerotization. Thus, Dox-A2 could represent a laccase-type PO. In *M. sexta*, 3 PO forms have been identified. The 1st is a granular form associated with pigment granules in the cuticle, the 2nd is a typical cuticular PO, and the 3rd is a hemolymph PO of different molecular weight. The cuticular PO does not cross-react with a polyclonal antibody prepared using the granular form.

A tyrosinase-type PO exists in the insect hemolymph as a proenzyme (proPO). ProPO is activated through the action of a cascade often called the proPO activating system, or ProPO cascade. This cascade can be activated in vitro by many things including detergents, isopropanol, fatty acids, chloroform, acid-base shock, cations, urea, microbial products, and abiotic particles. Ca^{2+} is a requirement for the activation. The kinetics of PO activity on various substrates can be affected by the way in which it is activated; thus characterization of activated enzymes as "diphenol oxidases" without monophenol oxidase activity should be carefully considered. Some of the putative "activators of PO" can actually activate a preceding step in the cascade. For example, in crayfish a fungal cell wall product activates a serine protease in crayfish hemocytes, which in turn activates the proPO. The proPO cascade of *B. mori* can also be activated by this fungal product; however, this is completely inhibited by the serine protease inhibitor, p-nitrophenol-p-guanidinobenzoate, and purified proPO from this species cannot be activated by these microbial products. Thus, studies using activators to assess PO type should be viewed with caution because they can act on 1 or more precursors in the pathway.

In vivo, proPO is probably activated by serine proteases. The first of these to be identified was purified as a cuticular prophenoloxidase activating enzyme and later identified as a serine protease. Incubation of proPO with the activator results in the loss of a short peptide fragment in *B. mori*. ProPO-activating serine proteases have been purified from several insects, including *H. cecropia* and *B. mori*, and their activity is inferred in many others. Serine protease PO-activators possibly exist as inactive precursors in some species that also must be activated, perhaps by additional serine proteases. Hemolymph of several species also contains protease and PO inhibitors that prevent PO activity. Because PO produces short-lived but reactive quinones that can be toxic in vivo, tight regulation of the activation of this system is essential.

ProPO activation can be mediated by cells or it can be humoral. In some insects, either all of the components or critical components of the pathway are contained in the hemocytes. Once hemocytes contact the invader they degranulate, or lyse, releasing the inactive components that then become activated. Alternatively, in some insects it is hypothesized that cells are not involved; the PO activating system components can exist in the plasma in an inactive form. Microbial products then react with the first component, causing a conformational change that stimulates further changes in the cascade, leading to PO activation. This postulated humoral path can be compared with the alternate pathway of the mammalian complement system because both can be activated in vitro by microbial surfaces and neither require cell mediation. In mammals, microbial cell wall products trigger the alternative pathway by providing a surface that protects factor C3b from its normal inactivation by a serum factor. A series of serine proteases are then generated in a cascade leading to the production of opsonizing or cytolytic factors. A similar pathway is postulated for those Diptera with small numbers of hemocytes that seem to melanize invaders without the benefit of hemocytes; however, proof of a humoral pathway without cellular involvement for PO activation is still lacking in insects. Cells could be involved in initiation of the response but in such a transitory way as to avoid observation. Indeed, during melanization of filarioid worms in *Aedes* mosquitoes, hemocytes have been observed to contact the surface of the worm within the first 5 minutes of exposure, whereupon they lyse, or degranulate, and melanization begins with little additional cellular involvement.

Finally, POs can be produced in other tissues besides the epidermis and hemolymph, such as the midgut. In a cockroach parasitized by an acanthocephalan, a subset of midgut cells is highly DOPA-reactive, whereas gut cells of unparasitized insects show no such response. Other tissues, including the thoracic muscle cells and Malpighian tubule cells, have also been reported to function in melanizing intracellular parasitic nematodes (Fig. 23.4).

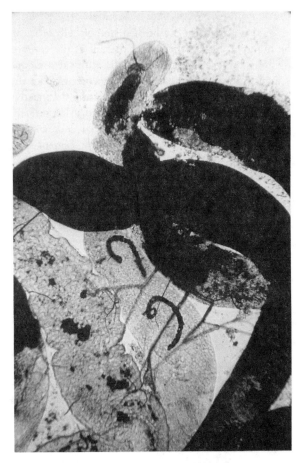

23.4 Melanized microfilariae of *Dirofilaria immitis* within the Malpighian tubules of *Aedes trivittatus*

Dopa Decarboxylase

Like PO, dopa decarboxylase (DDC) is important in sclerotization and melanization of eggs and cuticle and also occurs in the nervous system, where it generates the neurotransmitter dopamine. That it can also be important in immune response is demonstrated by studies showing that temperature-sensitive DDC mutants of *D. melanogaster* show a reduced ability to melanize parasitoids under high temperature regimes when DDC is nonfunctional. Enzyme activity is also elevated during filarial infections in mosquitoes.

Dopachrome Conversion Enzyme

Dopachrome conversion enzyme (DCE) occurs in *Ae. aegypti*, *D. melanogaster*, *B. mori*, *M. sexta*, and *H. cecropia* and mediates a structural rearrangement of dopachrome with the loss of a carboxyl group. The role of this enzyme is similar to dopachrome tautomerase, which has recently been identified in vertebrates as being important in melanin production. The type of melanin produced when this enzyme is functional has different properties from that produced by PO alone. Interestingly, dopachrome tautomerase in mice is 40% identical at the amino acid level to mouse tyrosinase, suggesting a gene duplication leading to an evolutionary split to the 2 functions. Nothing is known yet about the contribution of this enzyme to immune responses, although high levels of DCE activity in *Ae. aegypti* occur in hemolymph, regardless of immune status.

Encapsulation Responses to Human Pathogens in Vectors

Encapsulation has been identified in several systems of medical interest. For example, malaria parasites can be encapsulated in unsuitable hosts. This phenomenon was first observed by Sir Ronald Ross in 1898; the encapsulated sporozoites he noted are called "Ross's black spores." Melanized sporozoites have been observed both in the salivary glands and within the oocysts on the midgut. More recently mosquito strains have been identified in which both the entire oocyst (Fig. 23.5) as well as the earlier ookinete stage are melanized (Fig. 23.6). In the ookinete, this response is to a living parasite rather than to one that is dying or dead (which would be considered a secondary response). Ookinetes are encapsulated under the basal lamina of

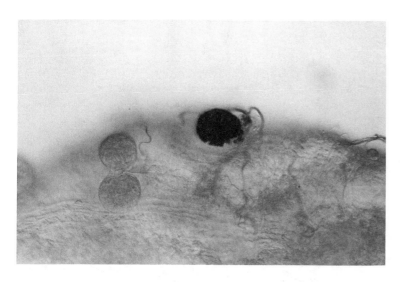

23.5 Light micrograph of melanized oocyst of *Plasmodium gallinaceum* on the midgut of *Aedes aegypti*

the midgut and are not directly in the hemocoel; thus the involvement of hemocytes in this response is not clear. Neither hemocytes themselves nor hemocyte fragments occur consistently near encapsulated parasites. Encapsulation could involve production of melanizing enzymes by the midgut cells or through a humoral form of the prophenoloxidase cascade. Incubation of infected mosquitoes with DOPA or dopamine results in heavy deposition of melanin around the encapsulated parasite in vesicular structures that seem to be confined to 1 cell in close proximity to the parasite. Melanized parasites are occasionally seen within gut cells (Fig. 23.7). This immune response occurs in a genetically selected resistant strain of the African malaria vector *An. gambiae* but not in a related susceptible strain. The differences between the 2 strains are caused by the influence of 2 or 3 genes. PO activity is different in the 2 strains and could contribute to reduced ability to encapsulate in the susceptible strain. To examine the underlying genetic differences, a homologue to the putative *Drosophila* phenoloxidase gene, Dox-A2, has been cloned from *An. gambiae*; however, no association between this gene and resistance has yet been determined. Thus, little is known about the underlying causes of this change in ability to respond to malaria parasites by the most important vector of malaria in Africa. Understanding the biochemical and genetic differences between these strains should provide much information about the molecular basis for resistance and provide a tool for studying genetic control of vectorial capacity.

The cellular and biochemical aspects of melanotic encapsulation also have been studied in several filarial worm–mosquito systems. The filarioid nematodes *Brugia malayi*, *B. pahangi*, and *Dirofilaria immitis* have been used with mosquitoes in the genera *Aedes* and *Armigeres* in attempts to clarify recognition and effector mechanisms responsible for resistance. Several detailed ultrastructural studies have illustrated the involvement of plasmatocyte-like hemocytes in this defense reaction. Although mosquitoes have a limited number of circulating hemocytes, during immune responses to nematodes these cells become activated, increase in numbers in the circulation, and secrete materials or lyse near the surface of the invading parasite (Fig. 23.8). At the same time, melanotic materials are formed that begin to encase the parasite and sequester it from the circulating hemolymph. In both *Ae. aegypti* and *Ae. trivattatus*, cell remnants are involved in the formation of a double membrane structure that completely surrounds the parasite, melanotic material, and cellular debris (Fig. 23.9). This membrane-like structure is believed to function in stopping the reaction and therefore the recruitment of additional hemocytes from a supply that is limited.

Studies using lectin-binding affinities and ^{125}I-labeling of cell surface molecules have shown that surface changes on hemocytes are associated with immune competence and activation in mosquitoes. It has not been determined whether any of these changes represent specific cell surface epitopes that might be related to signal recognition mechanisms. Hemocytes also seem to be the source of augmented PO activity

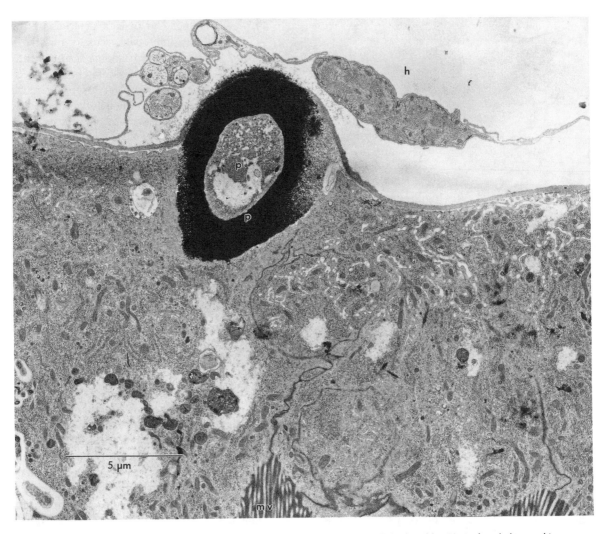

23.6 Encapsulated ookinete of *Plasmodium cynomolgi* between midgut cells and the basal lamina in *Anopheles gambiae*

during melanotic encapsulation reactions, and studies suggest that only 1 form of PO functions in both the hydroxylation of tyrosine as well as the oxidation of diphenols. In addition to PO activity, in vivo studies have demonstrated that dopa decarboxylase activity is significantly enhanced in the hemolymph during reactions against filarial worms; this increased activity occurs at the same time that hemolymph L-dopa levels are significantly elevated. It also is apparent that mosquito hemolymph possesses a high level of

dopachrome conversion enzyme, which can function in the conversion of dopachrome to 5,6-dihydroxyindole during the melanotic encapsulation of parasites. In summary, the biochemical pathways associated with melanotic encapsulation of filarial worms likely involve the production of o-quinones that serve as crosslinking molecules as well as the production of melanotic materials through eumelanin pathways (see Fig. 23.3).

Note that the chemistry required for the production of these melanotic materials is also involved in

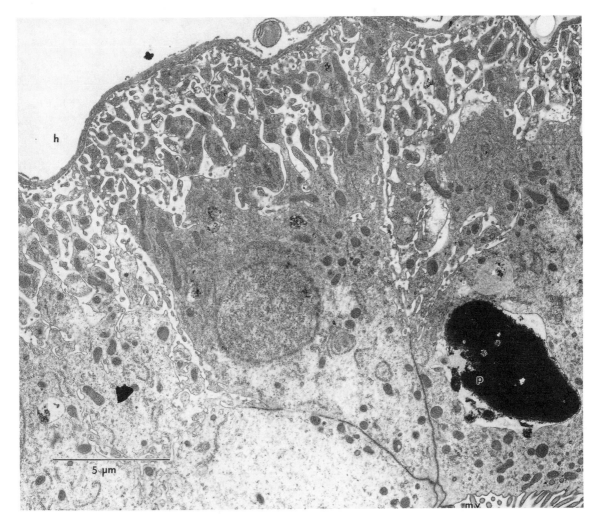

23.7   Encapsulated ookinete within a midgut cell in *Anopheles gambiae*

the tanning of the cuticle and eggshell chorion; there-fore, immune responses based on melanization reactions can determine the use of these molecules for other biological functions. It has been shown in *Ar. subalbatus* exposed to the filarial worm *B. malayi* that a melanotic encapsulation reaction against the parasite significantly delays the development and oviposition of eggs, likely because tyrosine and other molecules are used for defense and are not available for incorporation into developing eggs until destruction of the parasite is completed.

Although nothing presently is known concerning the genetic basis for encapsulation reactions of mosquitoes against filarial worms, the recent development of a saturated genetic linkage map based on restriction fragment length polymorphisms provides the opportunity to use quantitative trait loci mapping to identify those regions of the genome that influence immune responses in resistant mosquitoes (Chap. 26). This will prove invaluable when putative genes involved in resistance are identified, since their loci can be checked for correspondence with the mapped resistance sites.

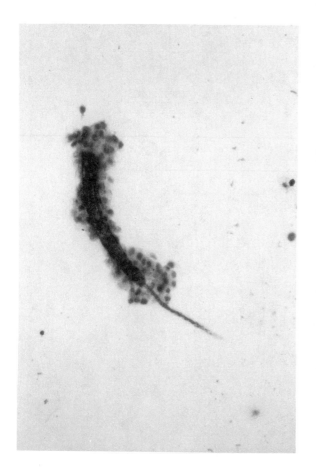

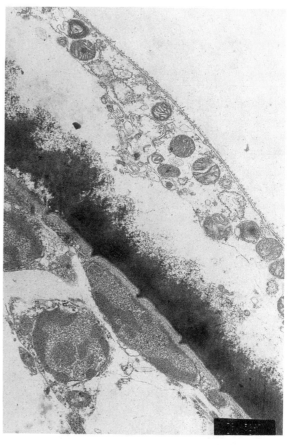

23.8 Microfilaria of *Dirofilaria immitis* sequestered in a classic melanotic encapsulation reaction in *Aedes aegypti*

23.9 Formation of "membranous structure" around encapsulated microfilaria in *Aedes trivittatus*

RECOGNITION

What aspect(s) of the foreign invader is recognized as foreign? And how is the invader recognized? These fundamental questions have not been adequately answered. Investigators have postulated that surface characteristics of pathogens and parasites are likely to be paramount in recognition, although released products might also serve. Surface characteristics would, of course, include carbohydrate, lipid, and protein moieties. Surface charge has also been identified as important, especially in the encapsulation of abiotic particles.

Responses to Abiotic Factors

Many studies have shown that insects are capable of responding to abiotic implants such as nylon fibers, glass beads, dye particles, and plastic. Similar results were found in a study of the mosquito *Ar. subalbatus*, which showed a strong encapsulation and melanization response to positively charged Sephadex beads but less response to negative and neutral beads after implantation into thorax and hemocoel. A 2-tiered system of recognition has been proposed to account for this type of observation. The 1st tier of recognition is based on surface charge and wettability (hydrophobicity); the molecules that are responsible for this response are unknown. The 2nd tier is more specific and is based on molecules that bind to specific surface molecules; this step could occur for biotics that more closely resemble the host in terms of charge and hydrophobicity.

Prophenol Oxidase Activating System

Some researchers have suggested that parts of the prophenol oxidase activating system are involved in immune recognition. The components involved may include small fragments released by serine protease cleavage that serve as opsonins or other unidentified factors. The evidence presented is that fungal laminarin or bacterial endotoxin increases hemocyte phagocytic capacity in a monolayer of *Galleria mellonella* hemocytes and that these microbial products also activate the PO system. Of course, it is possible that these microbial activators have multiple targets in vivo and can cause multiple responses within a cell population in vitro. In other words, laminarin can cause both stimulation of the hemocyte to phagocytose as well as the release of the PO cascade without the 2 being directly connected. Ultimately, purified components of the cascade will be needed to demonstrate the stimulation of phagocytosis.

Hemagglutinins or Lectins

Hemagglutinins are proteins that cause the agglutination of vertebrate red blood cells. This term is often confused with lectins, which are proteins or glycoproteins that specifically bind to carbohydrate moieties. The difference is mainly one of characterization. To identify something as a hemagglutinin, one need only show clumping of red blood cells; bivalent molecules such as immunoglobulins as well as lectins can serve this function. Lectins respond only to carbohydrates. They have been detected in all invertebrate phyla investigated. Many different functions have been suggested for invertebrate lectins, including (1) promoting the ingestion by hemocytes of self tissues on pupation of holometabolous insects, (2) sugar storage and transport, (3) calcium sequestration and transport, and (4) serving as immune recognition factors.

In insects, lectins have been found free in hemolymph, in the midgut, and in cell membranes and have been shown to be produced by the fat body and the hemocytes. Among the insects, lectins have been isolated and/or characterized from the stick insect, *Extatosoma tiaratum;* the grasshopper, *Melanoplus sanguinipes;* the cricket, *Teleogryllus commodus;* the giant silk moth, *H. cecropia;* the silkworm moth *B. mori;* the fall armyworm, *Spodoptera exigua;* the flesh fly, *S. peregrina;* the mosquito *An. gambiae;* and the blow fly, *Calliphora vomitoria.* However, tests of 25 different families of insects revealed only 3 with high titers of serum agglutinins. Often, detectable lectins appeared only after wounding or bacterial inoculation.

As immune molecules, one proposed function of lectins in hemolymph is to act as opsonins, mediating adherence and phagocytosis by hemocytes. Alternatively, the lectins can stimulate hemocytes to degranulate, resulting in coagulation or the release of components of the prophenoloxidase cascade. Lectins can bind to biologically relevant foreign particles, including bacteria, protozoans, and metazoan parasites, lending support to the opsonin hypothesis. In mollusks such a function is well documented; however, there has been conflicting evidence about whether insect lectins function primarily as opsonins. Some researchers have found that particles preincubated in sera with agglutinin activity were not phagocytosed as efficiently as saline-incubated controls, whereas other groups have found clear opsonizing functions in vitro and in vivo for purified lectins.

Sarcophaga lectin is a galactose-binding protein purified from the hemolymph of *S. peregrina* larvae. Normal larvae do not contain this lectin, but it is induced when the body wall is injured with a needle or when foreign substances such as sheep red blood cells are introduced into the body cavity. The gene for this well-characterized lectin has been identified. Its involvement in opsonization is not known, but it is clearly related to wound repair and immune responses.

The attachment of vertebrate erythrocytes to insect hemocytes in vitro in the absence of serum components suggests the presence of membrane receptors, possibly also lectins, involved in the recognition of nonself, or invader. It seems likely that a combination of both free and bound receptors coexist in any one species.

B-1,3, Glucan-Binding Proteins

Carbohydrates from fungal and algal cell walls containing (1-3) linked B-D glucopyranosyl residues (B-1,3,-glucans) induce activation of various defense processes in animals and plants. In arthropods, B-1,3-glucan binding proteins have been isolated from 2 insects, *Blaberus* and *Bombyx*, and a crayfish, and based on their activity these should be considered lectins. In the presence of B-1,3-glucan, these proteins enhance PO activity. In the crayfish, the binding proteins are found in hemocytes and also in the plasma. A receptor for this binding protein also has been purified from hemocytes of the crayfish. The binding protein binds to the B-1,3-glucan on the fungus and also to hemocytes. Hemocytes are then induced to spread and to partially degranulate, releasing components of the PO system.

Binding Proteins for Bacterial Cell Wall Components

Bacterial cell wall components, including peptidoglycan and lipopolysaccharide, have been examined for their ability to stimulate the immune system. Purified peptidoglycan can stimulate the release of antibacterial peptides from the fat body, and it is hypothesized that a receptor for this molecule occurs on the fat body cells. A soluble peptidoglycan-binding protein has been purified from silk moth hemolymph. Lipopolysaccharides of gram-negative bacteria (endotoxin in the free form) possibly stimulate the PO activating system and antibacterial protein synthesis, but this has not been documented in all insects tested. An LPS-binding protein has been purified from the hemolymph of the cockroach, *Periplaneta americana*. This protein recognizes specific oligosaccharides in LPS and is thus a lectin. In the arthropods *Limulus* and *Tachypleus* the interaction of LPS and LPS-binding proteins triggers the degranulation of hemocytes.

As noted above, hemolin is a member of the immunoglobulin superfamily that is expressed at high levels after bacterial inoculation. The Ig family contains 3 major groups, (1) the true immunoglobulins, functioning as antibodies; (2) the lymphocyte surface interaction molecules, including the T lymphocyte markers CD2 and CD8; and (3) the surface adhesion molecules associated with the nervous system (N-CAMs). In *H. cecropia* hemolin binds to bacterial surfaces, where it then forms a complex with 2 other hemolymph proteins. The complex formation, but not the initial hemolin binding, depends on the sugar residues of the bacterial LPS-core and on the presence of divalent cations. Hemolin has also been demonstrated on hemocyte and fat body surfaces in *Hyalophora* and in *M. sexta* binds to both bacterial and hemocyte surfaces, suggesting an opsonizing function. In *Manduca* hemolin inhibits hemocyte aggregation in vitro.

Hemagglutinins in Vectors

Hemagglutinating activity has been identified in several vectors. In *An. gambiae*, *Ar. subalbatus*, *Ae. aegypti*, and *Ae. togoi*, RBCs are agglutinated by hemolymph, and this is inhibited by several sugars. When microfilariae of *Brugia pahangi* and *B. malayi* are inoculated simultaneously with sugar inhibitors into the mosquito *Ar. subalbatus*, melanin deposition on the surface of the microfilariae is reduced. The effect of another parasitic nematode, *Onchocerca lienalis*, on the hemolymph of *Simulium ornatum* has been examined. Infected hemolymph was incubated with fresh *O. lienalis* or *B. pahangi*, and the motility of the worms found to be significantly attenuated. Hemolymph from *O. lienalis*–infected black flies also significantly increases the rates of agglutination of cat erythrocytes. Midgut trypanoagglutinins also have been identified in *Gl. palpalis palpalis* and *G. p. gambiensis*. The agglutinins were active only in the posterior midguts. Lectin secreted into the midgut lumen normally prevents the establishment of trypanosome infection but induces established midgut trypanosomes to mature. A 2nd lectin in the hemolymph is essential to complete the maturation process. Gut lectins in *Rhodnius prolixus* are also important to the establishment of *T. cruzi* in this insect.

EVASION OR SUPPRESSION OF THE IMMUNE SYSTEM

A wide variety of biotic agents can avoid the immune systems in their vectors, including nematodes, protozoa, bacteria, rickettsia, spirochetes, and viruses. Parasites and pathogens use a variety of methods to withstand the immune system. In vertebrates, *Yersinia pestis*, the agent of plague, grows an impenetrable coat of membrane proteins that neither complement nor cell-mediated responses can break through. No similar examples exist yet for vector-parasites; however, a 2nd strategy, immunosuppression, possibly operates in both vectors and vertebrates. Immunosuppressing parasites disable the host's immune system. For example, several parasites produce proteins that inhibit key elements of the complement system. Some mermithid nematode-infected locusts are killed from massive flagellate infections, but in locusts not infected with nematodes, flagellate numbers are controlled, suggesting that suppression occurs. Similar mechanisms can operate in vector-parasite relationships. For example, encapsulation of xenografts (tissue from another species) was reduced in *Triatoma* spp. when *Trypanosoma cruzi* was present. Because *T. cruzi* develops in the gut rather than the hemolymph, the significance of these observations is not clear. A 2nd example concerns *Bacillus thuringiensis*, which has been shown to produce antibacterial immune inhibitors that act by proteolytic cleavage of cecropins and attacins. Similarly, a fascinating symbiotic relationship has been observed. A bacterium, *Xenorhabditis nematophilus*, lives in symbiosis with a nematode and helps the nematode to kill insects. The nematode in turn helps the bacteria by making a proteolytic enzyme that selectively degrades the cecropins and the attacins. Because nonproteolytic, native inhibitors of serine proteases and phenoloxidases occur in the hemolymph of some insects, similar compounds could be produced by parasites.

Many other pathogens must evade detection. Parasites can distract or mimic. Distraction is exemplified by trypanosomes in humans, which have evolved a method to change surface antigens. As the immune system targets one antigen, the parasite has switched to a new one. This strategy is probably not found in insects that do not live long; however, parasites can also evade detection by mimicking host molecules. One example of mimicry in a vertebrate system concerns the alternative pathway of the complement system. In this pathway, a molecular fragment of the pathogen alone without a labeling antibody combines with a series of complement proteins to activate the

critical component, C5. To prevent activation by normal host proteins, a layer of carbohydrate molecules (sialic acid) coats most mammalian cells, which won't turn on complement. Several bacteria, such as the K1 strain of *E. coli*, cover themselves with long polymers of sialic acid and avoid the alternate pathway. An interesting example of molecular mimicry in insects concerns a parasitoid wasp using the caterpillar *Ephestia kuhniella* as host. These wasps inject viral particles along with their eggs, and the virus is capable of producing a hemolin-like protein. Because hemolin prevents hemocyte aggregation and could be a recognition molecule, the viral protein helps prevent encapsulation of the parasitoid eggs. Another example concerns filarial nematodes in aedine mosquitoes. The filarial nematode *B. pahangi* will not develop in *Ae. trivittatus* unless previously allowed to penetrate the midgut of a susceptible strain of *Ae. aegypti*. The parasite loses its high electronegative surface charge as it migrates through the gut, which can account for the reduced immune response, but it is unknown how this occurs. Several other examples also exist that suggest molecules related to those of the basal lamina cover a parasite, preventing recognition.

Alternatively, the pathogen can attempt to hide its identifying molecules altogether so that they do not interact with the immune system. This strategy is exhibited by intracellular parasites such as *Rickettsia* and malaria parasites in vertebrates and in *Salmonella*, which survives in macrophages despite the presence of defensins. In vectors, hemocytes can actually serve as host cells for some of the parasites/pathogens that develop in insects. For example, the spotted fever agent *R. rickettsii* multiplies within hemocytes of the vector tick *Dermacentor andersoni*, and *T. rangeli* lives in hemocytes of *Rhodnius prolixus*. The intracellular site of development for filarioid nematodes in mosquito vectors likely plays a role in removing them from contact with and recognition by circulating hemocytes.

FUTURE STUDIES

Recognition

Progress has been made in determining both the surface components of some organisms (fungi; B-1,3, glucans; bacteria; LPS; and peptidoglycan) that stimulate an immune response as well as the binding proteins that interact with them. Much less is known about how viral, nematode, or protozoan pathogens are recognized. Lectins seem to play an important role in parasite/vector interactions, but the extent of that role is not yet clearly defined.

Effector Systems

Once a pathogen is recognized as foreign, several coordinated systems can be activated to deal with the threat. These systems include the production of toxic compounds such as antibacterials as well as the mobilization of hemocytes to phagocytose, or enclosing in nodules or capsules. The biochemical components of the antibacterial and the melanin production pathways are being identified and characterized. However, many groups of vectors have not been examined yet, and some of these, especially the acarines, likely will respond to parasites with different biochemicals or with different emphases on the systems described. Additionally, the coordination of humoral and cellular responses has been shown in many insects. For example, microbial products can stimulate phagocytosis and nodule formation as well as the production of antibacterials and the PO cascade. Identification of the genes for many antibacterial proteins has provided the first glimpses of regulation of these coordinate responses, but much remains to be learned.

Signal Transduction

Both phagocytosis and encapsulation as well as the production of antibacterials by the fat body must rely on signal transduction. There are a variety of such processes that take place within plasma membranes, including: activation of ion channels; activation of adenylate cyclase; activation of phospholipase C, causing production of diacylglycerol and inositol phosphate; and activation of phospholipase A2, resulting in formation of prostaglandins and leukotrienes. Finally, protein phosphorylation by kinases represents the most common transduction pathway. Protein kinase can be activated by calcium, by cyclic AMP, by diacylglycerol, or by calcium-calmodulin–dependent processes. Receptors can contain both a recognition site and a transducer (e.g., a tyrosine kinase) located in different domains of the molecule. However, in many instances, receptors and effectors communicate by another class of proteins (G proteins), which act as switches connecting receptors to their intracellular effectors. With the identification of specific microbial binding proteins and their cellular receptors in insects and crayfish, work can proceed on understanding signal transduction in this context.

Cell-to-Cell Communication

Processes such as encapsulation and nodule formation require communication between the cells involved. Few studies in this area exist; however, a study of *M. sexta* suggested that eicosanoids might be important in cellular responses to bacteria. Eicosanoids are formed from C_{20} polyunsaturated fatty acids by the action of phospholipase A2 on membranes. Once generated, the fatty acids can be oxygenated in 2 ways. Products of both pathways are important in mammalian inflammatory responses. For example, cyclooxygenase pathway products affect macrophage locomotion, shape changes, and phagocytosis; lipoxygenase pathway products mediate chemotaxis, chemokinesis, and adherence responses of neutrophils. When eicosanoid synthesis is inhibited by injection of inhibitors into *Manduca*, bacterial clearance is also reduced; however, the effects of eicosanoid synthesis can be myriad, and the exact effects in vivo are unknown. It is possible that a general stress response has reduced the ability of these insects to respond to bacteria.

Cytokines are polypeptide mediators released by cells involved in vertebrate host defenses that are used to communicate with similar or different cells. Interleukin 1 (IL-1) and tumor necrosis factor are major immunoregulatory cytokines with many host defense–related properties. These molecules have been isolated and characterized from several invertebrate phyla by demonstrating biological activity in vertebrate bioassays. In some systems, IL-1 actually stimulates hemocyte phagocytosis and proliferation. Nothing is known yet about these polypeptides in insect immune responses.

Interactions with Other Systems

The cells and molecules constituting the immune system of insects can participate in other physiological processes as well. For example, during metamorphosis, new cuticle is created that requires the activity of phenol oxidase and DOPA decarboxylase for melanization and probably sclerotization. Additionally, special antibacterial substances are produced during this time; one type of cecropin, Cec C, is found only during metamorphosis. Hemocytes are also important in the identification of cells to be removed and replaced at metamorphosis.

In other systems there is overlap as well. For example, some of the catecholamines that are important melanin building blocks can also serve as neurotransmitters (especially dopamine). In mosquitoes, both phenoloxidase and DOPA decarboxylase activities increase after a blood meal. This is thought to be necessary for eggshell tanning because levels of DDC increase in the ovaries. The response of insects to wounding is also closely related to the immune system, and coagulation and melanization at the wound site are important protective measures.

The high degree of dual functionality reported from immune system components implies a high degree of differential regulation in response to different needs. Distinguishing between the genetic and biochemical methods by which regulation is accomplished has only begun for lysozyme and DDC in *Drosophila*. Much additional work remains to be done.

REFERENCES AND FURTHER READING

Ashida, M., and H.I. Yamazaki. 1990. Biochemistry of the phenoloxidase system in insects: With special reference to its activation. In: E. Ohnishi and H. Ishizaki, editors, *Molting and metamorphosis*. Berlin: Springer-Verlag. pp. 239–265.

Barracco, M.A., and C.T. Loch. 1989. Ultrastructural studies of the hemocytes of *Panstrongylus megistus* (Hemiptera: Reduviidae). *Memorias do instituto Oswaldo Cruz* 84:171–188.

Bayne, C.J. 1990. Phagocytosis and non-self recognition in invertebrates. *BioScience* 40:723–731.

Bhat, U.K.M., and K.R.P. Singh. 1975. The haemocytes of the mosquito *Aedes albopictus* and their comparison with larval cells cultured in vitro. *Experientia* 31:1331–1332.

Boman, H.G. 1986. Antibacterial immune proteins in insects. *Symp. Zool. Soc. Lond.* 56:45–58.

Boman, H.G., I. Faye, G. Gudmundsson, J.Y. Lee, and D.A. Lidholm. 1991. Cell-free immunity in *Cecropia*. A model system for antibacterial proteins. *Eur. J. Biochem.* 201:23–31.

Brunet, P.C.J. 1980. The metabolism of the aromatic amino acids concerned in the cross-linking of insect cuticle. *Insect Biochem.* 10:467–500.

Christensen, B.M. 1986. Immune mechanisms and mosquito-filarial worm relationships. *Symp. Zool. Soc. Lond.* 56:145–160.

Christensen, B.M., and D.W. Severson. 1993. Biochemical and molecular basis of mosquito susceptibility to *Plasmodium* and filarioid nematodes. In: N.E. Beckage, S.N. Thompson, and B.A. Federici, editors, *Parasites and pathogens of insects*. New York: Academic Press. pp. 245–266.

Christensen, B.M., and J.W. Tracy. 1989. Arthropod-transmitted parasites: Mechanisms of immune interaction. *Amer. Zool.* 29:387–398.

Drif, L., and M. Brehelin. 1983. The circulating hemocytes of *Culex pipiens* and *Aedes aegypti*: Cytology, histochemistry, hemograms and functions. *Devel. Comp. Immunol.* 7:687–690.

Drif, L., and M. Brehelin. 1993. Structure, classification and functions of insect haemocytes. In: J.P.N. Pathak, editor, *Insect immunity*. New Delhi: Oxford and IBH Publishing Co. pp. 1–14.

Dunn, P.E. 1986. Biochemical aspects of insect immunology. *Ann. Rev. Entomol.* 31:321–339.

Dunn, P.E. 1990. Humoral immunity in insects. *BioScience* 40:738–744.

Foley, D.A. 1978. Innate cellular defense by mosquito hemocytes. *Comp. Pathbiol.* 4:113–144.

Gotz, P. 1986. Mechanisms of encapsulation in dipteran hosts. *Symp. Zool. Soc. Lond.* 56:1–19.

Ham, P.J. 1992. Immunity in haematophagous insect vectors of parasitic infection. *Adv. Dis. Vector Res.* 9:101–149.

Hultmark, D. 1993. Immune reactions in *Drosophila* and other insects: A model for innate immunity. *Trends Gen.* 9:178–183.

Jones, J.C. 1967a. Effect of repeated haemolymph withdrawals and of ligaturing the head on differential counts of *Rhodnius prolixus* Stal. *J. Insect Physiol.* 13:1351–1360.

Jones, J.C. 1967b. Normal differential counts of haemocytes in relation to ecdysis and feeding in *Rhodnius prolixus*. Stal. *J. Insect Physiol.* 13:1133–1141.

Kaaya, G.P., and N.A. Ratcliffe. 1982. Comparative study of haemocytes and associated cells of some medically important dipterans. *J. Morphol.* 173:361–365.

Karp, R.D. 1990. Cell mediated immunity in invertebrates. *BioScience* 40:732–737.

Lackie, A.M. 1986. Evasion of insect immunity by helminth larvae. *Symp. Zool. Soc. Lond.* 56:161–178.

Lackie, A.M. 1988. Immune mechanisms in insects. *Parasit. Today* 4:98–105.

Luckhart, S., M.S. Cupp, and E.W. Cupp. 1992. Morphological and functional classification of the hemocytes of adult female *Simulium vittatum* (Diptera: Simuliidae). *J. Med. Ent.* 29:457–466.

Molyneux, D.H., G. Takle, E.A. Ibrahim, and G.A. Ingram. 1986. Insect immunity to Trypanosomatidae. *Symp. Zool. Soc. Lond.* 56:117–144.

Ratcliffe, N.A. 1986. Insect cellular immunity and the recognition of foreignness. *Symp. Zool. Soc. Lond.* 56:21–43.

Ratcliffe, N.A., and A.F. Rowley. 1979. Role of hemocytes in defense against biological agents. In: A.P. Gupta, editor, *Insect haemocytes.* Cambridge: Cambridge University Press. pp. 331–414.

Renwrantz, L. 1986. Lectins in molluscs and arthropods: their occurrence, origin and roles in immunity. *Symp. Zool. Soc. Lond.* 56:81–93.

Soderhall, K., and A. Aspan. 1993. Prophenoloxidase activating system and its role in cellular communication. In: J.P.N. Pathak, editor, *Insect immunity.* New Delhi: Oxford and IBH Publishing Co. pp. 113–129.

Sonenshine, D.E. 1991. *Biology of Ticks.* New York: Oxford University Press. 447 p.

Sugumaran, M. 1991. Molecular mechanisms for mammalian melanogenesis: Comparison with insect cuticular sclerotization. *FEBS* 293:4–10.

Vey, A. 1993. Humoral encapsulation. In: J.P.N. Pathak, editor, *Insect Immunity.* New Delhi: Oxford and IBH Publishing Co. pp. 59–67.

Wright, T.R.F. 1987. The genetics of biogenic amine metabolism, sclerotization, and melanization in *Drosophila melanogaster. Adv. Gen.* 24:127–221.

24. POPULATION BIOLOGY AS A TOOL FOR STUDYING VECTOR-BORNE DISEASES

William C. Black IV and Chester G. Moore

INTRODUCTION

To predict the course of an epidemic or, better yet, to predict its arrival, we must thoroughly understand the dynamics of disease transmission. In this chapter we describe the various biological components of vector populations that affect the rate of transmission of arthropod-borne diseases. The biotic factors discussed are chiefly birthrate, death rate, density, and age distribution. Migration rates, spatial distributions, and various genetic properties of populations also affect disease transmission and are discussed in Chapters 2 and 25.

Most basic treatments of population biology explore each biotic component individually. Excellent references that adopt this approach are Anderson and May (1982) and Bailey (1982). We explore instead many biotic factors simultaneously in the context of disease transmission models. These models are useful didactic tools that not only aid in learning about individual biotic components and how they interact but, in addition, illustrate their relative importance in the dynamics of disease transmission. These models are also important in designing optimal strategies for vector population suppression. The chapter ends with a discussion of the ways in which the biotic components of these models are actually estimated in field

populations using old "tried and true" methods as well as some new molecular methods.

SIMPLE MODELS OF DISEASE TRANSMISSION

We generally rely on mathematical models to describe the series of events in disease transmission because of the large number of factors involved and the ease of notation. However, a mathematical model is simply a shorthand statement of what we know and how we think various components are related to each other. Epidemiologists and other health professionals have tried to formulate mathematical models of disease transmission since the early part of the 20th century. It is interesting to note that the early models are very much like those we use today. It is the data that we fit into the models that have changed; we now know in many cases that what was thought to be a simple constant can be a variable composed of several interacting components. Let's examine briefly what we know (or think we know) about the transmission of a simple contagious disease.

The Reed-Frost Equation

For any communicable disease, there is a probability that contact between an infected and an uninfected susceptible individual during a specified time period will result in transmission of the disease organism. For some diseases, the probability is high (e.g., influenza), whereas for others it is low (e.g., leprosy) or requires special forms of contact (e.g., AIDS, gonorrhea, kuru). This value is called the probability of effective contact. We represent this value by P. The probability that any 2 individuals will *not* have effective contact is then $1 - P$.

At any time during an epidemic there are "cases," individuals who may or may not be ill but are infected with the disease organism and capable of transmission. Let's call the number of cases at some time t, C_t. Thus the probability that a given susceptible individual *does not* have contact with any of the cases in 1 time period is:

$$(1 - P)^{C_t} \qquad (1)$$

By similar reasoning, the probability that a given susceptible *does* have contact with *at least 1* of the cases during 1 time period is:

$$(1 - (1 - P)^{C_t}) \qquad (2)$$

If we know the number of susceptible individuals (let's denote them by S) at time t, then we can estimate the total number of cases that we expect to occur at time $t+1$ due to contacts with cases during time t. That value is given by:

$$C_{t+1} = S_t(1 - (1 - P)^{C_t}) \qquad (3)$$

Equation (3) is called the Reed-Frost equation. It is a recurrence equation, meaning that it describes what happens in 1 time period as a function of what has happened in the previous period. Note that all that we have done is to devise a shorthand statement of what was described in a somewhat "long-winded" fashion in the last few paragraphs. Cases at some future time depend on current susceptibles, current cases, and the likelihood they will come into "effective" contact.

Next let's look at how the equation works through a simple simulation and sees what it tells us. Assume that the probability of effective contact for a disease is 0.3. Assume also that the size of the susceptible population

at time $t = 0$ is 10. At this time a single case enters the population. Other than this initial case, the population is closed. There are no births, no deaths, and no immigration. Plugging these values into equation (3), the number of cases at time $t = 1$ is:

$$C_1 = 10 \, (1 - (1 - 0.3)^1) = 3$$

There are now 3 cases. The diseased individual contacts everyone in the population but only 3 become infected. If we want to continue this simulation through more time periods, we next must decide what to do with diseased individuals. If this is a fatal disease, we can simply drop them from the population. If this is a persistent infectious disease (e.g., schistosomiasis, giardiasis), the number of cases are cumulative and the number of diseased individuals in time $t = 1$ is 4 (the index case + 3 new cases). A 3rd possibility is that the diseased individuals in a time period are infectious within that time period and then become immune. We will make this last assumption because it best serves to illustrate components of the model; however, exploring the results of this model under the 2 earlier assumptions is instructive. The outcomes are very different.

Note that with an assumption of no mortality and acquired immunity the population remains closed; people don't leave even through death. Note also that we have created a 3rd category of people: immunes. These don't enter the model but leave the population of susceptibles. At time $t = 2$:

$$C_2 = 7 \, (1 - (1 - 0.3)^3) = 4.6.$$

We can repeat this process (this is called iteration) over 10 time periods to follow the course of the disease (Fig. 24.1). One case enters a population of 10 susceptibles and infects 3 people. Eventually all individuals are infected (i.e., become cases) and recover to become immune. The number of cases declines because all susceptibles are "used up." At the end of the simulation there are 11 immunes and no susceptibles. Everyone lives happily ever after.

Now let's see what the model can teach us about the probability of effective contact. Figure 24.2 (panels A, B, and C) shows us the progress of the disease in our

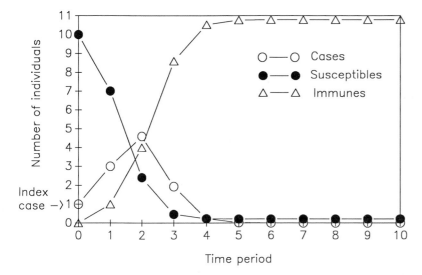

24.1 Iteration of the Reed-Frost model, equation (3), over 10 time periods. There is 1 index case that enters a closed population of 10 susceptible individuals at time $t = 0$. The probability of effective contact (P) is 0.3.

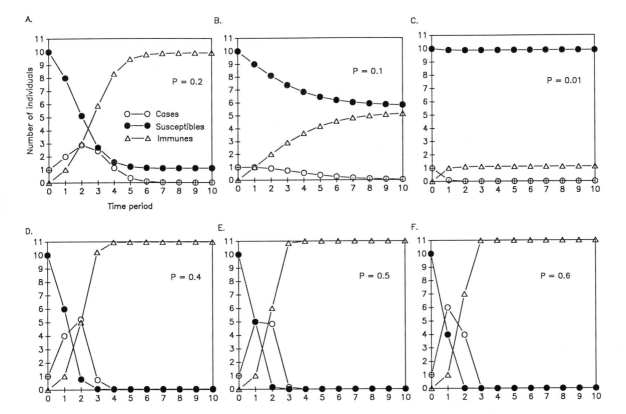

24.2 Iteration of the Reed-Frost model, equation (3), over 10 time periods with different probabilities of effective contact (P). (A) P = 0.2, (B) P = 0.1, (C) P = 0.01, (D) P = 0.4, (E) P = 0.5, (F) P = 0.6. Otherwise conditions are as in Figure 24.1.

closed population for decreasing values of $P = 0.2, 0.1,$ 0.01. As P decreases, the time required for transmission increases. The distribution of cases shifts to the right because it takes longer for transmission to occur. However, at $P = 0.1$, transmission levels off with 6 susceptibles and 5 immunes. No further transmission can occur. At $P = 0.01$, the probability of a case transmitting the disease to a susceptible is 1 in 100. There are only 10 susceptibles in the population, and no transmission occurs. The case enters and becomes immune without infecting anyone. Figure 24.2 (panels D, E, and F) shows progress of the disease for increasing values of $P = 0.4, 0.5, 0.6$. As P increases, the time required for transmission decreases. The distribution of cases shifts to the left because it takes less time for transmission to occur.

Interactions among recurrence equations can provide many interesting, nonlinear trends in the long-term progress of disease. We could "open" this population by allowing susceptibles to enter through immigration or birth. Furthermore, we could allow people to leave the population through mortality or emigration. Figure 24.3 shows iterations of the Reed-Frost model with a $P = 0.3$ through 50 time periods when the population receives 1 new susceptible every 2 time periods through immigration and 1 in every 10 cases leave the population by dying from the disease. Now we see

oscillations in numbers of susceptibles, cases, and immunes. The trends in the initial time periods are as in Figure 24.1. However, note that the number of susceptibles now begins to rise again from immigration, and the number declines as transmission occurs. The number of immunes rises, levels off, and then increases again. Immunes initially level off because transmission temporarily ceases; the number of susceptibles is not large enough for transmission to occur. Oscillations in susceptibles and cases eventually stabilize because the rate of transmission becomes constant. Increases in the susceptible population are offset by decreases caused by disease (i.e., they enter the immune population). Once the susceptible population reaches equilibrium, the number of cases becomes constant.

Vectorial Capacity

The Reed-Frost equation can be used, with slight modification, to describe the dynamics of vector-borne diseases (Fine 1981). The only place the disease vector affects equation (3) is in the "effective contact" component. The probability of effective contact depends on the average number of *potentially infective* bites per individual in the host population. Following Fine (1981), we call that quantity V/T where V is the total number of infective bites and T is the total size of the human population. Then equation (3) becomes:

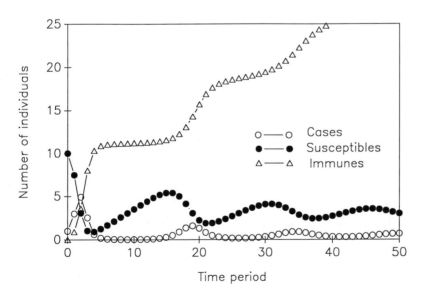

24.3 Iteration of the Reed-Frost model, equation (3), over 50 time periods. Conditions are as in Figure 24.1 except that the population is no longer closed. Susceptible individuals enter through immigration and some diseased individuals leave by dying.

$$C_{t+1} = S_t(1 - (1 - V/T)^{Ct}) \qquad (4)$$

We can derive a simpler formulation for the Reed-Frost equation because V/T is usually very small. For example, for arboviruses such as western equine encephalitis (WEE), eastern equine encephalitis (EEE), and Saint Louis encephalitis (SLE), V/T is probably in the range of 0.0001–0.00001, whereas for dengue it is probably between 0.01 and 0.001. Because

$$e^{-x} = 1 - x + (x^2/2) - (x^3/3) + \ldots .$$

where e is the base of the natural system of logarithms, we can write $e^{-x} = 1 - x$ if x^2 is small compared to x. If $(V/T)^2$ is small compared to (V/T), then equation (4) can be approximated as:

$$C_{t+1} = S_t(1 - e^{-(V/T)Ct}) \qquad (5)$$

This is a common form of the Reed-Frost equation used for examining the epidemiology of vector-borne diseases.

Estimating Vectorial Capacity

The value V is called the vectorial capacity. It is defined as the average number of potentially infective bites that will ultimately be delivered by all the vectors feeding on a single host in 1 day (Fine 1981). Equation (5) is the fundamental theorem of vector-borne disease dynamics. It draws together all we know (or think we know) about the vector-host-pathogen relationship and expresses it in a single value, the number of infective bites. Equation (5) is deceptively simple. When we start examining each of the component parts of V we find more layers—like peeling an onion. Equation (5) suddenly becomes highly complex.

Basically, V is the product of 3 components: feeding, survival rate, and length of the extrinsic incubation period (EIP) (Chap. 4) and is represented by:

$V =$
[Number of vectors feeding on the host per unit time] ×
[Probability the vector survives the EIP] ×
[Number of blood meals on people after EIP] (6)

The EIP is the period of time from ingestion of an infectious blood meal to the time of pathogen transmission capability.

Let's now take each of the 3 main segments and expand them until we find things we can actually measure in the laboratory or in the field. The measurable values are denoted below in italics.

Vector Density on Hosts

The number of vectors feeding is the product of several factors:

[Number of vectors feeding on the host per unit time] =
[Vector density in relation to the host (m)] ×
[Probability a vector feeds on a host in 1 day (a)] (7)

In turn:

a = [Feeding frequency] ×
[Proportion of meals on this species (Host index)] (8)

Probability of Surviving the EIP

This is simply the probability of surviving 1 day raised to the power of the length of extrinsic incubation.

[Probability the vector survives EIP] =
[probability of living 1 day (p)]^{[length of EIP in days (n)]} = p^n (9)

Number of Blood Meals Taken After EIP

This is the product of the feeding probability (see a, equation 8) and the expected duration of the vector's life.

[Number of blood meals on people after EIP] =
[Duration of vector's life after surviving EIP [1/–ln(p)]] ×
[Probability a vector feeds on a host in 1 day (a)]. (10)

Macdonald's Equation

Now that we have exposed the layers to find things we can measure, we use our notational shorthand to put everything into perspective. Vectorial capacity consists of the following more-or-less readily measurable quantities.

$$V = [ma] \times [p^n] \times [(a /-\ln(p)] \qquad (11)$$

The equation is still a little clumsy, and we usually combine the 2 *a* values and rearrange the equation as follows

$$V = \frac{m \times a^2 \times p^n}{-\ln p} \qquad (12)$$

A final quantity, *b*, is often incorporated into the equation. This is a measure of the proportion of vectors taking a meal from an infected host that actually become infective. It is a measure of the genetic and physiological "competence" of the vector. Vector competence was reviewed in Chapter 2. The full equation for *V* is:

$$V = \frac{m \times a^2 \times p^n \times b}{-\ln p} \qquad (13)$$

where: m = vector density in relation to the host
   a = probability a vector feeds on a host in 1 day (= host preference index × feeding frequency)
   b = vector competence, the proportion of vectors ingesting an infective meal that successfully become infective
   p = probability of vector surviving through 1 day
   n = duration of extrinsic incubation period (in days)
   $1/(-\ln p)$ = duration of vector's life in days, after surviving extrinsic incubation period

This equation arose from Garrett-Jones's (1964a) modification of Macdonald's original equation (Macdonald 1957) for case reproduction number. Macdonald pioneered the use of the model to study the dynamics of malaria transmission in Africa.

Table 24.1 explores how each component of the model affects vectorial capacity. The results demonstrate that of the many variables defined above, there are 3 that most strongly affect the magnitude of *V*. These are *a*, *n*, and *p*. Small changes in any 1 of these variables will cause large changes in *V*. *a* is important because it is squared; *n* is important because it is an exponent of *p*. But *V* is most sensitive to small changes in *p*. This latter point led Macdonald to predict that adulticides rather than larvicides would be most effective in reducing malaria transmission rates.

Vectorial Capacity of Populations Is Dynamic

Up to this point we have treated many of the biotic components of our models as static parameters; however, we need only consider the 1st component of Macdonald's equation, *m* (vector density in relation to the host), to sense the fallacy in this approach. It is well known that vector populations undergo large periodic fluctuations in size. We also know that daily survivorship and the age composition of vector populations change both geographically and seasonally. The vectorial capacity of populations is therefore a dynamic, fluctuating process that can only be estimated in the context of a particular population at a particular point in time. We need to understand the dynamics of vector density and age composition to completely appreciate the complexity of disease transmission.

Fluctuations in Vector Population Densities

Vector populations constantly fluctuate in density. The timing of these fluctuations is referred to as the seasonal phenology of a population. Density shifts can be a result of regular seasonal climatic changes in temperature, moisture, resources, or the emergence of new broods of adults. They also might arise through intraspecific and interspecific competition or predation by other species. Changes in density are important in disease epidemiology because, as we learned from Macdonald's equation, the vector-to-host ratio is a determinant of the vectorial capacity of a population.

There are 2 general elementary models for population growth: the exponential growth and logistic growth models. In the exponential growth model

$$N_{t+1} = N_t + rN_t = N_t + N_t(b_0 - d_0) \qquad (14)$$

where: N_t = number of vectors in a population at time t
   r = intrinsic rate of increase

TABLE 24.1 Changes in vector capacity (*V*) in Macdonald's equation as a function of changes in vector-to-host ratio (*m*), host preference index, days between blood meals, infected vectors that become infective (*b*), daily survivorship (*p*), and extrinsic incubation period (*n*)

	Original value	Original value + 10%	V	%ΔV	Original value − 10%	V	%ΔV
1. Vector:Host Ratio (*m*)	1000	1100	0.646	**10**	900	0.529	**−10**
2. Probability that a vector feeds on a host in one day (*a*)	0.25	(0.227–0.275)			(0.225–0.278)		
2a. Host preference index	(0.50)	0.55	0.711	**21**	0.45	0.476	**−19**
2b. Days between blood meals	(2.00)	2.20	0.485	**−17**	1.80	0.725	**23**
4. Proportion of vectors ingesting an infective blood meal that successfully become infective (*b*)	0.01	0.011	0.646	**10**	0.009	0.529	**−10**
5. Daily survivorship (*p*)	0.80	0.88	1.998	**240**	0.72	0.191	**−68**
Vector's life (in days) after surviving through the EIP	4.5	7.8			3.0		
6. EIP (*n*)	7.00	7.70	0.502	**−14**	6.30	0.687	**17**
Vector capacity (*V*)	0.587						

Note: Numbers in bold indicate the percent change in *V* for a 10% change in the independent variable. Changes in *V* are linear and directly proportional to changes in *m* and *b*. A 10% increase or decrease in these parameters causes a corresponding 10% increase or decrease in *V*. *V* changes in a nonlinear fashion relative to changes in host preference index, days between blood meals, and daily survivorship.

b_0 = individual birthrate, the number of off-spring 1 individual will give birth to on average per unit of time when the population is small

d_0 = individual death rate, the average number of deaths per individual per unit of time when the population is small.

This recurrence equation says simply that the change in population size at any point in time will be a function of the size of the population at the previous point in time multiplied by the difference between the rate that new individuals are born into the population and the rate that they leave the population through death. In "good" environments $b_0 > d_0$, $r \gg 0$, and the population grows, but in "bad" environments $d_0 > b_0$, $r \ll 0$

and the population declines. A model of exponential growth over 10 time periods (11 measurements) with r = 2.7 and starting from a single individual is shown in Figure 24.4. An r of 2.7 means that on average an individual produces 2.7 offspring per generation. This model explains the growth of a population over a short period of time and when a population is small; however, it is easy to see that a population would become infinitely large over a short period of time if this model was continued. The exponential equation therefore has limited utility in modelling changes in vector density over time.

It is more likely that populations will either go extinct because of resource depletion or that the population will reach some point at which it no longer grows because the death rate and birthrate have

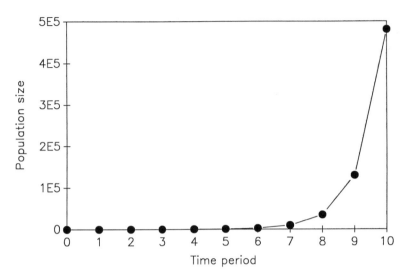

24.4 Plot of the exponential growth model, equation (14). The intrinsic rate of increase *(r)* was 2.7.

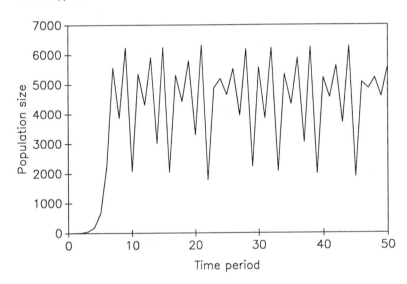

24.5 Plot of the logistic growth model, equation (15), Carrying capacity *(K)* was set to 5000. The intrinsic rate of increase *(r)* was 2.7.

begins, reproduces, and after a few generations the population begins to grow exponentially as described in equation (14). However, over time, resources become limited and the rate of growth slows down. Some time later, resources are insufficient to maintain growth, and births are offset by deaths; thus the population maintains itself in equilibrium. The density at which $N_{t+1} = N_t$ is called the carrying capacity of the environment. This scenario is modeled by the following equation:

$$N_{t+1} = N_t + r((K - N_t)/K)N_t \quad (15)$$

where K is the carrying capacity of the environment. This is called the logistic growth model and is shown in Figure 24.5 over 50 time periods with $r = 2.7$, $K = 5000$, and starting from a single individual. When N is low, $((K - N)/K)$ approximates 1, and equation (15) approximates equation (14). As N increases, $((K - N)/K)$ becomes less than 1, and the rate of population growth slows. As N approaches K, $((K - N)/K)$ approaches 0, and $N_{t+1} = N_t$. If the population exceeds K from a temporary increase in births or resources, then $((K - N)/K)$ becomes negative and the population declines to K. It is important not to think of K as a constant but rather to realize that K fluctuates around some mean value over time. Fluctuations in K can be regular because of seasonal changes in resource abundance (e.g., oviposition sites for mosquitoes during dry and wet seasons) or can be random and erratic when species are dependent on resources that are scarce in either time or space (e.g., head lice on schoolchildren).

become equal. A scenario commonly envisioned by population biologists is of a single pair of individuals or a single inseminated female arriving into a new region with abundant resources and few limitations to growth. Following oviposition a new generation

This seems to be a more realistic model of population growth than unlimited exponential growth. The extent to which births and deaths of a population are conditioned by its density is referred to as density dependence. The role of density dependence in natural populations is controversial. Some population biologists feel that species seldom reach the carrying capacity of the environment and that other factors, such as predation, interspecific competition, and disease intervene to regulate population size at values well below *K*. One clear example of a habitat where density dependence *can* be operational is in the artificial container habitat of some mosquitoes. Crowded larval habitats are often found in the field and produce smaller adult mosquitoes. Analysis of interspecific and intraspecific competition in vectors, especially in dipteran insect vectors, is an active area of research. The role of pathogens and predators in the regulation of vector population densities is the subject of Chapters 31 and 32.

There is also a wide variety of density-independent processes that influence population growth. These include environmental factors such as food availability, adverse weather, and extremes in temperature and relative humidity. Random factors include catastrophic reductions in populations through habitat destruction, large-scale meteorological disturbances (e.g., droughts and floods), and massive eradication programs.

Because of the many factors that influence density, seasonal changes in phenology are currently impossible to predict with even the most sophisticated models. This stands as one of the most challenging areas in developing predictive models of vector-borne diseases. There are many models of density-dependent and independent growth that are far beyond the scope of this chapter. Bellows (1981), Carey (1993), Charlesworth (1980), and Goodenough and McKinion (1992) provide detailed information on models and modeling. The review by Dye (1992) provides useful guidance for avoiding certain pitfalls in modelling vector-borne diseases.

Fluctuations in Age Structure

A seasonal change in density is only 1 factor that causes fluctuations in vectorial capacity. Fluctuations in the average age of individuals in a vector population are also important. The relative proportion of each age class in a population is referred to as the age structure of that population. Population biologists have shown that for many vector species, the proportions of a population consisting of eggs, immatures, and adults vary by time and location. Age structure is an important epidemiological factor because, as seen in our testing of Macdonald's equation, only older adults that have passed through the extrinsic incubation period are infective.

To follow or predict the age structure of a population, we begin by collecting information on the daily survivorship and fecundity of a species. To get a general idea about the pattern of survivorship in a cohort or generation of offspring, we could make a frequency histogram of the age at which individuals in a cohort die. This type of graph is called a survivorship curve. There are 3 basic types of such curves (Fig. 24.6): Type I curves occur in species in which most deaths occur at an age of senescence. This is the survivorship curve of humans in developed countries and is the survivorship curve for most of our domesticated plants and animals. Most of us live to an old age and then die. Domestic animals and plants grow to a certain age and are harvested or culled. In Type II curves, the probability of daily survivorship remains constant throughout life. A constant fraction of offspring is removed in each time period by predators, accidents, or other natural sources of mortality. For example, if the probability of daily survivorship is 0.9, then the probability that an individual survives through 2 days is $0.9 \times 0.9 = 0.81$, through 3 days is 0.73, and through 7 days is 0.48. This is the type of mortality that is most frequently seen or assumed among vector populations. Type III curves describe a pattern frequently found in species in the field. There is a high initial mortality among offspring (spores, seedlings, eggs), but the few that do survive stand a good chance of living to an old age.

Typically organisms with Type I survivorship curves produce fewer offspring that mostly survive to maturity (Chap. 2). The tsetse fly is a good example of a vector species with a Type I curve. Species with Type III curves tend to produce many offspring, and a small fraction of these survive to maturity. Many hard ticks produce 1000–5000 eggs (Sonenshine 1991), and very few survive the larval period.

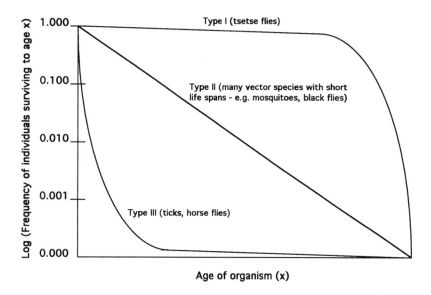

The y-axis is labeled "Log (Frequency of individuals surviving to age x)" with values 1.000, 0.100, 0.010, 0.001, 0.000. The curves are labeled: Type I (tsetse flies), Type II (many vector species with short life spans - e.g. mosquitoes, black flies), Type III (ticks, horse flies). The x-axis is labeled "Age of organism (x)".

24.6   Three types of survivorship curves. Species with Type I curves have low mortality at an early age and usually survive to a late average age of senescence. Species with Type II curves have a constant rate of mortality. Type III curves describe survivorship in species with high rates of mortality among offspring.

To obtain a complete life table we also need a lifetime fecundity curve. Three such curves for vectors are shown in Figure 24.7. Figure 24.7a shows the fertility curve for a female mosquito. Once she has molted to an adult, she mates, blood-feeds, and matures a batch of eggs. She oviposits, and then must take another blood meal to produce another batch of eggs. She can do this several times during her life. A trend that is seen in many insects is that the average size of the oviposition declines on successive batches of eggs. This type of fertility curve is typical for most dipteran vectors, most cockroaches, and soft ticks. The fertility curve for body lice or bed bugs is shown in Figure 24.7b. These insects feed continually on the host and produce eggs continuously throughout their lives. Figure 24.7c shows the fertility curve for a hard tick female that matures a large single batch of eggs and then dies.

Once survivorship and fecundity curves are estimated, a life table can be derived. Carey (1993) provides a detailed treatment of life-table construction. A life table for an imaginary mosquito is shown in

Table 24.2. It contains complete information on daily survivorship and fecundity. We assume that the maximum life span of this mosquito is 28 days long with 1 day spent as an egg, 7 days as a larva and pupa, and 20 days as an adult. The average egg survivorship is 0.5. The probability that a larva survives through 1 day is 0.6. The probability that an adult lives through a day is 0.9. A female usually oviposits once every 5 days and the average oviposition size in the first cycle is 120 eggs and declines by 20 eggs in the 3 subsequent cycles. This is therefore a Type II survivorship curve with a fecundity schedule like that in Figure 24.7a. With this information we are prepared to build a model to predict fluctuations in age structure and density of populations.

The Lewis-Leslie Model

The Lewis-Leslie age structure model is often used to simulate changes in population density and age structure in vector populations. The general form of the model in matrix notation is

$$M \times n_t = n_{t+1} \tag{16}$$

As with models discussed earlier, this is a system of recurrence equations. By iterating the system over several generations we can observe not only changes in seasonal phenology but the dynamics of age structure.

M is a square matrix that contains information taken directly from life tables in the form of 2 elements, f and p, for each age class where f is the fecundity of each age class and p is the probability of survival through that age class. The M matrix appears in Figure 24.8. Comparison with the life table in Table 24.2 indicates how the M matrix is derived. Fecundity values are placed across the top row. The 1st value greater

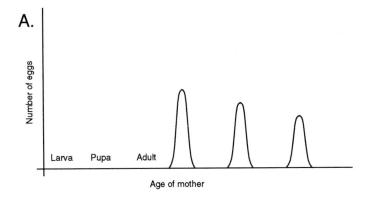

A.

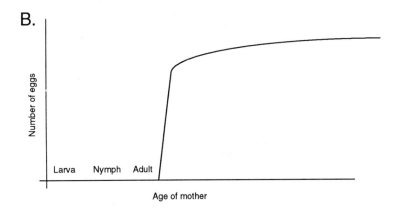

B.

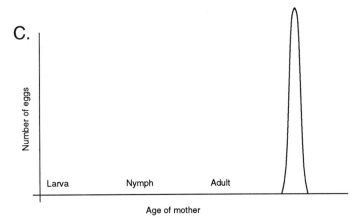

C.

24.7   Three types of fertility schedules in vectors. A is the schedule of reproduction in a species with multiple gonotrophic cycles. This is exhibited by most mosquito and muscid species. B describes fertility rates in species that produce offspring continuously throughout their life such as a soft tick or a body louse. C describes reproduction in species that produce a large batch of offspring, usually toward the end of their life, such as a hard tick.

TABLE 24.2 Life table of an imaginary mosquito (Daily survivorship is 50% in eggs, 60% in larvae, and 90% in adults.)

Life stage	Chronological age (days)	Probability of daily survival (p)	Fecundity (f)
Egg	0	0.5	0
Larva	1	0.6	0
	2	0.6	0
	3	0.6	0
	4	0.6	0
	5	0.6	0
	6	0.6	0
Pupa	7	0.6	0
Adult	8	0.9	0
	9	0.9	0
	10	0.9	0
	11	0.9	0
	12	0.9	120
	13	0.9	0
	14	0.9	0
	15	0.9	0
	16	0.9	0
	17	0.9	100
	18	0.9	0
	19	0.9	0
	20	0.9	0
	21	0.9	0
	22	0.9	80
	23	0.9	0
	24	0.9	0
	25	0.9	0
	26	0.9	0
	27	0.9	60
	28	0.9	0

Note: Each gonotrophic cycle requires 5 days. Each female oviposits 120 eggs during her first cycle and declining numbers in subsequent cycles. We assume that she passes through 4 gonotrophic cycles during her life. The egg stage lasts 1 day, larval development requires 6 days, and 1 day is required for adult development to occur in the pupal stage.

than zero appears in column 12. This corresponds with the 1st day of reproduction in the life table. Probability of daily survivorship appears below the principal diagonal of the M matrix. Egg survivorship appears in the 1st column on the 2nd row, survivorship of 1st day larvae appears in the 2nd column on the 3rd row. The n vector is the number of individuals in each age class at time *t*. This vector therefore records the age structure of the population at any point in time. By multiplying M by n, 2 things happen. The number of individuals at time *t* is multiplied by the probability of daily survival to give the number of individuals at *t* + 1 in the n_{t+1} vector. In this way the model tracks survivorship at each life stage. Secondly, the number of individuals reproducing (days 12, 17, 22, and 27) is multiplied by the fecundity in each of these life stages. This product records the number of new individuals introduced into the system at that time. These appear as eggs at the top on the n vector. In the next iteration these will become 1-day-old larvae; in the next iteration, 2-day-old larvae, etc. The number passing from 1 day to the next is determined by the probability of survivorship through that period. What enters into each new day (n_{t+1} vector) is a function of what survived from the previous day and new births from the reproductive age classes. This model could run indefinitely because new individuals are constantly regenerated through reproduction.

Iteration of the model over 30 days is shown in Figure 24.9. Note that adult density declines over the first 10 days as they die. Following day 5, the number of larvae increase because the eggs oviposited by the adults surviving to day 5 have hatched. These decline because of mortality over the next 5 days but increase again as the next batch of eggs hatch. On day 12, larvae from the first oviposition emerge, and the adult density increases. These fluctuations continue, and the census at 30 days is 8000 larvae and 300 adults.

Note that larval densities are greater than adult densities. Even though survivorship is 30% lower in larvae than adults, a large number of larvae are being produced, and they experience fewer days of mortality. Consideration of another model will help clarify this principle. In Table 24.3 the parameters of the model have been changed to match those of the tsetse fly.

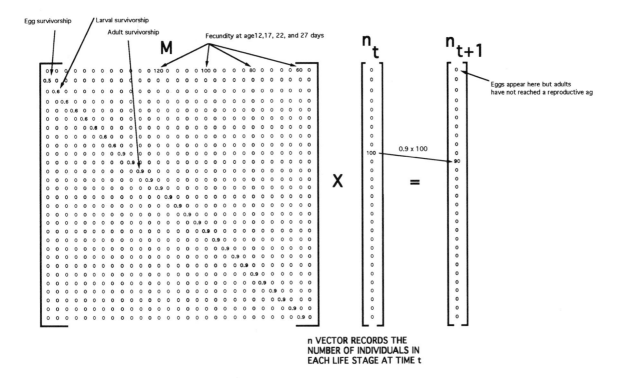

24.8   Leslie-Lewis M matrix and n vector for an imaginary mosquito. The components of the M matrix are as described in Table 24.2. The n vector indicates the population is initiated with 100 newly emerged individuals.

Recall that the tsetse fly doesn't oviposit but rather matures a single larva inside of its body and lays a fully developed 3rd instar larva that burrows into the soil and pupates. Egg, larval, and adult survivorship are therefore the same. The life table for this simulation is shown in Table 24.3.

Figure 24.10 shows the population size of larvae and adults through 30 weeks. Notice that larval and adult fluctuations trace one another very closely, because, unlike the mosquito system (Fig. 24.9), larval survivorship is totally dependent on adult survivorship and because the fecundity of the tsetse fly is so low.

An important result of iterating the Lewis-Leslie matrix over several generations is that the population will come to contain a constant proportion of each age class. When this occurs the population is said to have reached a stable age distribution (SAD). This is illustrated for our mosquito population in Figure 24.11, which shows the proportion of the population consisting of larvae and adults over a 200-day period. Notice that the magnitude of the oscillations stabilizes. Eventually in the absence of any perturbations they would become constant. The time required to reach a SAD is determined by the initial values of the model.

TABLE 24.3 Life table of a tsetse fly

Life stage	Chronological age (weeks)	Probability of daily survival (p)	Fecundity (f)
Larva	1	0.95	0
	2	0.95	0
Pupa	3	0.95	0
	4	0.95	0
Adult	5	0.95	0
	6	0.95	1
	7	0.95	0
	8	0.95	1
	9	0.95	0
	10	0.95	1
	11	0.95	0
	12	0.95	1
	13	0.95	0
	14	0.95	1
	15	0.95	0
	16	0.95	1
	17	0.95	0
	18	0.95	1
	19	0.95	0
	20	0.95	1
	21	0.95	0
	22	0.95	1
	23	0.95	0
	24	0.95	1
	25	0.95	0
	26	0.95	1
	27	0.95	0
	28	0.95	1
	29	0.95	0

Note: The female tsetse gives birth to a fully grown larva. A larva is produced at intervals of 14 days. The pupal stage lasts 2 weeks. The adult tsetse produces 12 larvae during her life.

Figure 24.12 follows the mosquito population over 100 days. It is easy to see the similarity between Figures 24.12 and 24.4 (the exponential model). Notice that in developing the Lewis-Leslie matrix no adjustments were made for density dependence. The model as we have developed it is an exponential growth model. We could introduce density dependence by making daily survival and fecundity values dependent on population density. Then we would expect to see population densities approximate a logistic model.

A point that is frequently overlooked in developing the Lewis-Leslie model is that age classes must be of equal length for the model to be accurate. For example, we could have made our mosquito model a 3-stage model with eggs, larvae, and adults and recorded survivorship and fecundity for these stages. But this model would be inaccurate because these stages vary in their lengths. Instead we have translated age classes to days. If a mosquito spends on average 7 days as a larva, we enter 7 larval periods into the model. A model using days as age classes predicts trends in field populations. We might predict on what days, weeks, months, or years the vectorial capacity of a population would be at its greatest; however, even a scale based on days is inaccurate because insects are not homeothermic. The time spent in each stage is dependent on temperature, with accelerated development at warmer temperatures. We might therefore adjust our time units to a product of time and temperature. A frequently used unit is day-degrees. Based on records of time and temperature, we could attempt to build a more predictive model. The nutritional resources of the larval habitat also will affect the duration of the larval stage. Similarly, ambient temperature and availability of hosts will affect the average length of the oviposition cycle.

Implications for Vector Control

It is important for people interested in suppressing vector populations to understand all of the factors that we have discussed before initiating control practices. Many models have been developed to examine and predict the outcome of control programs (e.g., the Garki project, Molineaux and Gramiccia 1980). Very sophisticated models employ factors such as density dependence and the presence of predators and parasites and indicate to the control-program managers what the outcome of insecticidal application is likely to be. Managers can use the programs to optimize the timing and placement of insecticidal control. An example of such a program that is easy to use and illustrates many

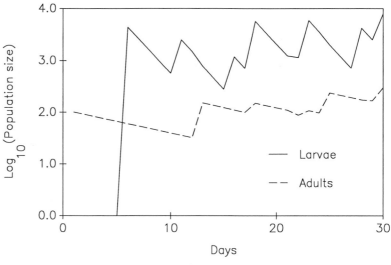

24.9 Iteration of the Leslie-Lewis matrix in Figure 24.8 over 30 days. Numbers of larvae and adults were obtained by summing over cells in the n vector for each time period.

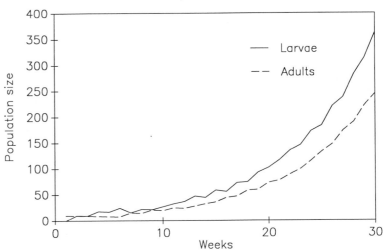

24.10 Iteration of the Leslie-Lewis matrix over 30 weeks. Components of the M matrix were as described in Table 24.3 for the tsetse fly.

of the principles discussed in this chapter is the fly management simulator (FMS) (Axtell 1992).

Usually in vector control we must accept that a population cannot be reduced to zero or eradicated. The cost might be too high or the amount of damage to the environment too great. Instead we ask: What is an acceptable economic threshold for a vector population? This is the population density at which damage caused by the species is at or below an economically acceptable level. This threshold varies for each species. In vector populations, economic thresholds can be

dictated by the vectorial capacity of a population and the severity of diseases transmitted. Examination of the Lewis-Leslie model provides an important insight into this issue of how to most efficiently reduce the vectorial capacity of a population. Figure 24.13 shows, using the same mosquito model described earlier, the relationship between the size of the adult population after 100 days and survivorship in eggs, larvae, and adults. Survivorship was varied from 1 to 0.1 for each stage and remained at 1 for the other 2 stages. Let's say that we had set the economic threshold to 1×10^6

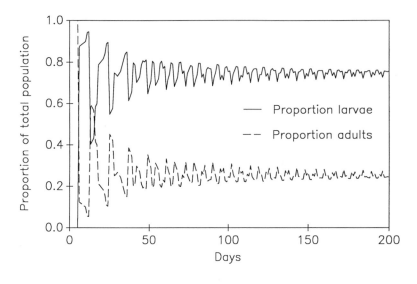

24.11 Approach to a stable age distribution. Plotted are the proportions of the total mosquito population consisting of larvae and adults in an iteration of the Leslie-Lewis matrix in Figure 24.8 over 200 days.

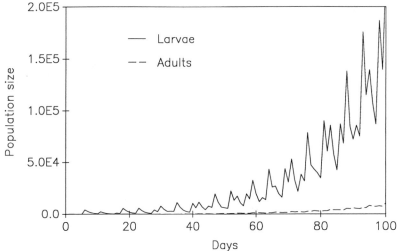

24.12 Exponential growth of larval and adult mosquito populations in an iteration of the Leslie-Lewis matrix in Figure 24.8 over 100 days.

adult mosquitoes. To achieve this level through ovicidal treatment would require reducing egg survivorship to 0.05. Adult survivorship would have to be reduced to approximately 0.35, but larval survivorship would only have to be reduced to 0.55 to achieve the same level of control. If we use insecticides to reduce the probability of daily survivorship and if the rate of insecticide used is proportional to the decrease in survivorship in each age class, it is easy to see that application of insecticides to kill larvae is the most efficient and environmentally least destructive way to obtain the

economic threshold. Fewer larvae must be killed to obtain the economic threshold.

This argument can be too simplistic if mortality is density dependent. For example, Agudelo-Silva and Spielman (1980) showed that in food-limited environments simulated larvicidal mortality (i.e., removal of a given percentage of the larval population) actually *increased* the number of adults that emerged. Hare and Nasci (1986) confirmed the foregoing observations using *Bacillus thuringiensis* subsp. *israeliensis* as a larvicide. Thus, the application of control measures in

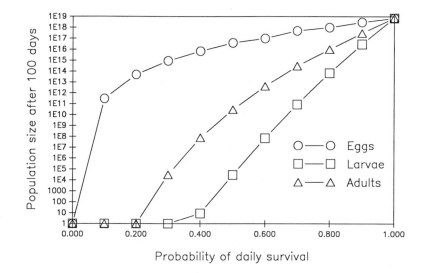

24.13   Effects of reducing the probability of daily survival *(p)* in eggs, larvae, and adults. Plotted are the final sizes of the egg, larvae, and adult populations in an iteration of the Leslie-Lewis matrix in Figure 24.8 over 100 days.

certain situations can eliminate naturally occurring mortality, with a net *increase* in total numbers (compensatory mortality).

These examples illustrate the importance of understanding the degree of density dependence before initiating vector control. When population densities are low, populations often grow exponentially in size. Individuals are often larger, healthier, and live longer (i.e., they have a large vectorial capacity); however, eventually the carrying capacity of the environment is reached and individuals must compete for resources. The size, viability, and fecundity of individuals decreases. At this point the population will either stabilize at the carrying capacity of the environment or undergo a drastic reduction in density. Thus, if a population is at its carrying capacity and we reduce population densities, we can create a healthier population with a greater vectorial capacity than if it had been left alone. Remember from our examination of Macdonald's equation that changes in vector-to-host densities had far less impact on vectorial capacity than changes in daily survivorship. Vectorial capacity of a population can be *increased* through control, or decreasing population densities can have little impact on vector capacity if it does not affect the probability of daily survivorship (Grimstad and Haramis 1984; Kay et al. 1989; Paulson and Hawley 1991; Grimstad

and Walker 1991). However, this pattern does not always appear (Nasci and Mitchell 1994; Dye 1992).

In addition to larval nutrition, adult nutritional status can affect mortality and the potential for disease transmission. Females of some mosquitoes are less susceptible to insecticides if they have recently taken a blood meal (Moore et al. 1990). This could result in the preferential selection of recently fed (and possibly infected) females by using improperly timed applications of adulticides in a vector control program.

It is also important to know how a population is regulated by parasites and predators. If in controlling a pest population predators and parasites are destroyed, it has been commonly observed that the target population will rebound to an even greater level than before control began. Furthermore, other nonpest species that were regulated by predators and parasites can suddenly reach densities that make them pests or even vectors. Pathogens spread most rapidly through dense populations; thus a population at carrying capacity can be more susceptible to decline caused by the epizootic spread of a pathogen. A population with a significant parasite or pathogen load that is at carrying capacity can be close to collapse. Under these circumstances, expensive and environmentally destructive control operations are unnecessary and can, in fact, be wasteful and injurious.

METHODS FOR MEASURING BIOTIC PARAMETERS THAT DETERMINE VECTORIAL CAPACITY

We have examined the biotic components that are important in regulating the vector capacity of populations. We have discussed how this knowledge can be used to design more efficient control strategies that are less destructive to the environment. We now discuss methods to estimate the biotic components of vectorial capacity.

THE HOST-BITING HABIT

Feeding Frequency

In species that require a single blood meal for each batch of eggs, the feeding frequency *(m)* is approximately equal to 1 divided by the length of 1 female reproductive cycle. This is either the time required for her to lay a batch of eggs following emergence as an adult or the time between ovipositions of separate egg batches. The cycle during which the ovaries mature to fully developed follicles is called the gonotrophic cycle (Detinova 1962). Thus, for a species with a gonotrophic cycle of 4 days, the feeding frequency is 1/4, or 0.25. We assume several things here. First, the gonotrophic cycle has constant length. Second, females lay their eggs as soon as ovarian development is complete. Third, females feed again on the same day that they oviposit (or there is a constant interval between oviposition and refeeding). Fourth, females take only 1 blood meal per gonotrophic cycle.

The feeding frequency is best determined by mark-release-recapture studies in which females coming to bite are marked and then released after feeding. Recaptures at subsequent biting catches provide exact measurements of the time between feeds. Another method, which requires sequential data on parous rates, is discussed in the section on daily survival rates.

Host Blood Index

Most vectors feed on more than 1 species of vertebrate. By collecting blood-filled females (and males in the case of some vectors), we can determine the relative importance of each host—or the "preference" of the vector.

It is absolutely essential that a representative (i.e., random) sample of all blooded individuals be collected. Specimens collected inside houses or stables can represent only those that have fed on the predominant host. For mosquitoes, vacuum sweeper collections of resting females frequently provide the most representative samples. Blooded specimens are usually uncommon, and very large samples must be collected to have sufficient data for statistical analysis.

The human blood index (HBI) (Garrett-Jones 1964b) is often used to make comparisons of host preference. This parameter is defined as the proportion of freshly engorged insects found to contain human blood. In studies estimating host preference indices, seldom are all potential vertebrate hosts present in equal numbers or equally available to the vector. Therefore, what appears to be a preference is really only an indication of the most common or easily accessible host species. The calculation of forage ratios (FR) and feeding indices (FI) can help to eliminate host density effects (Hess et al. 1978; Kay et al. 1979). FR adjusts the HBI by taking into account the number of available hosts. FI adjusts the HBI by taking into account the density of hosts, host size, age, and temporal and spatial concurrence between the host and vector. FR or FI values of 1 indicate no preference or avoidance of a host whereas values greater than 1 indicate host preference.

Identification of the source of blood meals is usually conducted by immunologic methods, such as micro-precipitin, ELISA (enzyme-linked immunosorbent assay), soluble antigen-fluorescent antibody, agar-gel diffusion, or related tests (Tempelis 1975). The most difficult problem in blood-meal testing is the preparation and standardization of antisera to the vertebrate host species under study (Washino and Tempelis 1983). Another method, hemoglobin crystallization, uses the morphology of crystals formed by the reaction of hemoglobin with different salt solutions to identify the host species. Precise conditions of temperature are required for crystal development, and large catalogs of crystal shapes must be maintained to permit identification.

Daily Survival

The birth, and death rates, discussed earlier in the context of the exponential and logistic models, are often immeasurable; it is more common to attempt to estimate the probability of daily survival. A number of techniques have been developed to estimate daily survivorship (p) because it is such a critical component of vectorial capacity (Gillies 1974). Four of the most promising techniques are reviewed here.

Mark-Release-Recapture Methods

In mark-release-recapture studies, large numbers of individuals of known age are marked by some means and released into the study population. The population is then sampled on consecutive days following the release and, it is hoped, some of the marked individuals are recovered. If the logarithm of the number of marked individuals is plotted against time following release, a straight line should result. The slope of the fitted regression line is an estimate of log p, the survival rate.

There are several assumptions made in mark-recapture studies. First, neither the survival nor the behavior of the marked animals is affected by the marking method. Second, the animals become completely mixed in the population at large. Third, the probability of capturing a marked individual is the same as that of capturing an unmarked individual. Fourth, sampling is at discrete time intervals, and the time spent in sampling is short relative to total time. There are several variations on the mark-recapture theme, and these are described in detail by Southwood (1978), Lounibos et al. (1985), and Service (1993). Conway et al. (1974) illustrated the use of mark-recapture in estimating *Aedes aegypti* densities in Tanzania.

Gonotrophic (Physiological) Age Grading

Much of the work on survival rates in mosquitoes and other biting flies has involved the use of changes in the ovarian status of the female (Detinova 1962). Early workers in this area were V.P. Polovodova and T.S. Detinova in Russia and D.S. Bertram in England.

As the female ages and passes through successive gonotrophic cycles, various changes occur in the ovaries and associated structures. If the time between various ovarian events can be determined (e.g., in laboratory experiments or by mark-release-recapture studies), then these physiologic "markers" can be used to tell the age of field-collected specimens. Two major events in the ovarian cycle are used: the unwinding of the ovarian tracheoles during the 1st gonotrophic cycle (Detinova method) and the formation of residual lumps or dilatations in the ovariolar pedicel following each oviposition (Polovodova method).

The Detinova method is by far the easier of the 2 methods, and for many species is the only reliable technique. The ovaries are removed from the abdomen and placed in a drop of water on a clean microscope slide. The water is allowed to evaporate, and the ovaries dry in place on the slide. As the ovaries dry, air is drawn into the tracheoles so that they are easily seen under normal light microscopy at 250x to 400x. In the nulliparous female (no eggs developed), the ends of the tracheoles are coiled, looking like a skein of knitting yarn. In the parous female, the tracheoles are extended as a result of the expansion of the ovary during an earlier gonotrophic cycle. The problem with this method is that individuals can only be classified as parous or nulliparous; in the Polovodova method several gonotrophic age classes are identifiable, and the number of prior gonotrophic cycles can be determined. Details on classifying individual insects into gonotrophic age classes is too detailed for this chapter. Use of the Polovodova method in the examination of age structure of muscid fly species is clearly illustrated in Tyndale-Biscoe and Hughes (1969), Krafsur and Ernst (1983), and Krafsur et al. (1985).

With both methods, very large numbers of individuals are required to produce an accurate estimate of parous rates. The survival rate is estimated from the parous rate by the equation

$$m = p^d \tag{17}$$

or

$$\log(p) = \log(m)/d \tag{18}$$

where: m = proportion parous
p = daily survival
d = length of gonotrophic cycle

This is a widely used method to estimate p. Not only is p critical in determining vector capacity, but it can be useful in determining whether control efforts are having an impact on daily survival. Estimation of parous rates in the face fly, *Musca autumnalis*, was used to test the efficacy of insecticidal ear tags by comparing p in treated versus control populations (Krafsur 1984).

There are several assumptions involved in using parous rates. First, we assume that the population has reached a SAD. Second, the sampling method provides an accurate cross-section of the general population. Third, the survival rate is not age dependent. Fourth, the length of the gonotrophic cycle is known and is constant. Assumption 1 is almost never true in temperate regions but can hold for some tropical species. However, the parous rate will accurately estimate p in temperate regions if calculated from the overall parous rate measured throughout a breeding season (Birley et al. 1983). It is well known that different sampling methods or sites provide radically different parity estimates, so that assumption 2 can also be violated. For example, Krafsur and Ernst (1983) showed that in horn fly (*Haematobia irritans irritans*) populations, parous rates were greatest among flies sampled from cattle bellies and nulliparous females were most frequent on cattle backs. Survival can, in fact, be age dependent (Clements and Paterson 1981), thus invalidating assumption 3. It is often impossible to estimate the length of the gonotrophic cycle without conducting mark-release-recapture studies; and the cycle length can change in response to temperature or other environmental stimuli. A method developed by M. Birley (Birley and Rajagopalan 1981) overcomes this latter problem but requires daily catches for periods of 2–3 weeks or more. The method uses cross-correlation analysis to estimate the primary or dominant cycle length.

Chronological Age

Daily growth layers in the cuticle and daily bands on the apodemes were 1st observed by Neville in the early 1960s (e.g., Neville 1963). Alternating light and dark bands are evident when sections through the cuticle are observed in polarized light microscopy. This banded pattern is caused by a circadian rhythm in the orientation of chitin rods in the protein matrix of the integument. Daytime deposition is unidirectional, whereas nighttime deposition rotates in a helicoidal fashion, giving rise to optically active material. By counting growth layers in the cuticle the chronological age of an insect can be determined.

An alternative technique was developed by Schlein and Gratz in 1972 and 1973. They showed daily bands on the apodemes and apophyses (infoldings of the integument) of *Anopheles*, *Aedes*, and *Culex* as well as *Glossina*, *Calliphora*, and *Sarcophaga* (Schlein 1979). Apodemes serve as muscle attachments and strengthen the skeleton. The muscle mass of an insect increases over the 1st few days of adult life; additional cuticle is laid down on the apodemes to handle the increase in muscle tissue. Electron microscope studies show that a daily variation in thickness of the apodemes gives rise to a banded appearance. The growth bands on apodemes are probably not the result of the same circadian changes in orientation of chitin rods as shown for cuticular growth lines. Instead, they probably result from differential stretching during the flight activity of the insect.

The Schlein-Gratz method requires a fairly elaborate and time-consuming staining process to make the bands visible. In addition (at least for *Culex pipiens*) the ages of known controls could not be determined with certainty. These factors are definite drawbacks for ecologically oriented work in which we would like to process large numbers of specimens to obtain statistical reliability.

Fortunately, another method has been found that is not only faster but provides more accurate results. Differential interference (Nomarski) microscopy causes structures of different composition, depth, or density to assume different shades or colors in a polarized light field. Because the bands have been shown by electron microscopy to vary in thickness, we can use Nomarski optics to see the bands. This method is faster than the Schlein-Gratz method because it requires little or no staining (Moore et al. 1986). It also offers greater resolution of the bands. Furthermore, Nomarski optics do not produce the halos that cause problems with techniques such as phase contrast microscopy.

As with the other techniques, this method has its own particular problems. In order to achieve statistical reliability, a series of coded, known-age controls should be included with each batch of field material. By doing this, it can be determined if readings on a given day or by a particular worker are biased. However, it is difficult to prepare known-age controls in an insectary. Presumably, this is caused by a lack of active flight during the normal activity period (and, therefore, the apodemes are not stretched and thickened at the appropriate times). Specimens with reasonably good band definition can be prepared if they can be reared outdoors in a large cage that permits normal daily flight activity.

Pteridine Quantification

Recently, molecular biology has provided another tool for chronological age determination in insects. Because of the large number of eye color mutants in *Drosophila melanogaster*, the biochemistry and metabolism of pteridines and ommochromes, the 2 major classes of eye pigments in insects, have been studied and understood for a long time. There are 5 major classes of pteridines. Listed in order of relative abundance they are: sepiapterin, biopterin, xanthopterin, isoxanthopterin, and pterine. They all share common biosynthetic pathways and utilize many of the same enzymes involved in ommochrome biosynthesis. Pteridines are synthesized in insect hemolymph, and while pteridines are found throughout the body, they are highly concentrated in the eye. They all absorb different wavelengths of light and most of them fluoresce. They function presumably to control the amount and wavelengths of light striking the ommatidia, the light-sensitive structure in the insect eye. All insects accumulate pteridine compounds in their eyes at a continuous rate as they age. No one understands why pteridines and other compounds accumulate in adult insect tissues rather than being excreted. Several workers have speculated that no mechanism for their excretion has evolved because the small amounts accumulated during the short life span of an adult are not deleterious. Most agree that pteridine accumulation is a natural process of aging in insects.

The general method for pteridine concentration determination involves grinding an insect head in a homogenization buffer, spinning down tissue debris in a microcentrifuge, and transferring the supernatant to a semimicro cuvette. A spectrofluorimeter is then used to quantify pteridine concentrations. Mail et al. (1983) reported a high correlation between pteridine amounts and chronological age in the stable fly. They reported a regression coefficient (r) of 0.97 (on a scale of 0–1), a value that is never seen with gonotrophic age grading (r = 0.5–0.8, depending on the species). They demonstrated that the rate of accumulation was temperature dependent; flies accumulated pteridines more rapidly at higher temperatures. Furthermore, the age of both sexes could be estimated. This allowed models to be built that incorporated temperature and pteridine amounts as independent variables to estimate chronological age. They tested their models in blind experiments with both males and females and were able to predict age within 1.9 days in females and 1.4 days in males. Lehane and Mail (1985) demonstrated that the technique also worked with the same accuracy in the tsetse fly and tested various other biotic and abiotic parameters to see how these affected pteridine accumulation. These factors included age, number of blood meals, total blood ingested, relative humidity, temperature, light intensity, the number of days a severed head was stored as well as the temperature, humidity, and lighting conditions under which it was stored. They found that body size and temperature affected pteridine amounts. The size was easily adjusted for by measuring the width of the head. Pteridine amounts were independent of light intensity, relative humidity, or nutritional status of the insect. With severed heads they found that only lighting conditions and relative humidity—not temperature—affected pteridine amounts. They demonstrated that severed heads could be kept at room temperature in light-safe vials with desiccant for 8 days before an appreciable decline in pteridine could be detected. This means that the time from which the head is severed until pteridines are measured is not critical and that the technique is therefore robust regarding many laboratory and field applications.

When the technique was used on recaptured insects that had been marked and released in the field, the regression coefficient declined to a range from 0.81–0.95 (Lehane and Hargrove 1988). This was compared with the gonotrophic age-grading technique on the same flies and found to be much more accurate. A decline in accuracy was observed because the researchers could not determine the temperature that was experienced by individual flies. A fly resting in the sun accumulates pteridines at a faster rate that a fly resting in the shade. Langley et al. (1988) demonstrated that this was not a major factor if flies were collected over finite intervals and the mean ambient temperatures were recorded. Temperature could be adjusted for and high correlation coefficients achieved. The use of pteridines in age grading is being expanded to other cyclorrhaphous flies. Krafsur et al. (1992) described its development in the horn fly. However, pteridine quantification has not been developed for mosquitoes or other vector groups even though it has been demonstrated that mosquitoes have pteridines. Spectrofluorimeters adapted for analysis of small volumes are required.

One of the major advantages of chronological methods is that they can be combined with gonotrophic data to establish the exact length of the gonotrophic cycle, time to the first blood meal, and many other characteristics of the population. A further advantage is that true horizontal (cohort) life tables can be constructed. This is particularly valuable in temperate regions in which rapid changes in recruitment or mortality can occur. It should be noted that mark-release-recapture methods also provide chronologic data. The advantage of techniques such as the apodeme or pteridine method is that essentially all specimens in a collection provide data, not just those with marks.

CONCLUSION

We have described the various biological factors in vector populations that affect the rate of transmission of arthropod-borne diseases. We have presented a variety of models to explore interactions among these factors and explain key concepts in population biology. These models also provide useful ways to learn about the dynamics of populations and provide clues to general strategies for reducing vector densities. *However,*

we emphasize that these models are only didactic tools and are largely inaccurate in their predictions concerning natural populations. For example, a significant part of this chapter centers on the use of Macdonald's equation. However, there are grave practical problems associated with measuring any and all of the components of the model. The interested reader is encouraged to consult references such as Dye (1992) to learn more about the problems associated with estimating the components of Macdonald's equation and ultimately the vectorial capacity of populations. Dye (1992) argues convincingly for taking a "comparative" rather than an "absolute" approach when estimating the importance of the biological factors affecting disease epidemiology. With the comparative approach, epidemiologists observe how disease prevalence and incidence change among populations that vary in the various factors we have discussed. Alternatively, observations can be made in a single population in which factors vary seasonally. The relative importance of each factor is judged by the degree to which variation in any 1 factor influences disease prevalence. Ultimately, this approach is more useful and informative than trying to obtain "absolute" estimates of these factors that are then incorporated into predictive models. In a final analysis, there is no substitute for empirical observations in understanding the dynamics of vector populations.

ACKNOWLEDGMENTS

We thank José Ribiero and Raymond E. Bailey for critically reviewing this chapter.

REFERENCES

Anderson. R.M., and R.M. May. 1982. *Population biology of infectious disease.* Dalem Conferences, Life Sciences Research Report #25. New York: Springer Verlag, 315 p.

Agudelo-Silva, F., and A. Spielman. 1980. Paradoxical effects of simulated larviciding on production of adult mosquitoes. *Am. J. Trop. Med. Hyg.* 33:1267–1269.

Axtell, R.C. 1992. Fly Management Simulator (FMS) User's Guide. Raleigh, NC: Department of Entomology, North Carolina State University.

Bailey, N.T.J. 1982. *The Biomathematics of Malaria.* Chas. London: Griffin and Co. 210 p.

Bellows, T.S. Jr. 1981. The descriptive properties of some models for density dependence. *J. Animal Ecol.* 50:139–156.

Birley, M.H., and P.K. Rajagopalan. 1981. Estimation of the survival and biting rates of *Culex quinquefasciatus* (Diptera: Culicidae). *J. Med. Entom.* 18:181–86.

Birley, M.H., J.B. Walsh, and J.B. Davies. 1983. Development of a model for *Simuliium damnosus* s.l. recolonization dynamics at a breeding site in the OCP area when contol is interrupted. *J. Appl. Ecol.* 20:507–519.

Carey, J.R. 1993. *Applied demography for biologists.* London: Oxford University Press. 206 p.

Charlesworth, B. 1980. *Evolution in age-structured populations.* London: Cambridge University Press. 300 p.

Clements, A.N., and G.D. Paterson. 1981. The analysis of mortality and survival rates in wild populations of mosquitoes. *J. Appl. Ecol.* 18:373–399.

Conway, G.R., M. Trpis, and G.A.H. McClelland. 1974. Population parameters of the mosquito *Aedes aegypti* (L.) estimated by mark-release-recapture in a suburban habitat in Tanzania. *J. Anim. Ecol.* 43:289–304.

Detinova, T. S. 1962. Age grouping methods in diptera of medical importance. WHO Monograph No.47. Geneva: World Health Organization. 216 p.

Dye, C. 1992. The analysis of parasite transmission by bloodsucking insects. *Ann. Rev. Entomol.* 37:1–19.

Fine, P.E.M. 1981. Epidemiological principles of vector-mediated transmission. In: J.J. McKelvey, B.F. Eldridge and K. Maramorosch, editors, *Vectors of disease agents.* New York: Praeger Scientific. pp. 77–91.

Garrett-Jones, C. 1964a. Prognosis for the interruption of malaria transmission through assessment of a mosquito's vectorial capacity. *Nature* 204:1173–1175.

———. 1964b. The human blood index of malaria vectors in relation to epidemiological assessment. *Bull WHO* 30:241–261.

Gillies, M.T. 1974. Methods for assessing the density and survival of blood-sucking Diptera. *Ann. Rev. Entom.* 19:345–62.

Goodenough, J.L., and J.M. McKinion, editors. 1992. Basics of insect modeling. ASAE Monogr. No. 10. St. Joseph, MI: Amer. Soc. Agric. Engin. 221 p.

Grimstad, P.R., and L.D. Haramis. 1984. *Aedes triseriatus* (Diptera: Culicidae) and La Crosse virus. III. Enhanced oral transmission by nutrient deprived mosquitoes. *J. Med. Entomol.* 21:249–265.

Grimstad, P.R., and E.D. Walker. 1991. *Aedes triseriatus* (Diptera: Culicidae) and La Crosse virus. IV. Nutritional deprivation of larvae affects adult barriers to infection and transmission. *J. Med. Entomol.* 28:378–386.

Hare, S.G.F., and R.S. Nasci. 1986. Effects of sublethal exposure to *Bacillus thuringiensis* var. *israelensis* on larval development and adult size in *Aedes aegypti. J. Amer. Mosq. Control Assoc.* 2:325–328.

Hess, A.D., R. Hayes, and C. Tempelis. 1978. The use of forage ratio technique in mosquito host preference studies. *Mosq. News* 28:386–389.

Kay, B.H., P. Boreham, and J.D. Edman. 1979. Application of the "feeding index" concept to studies of mosquito host-feeding patterns. *Mosq. News* 39:68–72.

Kay, B.H., J.D. Edman, I.D. Fanning, and P. Mottran. 1989. Larval diet and the vector competence of *Aedes aegypti, Culex annulirostris* and other mosquitoes (Diptera: Culicidae) for Murray Valley encephalitis virus. *J. Med. Entomol.* 26:487–488.

Krafsur, E.S., and C.M. Ernst. 1983. Physiological age composition and reproductive biology of horn fly populations, *Haematobia irritans irritans* (Diptera: Muscidae), in Iowa, USA. *J. Med. Entomol.* 20:664–669.

Krafsur, E.S. 1984. Use of age structure to assess insecticidal treatments of face fly populations, *Musca autumnalis* DeGeer (Diptera: Muscidae). *J. Econ. Entomol.* 77:1364–1366.

Krafsur, E.S., W.C. Black IV, C.J. Church, and D.A. Barnes. 1985. Age structure and reproductive biology of a natural house fly (Diptera: Muscidae) population. *Environ. Entomol.* 14:159–164.

Krafsur, E.S., A.L. Rosales, J.F. Robison-Cox, and J.P. Turner. 1992. Age structure of horn fly (Diptera: Muscidae) populations estimated by pterin concentrations. *J. Med. Entomol.* 29:678–686.

Langley, P.A., M.J.R. Hall, and T. Felton. 1988. Determining the age of tsetse flies, *Glossina* spp. (Diptera: Glossinidae): An appraisal of the pteridine fluorescence technique. *Bull. Ent Res.* 78:387–395.

Lehane, M.J., and J. Hargrove. 1988. Field experiments on a new method for determining age in tsetse flies (Diptera: Glossinidae). *Ecol. Ent.* 13:319–322.

Lehane, P.A., and T.S. Mail. 1985. Determining the age of adult male and female *Glossina morsitans* using a new technique. *Ecol. Entomol.* 10:219–224.

Lounibos, L.P., J.R. Rey, and J.H. Frank. 1985. *Ecology of Mosquitoes: Proceedings of a Workshop.* Vero Beach: Fla. Med. Entomol. Lab. 579 p.

Macdonald, G. 1957. *The Epidemiology and Control of Malaria.* London: Oxford University Press.

Mail, T.S.J. Chadwick, and M.J. Lehane. 1983. Determining the age of adults of *Stomoxys calcitrans* (L.) (Diptera: Muscidae). *Bull. Ent. Res.* 73:501–525.

Molineaux, L., and G. Gramiccia. 1980. The Garki project. Geneva: World Health Organization.

Moore, C.G., P. Reiter, and J.-J. Xu. 1986. Determination of chronological age in *Culex pipiens s.l. J. Amer. Control. Assoc.* 2:204–208.

Moore, C.G., P. Reiter, D.A. Eliason, R.E. Bailey, and E.G. Campos. 1990. Apparent influence of the stage of blood meal digestion on the efficacy of ground applied ULV aerosols for the control of urban *Culex* mosquitoes. III. Results of a computer simulation. *J. Am. Mosq. Control Assoc.* 6:376–383.

Nasci, R.S., and C.J. Mitchell. 1994. Larval diet, adult size, and susceptibility of *Aedes aegypti* (Diptera: Culicidae) to infection with Ross River virus. *J. Med. Entom.* 31:123–126.

Neville, A.C. 1963. Daily growth layers in locust rubber-like cuticle, influenced by an external rhythm. *J. Ins. Physiol.* 9:177–186.

Paulson, S.L., and W.A. Hawley. 1991. Effect of body size on the vector competence of field and laboratory populations of *Aedes triseriatus* for La Crosse virus. *J. Am. Mosq. Control Assoc.* 7:170–175.

Schlein, Y. 1979. Age grouping of anopheline malaria vectors (Diptera: Culicidae) by the cuticular growth lines. *J. Med. Entom.* 16:502–6.

Service, M.W. 1993. *Mosquito ecology: Field sampling methods*, 2nd ed. New York: Elsevier Applied Science. 988 pp.

Sonenshine, D.E. 1991. *Biology of ticks.* Vol. 1. New York: Oxford University Press. 447 pp.

Southwood, T.R.E. 1978. *Ecological methods with particular reference to the study of insect populations.* 2nd ed. New York: Chapman and Hall. 524 pp.

Tempelis, C.H. 1975. Host-feeding patterns of mosquitoes with a review of advances in analysis of blood meals by serology. *J. Med. Entom.* 11:635–53

Tyndale-Biscoe, M., and R.D. Hughes. 1969. Changes in female reproductive system as age indicators in the bushfly *Musca vetustissima* Wlk. *Bull. Entomol. Res.* 59:129–141.

Washino, R.K., and C.H. Tempelis. 1983. Mosquito host bloodmeal identification: Methodology and data analysis. *Ann. Rev. Entomol.* 28:179–201.

25. POPULATION GENETICS IN VECTOR BIOLOGY

Walter J. Tabachnick and William C. Black IV

INTRODUCTION

Population genetics is the study of genetic variation in natural populations and the factors that influence this variation. Population genetics is a critical area of study in arthropod vector biology. Understanding genetic variation in vector populations provides a foundation for understanding the role of the vector in disease epidemiology. The factors that shape genetic variation in vector species also influence variation in vector capacity and vector competence traits.

This chapter introduces basic population genetic concepts and addresses the following questions:

1. How does one measure and analyze genetic variation in populations of arthropod vectors?

2. What are the major factors that influence genetic variation in natural vector populations?

3. What can population genetics reveal about vector-borne disease epidemiology and how can it facilitate vector control?

We do not attempt to review the large body of work on vector population genetics. The examples used in this chapter represent a small portion of work in this field and focus primarily on the vectors with which the authors are most familiar. Table 25.1 represents a partial summary of the arthropod vectors that have been examined using population genetics analysis.

TABLE 25.1 Arthropod species that have been extensively studied for population genetic variation

Species	Reference
Aedes aegypti	Tabachnick 1991
Aedes albopictus	Kambhampati et al. 1991
Aedes triseriatus	Munstermann 1985
Aedes hendersoni	Matthews and Munstermann 1983
Aedes scutellaris group	Pashley et al. 1985
Amblyomma americanum	Hilburn and Sattler 1986
Anopheles gambiae group	Miles 1978; McLain and Collins 1989
Anopheles quadrimaculatus group	Lanzaro et al. 1990
Boophilus sp.	Sattler et al. 1986
Culex pipiens	Cheng et al. 1982
Culicoides variipennis	Tabachnick 1992a,b
Glossina morsitans	Gooding 1982
Ixodes scapularis	Wesson et al. 1993
Phlebotomus papatasi	Kassem et al. 1990
Simulium damnosum	Post and Crampton 1988

Population genetics has its foundations in the works of J.B.S. Haldane, R.A. Fisher, and S. Wright, each of whom developed the theoretical basis for the discipline in the 1930s. In the late 1930s and 1940s, the field was integrated with evolutionary and systematic biology through the works of T. Dobzhansky and later E. Mayr, G.L. Simpson, and L.E. Stebbins. In the 1950s J.B. Kitzmiller and G.B. Craig Jr. recognized the importance of population genetics for understanding arthropod disease vectors. However, work on vector population genetics actually began with Craig's analysis of morphologic mutants in populations of *Aedes aegypti* in the early 1960s. Despite early attempts, the difficulty of population genetic analyses using morphological variants prevented much progress. A major breakthrough occurred with the advent of isozyme electrophoresis and its first application to *Drosophila pseudoobscura* populations in 1966 by R.C. Lewontin and J.L. Hubby. Soon after, L. Bullini and colleagues at the University of Rome studied species of *Aedes*. G.B. Craig and L.E. Munstermann at the University of Notre Dame began population genetic studies of African *Ae. aegypti*. W.J. Tabachnick and J.R. Powell at Yale University also analyzed populations of *Ae. aegypti* from throughout the world. Studies of the *Culex pipiens* complex were conducted by M.L. Cheng at the University of California–Los Angeles and S. Miles at the London School of Tropical Medicine and Hygiene. Research principally with *Ae. aegypti* has proceeded to the present, and other species of *Aedes* have also accumulated a large body of information primarily through the efforts at the University of Notre Dame by Craig, K.S. Rai, L.M. Munstermann, W.C. Black, S. Kambhampati, and others. Population genetic studies of several species of *Anopheles* have been conducted by M. Coluzzi, University of Rome; A. Cockburn, J. Seawright, S. Narang, and G. Lanzaro, USDA-ARS (U.S. Department of Agriculture–Agricultural Research Service) and Fort Collins, US-CDC (U.S. Centers for Disease Control and Prevention). Population genetics of other arthropod vectors, including many species of mosquitoes, *Glossina*, Plebotomines, Ceratopogonids, and ticks, are currently being investigated.

CHARACTERIZING GENETIC VARIATION IN NATURAL POPULATIONS OF ARTHROPOD VECTORS

Techniques

Much of population genetics was initially theoretical because only morphologic mutants were available, and these often segregate as recessive markers. Empirical studies awaited the advent of techniques that allowed both alleles in an individual to be identified. A list of available techniques and the genotype information they provide for population genetic analyses is shown in Table 25.2.

TABLE 25.2   Methods used to identify genetic variation in natural populations

1. Morphologic mutants—mostly recessive

2. Chromosomal inversions—codominant

3. Isozyme (allozymes)—codominant

4. DNA markers

   a. Restriction fragment length polymorphisms (RFLPs)—codominant

   b. Arbitrarily amplified DNA (RAPD-PCR, AP-PCR)—mostly dominant

   c. Simple sequence length polymorphisms (SSLPs)—codominant

5. Nucleotide sequencing—codominant when cloned

Note: When both alleles are detected by a certain method, they are said to segregate as codominants. The dominant or codominant phenotypes associated with alleles detected by each method are provided.

Analyses of chromosomal structural variants, principally chromosome inversions, have been most used in studies of various species of *Anopheles*. M. Coluzzi studied the population genetics of the *Anopheles gambiae* complex through an analysis of inversion polymorphisms in polytene chromosomes (Coluzzi and Sabatini 1969). Certain specific inversions are associated with indoor resting *An. gambiae* and can play a role in controlling aspects of vector capacity. Chromosomal studies have also been used extensively to study species of *Simulium* (Dunbar and Vajime 1981).

By far the most extensive amount of population genetic data has been gathered through the use of isozyme electrophoresis. Recent methods for analyzing genetic variation in natural populations of vectors focus directly on the use of DNA markers. Chapter 14 introduced RFLPs, RAPDs, and SSLPs as gene markers. The use of this technology is only beginning to be applied to vector populations. All of the above techniques, except RAPD-PCR and AP-PCR, are similar in that they enable one to identify genotypic variation by visualizing individual alleles and therefore discriminate heterozygotes from homozygotes.

We will use the method of isozyme electrophoresis to illustrate how to identify population genetic variation. In isozyme electrophoresis, a homogenate of an individual arthropod is separated by electrophoresis on some type of supporting media, e.g., acrylamide, cellulose acetate, or starch gels. When proteins are loaded into these supporting media and an electrical field is applied, they differentially migrate according to size, conformation, and net electric charge, which is dependant on the amino acid content. Enzymes with different numbers of basic or acidic side groups migrate differently in the electric field. Once electrophoresis is completed, the gel contains all of the proteins from the individual fractionated by charge and size.

Specific enzymes can be visualized in the gel using a histochemical activity stain. This stain contains the substrate and cofactors for the particular enzyme, along with a dye that precipitates when the substrate is acted upon. The dye precipitates in the region of the gel containing the specific enzyme. Variants of a specific enzyme are called isozymes, and allelic variants at a single enzyme locus are called allozymes.

The allozyme pattern on a gel is a direct representation of the genotype of the individual at the locus encoding the isozyme. Figure 25.1 demonstrates the relationship between allozyme phenotype and genotype. Individual alleles can be visualized so that heterozygotes can be distinguished from homozygotes. The genetic basis for the electrophoretic variants can

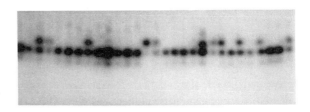

25.1 *Culicoides variipennis* electrophoretic variation for phosphoglucomutase (PGM)

be tested through appropriate genetic crosses. Allozyme loci have been placed on linkage maps of *Ae. aegypti* and *Ae. triseriatus* by L.E. Munstermann.

Figure 25.1 shows a representative starch gel that has been stained for the enzyme phosphoglucomutase (PGM). Each lane is 1 individual of a sample of 29 individual *Culicoides variipennis* that have been subjected to electrophoresis. Because variation in PGM in *C. variipennis* is controlled by a single locus, no diploid individual can have more than 2 PGM allozymes. However, populations of *C. variipennis* can contain several different PGM allozymes (multiple alleles) which, by convention, can be designated according to their migration rate after electrophoresis relative to a usually common PGM allozyme (designated the "100 allozyme"). Accordingly, the 78 band migrates 78% relative to the 100 band. Approximately 70–80 different enzymes can be identified (Murphy et al. 1990) through activity staining. Depending on the insect, between 10 and 20 isozyme loci can be analyzed in an individual.

MEASUREMENTS OF ALLELIC AND GENOTYPIC FREQUENCIES

Once a sample of individuals in a population has been characterized for variation at any locus, it is possible to calculate the frequency of different genotypes at that locus and the allele frequencies in the population. In the PGM example, the number of different genotypes in the sample are counted, disregarding the 2 heterozygous controls, to determine genotypic frequencies. In the sample of 27 individuals, there were 1, 78/78; 8, 78/100; and 18, 100/100. Therefore, the respective genotypic frequencies are 0.037 (1/27), 0.296 (8/27), and 0.667 (18/27).

Another measure of genetic variation in populations is the allelic frequencies at each locus. Historically, the gene frequencies of each allele at a locus have been termed p, q, r, s . . . , or $p1$, $p2$, $p3$ . . . pi. To determine gene frequencies, the number of occurrences of each allele in the population is counted and divided by the total number of alleles sampled (twice the number of individuals sampled in a diploid species), as is illustrated in the PGM data in Table 25.3. One measure of genetic variation is the observed frequency of heterozygotes (Het_{obs}), which is the total number of heterozygotes divided by the number of individuals sampled.

TABLE 25.3 Calculation of gene frequencies from the observed genotypes in a population (data shown in Fig. 25.1)

	78/78	78/100	100/100
Observed number of occurrences	1	8	18
Gene frequency: 78 = p = (2 + 8) / 54 = 0.185			
Gene frequency: 100 = q = (36 + 8) / 54 = 0.815			
Het_{obs}:= 8/27 = 0.296			

Note: Alleles are scored twice in a homozygote and once in a heterozygote.

Hardy-Weinberg Equilibrium Law

An excellent starting place for addressing factors responsible for the genetic structure of populations is the Castle-Hardy-Weinberg Equilibrium first proposed in the early part of the 20th century. (For reasons that are not clear, Castle's name is usually not used when discussing this principle.) The proposition can be stated as follows: In a large, randomly mating population in the absence of selection, migration, and mutation, gene and genotypic frequencies remain constant from generation to generation. This statement summarizes the factors that are responsible for causing gene and genotypic frequencies to change in any population as:

1. Mating—nonrandom mating between genotypes causes change in genotypic frequencies.

2. Population size—small populations are subject to greater random shifts in gene frequencies due to sampling effects.

3. Migration—differential migration of individuals with novel genotypes into and from populations changes allele frequencies.

4. Mutation—mutation rate affects gene frequencies.

5. Selection—genes can vary in their fitness effects among individuals. Selection changes genotype and allele frequencies.

We can examine genotype frequencies to determine if a sample from a population conforms to Hardy-Weinberg equilibrium. The equilibrium can be viewed as a null hypothesis regarding these 5 factors. If any of them significantly affect genotypic frequencies, the frequencies will not be in equilibrium. To understand the basis of the equilibrium, consider a particular locus in which there are 2 alleles (A_1 and A_2) in the population with frequency p and q. When the frequency of the alleles in each sex are equal, random mating between the sexes results in the random union of gametes. Genotypic frequencies in the next generation are a function of allelic frequencies in the parental gametes and are predicted as:

		Sperm	
		p (A_1)	q (A_2)
Eggs	p (A_1)	p^2	pq
	q (A_2)	pq	q^2

The genotypic frequencies, A_1A_1, A_1A_2, and A_2A_2, for the next generation are then p^2, $2pq$, q^2, respectively. Note that $p + q = 1$ and that the Hardy-Weinberg expected genotypic frequencies for any generation can be obtained by the binomial expansion of the gene frequencies $(p + q)^2$. The gene frequencies can be calculated from the genotypic frequencies as

$$p = p^2 + pq = p^2 + p(1-p) = p$$

and

$$q = q^2 + pq = q^2 + q(1-q) = q$$

Therefore, under random mating and in the absence of the other 5 factors, the gene and genotypic frequencies remain constant from generation to generation. The same situation occurs when more than 2 alleles are found in a population at any locus. The Hardy-Weinberg expected genotypic frequencies are the expansion of :

$$(p + q + r \ldots)^2 = p^2 + 2pq + q^2 + 2pr + r^2 + 2qr \ldots$$

Because these are frequencies, the total of each expression must be 1.

To determine whether any population is in Hardy-Weinberg equilibrium, a number of individuals are sampled and genotypic and allelic frequencies are estimated. The observed and expected numbers are compared using a nonparametric test such as chi square (X^2). The degrees of freedom are calculated as $n(n - 1)/2$ where n is the number of alleles. Table 25.4 shows an example of a test for Hardy-Weinberg equilibrium using the PGM example.

$$X^2 = (obs - exp)^2/exp =$$
$$(1 - 0.924)^2/0.924 + (8 - 8.142)^2/8.142 +$$
$$(18 - 17.934)^2/17.934 =$$
$$0.006 + 0.002 + .0002 = 0.010$$

In Table 25.4, there are 2 alleles and 1 degree of freedom; the probability of obtaining this result due to chance alone is >0.05. There is no significant difference between the observed and expected; the population sample is in Hardy-Weinberg equilibrium.

Another indicator of genetic variation in natural populations is the expected heterozygosity (Het_{exp}) under Hardy-Weinberg equilibrium. This can be calculated as:

$$1 - \Sigma p_i2$$

In our example, this is $1 - (0.034 + 0.664) = 0.302$. A more accurate description of a population is obtained when many different loci are analyzed and the mean of the Het_{exp} is calculated as the average expected heterozygosity.

When testing if a population is in Hardy-Weinberg equilibrium, it is often assumed that the sample of individuals comes from a single randomly mating or panmictic population. If a single sample is actually a mixture of 2 genetically different populations, the sample may not meet Hardy-Weinberg expectations. As an example, suppose there are 2 populations, one entirely AA, the other entirely BB. Note there are no AB heterozygotes in either population. However, when we sample, we believe there is only a single population, and assuming we sample both populations equally, then we will observe genotypic frequencies AA = 0.5 and BB = 0.5, and therefore $p = q = 0.5$. According to Hardy-Weinberg expectations, there should be $2pq = 0.5$ AB heterozygotes; yet there are none. The reduced observed heterozygosity, due purely to sampling more than 1 population simultaneously, has been termed the Wahlund Effect. The magnitude of the Wahlund Effect depends on the extent of the genetic differences between the populations. The greater the gene frequency differences, the greater will be the decreased Het_{obs} relative to Het_{exp}.

The concept of the Wahlund Effect has been used in studies of several arthropod vectors. In particular, decreased heterozygosity has prompted several investigators to reexamine presumed single population samples and to propose different species. G. Lanzaro used such an approach in an analysis of *An. quadrimaculatus* populations that resulted in the discovery of cryptic species in this group (Lanzaro et al. 1990).

TABLE 25.4 Testing a population for Hardy-Weinberg equilibrium

	78/78	78/100	100/100
Observed	1	8	18
Expected genotypic frequencies	$(0.185)^2 = 0.034$	$2 \times 0.185 \times 0.815 = 0.302$	$0.815^2 = 0.664$
Expected numbers	$27(0.034) = 0.924$	$27(0.302) = 8.142$	$27(0.664) = 17.934$

FACTORS THAT INFLUENCE GENETIC VARIATION IN NATURAL POPULATIONS

Random Mating

When genotypes within a population do not mate at random with one another, it is referred to as assortative mating. Individuals with a similar or identical genotype mate preferentially in positive assortative mating. Alternatively, individuals with dissimilar genotypes preferentially mate in negative assortative mating. Positive assortative mating is more common. The effects of positive assortative mating on the genotypic frequencies of a population are shown in Table 25.5. The general effect of positive assortative mating within a population is the reduction in the number of heterozygotes in each generation; thus in each generation the heterozygotes approach zero. In this example, positive assortative matings do not change the gene frequencies, and the population ends up with 0.5 AA and 0.5 BB individuals with $p = q = 0.5$. There is some evidence that certain chromosomal inversion types in the *An. gambiae* complex mate preferentially.

TABLE 25.5 Positive assortative mating and genotypic frequencies in a population with $p = q = 0.5$ and genotypic frequencies of 0.25 AA, 0.5 AB, and 0.25 BB

Mating	AA × AA	AB × AB	BB × BB
Frequency of mating	1/4 × 1/4	1/2 × 1/2	1/4 × 1/4
Segregation in offspring	All AA	1/4 AA, 1/2 AB, 1/4BB	All BB
Genotypic frequency after 1 generation	1/4 + 1/8	1/2 − 1/4	1/4 + 1/8

There are no examples of arthropod vectors that mate by negative assortment. An extreme example occurs between sexes where XX (or the female determining genotype) mate only with XY; XX × XX and XY × XY never occur.

Inbreeding is the mating between relatives and is similar in effect to positive assortative mating. When relatives mate, it is likely that they share characteristics and similar alleles with higher frequency than mates chosen from the population at random. Self-fertilization in plants, the mating of identical twins, or the mating of siblings (sibs) are extreme examples of this. Inbreeding can be forced upon a population by limited dispersal capabilities or limited resources. In contrast with positive assortative mating, inbreeding occurs without preference to genotype, but the result is also an increase in homozygosity. Because relatives can be a smaller sample compared to the general population, inbreeding can also be viewed as mating within small populations. The rate with which homozygosity increases is a function of the degree of relatedness among mates. Homozygosity increases most rapidly with parent-offspring or sibling matings and less rapidly when matings are among, for example, first cousins.

Population Size

The Hardy-Weinberg equilibrium assumes infinite or very large constant population size. However, we know that natural populations fluctuate greatly in size and that local populations can approach or reach extinction. Small population sizes can change both gene and genotypic frequencies. The effect of small population size on genetic variation is often unappreciated by many biologists. Small population size increases the probability that gene and genotypic frequencies will shift by random chance and can be thought of as a sampling phenomena. With a 2-allele locus, the variance of any series of samples is $Var(p) = Var(q) = pq/(2N)$, where N is the number of individuals sampled. The square root of the variance is the standard deviation. Table 25.6 demonstrates the relationship of small population size and chance changes in gene frequencies. As the population size decreases, the standard deviation in the gene frequencies for the next generation increases because of chance alone.

Figure 25.2 represents a starting large population of 5000 organisms in Hardy-Weinberg equilibrium and with gene frequencies equal to 0.5. Assume that the population randomly breaks up into 100 groups of 50 organisms prior to mating. Chance alone causes some of these small groups to have gene frequencies above and below 0.5. Given the standard deviation in gene

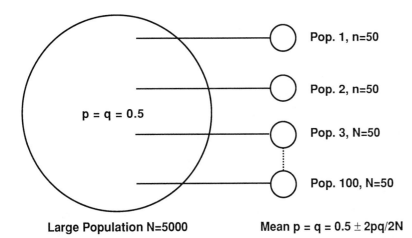

Large Population N=5000 **Mean p = q = 0.5 ± 2pq/2N**

25.2 A large randomly mating population subdivided into 100 populations of 50 individuals each

TABLE 25.6 The effect of small population size on gene frequencies in a population where $p = q = 0.5$

Population size	Variance	Standard deviation
1000	0.000125	0.011
100	0.00125	0.035
50	0.0025	0.05
10	0.0125	0.112

frequencies in Table 25.6 and assuming allelic frequencies are normally distributed around the mean of 0.5 in the subpopulations, we can anticipate that 32% of our samples will be more than 1 standard deviation above or below the mean, and that 5% and 2% of the samples will be 2 and 3 standard deviations above or below the mean, respectively. Although the mean of all samples must be 0.5, there will be samples from our large initial population with a gene frequency of 0.35 (−3 standard deviations) and 0.65 (+3 standard deviations). Instead of dividing up our large population into 100 groups of 50, assume that in each generation only 50 individuals are selected at random to be parents of the next generation and this continues for 100 generations. During any single generation, the gene frequencies will change by a predictable magnitude, and during some generations the change will be as large as 3 standard deviations from whatever the starting frequency is in the

previous generation. There will be considerable fluctuation in gene frequencies, even in samples of 50.

The effect of chance caused by small population size is predictable in magnitude, but is not predictable in direction. Changes in frequencies over time resulting from random chance are referred to as genetic drift.

Genetic drift affects the observed heterozygosity of the population. In a population in Hardy-Weinberg equilibrium where $p = q = 0.5$, the heterozygosity is $2pq = 0.5$, or the maximum expected heterozygosity. To verify this, recalculate heterozygosity with p slightly less than or greater than 0.5. Through genetic drift, frequencies either decrease or increase by some probability depending on the sample size, N. Hence, heterozygosity decreases due to genetic drift in small populations. Eventually, gene frequencies will fluctuate to such extremes that a particular gene becomes the only allele in the population ($p = 1$). When this happens, the allele is said to be fixed in the population because in the absence of migration there will be no further fluctuations in the frequency of that allele. In each generation even starting from a $p = q = 0.5$, there is a finite probability that any allele will be lost completely or be fixed in the population. In subsequent generations, loss or fixation eventually occurs, and the gene frequencies can no longer fluctuate from chance alone because variation at the locus does not exist. In each generation more extreme gene frequencies are possible, and eventually the populations approach homozygosity.

When a new isolated population arises from a limited number of individuals, there is often a shift in gene frequencies. Assume that, each generation 50 individuals, in our example from our large population, move off together by chance and begin or found a new population. By chance alone, the new population can differ from the starting large population. This chance effect caused by colonization has been termed the founder effect.

Many vector species probably occur with population sizes that because of seasonal fluctuations such as heat, freezing, and desiccation, or control efforts become small. At these times, random chance and genetic drift can have significant consequences on gene frequencies. *Ae. aegypti* populations, particularly on many Caribbean islands, demonstrated this effect (Tabachnick 1991). Islands such as Jamaica, Puerto Rico, Martinique, Barbados, and Aruba have extensive mosquito control activities directed against *Ae. aegypti*. These control activities cause reduced mosquito population size. However, mosquito population sizes fluctuate because control activities are often discontinued until the mosquitoes become abundant. The gene frequencies at many isozyme loci show little correlation between island populations of *Ae. aegypti*, as predicted, given the genetic drift that is independently occurring on each island. Black et al. (1988a) observed an extreme founder effect in the newly introduced population of *Ae. albopictus* in the United States. Most *Ae. albopictus* populations throughout the world segregate for 5–6 alleles at the esterase–6 locus; however, populations in Florida, Tennessee, and Indiana were found to be fixed for a single allele. Phlebotomine sand flies exist in small population groups and because of their limited dispersal ability have genetic structures that are greatly influenced by genetic drift (Kassem et al. 1990). The effects of small population size with accompanying genetic drift represent an important component to understanding genetic variation in natural populations of arthropod vectors. Unlike positive assortative mating, which only effects a single locus, small population size and drift affect the entire genome, including those traits that are important to vectorial capacity and competence. Arthropod vectors of disease are different from many other organisms because they are often directly subject to human efforts to control populations. The efforts to reduce populations through vector control play a major role in changing gene frequencies through genetic drift.

Migration

When 2 populations differ in gene frequencies and exchange migrants, the gene frequencies in each population change depending on the proportion of migrant individuals. If a population of all AA individuals receives immigrants from a population of all BB individuals, the frequency of A will decline depending on the numbers of BB immigrants. If the 2 populations exchange migrants continually, migration will cause the 2 populations to have similar gene frequencies. The exchange of mating individuals among populations is referred to as gene flow. Gene flow causes populations to become genetically similar.

The proportion of migrants relative to the total population is called the migration rate *(m)*. Migration rate determines how quickly migration will cause populations to become genetically similar. *m* is an important parameter for arthropod disease vectors because it estimates the potential for the spread of an arthropod-borne pathogen from one population to another.

F-Statistics

One way to estimate *m* is to partition the levels of variation among populations using Wright's F-Statistics. Even though we often refer to individuals in a broad geographic area as members of a population, we frequently observe that individuals exist as clusters—mosquitoes distributed around larval breeding sites, fleas in a rodent burrow, or ticks clustered on vertebrate hosts. These clusters of individuals (I) are called subpopulations (S) within a total population (T). Departures from random mating within and among subpopulations create hierarchical "structuring" in the total population. Wright introduced 3 F-statistics (F_{IS}, F_{ST}, and F_{IT}) as a means of describing the breeding structure of natural populations (Table 25.7).

Nonrandom mating *in* subpopulations is described by F_{IS}, which is the average over all subpopulations of the correlation between uniting gametes relative to

TABLE 25.7 Calculation of F-statistics by partitioning heterozygosity

$$F_{IS} = (H_S - H_I)/H_S$$
$$F_{ST} = (H_T - H_S)/H_T$$
$$F_{IT} = (H_T - H_I)/H_T$$

where:

H_I = Average H_{obs} among subpopulations

H_S = Average H_{exp} among subpopulations
$= 1 - \Sigma p^2_{i,s}$ where $p_{i,s}$ = frequency of the ith allele in subpopulations

H_T = Total expected heterozygosity on the ioverall population
$= 1 - \Sigma \bar{p}_i^2$ where $\bar{p}_i$ = the average frequency of the ith allele among all subpopulations

those of their own subpopulation (Wright 1980). Two gametes are said to be correlated if they share 2 alleles that are identical by descent, meaning that the 2 alleles are derived from the same allele in an ancestral parent. This occurs more often in a system with severe inbreeding or in small isolated subpopulations than in an outbred species with a large effective population size. F_{IS} is calculated as $1 - (Het_{obs}/Het_{exp})$ where Het_{obs} and Het_{exp} are as previously defined. If Het_{obs} and Het_{exp} are equal, $F_{IS} = 0$, the population is in Hardy-Weinberg equilibrium, and there is no correlation between uniting gametes. Inbreeding leads to an excess of homozygotes, or conversely a deficiency in heterozygotes. Thus, $F_{IS} > 0$, the subpopulation is not in Hardy-Weinberg equilibrium, and there is a correlation between uniting gametes. F_{IS} can be less than 0 because it is a correlation and occurs under circumstances that cause excess heterozygotes as discussed previously. The correlation is negative because uniting gametes are more likely to carry alleles that are *not* identical by descent.

Nonrandom mating *among* subpopulations is described by F_{ST}, which is the correlation between random gametes within a subpopulation relative to the gametes within the entire population. F_{ST} is positive when there is restricted gene flow among subpopulations because random gametes from a subpopulation

bear alleles that are more often derived from a common ancestor than gametes from the total population. Genetic drift, founder effects, or local selection cause uniting gametes within a subpopulation to be correlated. F_{ST} is a standardized variance in allele frequencies among populations. Wright described it as the ratio of the observed variance (s^2) in allele frequencies among subpopulations relative to the maximum possible variance under complete isolation of subpopulations. The maximum variance, as discussed previously, is $p(1 - p)$, and F_{ST} can be calculated as $s^2/p(1 - p)$. F_{ST} can also be calculated as $1 - (H_{exp}$ in subpopulations/H_{exp} in the total population) where H_{exp} in subpopulations is the average H_{exp} described earlier, and H_{exp} in the total population is calculated using the same procedure but with the unweighted average allele frequency among subpopulations. Thus, there is a decrease in heterozygosity among subpopulations resulting from the Wahlund Effect discussed earlier.

To summarize nonrandom mating in the entire population, Wright introduced F_{IT} as the correlation between gametes that unite to produce individuals relative to gametes of the total population. This correlation results from nonrandom mating within populations already discussed and summarized in the term F_{IS} and nonrandom mating among subpopulations described by F_{ST} so that $F_{IT} = F_{IS} + F_{ST} - (F_{IS} \lozenge F_{ST})$. F_{IT} is an inbreeding coefficient in the total population resulting from inbreeding within subpopulations and the Wahlund Effect among subpopulations. Alternative ways of calculating F-statistics for particular alleles and loci are summarized in Black and Krafsur (1985).

Estimating Migration

The F-statistic used for determining m is F_{ST}, and Table 25.8 shows how to calculate this statistic from gene frequency data. F_{ST} is related to m as $F_{ST} = 1/(1 + 4Nm)$, or $Nm = (1 - F_{ST})/4F_{ST}$. The value Nm is the product of a potentially large number, population size N, and a potentially small frequency, migration rate m. However, m = number of migrants/N, hence Nm is the absolute number of migrants irrespective of population size. In Table 25.8, $Nm = 0.612$. Thus gene frequency differences between these subpopulations are maintained by approximately 1 individual migrant every 2 generations, regardless of the sizes of the populations. A graph of F_{ST} as a function of Nm is shown in Figure 25.3. This graph illustrates a basic principle of population genetics: very little migration is required to maintain genetic homogeneity among subpopulations. As Nm approaches 10, F_{ST} rapidly drops to 0.

M. Slatkin (1985) developed another method to estimate Nm using the frequency of private alleles in subpopulations. Private alleles are those alleles that are found in only 1 subpopulation. Slatkin estimates Nm using $\ln[p(1)] = a\ln[Nm] + b$, where $p(1)$ is the average frequency of private alleles, $a = 0.505$, and $b = 2.44$ for sample sizes of 25 (corrections for other sample sizes are obtained by dividing Nm by the actual sample size of 25). The biting midge, *C. variipennis* (see Chap. 8) had $Nm = 2.15$ and 6.95 using F_{ST} and Slatkin's method, respectively, among populations in Colorado. The estimated number of individuals

TABLE 25.8 Example of calculating F_{ST} from population gene frequency data

| Subpopulation | Allele frequency (p) / locus | | | |
	1	2	3	4
1	0.3	0.2	0.5	1.0
2	0.25	0.5	0.1	0.5
3	0.5	0.1	0.6	0.0
4	0.7	0.3	0.2	0.0
$\bar{p}$	0.438	0.275	0.350	0.375
$H_S = (2p_i(1-p_i))/4$	0.429	0.355	0.370	0.125
$H_T = 2\bar{p}(1-\bar{p})$	0.429	0.399	0.455	0.469
F_{ST}	0.129	0.110	0.187	0.733
$F_{ST} = 0.290$				

migrating between populations only a few hundred meters from one another was small compared to the estimated thousands of individuals present. The estimated number of migrants refers only to individuals actually exchanging genes, not simply dispersal. On the basis of such small numbers of migrants and the observation of <1% infected insects in the field, it is more likely that the spread of bluetongue virus occurs via infected hosts, not by infected insects (Tabachnick 1992b). Such Nm estimates are directly applicable to models of the spread of introduced genes from one vector population to another. Kambhampati et al. (1989) used the F_{ST} estimates to show an increase in Nm among *Ae. albopictus* subpopulations in Houston between 1986 and 1988.

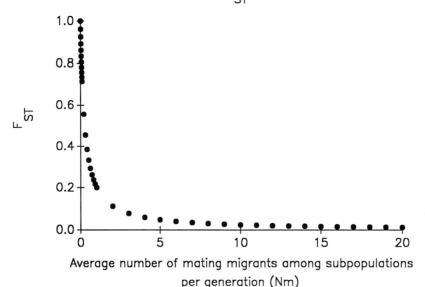

Relationship between the effective migration rate (Nm) and genetic differentiation (F_{ST}) among subpopulations

Average number of mating migrants among subpopulations per generation (Nm)

25.3 The relationship between F_{ST} and Nm.

Often we find a hierarchical structuring to populations. We might sample mosquitoes in a tire yard and call this our basic sampling unit. However, there are often multiple tire yards within a city, several cities within a county, multiple counties within a state, many states within a country. We might be interested in the migration rate within and across these boundaries. Boundaries constructed by humans are artificial, and hierarchical structuring might be identified across habitats such as forests within and among eastern and western regions of a continent, breeding sites within river valleys, and among valleys within a region. We might also be interested in how human activities intervene in the breeding structure of populations. We might consider how much migration exists within and among subpopulations, within abatement districts that differ in insecticidal application procedures, or across herds of cattle (some treated with insecticides, others untreated).

Epidemiologists are often interested in migration across these potential barriers. This problem is circumvented by sampling within the different hierarchies in the field. One would sample several tire yards within a city, in several cities within a county, and in several counties within a state, and finally among states. Wright's F_{ST} can be partitioned into different components and Nm estimated using F_{ST} among tire yards within a city, among cities within counties, among counties within a state, and among states. The approach has been termed nested spatial sampling and has been used in a number of different studies (Black et al. 1988a; Kambhampati et al. 1989).

Mutation

The mutation of alleles into variant forms is the ultimate source of new genetic material. The effect on genetic variation is dependent on the mutation rate (u), which for allozymes is usually estimated on the order of 10^{-6} per locus per generation. Mutation rates alone are not believed to be high enough to play a major role in the population genetics of a species. However, mutation rates in noncoding regions, especially in highly repetitive sequences with simple repeat structures, are known to be greater, and mutation rates cannot be ignored when using these in population studies. Mutation rates in these regions are probably greater because they do not code for a gene product and are, therefore, not constrained by selection. However, if they occur as tandem repeats, specific molecular events can cause them to mutate at a greater rate. The intergenic spacer (IGS) in the ribosomal DNA (rDNA) cistron is discussed later as an example of this.

Selection

Natural selection can play an important role in causing genetic variation among populations whenever genotypes differ in the fitness (W) they confer to the individual. Evolutionary biologists define W in terms of the relative fitness of one genotype compared to other genotypes in the population. A simple way to view the relative nature of W is to consider 3 genotypes in a population and to assign the probability of each genotype surviving to reproduction (viability). The fitnesses relative to each other can be defined by setting the most fit genotype to one and comparing the other relative fitnesses as:

Genotype	AA	AB	BB
Viability	0.75	0.75	0.5
W	.75/.75 =1.0	1.0	.5/.75 = 0.67

Because the BB genotype has W = 0.67 relative to the other genotypes in the population, it is the least fit genotype, and its frequency and the frequency of B will decline in this population. Consider an alternative case in which the heterozygote has the greatest relative fitness. A well-known example of this occurs with the human β globin and resistance to *falciparum* malaria in West Africa. Three alleles in the β globin gene are denoted A, C, and S. Homozygotes for S have sickle cell disease that causes severe anemia and greatly reduced life span. When red blood cells of SS individuals experience low oxygen tension in the peripheral circulatory system, they tend to collapse and form a sickle shape. There is an abnormal tertiary structure of the globin protein that causes the hemoglobin to form long sharp crystals under low oxygen tension; these crystals pierce and kill the malarial trophozoites in the red blood cell. Malaria is a major cause of mortality in Africa. Individuals (especially children) that are AA homozygotes are susceptible to mortality from malaria.

AS homozygotes are resistant to mortality from malaria, and their red blood cells do not sickle in the peripheral circulatory system. Cavalli-Sforza and Bodmer (1971) set the fitness of AS to 1 and estimated the relative fitness of AA to be 0.89 in the presence of malaria and the relative fitness of SS to be 0.20 due to sickle cell anemia. Selection leading to highest fitness in the heterozygote is referred to as overdominance, or balancing selection. Note that this type of selection maintains 2 alleles, even potentially deleterious alleles, in the population. There are numerous other types of selection that are beyond the scope of this chapter. These include selection against heterozygotes, selection with dominance or additive effects among alleles, and frequency dependent selection.

Determining the fitnesses of specific genotypes is not easy; indeed, some would argue it is impossible. The rate with which selection can act is proportional to the fitness differences between genotypes, and such differences are dependent on the environment in which the population is found. Furthermore, the effect of the gene in question must be isolated from the effects of other genes, which becomes a problem when closely linked genes influence fitness. For example, the frequency of phosphoglucomutase alleles in *Cx. pipiens* populations in the central valley of California correlate with temperature. Although this might indicate selection at this locus, selection at closely linked loci results in the same observation. Overwintering larval populations of *Culicoides variipennis* show seasonal cycles of gene frequencies at 2 isozyme loci, which also suggests either the action of selection at the loci or selection operating on closely linked loci. There is little direct evidence that any of the molecularly based markers commonly used in population genetics, including RAPDs, RFLPs, SSLPs, and inversions, have a measurable effect on fitness. Many of these markers are considered to be neutral in their impact on fitness, and variation in their frequencies among populations is most likely caused by migration, mutation, population size, and drift.

With the exception of selection for and against genes that condition resistance to insecticides, on which selection is expected to have a large effect, no research exists on the fitness of specific genes and genotypes in arthropod vectors. The relative fitness of insecticide-susceptible and -resistant genotypes has been estimated in treated and untreated environments. Wood and Bishop (1981) estimated fitness of resistant homozygotes in both *An. culifacies* and *An. stephensi* to DDT, dieldrin, and malathion. In the insecticide environments, the fitness of resistant genotypes were from 1.3–6.1 relative to susceptible genotypes. Fitness in untreated environments were 0.44–0.97. Such studies enable management practices to reduce the development of resistant populations. Once vector capacity genotypes are identified, experiments on fitness will be necessary to determine causes of observed variation within and among populations.

A long-standing question in evolutionary biology and population genetics, called the selectionist-neutralist debate, concerns the origin and significance of biochemical and molecular polymorphisms. Are there differences in relative fitness among allozyme genotypes? Selectionists believe that allozyme genotypes differ in fitness. They believe that many mutations have occurred at a particular genetic locus; however, the majority are lethal or deleterious. Rare mutations occur that confer greater fitness, are adaptive, and increase in frequency. Selectionists argue that many allozymes are maintained through overdominance. One allele confers greater fitness in one habitat whereas another confers greater fitness in another habitat; a heterozygote can have the highest fitness because it can use resources in both habitats.

Neutralists agree that most mutations are deleterious; however, they believe that there are many mutations that become established in populations that have no effect on fitness. Some argue that there are so many gene products in an organism interacting in such complex ways to influence fitness that it is hard to believe, outside of a deleterious or lethal mutation, that any single locus can significantly affect fitness. Neutralists believe that neutral alleles become established in populations through genetic drift, and that their frequencies are not determined by adaptive mechanisms. The father of the neutralist school, M. Kimura, showed that the probability of a new, neutral allele eventually becoming fixed in a population is 1/2N, where N is actual population size (Kimura 1983). He found that these are fixed in $4N_e$ generations where N_e is the effective population number but will be lost in $(2N_e/N)\ln(2N)$ generations. The second term is always smaller than the first. Therefore, in populations with small subpopulations, neutral alleles have a finite probability of fixation. However, it takes longer for them to be fixed rather than to be lost, and as a result, most will be lost. The selectionist-neutralist debate is difficult to resolve empirically because of the difficulty associated with separating the effects of a single gene from the genetic background in which it occurs. Experimental approaches to estimating fitness are available (Endler 1986; Manly 1985) but are beyond the scope of this chapter.

Interactions of Evolutionary Factors

The many factors that we have outlined interact with one another in populations. Wright developed a model in which selection, migration, and drift interact in shaping the breeding structure of natural populations (see Wright 1980). This is referred to as an adaptive landscape model in Wright's shifting balance theory.

Figure 25.4 shows a plot of the average fitness of individuals in a population in which 3 genotypes are segregating and where, as in the malaria resistance–sickle cell balance discussed earlier, the heterozygote has the highest W. If the relative fitness of the 2 homozygous genotypes is equal, then the maximum average fitness occurs when the frequency of heterozygotes is greatest or when $p = q = 0.5$. Note that when the relative fitness of the 2 homozygote classes is not equal (as in the malaria resistance–sickle cell balance), then the maximum fitness will not occur at $p = q = 0.5$. The relationship between gene frequency and average W is an adaptive landscape.

Now let us consider 2 loci that interact with one another to influence fitness. Although there are 9 possible genotypes, assume that the genotypes with the highest fitnesses are AAbb, AaBb, and aaBB, and the low fitness genotypes are aabb and AABB. Figure 25.5 shows an adaptive landscape for the interactions between these 2 loci where a "+" represents a peak for a genotype with high fitness and a "–" represents a valley for a low fitness genotype. It is important to note that although selection will act to maximize the average fitness of the population, individuals with lower fitness genotypes will continually arise as offspring of the most fit individuals in the population because all 4 alleles are still segregating in these individuals. High-fitness genotypes are selected, whereas low-fitness genotypes are selected against, meaning that individuals of lower fitness will not survive to reproduce or will produce fewer offspring. As a result, if the gene frequencies of the population are such that the initial genotypic frequency is at the base of a peak, selection,

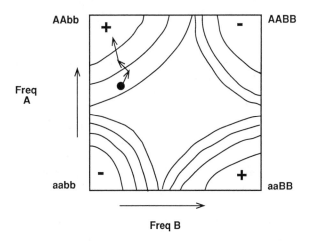

25.4 An example of an adaptive landscape, plotting the relationship between gene frequency and average, W

25.5 An adaptive landscape showing fitness relationships of different genotypes, fitness peaks, and fitness valleys

by itself, will move the population up this peak (see Fig. 25.5). Selection cannot change the population to a lower fitness by moving through a valley. Selection is opportunistic, and the peak for the population is often not the highest peak or the most optimal. The effect is to select the population for the nearest local peak, which can be determined strictly by past history and chance. Thus, biologists should not attempt to seek optimality stories in every observable trait.

Wright's shifting balance theory incorporates the interactions of migration, selection, and drift into a comprehensive theory showing how different fitness peaks can be tested and explored in any population or species. Although selection by itself cannot move populations to different peaks, drift can allow new combinations of genes to arise so that populations can "explore" different fitness peaks. In small subpopulations, genetic drift can allow the movement of a subpopulation to the base of a new, higher peak, where selection can then push the subpopulation to this peak. Because this subpopulation now has the highest fitness, individuals from this subpopulation spread to other subpopulations, and soon the entire population reaches a new adaptive peak.

The adaptive landscape changes if the environment changes because fitnesses are directly related to the environment of the population. Wright's shifting balance theory is an important model. Although it has not been completely explored to determine its full applicability to natural populations, it does provide a way to discuss interactions.

The roles of migration, drift, selection, and their interactions remain to be explored in arthropod vectors. Estimates of these important population parameters are necessary to understand vector evolution, vector-pathogen interactions, and the effects of insect control strategies on vector breeding structure. There is some debate concerning the coevolution of arthropods and various pathogens that they vector. Coevolution occurs when there is a reciprocal relationship, such that a change in species A causes a change in species B, which causes species A to change. The demonstration of coevolutionary relationships provides a mechanism to understand why specific species serve as vectors of specific pathogens.

We emphasize that adaptation is not necessary to explain all genetic variation in a population or species. The processes of genetic drift, mutation, and migration are extremely important. The association of a particular arthropod with a particular arbovirus or other pathogen may have little to do with adaptation. Past history of the species, random chance, and chance mutation can be factors. If coevolution is a major factor in vector-pathogen relationships, specific traits responsible for interactions must be identified and their fitness determined to demonstrate that variants of the pathogen affect the fitness of genotypes in the vector population. Variants in the vector also must influence the fitness differences between variants of the pathogen.

DETERMINING GENETIC RELATIONSHIPS BETWEEN POPULATIONS

Gene frequencies can be used to estimate the overall genetic relatedness among populations. A variety of measures are available to estimate the genetic similarity and hence the genetic distance using observed gene frequencies of any pair of populations. We present only 1 of many measures of genetic relatedness, the genetic distance (D) value of M. Nei (1972). The determination of the genetic similarity, I, of any population pair is illustrated for 2 populations, where the allele frequencies at locus k are Population A: *a1, a2, a3, . . . ai* and Population B: *b1, b2, b3, . . . bi*. The genetic similarity is calculated as

$$I = \Sigma a_i b_i / \sqrt{\Sigma a_i^2 \Sigma b_i^2}$$

Examples of calculations are shown in Table 25.9. The genetic similarity for each locus sampled is calculated and then used to estimate the overall similarity using

$$I = I_{ab} / \sqrt{I_a I_b}$$

where I_{ab}, I_a, I_b = arithmetic averages over all loci of $\Sigma a_i b_i$, Σa_i^2, Σb_i^2, respectively.

The genetic distance between any pair of populations is $D = -\ln(I)$.

TABLE 25.9 Estimating Nei's genetic distance (D) and genetic similarity (I)

Population		
1.	A: $a_1 = 1.0$ B: $b_1 = 1.0$	$I = 1 \times 1 / \sqrt{1^2 + 1^2} = 1$
2.	A: $a_1 = 1.0$ $a_2 = 0.0$ B: $b_1 = 0.0$ $b_2 = 1.0$	$I = \dfrac{(1 \times 0) + (0 \times 1)}{\sqrt{(1^2 + 0^2)(0^2 + 1^2)}} = 0$
3.	A: $a_1 = 0.1$ $a_2 = 0.9$ B: $b_1 = 0.8$ $b_2 = 0.2$	$I = \dfrac{(0.1 \times 0.8) + (0.9 \times 0.2)}{\sqrt{(0.1^2 + 0.9^2)(0.8^2 + 0.2^2)}}$ $= \dfrac{0.26}{0.75} = 0.35$

Because the 2 populations in Table 25.9 differ for all 3 loci, to calculate the overall I and D values between them:

$$
\begin{aligned}
I_{ab} &= (1 + 0 + 0.26)/3 = 0.42 \\
I_a &= (1 + 1 + 0.82)/3 = 0.94 \\
I_b &= (1 + 1 + 0.68)/3 = 0.89 \\
I &= 0.42/\sqrt{0.94 \times 0.89} = 0.459 \\
\text{Thus } D &= -\ln 0.459 = 0.779.
\end{aligned}
$$

Genetic distance values have been determined among populations and species of many different arthropod disease vectors. Often when there are many different population or species comparisons, it is useful to view genetic relationships diagrammatically in the form of a dendrogram. One method of converting genetic distance or similarity values into dendrograms is the unweighted pair-group method with arithmetic mean (UPGMA). The following is a genetic distance matrix, showing all the genetic distance (D) values between every pair of 4 different populations:

	A	B	C	D
A	—	0.1	0.01	0.05
B		—	0.12	0.07
C			—	0.08
D				—

Using the UPGMA method, a tree is constructed by first joining the 2 populations or species with the smallest distance. Therefore, populations A and C are joined at distance D = 0.01. Next one constructs a new matrix using the now previously joined species as 1 unit, with its distance to the next unit as its average from all populations within the unit. Population D's average distance from the A and C unit is 1/2(0.05 + 0.08) = 0.065. B's distance from the new unit (A,C,D) is 1/3(0.1 + 0.12 + 0.08) = 0.1. The resulting dendrogram with the nodes at 0.01, 0.065, and 0.1, respectively, is illustrated in Figure 25.6.

When calculating genetic distances among subpopulations, often certain loci contribute more to the overall variation than other loci. This can also be observed when calculating F-statistics, and estimates of migration rates can be greatly influenced by single loci. Furthermore, the dendrograms derived from separate loci are not always congruent. There are no simple explanations for this phenomenon. If all loci were neutral and all alleles were sampled equally from subpopulations, genetic distance estimates from the various loci should be equal and dendrograms should be congruent. The fact that this is rarely seen suggests confounding effects of selection, genetic drift, and migration in shaping the breeding structure of natural populations. A FORTRAN computer program, BIOSYS–1 performs most of the analyses described in this chapter (Swofford and Selander 1981), including derivation of F-statistics and dendrograms using individual loci. Thus, contributions of individual loci can be identified.

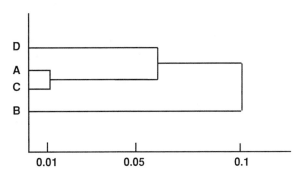

25.6 The resulting dendrogram, based on the genetic distances between units A, B, C, and D above

There are many examples of using genetic relationships to understand the evolution of arthropod vectors and to provide information concerning vectors' roles in disease epidemiology. More than 100 populations of *Ae. aegypti* have been analyzed worldwide for genetic variation using isozyme markers (Tabachnick 1991). Genetic relationships demonstrated that there were 2 subspecies, a domestic *Ae. aegypti aegypti* and the sylvan *Ae. aegypti formosus*. The domestic form is more often associated with disease transmission, particularly in the Caribbean area, where it is the predominant vector of dengue viruses. The structure of genetic relationships between populations in different geographic regions is consistent with the migration of *Ae. aegypti aegypti* from its ancestral home in Africa to other regions of the world as a consequence of human transport, most likely shipping. The average genetic distance between the *Ae. aegypti* subspecies is about one-fifth that found between subspecies for many other insect species. Several studies demonstrate the direct relation between the time of separation of 2 populations or species and the magnitude of genetic distance. The longer the time of separation, the greater the genetic differences that accumulate. In the case of *Ae. aegypti*, the low D values are consistent with a short time since the origin of the domestic form. Because the domestic form is adapted to oviposition in human water storage containers, its origins probably occurred in the relatively recent past when humans began storing water. Kambhampati et al. (1991) used genetic distance analysis to verify that the newly introduced U.S. and Brazilian populations of *Ae. albopictus* originated in Japan.

Analyses of genetic distance values have also proved to be useful in understanding *C. variipennis* and the epidemiology of the bluetongue viruses. A survey of *C. variipennis* populations in the United States and an analysis of their genetic relationships demonstrated the existence of at least 3 different subspecies. Extensive epidemiologic surveys have shown that bluetongue disease has never been reported in the northeastern region of the United States despite the presence of *C. variipennis* and suitable domestic ruminant hosts. The information is consistent with the view that the subspecies of *C. variipennis* present in the northeastern region of the United States is not an efficient vector. Such information can be used to declare this region as bluetongue free. Thus, the unrestricted movement of livestock and animal germplasm from this region of the United States to bluetongue-free countries would be possible, thereby resulting in economic gain for U.S. industries.

DNA-BASED MOLECULAR POPULATION GENETICS

Genetic Markers

The use of DNA-based molecular markers is only beginning to be applied to vector population genetics. Many of the new techniques have the advantage, compared with isozyme electrophoresis, of being able to assess genetic variation at the nucleotide level. Variation in isozyme mobility is an indicator of nucleotide variation. However, 2 isozymes with the same migration rate may not be the products of equivalent alleles. Hence, isozyme electrophoresis underestimates genetic variation. Assays of variation at the DNA level, either through restriction-site polymorphism or direct sequencing, provide a more accurate measure of variation. In addition, isozyme markers are limited in number whereas nucleotide variation can be sampled throughout the genome as long as appropriate probes, primers, or clones are available.

Ribosomal DNA

The structure and function of the ribosomal DNA cistron is described in Chapter 26. rDNA genes occur as 100–5000 tandem repeats. Each repeat contains 18s, 5.8s, and 28s rRNA genes alternating with a large IGS region. Because of the tandem repeat structure, the rDNA genes form a multigene family. A curious feature of multigene families is that members exhibit homogeneity within species. If a mutation is found in 1 gene member, it is often distributed among all members. Even noncoding regions that diverge rapidly among closely related taxa are conserved within a species. This is inconsistent with a hypothesis of independent evolution and suggests instead that some mechanism constrains members to evolve in concert. This observation of concerted evolution suggests the operation of molecular drive (Dover 1982). Mutations can spread throughout a multigene family principally through the processes of unequal crossing over and gene conversion. Through molecular drive, variants become established and potentially fixed in a population or species in a manner operationally distinct from selection and genetic drift.

In this section, we focus on the IGS because it is this region that usually varies in size and sequence within a species. Whereas the rRNA coding regions are central to the construction and functioning of the ribosome and conserved within species, the IGS frequently varies intraspecifically in sequence and length and does not appear to be under the same intensity of selection. The IGS frequently consists of tandem direct or nested repeats that vary in size. Unequal crossing over, gene conversion, and slippage replication within and among these repeats can cause the IGS to vary in length within an individual and within a species. The patterns of IGS size variation are species specific and dependent upon forces operating at molecular and population levels, for example, repeat patterns within the IGS, copy numbers, chromosomal locations, and effective population size.

A number of studies have attempted to use the size of the entire IGS or subrepeats within the IGS to determine genetic distances among populations. Restriction enzymes that cut in the 5' end of the 18s and the 3' end of the 28s are used, or alternatively an enzyme is employed that cuts within a tandem repeat in the IGS. This DNA is subjected to Southern analysis and probed with a homologous IGS probe. Many bands are often revealed on the autoradiograph due to the many IGS copies in an individual, but certain bands predominate, thus indicating a prevailing spacer or subrepeat. Studies have shown enormous variation in the size and numbers of bands among individuals in a subpopulation. Furthermore, individuals within subpopulations usually share more bands than individuals from different subpopulations, even those within close proximity.

Because the processes of concerted evolution are complex, there are no models with which to estimate genetic distance. Instead, multivariate techniques that make few assumptions concerning the genetics of multigene families must be used. Black et al. (1988b) used canonical discriminant analysis and the derived Mahalanobis distances to test for differentiation of *Ae. albopictus* populations based on IGS spacer and subspacer lengths. Populations that shared more bands were judged to be similar. Nested spatial sampling and hierarchical cluster analysis were used to partition variation in spacer lengths among various populations. No relationship was observed between statistical distance and geographic distance, and 80% of the total variation in spacer sizes occurred among individuals within a population. The results indicated that concerted evolution occurs quickly within populations, thereby resulting in unique sets of predominant spacers. Because this occurs independently in every population and is not strongly influenced by genetic drift, migration, and probably selection, there is no relationship between genetic distance and geographic distance.

These same patterns have been observed in studies of other vector species. Although all of the data gathered to date supports the notion of rapid concerted evolution of IGS lengths and subrepeats within mosquito populations, this precludes the effects of migration and genetic drift. Although much local genetic differentiation is found in mosquito populations, supported by observations with isozymes, no useful way exists to use rDNA information in population genetic studies in which information on migration or genetic distance are desired. rDNA variation has proven to be useful as a fingerprinting tool in insects, although it has not been employed in this way in any vector species.

Mitochondrial DNA

Mitochondrial DNA (mtDNA) offers another molecular marker for population genetics. MtDNA is primarily maternally inherited. Unlike nuclear markers, there is no recombination among genomes of different maternal clones. Studies of intraspecific variation in mtDNA have shown that one or more maternal clones often characterize local populations. The presence of these clones outside of their typical ranges provides information on gene flow and dispersal. The number of maternal clones in populations provides information on the number of females founding new populations, and thus evidence for population bottlenecks. Because of this sensitivity, it is possible to map distributional and founding events of populations through their matrilineality. This makes it possible to trace maternal lineages and to determine the phylogenies of existing populations independent of founder effects and selection or adaptation. Such evidence cannot be obtained as easily from studies of genomic systems experiencing recombination or biparental inheritance. MtDNA evolves at a rate approximately 10 times faster than nuclear DNA, and therefore, intraspecific variation is frequently detectable.

To date, mtDNA has not proven to be very useful in understanding the population structure of vectors. Kambhampati and Rai (1991) examined RFLP variation among 17 worldwide populations of *Ae. albopictus* and found 99% of fragments were shared among the populations. Mitchell et al. (1992) found similarly low variability in mtDNA RFLPs in the 4 sibling species of the *An. quadrimaculatus* species group. This low variability suggests either that populations were too recent in origin to have accumulated differences or that the mtDNA in Culicidae evolves slowly.

RAPD-PCR and AP-PCR

Techniques that employ the polymerase chain reaction (PCR) to amplify arbitrary regions of genomes have recently been described. These are technically simple, do not

STEP 1. PRIMER ANNEALING

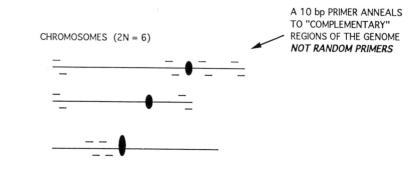

CHROMOSOMES (2N = 6)

A 10 bp PRIMER ANNEALS TO "COMPLEMENTARY" REGIONS OF THE GENOME *NOT RANDOM PRIMERS*

STEP 2: PRIMER EXTENSION - TAQ POLYMERASE

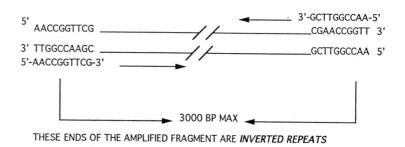

5' AACCGGTTCG ————————//———— 3'-GCTTGGCCAA-5'
                                   CGAACCGGTT 3'
3' TTGGCCAAGC ————————//———————GCTTGGCCAA 5'
5'-AACCGGTTCG-3' ————————→

←———————— 3000 BP MAX ←————————

THESE ENDS OF THE AMPLIFIED FRAGMENT ARE *INVERTED REPEATS*

INVERTED REPEAT DNA SEQUENCES ARE FOUND IN:
A) HETEROCHROMATIC REGIONS
   TELOMERES
   CENTROMERES
B) THE ENDS OF TRANSPOSABLE ELEMENTS

AMPLIFIED REGIONS ARE NOT RANDOMLY LOCATED

STEP 3: AMPLIFICATION BY PCR

25.7 The mechanism of RAPD-PCR

require the use of radioactive nucleotides, and DNA-based polymorphisms can be visualized in a 24 hour period. Because the techniques employ PCR, they also enable entomologists to examine genetic variation in small arthropod vectors (e.g., Ceratopogonidae, or mites). RAPD-PCR is an acronym from random-amplified polymorphic DNA amplified by PCR. By contrast, AP-PCR stands for arbitrarily primed DNA amplified by PCR. Both techniques employ single primers to amplify arbitrary regions of the genome. The mechanism of RAPD-PCR is shown in Figure 25.7.

An agarose gel showing RAPD-PCR amplified products from *C. variipennis* appears in Figure 25.8. Polymorphisms at loci amplified by arbitrarily primed PCR are usually expressed as dominant markers. The phenotype of an individual that is homozygous or heterozygous for an amplifiable sequence produces a fragment of a specific molecular weight. In contrast, a homozygous recessive individual does not produce that fragment. In many studies, often greater than 95% of polymorphisms at RAPD-PCR loci segregated as recessives.

The dominance of most RAPD-PCR alleles presents a problem for population genetics studies. Mating patterns in populations cannot be studied because testing for Hardy-Weinberg equilibrium requires identification of both alleles at a locus. If we make the assumption that a population is in Hardy-Weinberg equilibrium, then the frequency of the recessive allele (q) can be calculated as the square root of the frequency of homozygous recessive (blank) individuals (q^2). Under this assumption, the techniques discussed that utilize allele frequencies can be applied to studies of RAPD-PCR variation. RAPD-PCR has been used for population genetic studies of vectors (Ballinger-Crabtree et al. 1992) and in fingerprinting studies to estimate the numbers of full sibling families at oviposition sites (Apostol et al. 1993).

CONCLUSIONS

Population genetic studies of arthropod vectors have improved our understanding of the dynamics of vector populations in general and genetic relationships among these populations in particular. This knowledge has and will continue to increase our ability to

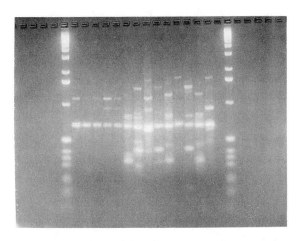

25.8   RAPD-PCR results using individual *C. variipennis*

understand and more efficiently control arthropod-borne diseases. The application of molecular genetic technologies to study variation at the nucleic acid level offers exciting new tools for vector population biology.

REFERENCES AND FURTHER READING

Apostol B. L., W.C. Black, B.R. Miller, and B.J. Beaty. 1993. Estimation of the number of full sibling families at an oviposition site using RAPD-PCR markers: applications to the mosquito *Aedes aegypti. Theor. Appl. Genet.* 86:991–1000.

Ballinger-Crabtree, M.E., W.C. Black, and B.R. Miller. 1992. Use of genetic polymorphism detected by RAPD-PCR for differentiation and identification of *Aedes albopictus* subspecies and populations. *Am. J. Trop. Med. Hyg.* 47:893–901.

Black, W.C. IV, and E.S. Krafsur. 1985. A FORTRAN program for analysis of genotypic frequencies and description of the breeding structure of populations. *Theor. Appl. Genet.* 70:484–490.

Black, W.C. IV, J.A. Ferrari, K.S. Rai, and D.A. Sprenger. 1988a. Breeding structure of a colonizing species: *Aedes albopictus* in the United States. *Heredity* 60:173–181.

Black, W.C. IV, D.K. McLain, and K.S. Rai. 1988b. Patterns of variation in the rDNA cistron within and among populations of the mosquito, *Aedes albopictus* (Skuse). *Genetics* 121:539–550.

Cavalli-Sforza, L.L., and W.F. Bodmer. 1971. *The genetics of human populations.* San Francisco: W.H. Freeman.

Cheng, M.L., C.S. Hacker, S.C. Pryor, R.E. Ferrell, and G.B. Kitto. 1982. The ecological genetics of the *Culex pipiens* complex in North America. In: W.W.M. Steiner et al., editors, *Recent developments in the genetics of insect disease vectors.* Champaign, IL: Stipes Publishing. pp. 581–687.

Colluzi, M., and A. Sabatini. 1969. Cytogenetic observations on the saltwater species, *Anopheles merus* and *Anopheles melas* of the gambiae complex. *Parassitologia* 11:177–187.

Dover, G. 1982. Molecular drive: A cohesive mode of species evolution. *Nature* 299:111–117.

Dunbar, R.W., and C.G. Vajime. 1981. Cytotaxonomy of the *Simulium damnosum* complex. In: M. Laird, editor, *Blackflies: The future of biological methods in integrated control.* London: Academic Press. pp. 31–43.

Endler, J.A. 1986. *Natural selection in the wild.* Princeton: Princeton University Press.

Gooding, R.H. 1982. Classification of nine species and subspecies of tsetse flies (Diptera: Glossinidae: *Glossina* Wiedemann) based on molecular genetics and breeding data. *Can. J. Zoology* 60:2737–2744.

Hartl, D.L., and A.G. Clark. 1989. *Principles of population genetics.* 3rd ed. Sunderland, MA: Sinauer Associates.

Hilburn, L.R., and P.W. Sattler. 1986. Electrophoretically detectable protein variation in natural populations of the lone star tick, *Amblyomma americanum* (Acari: Ixodidae). *Heredity* 56:67–74.

Kambhampati, S., W.C. Black IV, and K.S. Rai. 1991. Geographic origin of U.S. and Brazilian *Aedes albopictus* inferred from allozyme analysis. *Heredity* 67:85–94.

Kambhampati, S., W.C. Black IV, K.S. Rai, and D.A. Sprenger. 1989. Temporal variation in the genetic structure of a colonizing species: *Aedes albopictus* (Skuse) in the United States. *Heredity* 64:281–287.

Kambhampati, S., and K.S. Rai. 1991. Mitochondrial DNA variation within and among populations of the mosquito *Aedes albopictus. Genome* 34:288–292.

Kassem, H.A., D.J. Fryauff, B.M. El Sawaf, M.G. Shehat, and N.F. Shoumar. 1990. Electrophoretic comparison of the *Leishmania* vectors *Phlebotomus papatasi* and *P. langeroni* (Diptera: Psychodidae). *J. Med. Entomol.* 27:592–601.

Kimura, M. 1983. The neutral theory of molecular evolution. Cambridge: Cambridge University Press.

Lanzaro, G.C., S.K. Narang, and J.A. Seawright. 1990. Speciation in an anopheline (Diptera: Culicidae) mosquito: Enzyme polymorphism and the genetic structure of populations. *Ann. Entomol. Soc. Am.* 83:578–585.

Manly, B.F.J. 1985. *The statistics of natural selection.* London: Chapman and Hall.

Matthews, T.C., and L.E. Munstermann. 1983. Genetic diversity and differentiation in northern populations of the tree-hole mosquito *Aedes hendersoni* (Diptera: Culicidae). *Ann. Entomol. Soc. Am.* 76:1005–1010.

McLain, D.K., and F.H. Collins. 1989. Structure of rDNA in the mosquito *Anopheles gambiae* and rDNA sequence variation within and between species of the *Anopheles gambiae* complex. *Heredity* 62:247–256.

Miles, S.J. 1978. Enzyme variation in the *Anopheles gambiae* Giles group of species (Diptera: Culicidae). *Bull. Ent. Res.* 68:85–96.

Mitchell, S.E., S.K. Narang, A.F. Cockburn, J.A. Seawright, and M. Goldenthal. 1992. Mitochondrial and ribosomal DNA variation among members of the *Anopheles quadrimaculatus* (Diptera: Culicidae) species complex. *Genome* 35:939–950.

Munstermann, L.E. 1985. Geographic patterns of genetic variation in the treehole mosquito. In: L.P. Lounibos, J.R. Rey, and J.H. Frank, editors, *Ecology of mosquitoes: Proceedings of a workshop.* Vero Beach, FL: Florida Medical Entomology Laboratory. pp. 327–343.

Murphy, R.W., J.W. Sites Jr., D.G. Buth, and C.H. Haufler. 1990. Proteins 1: Isozyme electrophoresis. In: D.M. Hillis and C. Moritz, editors, *Molecular sytematics.* Sunderland, MA. Sinauer Associates: pp. 45–126.

Nei, M. 1972. Genetic distance between populations. *Am. Nat.* 106:283–292.

———. 1975. *Molecular population genetics and evolution.* New York: American Elsevier,

Pashley, D.P., K.S. Rai, and D.N. Pashley. 1985. Patterns of allozyme relationships compared with morphology, hybridization, and geological history in allopatric island dwelling mosquitoes. *Evolution* 39:985–987.

Post, R.J., and J.M. Crampton. 1988. The taxonomic use of variation in repetitive DNA sequences in *Simulium damnosum* complex. In: M.W. Service, editor, *Biosystematics of haematophagous insects.* Oxford: Clarendon Press. pp. 245–255.

Sattler, P.W., L.R. Hilburn, R.B. Davey, J.E. George, and J.B.R. Avalos. 1986. Genetic similarity and variability between natural populations and laboratory colonies of North American *Boophilus* (Acari: Ixodidae). *Ann. Entomol. Soc. Amer.* 72:95–100.

Slatkin, M. 1985. Rare alleles as indicators of gene flow. *Evolution* 39:53–65.

Swofford, D.L., and R.B. Selander. 1981. BIOSYS–1: A FORTRAN program for the comprehensive analysis of electrophoretic data in population genetics and systematics. *J. Heredity* 72:281–283.

Tabachnick, W.J. 1991. Evolutionary genetics and arthropod-borne disease: The yellow fever mosquito. *Am. Entomol.* 37:14–24.

———. 1992a. Genetic differentiation among North American populations of *Culicoides variipennis* (Diptera: Ceratopogonidae), the North American vector of bluetongue virus. *Ann. Entomol. Soc. Am.* 85:140–147.

———. 1992b. Microgeographic and temporal patterns of genetic variation in natural populations of *Culicoides variipennis* (Diptera: Ceratopogonidae). *J. Med. Entomol.* 29:384–395.

Wesson, D.M., D.K. McLain, J.H. Oliver, J. Piesman, and F.H. Collins. 1993. Investigation of the validity of species status of *Ixodes dammini* (Acari: Ixodidae) using ribosomal DNA. *Proc. Natl. Acad. Sci. USA* 90:10221–10225.

Wood, R.A., and J. A. Bishop. 1981. Insecticide resistance: genes and mechanisms. In: J.A. Bishop and L.M. Cook, editors, *Genetic consequences of man-made change.* London: Academic Press. pp. 97–127.

Wright, S. 1980. Genic and organismal selection. *Evolution* 34:825–843.

26. MOLECULAR TAXONOMY AND SYSTEMATICS OF ARTHROPOD VECTORS

William C. Black IV and Leonard E. Munstermann

DEFINITIONS

Taxonomy is the theory and practice of classifying organisms (Mayr and Ashlock 1991). It is a science that originated more than 2 centuries ago and thus draws from extensive accumulated information on morphology, biogeography, and habitat distributions of a large proportion of extant species. This information base has permitted the construction of thousands of keys for species identification; however, as knowledge of biological species has become more detailed, morphological characters have not always proved sufficient for correct classification. This chapter discusses taxonomic groups in which identification has been difficult or impossible with morphological characters and, in these cases, emphasizes the molecular taxonomic approach to classification. Molecular taxonomy is the classification and identification of organisms based on protein or nucleic acid characters rather than morphological characters.

Correct species identification is critical to medical entomologists during suppression of disease outbreaks and in associated epidemiological and ecological studies. There are a variety of circumstances in which a molecular approach to taxonomy can improve the speed and accuracy of vector species identification.

Systematics is the study of evolutionary relationships among taxa. Molecular systematists study evolutionary relationships using molecular characters.

Proteins and nucleic acid sequences provide large numbers of characters for phylogenetic analysis in addition to the morphological characters usually studied in a group. Molecular systematics has been and continues to be a powerful tool in the study of evolutionary relationships among hematophagous arthropod taxa, providing important clues on the genetic relationships among different groups as well as information on evolutionary origins.

When objective phylogenies derived through molecular systematic investigations are examined in the context of the hosts, habitats, or biogeographical distributions of vector species, valuable information on the modes of speciation can be derived. Examination of derived molecular phylogenies in both vectors and pathogens allows the testing of hypotheses concerning host-parasite cospeciation.

OVERVIEW

We begin by giving several examples of medically important taxa that have proven to be troublesome for separation by morphological analysis, and we indicate how these species groups have thwarted epidemiological and ecological studies. The ways in which molecular taxonomy can overcome these difficulties are described. Different molecular and biochemical techniques are described the taxonomic procedures to follow in testing their validity are listed. We end with a discussion of applications of molecular systematics in medical entomology.

WHY BOTHER WITH MOLECULAR TAXONOMY?

Medical entomologists and epidemiologists are often called upon to identify the vectors involved in the outbreak of an arthropod-borne disease. Once a correct identification has been made, control programs can interrupt disease transmission by accessing critical information on adult and larval habitats, host preference, ecology, vector competence, histories of earlier epidemics, and ultimately the control tactics that are appropriate for that species. In prevention and abatement programs, monitoring of vector or reservoir populations for the prevalence of infected individuals requires correct species identification. Furthermore, prevention and control is often focused directly on the vector species of concern (species sanitation). Certainly, research on the ecology and geographic and seasonal distributions of vector species also requires accurate identification.

The number of hematophagous arthropod species is vast (Table 26.1). Each of the groups listed contains genera whose member species are often difficult to separate based on morphology. The taxonomic problems in many of these groups is summarized in a recent series of reviews (Service 1988). The taxonomy of arthropod vectors can be a daunting task, requiring extensive time, training, and experience. This can severely limit the scope of epidemiological or ecological studies with these species, to say nothing of the inability to react quickly in control or abatement programs.

Often the species composition in a geographic region is well known, and correct identifications are obtained without the need of highly trained taxonomists. For the bulk of identifications, the morphological characters are clear, and the species designation is conclusive; however, for some taxa, problems in identification can arise. For example, sibling species or species that can be easily distinguished only during a single life stage may be present. Moreover, minute arthropods require careful preparation before identification is possible.

TABLE 26.1   Numbers of species in the major arthropod groups that are reported to feed on vertebrates (modified from Crosskey 1988)

Order or suborder	Group	Number of species described worldwide
Class Insecta		
Anoplura	sucking lice (all families)	490
Mallophaga	chewing lice (all families)	3000
Hemiptera	bed bugs (Cimicidae)	108
	kissing bugs (Reduviidae, Triatominae)	120
Diptera	biting midges (Ceratopogonidae)	1300
	mosquitoes (Culicidae)	3600
	sand flies (Psychodidae, Phlebotominae)	700
	black flies (Simuliidae)	1460
	horse and deer flies (Tabanidae)	3500
	filth flies (Muscidae, Glossinae)	23
	(Stomoxyinae)	49
	louse flies (Hippoboscidae)	|
	bat flies (Nycteribiidae)	|— 600
	bat flies (Streblidae)	|
Siphonaptera	fleas (all families)	2200
All orders	17,150	
Subclass Acari		
Ixodida		
	Ixodidae	660
	Argasidae	140
Mesostigmata		4500
Prostigmata		10,500
Astigmata		10,000
All orders		25,800

Note: Tick and mite species were estimated by the current authors with assistance from Dr. Hans Klompen.

Species Complexes

We define biological species as reproductively isolated gene pools, following Mayr and Ashlock (1991). When 2 populations become reproductively isolated through either geographic separation or as a consequence of the evolution of prezygotic or postzygotic isolation mechanisms, they often accumulate morphological differences. Occasionally these differences are subtle or they appear as continuous grades rather than discrete discontinuities among taxa. Such character differences are difficult to use in routine identification. Closely related species that are reproductively isolated but that appear as a single species even to specialists are often referred to as cryptic or sibling species. The group of cryptic species is referred to as a species complex. The problem of cryptic species would be academic if it were not for the fact that closely related species can differ greatly in their vector competence, preferred host, larval habitat, and adult feeding behavior.

The most striking historical example is the *Anopheles maculipennis* species complex. Before the 1920s this complex was described as a single species with a broad Palearctic range. At that time, malariologists in Europe had known that the distribution of malaria was largely coastal and did not coincide with the widespread and often dense inland distribution of *An. maculipennis*. This phenomenon came to be known as anophelism without malaria. The first description of a distinct taxon within *An. maculipennis* appeared in 1924 when Van Thiel described *An. atroparvus* in Holland as a short-winged, nonhibernating form of *An. maculipennis* and determined that this was the species responsible for indoor malaria transmission during winter in "malaria houses." In 1926, Falleroni found 2 colors of eggs within *An. maculipennis* collected in Italy. The race associated with the dark gray eggs was described as *An. labranchiae,* and the race with the silvery white eggs was *An. messeae.*

In the 1920s the development of the precipitin test permitted the identification of a blood meal with respect to its animal source. By the 1930s, this method had been used to demonstrate that *An. maculipennis* was zoophilic (feeding preference for animals other than humans) in malaria-free regions but was anthropophilic (feeding preference for humans) in malarious regions. When feeding preference was analyzed in Falleroni's species, only *An. labranchiae* was anthropophilic, and hence the only one responsible for malaria transmission. Further investigation divided the dark gray egg taxon into *An. labranchiae, An. atroparvus,* and *An. sacharovi.* The silvery egg taxon was subdivided into *An. maculipennis, An. messae, An. melanoon,* and *An. subalpinus.* These 7 taxa were found to be partially or fully reproductively incompatible, indicating that they were suitably delineated, biological species. Later, distinctive differences among them were identified in mating patterns and in inversion polymorphisms in the polytene chromosomes of the larval salivary gland. After the taxonomy of this group was clarified, a study of species distributions became possible. Generally, the 7 species occupy disjunct geographic regions, although several do overlap in distribution. Of the 7, only 2, *An. labranchiae* and *An. sacharovi,* are important malaria vectors throughout their ranges. *An. sacharovi* is the only species that can be identified as an adult; the others must be identified on the basis of egg morphology or polytene chromosomes.

The primary vectors of malaria and lymphatic filariasis in Africa are mosquitoes in the *Anopheles gambiae* complex. Inland, the larvae are found in small sunlit, freshwater pools throughout most of the species range. However, along the coasts these larvae can be found as well in brackish intertidal swamps. Larvae occurring in coastal habitats were morphologically indistinguishable from larvae collected at inland sites, but adults and eggs obtained by rearing these larvae were distinct. Coastal forms were separated from *An. gambiae* s.l.[1] as 2 species, *An. merus* in East Africa and *An. melas* in West Africa. Subsequently, in the 1960s, investigations of the inland forms were initiated with genetic approaches, hybridization, and polytene chromosomes. George Davidson examined the fertility in single F_1 crosses from field-collected *An. gambiae,* and Mario Coluzzi, the inversion polymorphisms in the larval salivary glands chromosomes. Through their discoveries, *An. gambiae* s.l. was subdivided into 4 species: and *An. gambiae* s.s. (former species A), *An. arabiensis* (species B), *An. quadriannulatus* (species C), and *An. bwambae* (species D).

Years of intensive field collections have determined that *An. gambiae* s.s. and *An. arabiensis* are widespread throughout Africa. They are often sympatric and are the 2 most important vectors of malaria and bancroftian filariasis. *An. gambiae* s.s. is more anthropophilic and endophilic (preferring to feed indoors) than *An. arabiensis*. *An. quadriannulatus* is zoophilic and not a vector of either malaria or filariasis. *An. bwambae* is now found only in mineral water springs at the base of the Ruwenzori Mountains, Bwamba County, Uganda.

The *Labranchiae* and *Gambiae* complexes are the best-known complexes in *Anopheles* for both historical and medical reasons; however, more recently, numerous other examples have been documented in this genus as well as in *Aedes* and *Culex*. The 2 subspecies of *Ae. aegypti* differ markedly in their vector competence for flaviviruses, filarial worms, and bird malaria. The *Cx. pipiens* complex has been formally separated into 2 species, *Cx. pipiens* s.s. and *Cx. quinquefasciatus*. However, the mosquito literature still abounds with references to "varieties," "crossing types," "subspecies," and even other "species" in this very difficult complex.

The family Simuliidae (black flies) (Chap. 7) contains several species complexes in both the New and Old worlds. Many of these complexes contain species that are major vectors of onchocerciasis (river blindness). The presence of excellent larval salivary polytene chromosomes permitted the discovery and definition of many black fly species complexes; this approach has remained the most rigorous means of species identification within complexes. The *Simulium damnosum* complex, prevalent in Africa, has been studied most extensively.

Tsetse flies (Muscidae: Glossinae) consist of several species complexes (e.g., *Glossina morsitans*) that vary in geographic distribution and host-seeking behavior. At the microgeographical level, the human body louse, *Pediculus humanus humanus*, and head louse, *Pediculus humanus capitis*, are subspecies that are indistinguishable by morphological characters, but that clearly differ in behavior, microhabitat distribution, and vector competence for louse-borne typhus. The tick vector of the relapsing fever spirochete in Africa, *Ornithodoros moubata*, is a complex of at least 6 species that differ in geographic distribution and host preference. Other tick species complexes include the *Rhipicephalus sanguineus* group and the *Hyalomma marginatum* group.

These examples of species complexes share 2 important features. First, members of species complexes can differ dramatically in their vector potential. Second, in almost every case, identification of species within the complex requires access to specific developmental stages, detection of subtle morphological differences, or specialized techniques. These identifications often require time-consuming, laborious, and often expensive determinations by skilled specialists.

Morphologically Similar Species

Closely related, morphologically similar species usually can be separated if adequate keys are available. However, congeneric species are often difficult to separate at all life stages. For example, the 5 members of *An. maculipennis* complex can be distinguished only as eggs. *Aedes* in the subgenus *Ochlerotatus* consists of many boreal species that can be distinguished easily only as 4th instar larvae. Keys for early instars and pupae are generally nonexistent. The best characters are found in the genital structures of adult males. Unfortunately, these require slide mounts and examination with a compound microscope; furthermore, the males are less well represented in most collections. Identification of adult females is hampered by loss of diagnostic scales or setae as a result of aging or the collection process.

Many species of ticks and hematophagous mites can be separated only as nymphs or adults. Larval keys are rare. Some species cannot be distinguished in both sexes. For example, *Boophilus annulatus* and *B. microplus*, the primary vectors of babesiosis in cattle, can be separated only by the presence or absence of a caudal appendage in males. Morphological characters in the females are not dependable, and immatures cannot be identified at all.

The fact that morphologically similar species can be separated only during 1 stage of development severely limits the types of epidemiological or ecological studies in these groups. In general, these organisms must be collected and retained alive in the laboratory for identification when the specimen matures to an identifiable stage. Alternatively, specimens must be mated and reared through another generation if identification of an earlier stage is required.

Small Species

Many arthropod vectors are small and require preservation, clearing, and mounting for microscopic analysis of characters. This is true for most medically important mites, chewing and sucking lice, biting midges, sand flies, black flies, and fleas. Any microorganisms associated with species in these groups are usually destroyed during sample preparation. This results in lost information on pathogens transmitted by the mounted specimen. Information on biological control organisms present in or on mounted specimens is also destroyed. Furthermore, genetic information that might be useful in population studies is lost.

THE MOLECULAR APPROACH TO TAXONOMY

We begin with the premise that molecular taxonomic approaches are appropriate only when taxonomic ambiguities from factors outlined earlier. Under these circumstances, molecular taxonomy can improve the quality of ecological and epidemiological studies because: (1) members of species complexes can be identified, (2) morphologically similar species can be identified at any life stage, (3) current technology allows visualization of biochemical and protein markers in small arthropods, and (4) the remainder of the specimen or specimen homogenate can be used for identification of associated microorganisms, whether they be pathogens or potential biological control agents, and for estimation of genetic variation in population genetics studies.

We emphasize that the practice of developing molecules as taxonomic tools is neither quick nor trivial. Molecular taxonomy requires the same rigor and careful attention to intraspecific variation that has been practiced for centuries with morphologically based taxonomy.

The fundamental difference between molecular and morphological characters is that the former consists of an array of identifiable single gene or base pair differences, whereas the latter is the product of a variety of genetic components, including developmental genes, structural genes, and epistatic interactions among multiple loci. Environmental effects and interactions between the environment and different genotypes can also affect morphological variation.

Methods in Molecular Taxonomy

A variety of technologically advanced methods that have proven to be useful in addressing taxonomic ambiguities will *not* be discussed in this chapter. These include fine-scale morphological investigations using scanning electron microscopy, banding patterns of polytene chromosomes (cytotaxonomy), cuticular hydrocarbons, and immunology. Although each has played an important role in specific insect groups, treatment of these approaches is beyond the scope of the present chapter. Service (1988) serves as an excellent review of these methods and their applications. In the following sections, we explore 2 levels of molecular methodologies at the posttranslational level of the protein (amino acid substitutions) and pretranscriptional level of nucleic acids (base-pair substitutions, deletions, and insertions).

PROTEINS AS TAXONOMIC MARKERS

Isozyme electrophoresis was first used as a tool for recognizing species differences in the middle 1960s. Since then, it has been the method of choice in uncovering intraspecific variability, genetic mapping, and routine species identification in plant and animal taxa spanning the phylogenetic spectrum.

The principle of isozyme electrophoresis consists of separating proteins on the basis of electrical charge. In an electric field, proteins of highest charge move fastest toward the pole of opposite charge. In a homogeneous gel matrix, the proteins of identical charge move together at the same rate toward the pole. Because of their aqueous solubility and intrinsic levels of amino acid variability, enzymes have proven the most serviceable of proteins in taxonomy and population genetics. For a successful separation of the enzyme and visualization on a gel, the following conditions must be met:

1. Enzymes must retain their activity after electrophoresis. Therefore, the organism must be kept

alive or frozen at temperatures lower than −40°C. Enzymes are generally fractionated on native gels that are chilled during the electrophoretic process to avoid denaturation from heating.

2. The buffer, gel pore size, and electrical field must be carefully standardized to permit an ordered migration of proteins through the gel.

3. Following electrophoresis, a gel contains a huge variety of insect proteins fractionated by size and charge. The activity of a particular enzyme is visualized by soaking the gel in a histochemical stain containing that enzyme substrate and linked through various chemical reactions to a dye. The location of the enzymatic reaction on the gel is visualized by precipitation of the dye. Specific activity can be visualized only for enzymes in which a histochemical stain has been developed.

Protein Electrophoresis

The amino acids that contribute most to an enzyme's charge are those with unbalanced numbers of carboxyl (—COOH) and amino (—NH$_2$) side groups. At a pH greater than the isoelectric point of a protein, the hydrogen ions dissociate from the carboxyl groups, leaving the protein with a net negative charge. In an electric field, these proteins migrate to the cathode. In a mixture of enzymes with a difference of a single carboxyl group (addition or subtraction of an aspartic acid or glutamic acid), the enzymes are readily separated on a gel when subjected to an electric field (Fig. 26.1).

The operational application of electrophoresis involves 2 steps. The 1st consists of the mechanics of the process, and the 2nd is the interpretation and translation of the banding patterns into numerical data. The mechanics of electrophoresis can be delineated into 5 stages: gel preparation, specimen preparation, enzyme separation, enzyme visualization with histochemical staining, and gel archiving. Interpretation requires measurement of band movement, converting band morphologies into genotypes, estimating allele frequencies, and comparing species by genetic distances values and dendrograms. Procedures for this last step are discussed in Chapter 25.

Gel Preparation

Three types of gels form matrices sufficient for separation of enzymes in electrophoresis: starch, polyacrylamide, and cellulose acetate. The most popular and widely applied has been the starch gel; the electrophoretic apparatus is inexpensive and thick slabs are readily sliced for multiple enzyme assays and easy to use. Starch gels suffer during long-term storage and, for some enzymes, provide resolution of lesser quality. Starch gel electrophoresis procedures are summarized in Hillis and Moritz (1990) and will not be discussed in this chapter.

Small quantities of enzyme can be visualized on cellulose acetate gels, and this technique is excellent for very small organisms. Although the gels are easy to preserve, they are generally quite small, and resolution of closely migrating forms can be difficult. Cellulose acetate gel electrophoresis (CAGE) is reviewed in Richardson et al. (1986), and Kazmer (1991) described a system for analysis of small arthropods using CAGE with isoelectric focusing.

Polyacrylamide gels were among the first matrices to be used for separating proteins, but they lost popularity because of the difficulty in slicing the slabs for multiple assays, the toxicity of acrylamide, and the high cost of the electrophoretic apparatus. In recent years, polyacrylamide gel electrophoresis (PAGE) has become more prevalent. New commercial PAGE systems allow electrophoresis to be performed on multiple gels simultaneously. Thinner gels offer greater resolution and require small samples. Specific details on the pouring, loading, and running of native PAGE gels (used and preferred by both authors) are provided in Table 26.2 because general methods for preparation of native PAGE gels are not provided in any general references.

Histochemical Staining

Histochemical stains for a hundred or more enzymes appear in Hillis and Moritz (1990) or Harris and Hopkinson (1976). Although Singh and Rhomberg (1987) reported on genetic variability in 117 enzyme loci in *Drosophila melanogaster*, only 30 or fewer are routinely examined in a typical electrophoretic study. The most useful enzymes have been esterases, glycolytic pathway

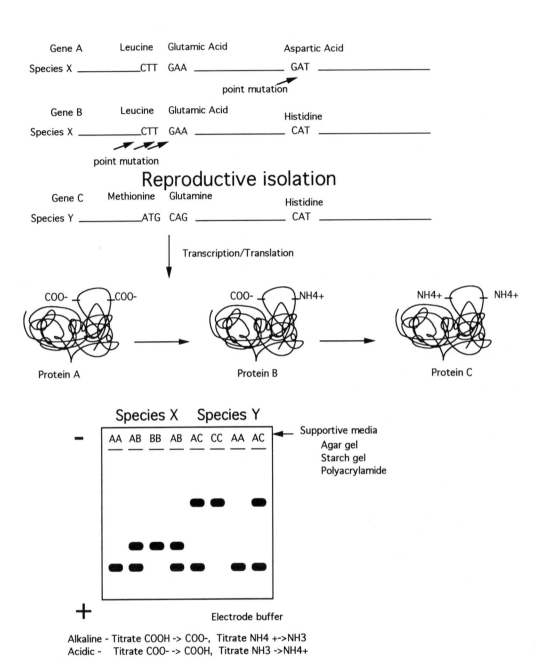

26.1 Genetic polymorphisms revealed by protein electrophoresis on a denaturing gel. Point mutations in the gene that cause nonsynonymous substitutions produce proteins with altered amino acid sequences. When these substituted amino acids carry different charges, the mobility of the protein in an electrical field will be altered. Different types of substitutions will be detected under different pH conditions during electrophoresis.

TABLE 26.2 Instructions for pouring, loading, and running native PAGE gels

Tris-citrate (TC) buffer

To make 1 L of 40X TC Buffer, dissolve 94.1 g (0.78 M) Tris and 45 g of citric acid (monohydrate) into 700 ml distilled water. After all salts are dissolved, titrate the solution to pH 7.1 with 1 M citric acid and bring the entire solution to volume. Dilute this buffer 1:39 with distilled water to make the electrode buffer.

Tris-borate-EDTA (TBE) buffer

To make 1 L of 10X TBE Buffer, dissolve 98.3 g (0.81 M) Tris, 12.5 g (0.20 M) boric acid, and 5.58 g (15 mM) EDTA (disodium) in enough distilled water to bring the volume to 1 L. The pH should be 8.8–9.0, and no adjustment in pH is necessary. Dilute this buffer 1:9 with distilled water to make the electrode buffer.

Acrylamide stock

To make 1 L of acrylamide stock solution, dissolve 380 g acrylamide and 20 g N,N,-bis-acrylamide in 900 ml distilled water. After all salts are dissolved (30–40 minutes), filter the solution through 3–4 layers of Whatman #1. Bring to 1 L volume.

To pour 100 ml of polyacrylamide gel solution:

(1) Pour 12.5 ml of the acrylamide stock solution into a beaker with either 5 ml of the TC concentrate and 82.5 ml distilled water or 10 ml of the TBE concentrate and 77.5 ml distilled water. (2) Mix briefly and then degas the gel solution by applying vacuum for 5 min until bubbles no longer form. (3) Add 500 µl Photo-flo®, 150 µl TEMED—N,N,N'N'-tetramethyl-ethylenediamine and stir briefly. (4) Add 500 µl of 10% (w/v) ammonium persulfate and stir briefly. The gels must be poured immediately and Teflon® slot formers (combs) placed in position at the top of the gel before polymerization. These slots act as wells into which insect homogenates will be loaded. The gel must set for approximately 1 hr before the combs can be removed. A "prerun" at 200V is performed after polymerization to remove catalysts and to stabilize the buffer through the gel.

Specimen preparation

From 0.5–2 mg of tissue are sufficient to resolve enzymes in 12–16 or more gels. Single specimens (in the case of sand flies, *Culicoides*, or mosquitoes) are placed in a 25 µl loading buffer (20% sucrose, Triton X–100 [0.5%]), Tris-citrate pH 7.0 electrode buffer, and bromophenol blue tracking dye (trace amount). The specimen is homogenized with a pestle fitted to the tube, and the tubes centrifuged in a microfuge (3 min, 12,000 × g). The supernatant is removed from the tube with a 25 µl gas chromatography syringe and 1–2 µl placed in 1 well of each gel. The high density provided by the sucrose solution causes the homogenate to sink to the bottom of the well. Specimens are kept at 0–4°C throughout this preparation to insure enzyme stability.

Electrophoresis

After the specimens are loaded, electrode buffer previously cooled to 0°C is circulated around the gel plates to maintain an even and cold environment. Constant voltage is applied to suit the desired length of the separation time. Usually around 300V are sufficient with either buffer system to complete enzyme separation in 2½ – 3 hr. The gels are then removed to trays for histochemical staining.

---

enzymes, and a handful of esterases, phosphatases, kinases, proteases, and transaminases.

Although several basic strategies are applied to identify the position of each enzyme, the general scheme is as follows: (1) A gel is placed in a shallow pan or tray with the appropriate stain. This usually consists of the enzyme substrate and required cofactors (e.g., magnesium). (2) The action of many of these enzymes (e.g., the dehydrogenases) removes a proton that is passed to a cofactor, usually NAD or NADP. (3) These are reduced in situ to NADH or NADPH. (4) To produce a band at the site of the enzyme activity, a water-soluble tetrazolium dye is reduced, in turn, by NADH or NADPH. The reduced dye is water insoluble, and a colored precipitate is immediately formed at the site of enzyme activity. After a few minutes to a half an hour, the gels are fixed in a methanol-acetic acid fixative until ready to hydrate and dry. An activity stain for phosphoglucomutase, a glycolysis enzyme, is illustrated in Figure 26.2.

Data Quality Control and Storage

Complete records of the migration patterns are essential for interpreting results or reestablishing electrophoretic conditions. Every newly initiated study necessarily requires comparisons from many gels. The conditions for each electrophoretic run should be kept as constant as possible throughout a study, although some day-to-day variation is inevitable. To control for this variation, homogenates from standard laboratory strains are loaded on all gels. The mobility of enzymes of other species is measured with respect to this reference standard.

The migration of bands can be recorded on data forms for later comparison. However, differences among bands on the same and different gels can be subtle and it is often desirable to have a permanent record of the gel. This can be accomplished by photographing the gel or transferring the gel to filter paper and drying it on a gel dryer. Preserving gels between dialysis membranes is an inexpensive alternative (Table 26.3).

Biochemical Taxonomy

Biochemically based dichotomous keys for identifying mosquito species are rare. Most studies have compared only a few species in a closely related group where, in most cases, formal keys are unnecessary. Unfortunately, the deficiency in electrophoretic keys has impeded the recognition and application of electrophoresis as a general identification technique. Moreover, as larger numbers of species are compared, more enzyme assays per individual specimen become necessary to identify the specimen. Fortunately, improved

technology has mitigated the latter problem, both in terms of increased sensitivity and in cost.

Within the Culicidae, several studies stand out as comprehensive in yielding information both on population genetic structure and contributing to taxonomy. The worldwide study on the genetic structure of *Ae. aegypti* by Tabachnick and coworkers ranks among the best in terms of numbers of populations sampled, sample sizes per population, and the substantial number of enzyme systems applied. This work examined the interface between population genetics and systematics and demonstrated the substantial substructuring that can occur in a species with a worldwide distribution. These studies provided a model and guidelines for rational use of electrophoretic techniques in investigations of new insect groups (Tabachnick 1991).

Using single or several electrophoretic enzyme phenotypes for distinguishing mosquito sibling species has a fairly long history. Among the first enzymes to be used was alkaline phosphatase for separating the sibling species pair *An. labranchiae–An. atroparvus*. Somewhat later the enzyme phosphoglucomutase was examined in a number of European mosquito species. Subsequently, multiple enzyme assays were applied to a species set that included 6 European species of the *An. maculipennis* complex, 3 of the *Ae. mariae* complex, and several other species groups (Bullini and Coluzzi 1982). North American researchers described diagnostic isoenzymes for members of the *Ae. triseriatus* group, *Ae. atropalpus* group, *Ae. scutellaris*, and local *Culex* species. However, formal electrophoretic keys were rarely presented, with the exception of those for 9 species of the *Annulipes* group (Munstermann 1988) and 4 species of the *Communis* species group (Brust and Munstermann 1992).

The initial biochemical key for mosquitoes was developed by Miles (1979) for 5 of the species of the *An. gambiae* complex. Miles's keys have proven to be of exceptional value under local conditions and have been extensively applied for *An. gambiae* identifications in Tanzania and the Grand Comoros Island. The recent discovery of a sibling species complex in *An. quadrimaculatus* s.l. resulted in a key based on enzymatic characters alone (Narang et al. 1989).

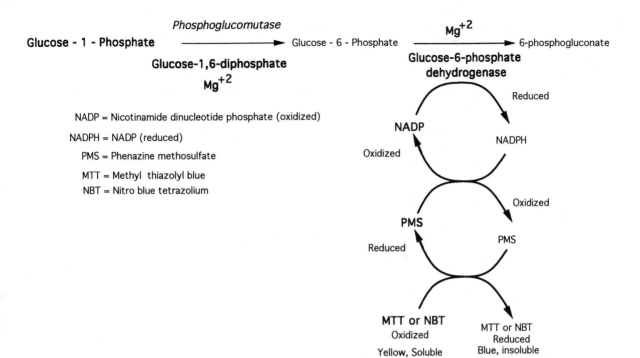

Phosphoglucomutase

Glucose - 1 - Phosphate $\xrightarrow{\hspace{2cm}}$ Glucose - 6 - Phosphate $\xrightarrow{\hspace{1cm}Mg^{+2}\hspace{1cm}}$ 6-phosphogluconate

Glucose-1,6-diphosphate
Mg^{+2}

**Glucose-6-phosphate
dehydrogenase**

NADP = Nicotinamide dinucleotide phosphate (oxidized)

NADPH = NADP (reduced)

PMS = Phenazine methosulfate

MTT = Methyl thiazolyl blue

NBT = Nitro blue tetrazolium

Reduced

NADP

NADPH

Oxidized

Oxidized

PMS

PMS

Reduced

MTT or NBT
Oxidized

Yellow, Soluble

MTT or NBT
Reduced

Blue, insoluble

26.2   Steps in the activity stain for phosphoglucomutase. Items in bold are components that are added to the stain mixture. All other items are reaction products. This series of reactions is initiated at the locations on the gel in which phosphoglucomutase occurs. The location of the reaction is visualized by the presence of reduced, blue insoluble MTT, or NBT dye.

Advantages and Disadvantages of Protein Electrophoresis

These studies have clearly demonstrated the utility of protein electrophoretic techniques for taxonomic problems involving closely related species. When larger numbers of more distantly related species are studied, electrophoretic methods can have definite advantages over morphological methods of identification under some circumstances. However, correct identifications depend on the extent of prior information available on population structure of each species being identified.

A disadvantage of protein electrophoresis relative to analysis of nucleic acids described later is that the expression of proteins can differ in amount or in the patterns of expression across life stages. Less enzyme is expressed in earlier life stages (correlated with insect volume) and, occasionally, different forms of the enzyme (isozymes) are expressed. This could require

developing keys specific for each stage of development. Perhaps the major disadvantage of using proteins in taxonomic work is that they are very easily degraded, and enzyme activity is rapidly lost. Protein instability necessitates either maintaining collected specimens alive and in good condition awaiting return to the laboratory or storage of specimens at low temperatures (−40°C) in the field. In contrast, dried specimens and material preserved in alcohol are frequently used for nucleic acid analyses.

MOLECULAR TAXONOMY WITH NUCLEIC ACIDS

A eukaryotic genome consists of a complex mixture of unique and repetitive gene sequences. Some of these sequences code for proteins whereas others code for ribosomal and transfer RNAs involved in transcription and translation. Noncoding regions can contain

TABLE 26.3   Storage of PAGE gels using dialysis membranes

Equipment

Two 0.125–0.25 inch-thick plexiglass frames. Outside dimensions should be 2 inches wider and taller than the gel. A square is cut from the center of each piece of plexiglass such that the frame will fit evenly around the entire gel with a minimum of 0.25–0.50 inches to spare along all edges of the gel.

2 dialysis membranes cut to the outside dimensions of the frame

6 Black spring steel clamps with chrome handles

Procedure

1. Rinse fixative (1:5:5 glacial acetic acid, methanol, water) from gels and submerse in deionized water for at least 20 min.

2. Cut 2 sheets of dialysis membrane to size of frame, 2 sheets per gel.

3. Rinse a sheet of dialysis membrane in deionized water and place over lower frame, making sure no bubbles are between frame and membrane.

4. Place trimmed gel carefully on wet membrane with no bubbles between gel and membrane.

5. Make labels on laser printer, 16 pt. type font. Label should list gel code number and enzyme system. Photocopy printer output onto transparency sheets.

6. Place transparent label at upper left of gel: gel number and enzyme.

7. Rinse 2nd dialysis sheet, place over gel to edges of frame, and remove all bubbles.

8. Clamp the frames together with the 6 spring steel clamps, 2 at each the base and the top and 1 on each side.

9. Allow to dry under an incandescent lamp.

10. Remove the dried gel and membrane. Trim and place in a notebook.

regulatory elements, serve a structural purpose in the genome, or be merely "parasitic" or "junk" DNA. For the purposes of molecular taxonomy we focus on those sequences that mutate or evolve quickly. Noncoding regions are often targeted for use in molecular taxonomy because they are less constrained by selection than coding regions. These are most likely to vary among closely related species. Noncoding repetitive regions are especially useful as species diagnostic probes because they are easier to detect in hybridization assays due to high copy number and the fact that they diverge quickly among closely related species for reasons outlined later. Sequences chosen as diagnostic tools can vary either in their presence or absence among species or in their nucleic acid sequences depending upon the technique chosen for identification.

We focus on techniques that are fast, inexpensive, and do not require extensive technical training. Appropriate technologies fall into 2 general categories: (1) protocols involving hybridization of species-specific probes to the target DNA from unknown field specimens and (2) techniques employing the polymerase chain reaction (PCR) to amplify either targeted or arbitrary regions of the genome from unknown field specimens that can then be analyzed to identify the species. The strengths and weaknesses of each approach are discussed.

Specimen Preparation

The amount of time spent in specimen preparation varies enormously depending on the detection techniques to be employed. Perhaps the most rapid technique is the "squash blot," in which many insects (or parts of many insects) are simultaneously crushed directly onto nitrocellulose or nylon filters to be probed with species-specific markers (Gale and Crampton 1987; 1988). Similarly, some investigators using PCR report success using "parts" (e.g., legs, heads, or abdomens) of arthropods snipped off and placed directly into the PCR reaction. Scott et al. (1993) demonstrated successful PCR amplification with a single mosquito leg.

Although squash blots or PCR with insect parts can be completed rapidly, investigators often want to store DNA from specimens over longer periods of time for use in other analyses. A variety of procedures can be used to isolate DNA from individual insects. Kawasaki (1990) described a rapid method in which a specimen is crushed in a homogenization buffer, heated briefly at 95°C to denature nucleases, and then briefly spun on a microcentrifuge to pellet debris. The method is quick and reliable, but the extracted DNA is stable only for a few days, regardless of the storage method. The DNA is sufficiently pure for use in PCR, but we suspect that it would be extremely unstable in other procedures. Rapid procedures involving chelating resins such as Chelex® have also been described; however, lack of stability over long periods is of concern with these as well. Instability is probably attributable to residual nuclease activity following heating or proteinase procedures.

Three general methods for stable DNA extraction from individual insects are described in the literature. Technical details for a sodium dodecyl sulphate (SDS)–extraction procedure are frequently attributed to Coen et al. (1982). When isolation procedures used in different laboratories are compared, this original procedure differs markedly from what is actually used; nevertheless, the general principle is the same in all cases. The method is safe and inexpensive (Table 26.4). A second commonly used procedure employs overnight lysis and phenol/chloroform extraction (see Ballinger-Crabtree et al. 1992 for details). A CTAB (Cetyltrimethylammonium bromide) procedure followed by phenol/chloroform extractions is also frequently used and is described in depth in Hunt and Page (1992).

DNA Hybridization

In hybridization assays a labeled, single-stranded, species-specific piece of DNA (the probe) is mixed with single-stranded target DNA that has been immobilized on a nylon or nitrocellulose filter. The target DNA originates from field-collected individuals of unknown species identity. The mixture is incubated for a short period at a temperature that is sufficiently high and in a salt concentration that is sufficiently low to insure that the probe and target strands can hybridize. The temperature and salt conditions control the stringency of a hybridization reaction. Stringency of the hybridization must be sufficiently great that the probe does not hybridize to arbitrary regions of the target genomic DNA but sufficiently low to allow good hybridization between the probe and the complementary target sequence. Generally, stringency conditions are adjusted so that the probe will hybridize only to regions that are 90% complementary in sequence. Following hybridization, the filter containing the immobilized target DNA is washed in a series of low-, medium-, and high-stringency washes and dried. The washes remove all of the probe that has not bound to a complementary piece of target DNA. Hybridization events are detected by exposure of the filter to X-ray film for radioactively labeled probes or through enzyme detection for probes labeled with specific ligands. Results are recorded as the presence or absence of a hybridization signal at each location on the filter where target DNA was placed. The filter is next "stripped" of the label at a high temperature or by soaking in a alkaline solution to disrupt base pairing between the probe and the target DNA. The filter can then be tested again by hybridization with another probe. The general steps involved in hybridization assays are listed in Table 26.5.

What Should Be Used for a Species-Specific Probe?

Strategies that have been adopted for isolating species-specific probes are reviewed in Post et al. (1992). Procedures are discussed and illustrated in Post and Crampton (1988). The tactic that is most commonly

TABLE 26.4 Modification of the Coen et al. (1982) procedure for obtaining stable template DNA for species identification

---

Grinding buffer: Make up grinding buffer and store frozen in 1 ml aliquots.

0.1 M NaCl

0.2 M sucrose

0.1 M Tris-HCl (pH 9.1)

0.05 M EDTA

0.05% SDS

1. Place individual insects in 1.5 ml tubes with 25 µl grinding buffer. Grind with at least 10 turns of a pestle (we use the Kontes blue plastic pestles). Don't stop grinding until you can't see any insect parts. Wash the pestle with an additional 25 µl grinding buffer. Place the contaminated pestle in 1M HCl. Before these are used again they should be rinsed several times, washed in soapy water, rinsed in distilled water, and autoclaved.

2. Briefly microfuge to get all homogenate down into the bottom of the tube. This is important!

3. Incubate homogenate at 65°C for 30 min.

4. While tubes are still warm, add 7µl 8M KAc. Mix by tapping.

5. Incubate on ice for a minimum of 30 min to precipitate SDS.

6. Centrifuge at 14,000 to 17,000 Xg for 15 min in a microcentrifuge. Transfer supernatant to fresh 1.5 ml tubes. Try not to carry over any SDS precipitate.

7. Add 100 µl 100% ethanol (EtOH) and incubate at room temperature for 5 min to precipitate nucleic acids (you may also stop at this point, putting the tubes in −20°C overnight). Microfuge at 14,000–17,000 Xg for 15 minutes.

8. Carefully remove EtOH. Add 100 µl 70% EtOH, centrifuge. Carefully remove the EtOH so that the DNA pellet remains in tube. The pellet will often appear as a smear and as often you may not see anything at all. Do not be discouraged! Add 100 µl 100% EtOH and centrifuge. Carefully remove the EtOH. Air dry the pellets or use a Speed Vac®.

9. Resuspend the pellet in 100 µl TE (0.05 M Tris-HCl, EDTA pH 8.0). This DNA will be stable in the refrigerator or freezer for up to 6 months and often longer.

Note: These modifications seem to have originated in Dr. Pat Roman's laboratory at the University of Toronto. This procedure is written for mosquitoes, but we have used it with many different types of arthropods.

used is illustrated in Figure 26.3. Individual genomic libraries are constructed for each of the various species in a complex. These libraries are then lifted to a set of replicate filters and probed with labeled whole genomic DNA from each complex member.

This tactic accomplishes 2 things. First, only clones that contain repetitive DNA give a strong hybridization signal. Second, a repetitive clone that contains species-specific sequences or differs greatly in copy number among subspecies hybridizes differentially on replicate filters that have been probed with DNA from the different species.

A clone with high copy number in 1 species but that gives little or no hybridization signal when probed with genomic DNA from other species is a good candidate for a species-specific probe. This clone

TABLE 26.5 General conditions for the performance of hybridization assays in molecular taxonomy

1. Target DNA is placed onto a nylon or nitrocellulose filter either through squashing part or all of an insect directly onto a filter sitting on filter paper saturated with 10% SDS (sodium dodecyl sulphate) or by placing extracted DNA directly onto a fresh hybridization filter.

2. Target DNA is denatured by setting the hybridization filter on filter paper saturated with 0.1 M NaOH/ 1.5M NaCl for 5 min. The hybridization filter is blotted dry and neutralized by placing it on filter paper saturated with 0.5 M Tris-HCl pH 7.0/3.0 M NaCl for 5 min. The hybridization filter is blotted dry and baked for 2 hr at 80°C under vacuum to adhere the DNA to the filter.

3. Baked filters are sealed in a plastic bag with 10 ml of prehybridization solution (50% deionized formamide, 0.2% polyvinyl-pyrrolidone (M.W 40,000), 0.2% bovine serum albumin, 0.2% ficoll (M.W. 400,000), 0.05M Tris-HCl pH 7.5, 1.0% SDS, 1.0M NaCl, 0.1% sodium pyrophosphate, and 10% Dextran sulfate (M.W. 500,000) and 100 µg/ml denatured and sonicated calf thymus DNA. The filter is prehybridized at 42°C for 6 hr or overnight.

4. The probe DNA is labeled with CTP or ATP (cytosine or adenosine triphosphate) (labeled with ^{32}P or biotin using nick translation or random primer labeling. The labeled probe is mixed into 1 ml of 100 µg/ml denatured and sonicated calf thymus DNA and the solution is boiled for 10 min to denature the probe. This is then placed directly into 3 ml of the prehybridization buffer described in Step 3. The bag is opened and the probe solution is placed in the bag with the prehybridization solution and filter. The bag is resealed, and hybridization proceeds for 24 hr at 42°C.

5. Following hybridization, the filter is washed twice for 5 min in 1X wash buffer (0.3 M NaCl, 0.06M Tris-HCl (pH 8.0), 2 mM EDTA) at room temperature, twice in 1X buffer with 1% SDS for 30 min at 60°C and twice in 0.1X wash buffer for 30 min at room temperature. The filter is allowed to dry at room temperature. For radioactively labeled probes, filters are loaded into X-ray cassettes with film and exposed overnight. For probes labeled with ligands, enzyme detection is used following the manufacturer's instructions.

Note: Detailed recipes and instructions appear in Sambrook et al. (1989).

is isolated, purified, labeled, and tested as a probe on filters containing DNA from each species in the complex. The ideal species-specific probe should hybridize strongly with only 1 member of a species complex. Probes that hybridize moderately with other species should be avoided as should probes that hybridize weakly or inconsistently with the target taxa. Recently, a number of subtractive hybridization techniques have been described for isolating species-specific sequences (Clapp et al. 1993). These offer a more rapid and effective way to isolate species-specific probes and could supplant the library screening techniques.

All of these procedures are biased toward obtaining repetitive DNA clones. This bias is beneficial because using repetitive probes ensures a strong hybridization signal when screening field-collected material. This is important in identifying small arthropods. More important, repetitive elements undergo concerted evolution through a series of mechanisms collectively known as molecular drive (Figure 26.4). During the process of speciation, populations become reproductively isolated and begin accumulating unique sequences. Mutations within repetitive regions of the genome have been shown to evolve in a concerted fashion rather than independently. Thus, a mutation found in 1 repetitive element is distributed throughout all elements. Dover (1986) discussed the many molecular mechanisms (chiefly unequal crossing over, gene conversion, and slippage replication) that can explain this commonly observed phenomenon. Therefore, repetitive elements can diverge in sequence and abundance rapidly following reproductive isolation of populations.

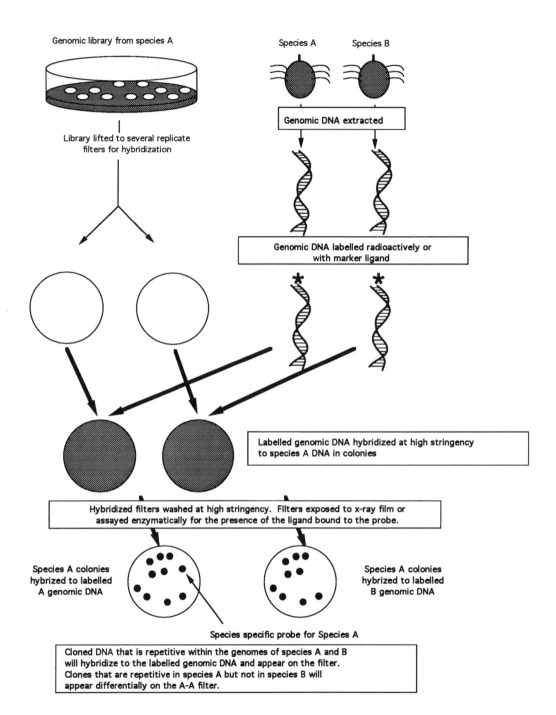

Genomic library from species A

Library lifted to several replicate
filters for hybridization

Species A   Species B

Genomic DNA extracted

Genomic DNA labelled radioactively or
with marker ligand

Labelled genomic DNA hybridized at high stringency
to species A DNA in colonies

Hybridized filters washed at high stringency. Filters exposed to x-ray film or
assayed enzymatically for the presence of the ligand bound to the probe.

Species A colonies
hybrized to labelled
A genomic DNA

Species A colonies
hybrized to labelled
B genomic DNA

Species specific probe for Species A

Cloned DNA that is repetitive within the genomes of species A and B
will hybridize to the labelled genomic DNA and appear on the filter.
Clones that are repetitive in species A but not in species B will
appear differentially on the A-A filter.

26.3   Protocol for identification of species-specific probes in genomic libraries. Adapted from Post and Crampton (1988).

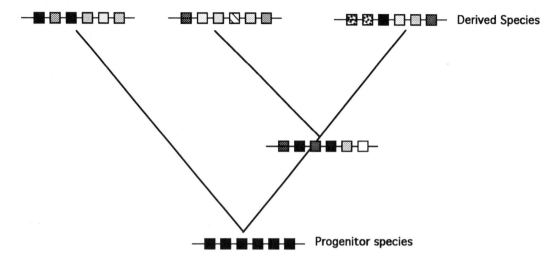

A. **Independent evolution** among members of a multigene family. All members evolve independently of one another in species derived from the progenitor species.

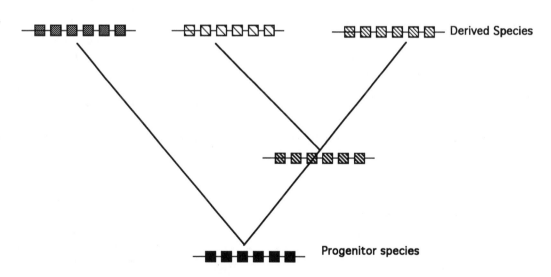

B. **Concerted evolution** among members of a multigene family. All members evolve in concert as new species arise from the progenitor species.

26.4 Concerted evolution is commonly observed among members of a multigene family. New variants that arise following speciation are not confined to one member of the multigene family but spread through the family as a result of several molecular processes, chiefly unequal crossing over and gene conversion.

These principles and techniques have been successfully applied in developing species-specific probes in a number of complexes including, for example, the *An. gambiae* complex (Gale and Crampton 1988; Hill et al. 1991a,b; Post et al. 1992). Panyim et al. (1988) report the use of this technique in isolation of a species D–specific probe in the *An. dirus* complex. Post and Crampton (1988) developed markers to identify members of the *Simulium damnosum* complex. Hill et al. (1991a,b; 1992) report a refinement in which oligonucleotides identified through sequencing of species-specific clones are used as probes. They further describe the use of these with enzymatic reporter systems.

Advantages and Disadvantages of DNA Hybridization Techniques

Minimal preparation of the field-collected specimen is needed for hybridization screening, and the method has proved to be sensitive in all cases discussed. Furthermore, less time is needed to visualize results in hybridization assays as methods have improved. Hill et al. (1992) reported on a hybridization assay system using nonradioactive, synthetic DNA probes that allow species identification in fewer than 48 hours.

Disadvantages are that species-specific probes are often difficult and expensive to isolate. Construction of genomic libraries is expensive and time-consuming but is a one-time investment. In the future, subtractive hybridization procedures may obviate this need. There is a major operational disadvantage of this approach. If there are several species in a complex, multiple stripping, prehybridization, and reprobing steps are required to identify all species that potentially exist on a filter. Duplicate filters can be made by placing insects between 2 filters prior to crushing them, thus allowing simultaneous probing of 2 membranes. Nonradioactive approaches that use species-specific oligonucleotides also could prove useful in reducing the number of separate hybridizations required for a group of insects. Each probe can be labeled with a different ligand (e.g., biotin, digoxigenin) that binds to reporter molecules (e.g., streptavidin-labeled alkaline phosphatase or horseradish peroxidase) that yield different colors in their respective reactions. Alternatively, with fluorescence detection methods, oligonucleotides can be labeled with different fluorescent molecules that appear as different colors under varying wavelengths of light. Either approach would require only a single hybridization reaction. Development of nonradioactive techniques also allows application of these techniques in situations in which radioactive labeling is not feasible.

Techniques Based on the Polymerase Chain Reaction

The polymerase chain reaction is a procedure developed in 1985 that has revolutionized molecular genetics (Saiki et al. 1985). The power of PCR is that it can quickly amplify a gene sequence represented once or only a few times in a large and complex mixture of genes. Starting with a sample of the total DNA from an organism, within 2–3 hours a particular region of the genome can be amplified over 1–100 million times. The steps involved in a generalized PCR procedure are outlined diagrammatically in Figure 26.5. PCR reactions are generally done in small (500 µl) microcentrifuge tubes. From 25–100 µl of a PCR reaction mixture is placed in the tube. The reaction mixture generally contains 10 mM Tris-HCl (pH 8.5–9.0), 50.0 mM KCl, 1.5mM $MgCl_2$, 1% Triton X–100, 0.01% gelatin (w/v)), 200 mM dNTPs, 1 mM of each primer, and 1 unit of a thermostable DNA polymerase such as *Taq* polymerase. Template DNA (1–10 ng) is placed in the reaction mixture and the entire contents of the tube overlaid with oil and placed on a thermal cycler. The thermal cycler is generally a metal block that holds many PCR reaction tubes. The temperature of the block can be programmed to follow a precise cycle of heating and cooling.

The 1st step of the PCR process involves melting the double strand template DNA to single strands at a temperature of 95–98°C for 0.5–1 min. For the 2nd step, the temperature of the reaction is lowered to a point at which a pair of flanking oligonucleotide primers can anneal to the template DNA. The flanking primers are designed to anneal with high specificity to conserved sequences that flank a gene. If the annealing temperature is too high, the primers will not anneal; if the temperature is too low, the primers will anneal nonspecifically to various regions of the genome and give several false products. The annealing step is

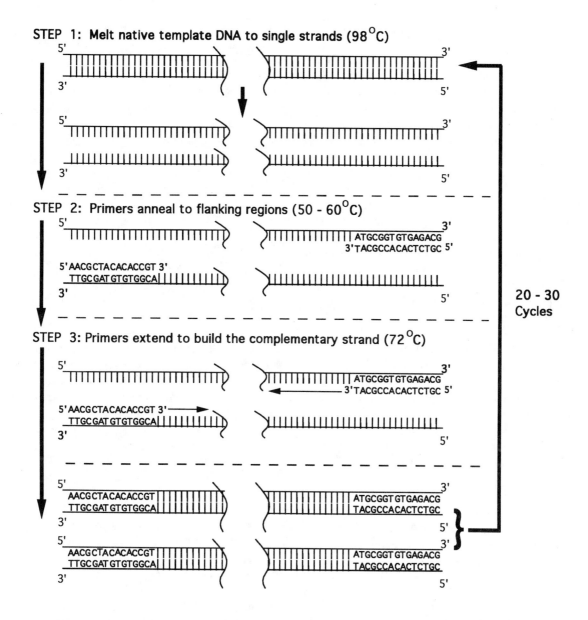

STEP 1: Melt native template DNA to single strands (98°C)

STEP 2: Primers anneal to flanking regions (50 - 60°C)

20 - 30
Cycles

STEP 3: Primers extend to build the complementary strand (72°C)

Two copies of the original template are now present. The temperature is raised to melt the DNA strands (Step 1), lowered to allow the primers to anneal (Step 2) and then raised to 72°C to allow extension (Step 3). At the end of the second round of thermal cycling there are 4 double stranded DNA molecules. The cycling among steps 1, 2 and 3 is repeated 20-30 times. The number of molecules is doubled in each cycle so that 2^{20} or 2^{30} copies of the original molecule are produced.

26.5 Steps involved in the polymerase chain reaction (PCR)

allowed to proceed for 0.5–1 min. The 3rd and final step involves raising the temperature to 72°C. This is the optimal temperature for the thermostable DNA polymerase and permits rapid extension of the primer to build a DNA strand that is complementary to the template strand to which the primer annealed. The extension step is allowed to proceed from 2.5–3 min. At the end of the extension step, the number of double stranded DNA molecules is doubled. The thermal cycler then returns to the melting temperature to melt the newly synthesized strands, the temperature is lowered to allow primer annealing, and then raised to promote extension. This cycle is repeated 20–30 times. Because the number of DNA molecules is doubled at each step, at the end of the thermal cycling there will be 2^{20}–2^{30} (10^6–10^9) molecules.

Prior to PCR, cloning a gene from an organism required construction of a genomic library, screening the library with a homologous probe, isolating clones that cross hybridized with the probe, purifying these clones, and then analyzing them. This procedure required months. In contrast, PCR directly amplifies a sequence in a few hours using oligonucleotide primers that anneal to conserved regions that flank a target gene sequence. The amplified gene is visualized on an agarose gel and can then be cloned, analyzed with restriction enzyme digestion, or even sequenced directly. Genes that were previously analyzed using Southern blots and hybridization with gene-specific probes can now be analyzed directly following PCR amplification. Furthermore, PCR is becoming a widely used and highly sensitive diagnostic tool. A small amount of DNA or RNA from a pathogen can, if present, be amplified directly from host tissue.

Modifications of the original PCR procedure are now found in all fields of genetics, including genome mapping (Chap. 13), population genetics (Chap. 25), and gene expression (Chap. 15) as well as molecular taxonomy and systematics. PCR in species diagnostics is powerful; it can amplify a DNA sequence from a minute amount of template DNA collected from field specimens. The amplified DNA can then be analyzed using the methods described below to determine species identity. The technique is extremely useful for small arthropods. It also permits the investigator to retain much of the carcass to be examined for pathogens, parasites, potential biological control agents as well as gut contents, age, and other characters important in epidemiological and ecological studies. Amplified regions need not be repetitive (although these regions are frequently useful), and this increases the number of possible genes or regions that can be exploited for identification. Two categories of PCR techniques are used. Some PCR techniques amplify a specific "targeted" region of the genome using primer pairs that flank that region. Alternative techniques use a single primer and low annealing temperatures to amplify arbitrary regions of the genome.

PCR Amplification of Specific Regions (Targeted PCR)

The goal in designing targeted PCR systems for taxonomy is to identify regions of the genome that have species-specific sequences or are species-specific in size. The general tactic adopted is outlined in Figure 26.6. Complete sequence information in the chosen region from all species that we wish to differentiate is necessary. This can require cloning them from a library or PCR amplification of these regions using primers that anneal to flanking sequences that are conserved across distant taxa. These cloned or amplified regions are then sequenced. When complete sequence information is available, we design primer A so that it always anneals to a conserved sequence in the region and then design a species-specific primer B that anneals to a region unique to a species. Ultimately, the PCR reaction contains multiple B primers, each complementary to only 1 member of the complex. A further requirement for detection is that each amplified product be unique in size.

During the PCR reaction, primer A will anneal with template DNA from all species; however, primer B, if designed correctly, will only anneal to the flanking region in the species with the complementary sequence. Geometric amplification occurs only if both primers can anneal to DNA of the target species. The PCR reaction mix contains all primers, but only those complementary to the template from the unknown field specimens will result in amplification. Furthermore, they will amplify a fragment that is unique in

1) Amplify genomic region containing species specific sequences in each member of the species group.

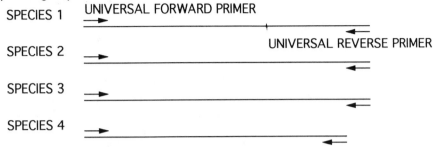

SPECIES 1   UNIVERSAL FORWARD PRIMER

                                              UNIVERSAL REVERSE PRIMER

SPECIES 2

SPECIES 3

SPECIES 4

2) Obtain complete nucleotide sequences in all species. Locate sequences that are species specific and are located in regions that will produce products of a detectably different size.

3) Build a primer that is complementary to the species specific region for each species.

4) Perform PCR with a mixture of the 5 primers. The universal forward primer and 4 reverse, species specific primers.

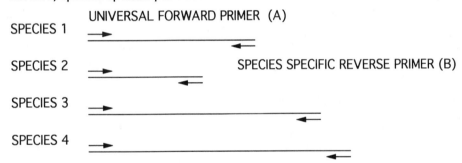

UNIVERSAL FORWARD PRIMER (A)

SPECIES 1

SPECIES 2   SPECIES SPECIFIC REVERSE PRIMER (B)

SPECIES 3

SPECIES 4

5) Separate products of PCR reaction on agarose gels. Stain gel with ethidium bromide and visualize bands under ultraviolet light. Each species produces a band that is unique in size

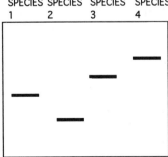

SPECIES SPECIES SPECIES SPECIES
  1   2   3   4

26.6 Steps in developing species-specific primers for targeted PCR amplification as a tool for discriminating closely related species

size for each species. This size difference can be visualized on ethidium bromide-stained agarose gels following electrophoresis of the amplified product. Two excellent references on recent applications of this technique in differentiation of members of the *An. gambiae* complex are Paskewitz and Collins (1990) and Scott et al. (1993).

Most recently, Hiss et al. (1994) developed a technique based on single strand conformation polymorphism (SSCP) (Orita et al. 1989) analysis of PCR products that circumvents the need for the identification and design of species-specific primers. This is illustrated in Figure 26.7. With this procedure, PCR is performed using universal primers. Following amplification, the double-stranded product is melted to single strands at 95°C for 5 min and then placed immediately into an ice bath (0–4°C) so that single strand duplexes are formed from intrastrand base pairing. The conformation of the single strand duplexes is extremely sensitive to the primary DNA sequence. Orita et al. (1989) reported that up to 95% of all point mutations in a gene affect its single strand conformation. Hiss et al. (1994) emphasized the use of rDNA genes for SSCP because the rRNA product is known to form secondary stem structures throughout the molecule in vivo and is thus likely to be more sensitive to point mutations that affect intrastrand pairing; however, it is likely that other types of genes will work as well.

Variation in the conformation of the intrastrand duplexes is visualized in a gel retardation assay. Following PCR, and the heating and rapid cooling process, the chilled products are loaded onto a 5% polyacrylamide 1X TBE (0.09 M Trisborate, 0.02 M EDTA) gel containing 5% glycerol and fractionated at room temperature for 16 hr, using low amperage to insure no increases in temperature that could disrupt the intrastrand pairing conformation. The gel is then removed and the products are visualized using silver staining. Application of this technique to ticks is illustrated in Figure 26.8. SSCP analysis uses the same types of vertical polyacrylamide gel apparatus as described for protein electrophoresis.

What Are Candidate Regions of the Genome for a Targeted PCR Approach?

From our discussion of species-specific probes it is clear that repetitive DNA sequences are often species-specific. Although it might be possible to design species-specific primers in these regions, repetitive regions frequently vary more in number than in kind among closely related taxa. Thus, a great deal of sequencing and searching would be necessary to identify species-specific sequences in repetitive regions. Furthermore, PCR is so sensitive that if a repetitive region occurred even in a few copies in a nontarget species, the primers would no longer be specific. Standard PCR is not quantitative; the numbers of copies in the initial template DNA are not reflected in the amount of product at the end of the reaction.

In looking for regions containing species-specific sequences, multigene families are a good alternative to dispersed or localized repetitive regions of genomes. Members of multigene families are frequently distributed in an array of tandem repeats. Conserved coding regions of family members are frequently separated by noncoding, spacer regions. Examples of multigene families that have this structure are the ribosomal RNA genes, the histone genes, globin genes, and actin and myosin genes. Each of the multigene families has conserved coding regions that flank often variable, noncoding regions. A conserved primer (Primer A, Fig. 26.6) can be constructed in conserved areas of the coding region whereas species-specific primers (Primer B, Fig. 26.6) can be designed in the more variable noncoding regions. A multigene family that has been used in this way is the rDNA cistron that codes for the RNA components of ribosomes. Excellent reviews of insect rDNA are in Beckingham (1981) or Gerbi (1985). The anatomy of the rRNA cistron is outlined in Figure 26.9. The rDNA genes occur as 150–1000 tandem repeats in arthropods. Each repeat contains 18S, 5.8S, and 28S rRNA genes alternating with a large intergenic spacer (IGS) region. Located between the 18S and 5.8S genes is the 1st internal transcribed spacer (ITS1), and between the 5.8S and the 28S genes is the ITS2. Each member of the rDNA multigene family is connected

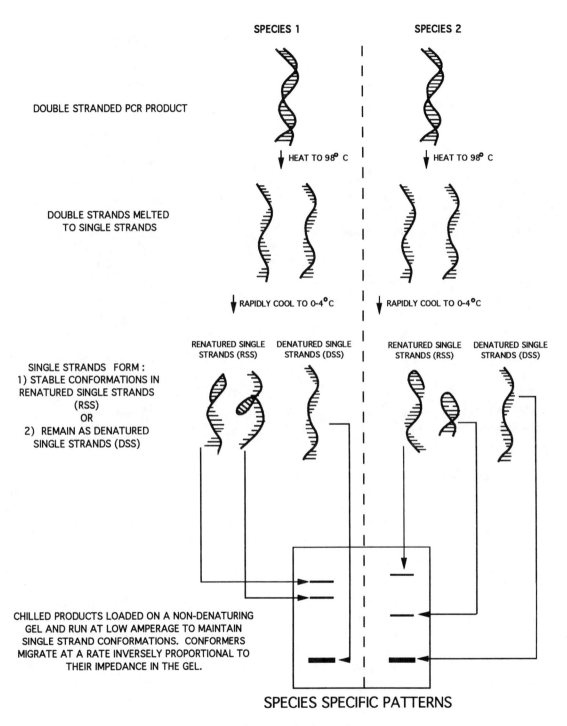

26.7 Steps in the detection of single strand conformational polymorphisms

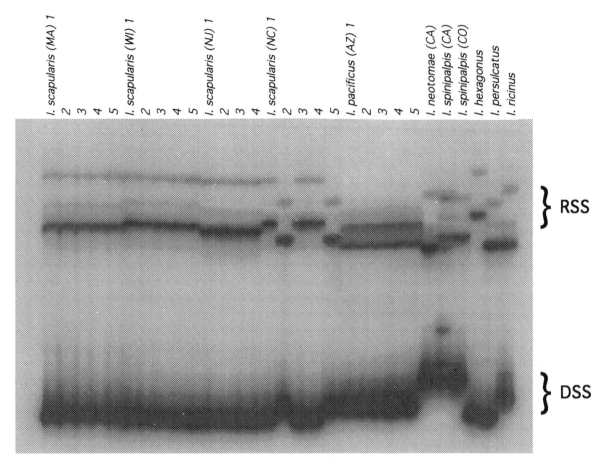

26.8 Autoradiograph of a 16S mitrochondrial rDNA PCR-SSCP gel. Procedures are described in Figure 26.7 and the text. The first 5 lanes are *Ixodes scapularis* from Massachusetts, the next 5 lanes are the same species from Wisconsin, the next 4 individuals are the same species from New Jersey, and the final 5 *Ixodes scapularis* are from North Carolina. *I. pacificus* individuals from Arizona appear in the next 5 lanes followed by *I. neotomae* from California, and *I. spinipalpis* from California and Colorado. The final 3 contain PCR-SSCP products from the species indicated.

by the IGS that is 3–5 kb or greater in length. The IGS frequently contains tandem direct or nested repeats that vary in size. Although the rRNA coding regions are central to the construction and functioning of the ribosome and conserved within species, the ITS regions and the IGS frequently vary intraspecifically in sequence and length and do not appear to be under the same intensity of selection. Members of this multigene family seem to evolve through concerted evolution and molecular drive discussed previously.

Species-specific primers for the 5 common members of the *An. gambiae* complex have been developed using primers in the rDNA IGS. The conserved primer (Primer A, Fig. 26.6) was located in the 3' end of the 28S molecule. Approximately 2 kb of sequence information from the flanking IGS regions was obtained in each member of the complex and from this 4 species-specific primers (Primer B, Fig. 26.6) were designed. These were located so that they amplify different size fragments in each species (Paskewitz and Collins 1990; Scott et al. 1993).

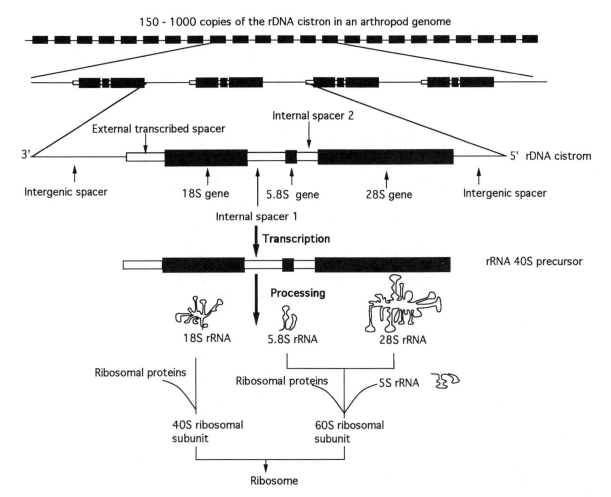

26.9 The genes that code for the RNA component of the ribosome are coded for by the rDNA cistron. Individual rDNA cistrons form members of rDNA multigene family. These members are distributed as tandem repeats in one or more locations in the genome of an organism. The rDNA cistron alternates between conserved rRNA coding genes, variable internal transcribed spaces, and a highly variable intergenic spacer.

Advantages and Disadvantages of Targeted PCR

There are many advantages to this technique. Little initial intact template DNA is required because the process utilizes PCR. Some laboratories work with single parts of arthropods, leaving the rest of the carcass for pathogen isolation or testing for associated biological control agents. PCR-based procedures work well with small arthropods. Specimens in alcohol or dried specimens can usually be used. Primers, or at least primer sequences, can be sent to other laboratories. Reaction conditions can be standardized to promote reproducibility across laboratories. The precautions to take when setting up a PCR laboratory and the techniques used to set up PCR reactions are easily learned. There is minimal concern with contamination from distant taxa because primers are species-specific. This is of concern with the arbitrarily primed PCR methods in which DNA from pathogens, parasites, and phoretic organisms can potentially produce contamination.

The few disadvantages of this approach are that the thermal cycler and electrophoresis equipment are fairly expensive (minimum investment is about $6,000 in 1994 dollars). Development of primers requires knowledge of complete sequence information of target taxa and closely related species. This is becoming faster and easier with increased information on primers with broad taxonomic applications and techniques involving automated sequencing and cycle sequencing; however, even sequence information is no longer necessary with the SSCP-based procedures described. In all PCR-based techniques there is always the danger of minute amounts of contaminating template DNA being passed among tubes, and this is a danger when working with groups of individuals. A negative control, a tube containing all components of a reaction and handled simultaneously and in an identical manner to all treatment tubes, should always be processed and examined for contamination.

PCR Amplification of Arbitrary Genomic Regions

Recently 2 closely related techniques have been described that employ PCR to amplify arbitrary regions of a genome using a single primer. Williams et al. (1990) developed a technique, random amplified polymorphic DNA (RAPD) PCR, that uses a 10 oligonucleotide primer of random sequence but with a minimum guanine-cytosine content of 60%. Welsh and McClelland (1990) invented an analogous technique called arbitrarily primed (AP) PCR that employs a longer primer but with no known similarity to sequences in the template DNA (e.g., the universal M13 sequencing primer). In both techniques a relatively low annealing temperature (37–40°C) is used that allows the primer to anneal to arbitrary regions of the genome that are not fully complementary to the primer. A low annealing temperature is maintained throughout all cycles in RAPD-PCR but is used in only the initial cycles with AP-PCR. A general mechanism for arbitrarily primed PCR is described in Fig. 26.6. The product of either of these processes is a

series of bands up to 2 kb in size that vary in their presence or absence among and within species.

Products from arbitrarily primed PCR reactions are visualized and compared on ethidium bromide–stained agarose gels following electrophoresis. This approach has shown that banding patterns are diagnostic for species. Wilkerson et al. (1992) demonstrated that RAPD patterns are species-specific in *An. gambiae* and in *An. arabiensis*. RAPD-PCR patterns were diagnostic for subspecies of *Ae. aegypti* (Ballinger-Crabtree et al. 1992). Kambhampati et al. (1993) used them as species diagnostic markers in the *Ae. scutellaris* group.

The advantage of arbitrarily primed PCR over amplification of specific regions is that no sequence information or expensive designing of primers is required. In practice only 1 or a few primers must be examined to derive a specific pattern. The patterns that are produced are highly species-specific. This advantage exacts a price, however, because microscopic examination of field-collected material usually reveals the presence of pathogens, parasites, symbionts, or simply phoretic microorganisms. The low annealing temperatures used in arbitrarily primed PCR allow the primers to anneal to any template. Amplified bands can arise from the target taxon or from contaminants.

Banding patterns resulting from RAPD- or AP-PCR can often be complex in a taxon and difficult to score and compare among taxa. This contrasts with targeted PCR in which sizes of amplified products are easily compared on agarose gels or with PAGE gels following SSCP analysis. Banding patterns are influenced by the quality of DNA so that alcohol or dried preserved specimens cannot be used reliably. Many factors before and during the reaction can affect banding patterns so that there must be extensive standardization within and among laboratories. Black (1993) reviewed the uses and abuses of this technique in insect genetics.

WHAT'S BEST?

All of the techniques that have been described have unique advantages and disadvantages. Protein analysis is rapid and inexpensive but requires the availability of refrigerated protein electrophoresis equipment. Protein instability demands that field material be kept alive or preserved frozen. Furthermore, protein banding patterns are often specific to the life stage under analysis. Hybridization assays with species-specific probes offer a rapid and inexpensive means to screen a large number of squash-blotted individuals simultaneously. Hybridizations require the least amount of specialized (and expensive) equipment. Primers labeled with specific ligands for detection with linked enzyme assays or flourescence detection offer the potential for simultaneous detection of all probes in a single hybridization; however, considerable work is involved in identifying and developing species-specific probes.

All PCR processes are rapid, highly sensitive, and specific. PCR techniques require the availability of a thermal cycler and agarose gel electrophoresis equipment and depend upon refrigeration to maintain nucleotides and polymerases. Furthermore, setting up PCR reactions involves many manipulations of individual insects and solutions. In contrast to squash blots, these techniques require not only a great deal of pipetting but also deplete plastic microcentrifuge tubes and pipette tips. These practical considerations aside, targeted PCR amplification of specific regions using a mixture of species-specific primers shows great promise as a molecular taxonomic tool; however, as with species-specific probes, considerable effort is required to identify and design species-specific primers. SSCP analysis of targeted PCR products does not require the identification and design of species-specific primers or probes but does require vertical PAGE equipment. SSCP analysis promises to become a useful technique in molecular taxonomy if only for rapidly analyzing candidate genes for their species-specificity. All 4 techniques discussed are superior to arbitrarily primed PCR because they require almost no data analysis and are not subject to extraneous banding from environmental sources of contamination.

It is important to point out that PCR- and hybridization-based diagnostics are being developed for many vector-borne pathogens. PCR and hybridization techniques are widely used in arbovirology. Delves et al. (1989) and Hughes et al. (1990) described techniques for detection of *Plasmodium falciparum* with hybridization techniques in field-collected mosquitoes to study sporozoite prevalence in members of species complexes.

Barker et al. (1992) described a PCR assay for *P. falciparum*. PCR diagnostics are available now for *Leishmania* (Lopez et al. 1993), *Trypanosoma cruzi* (Breniere et al. 1992), and *Rickettsia tsutsugamushi* (Sugita et al. 1993), to provide just a few examples. These diagnostics can be integrated with the techniques described in this chapter to develop an integrated molecular approach to epidemiology. Field-collected arthropods can be identified to species and tested for the presence of pathogens to determine prevalence rates in different species and races. At the same time, information on genetic relationships among vector and pathogen populations can be obtained.

INTRASPECIFIC VARIATION IN MOLECULAR TAXONOMY

Is the Chosen Marker Species-Specific?

Good taxonomic practice dictates that the amount of intraspecific information in a character be estimated, described, and incorporated into the taxonomic description of a species. A taxonomic character that appears to be useful for separation of taxa in 1 geographic region may overlap taxa in another region. It is important when developing molecular markers to sample populations from diverse geographic and temporal settings and to examine variation in pattern or sequence among these collections. The question should be asked: Is the amount of variation within the species less than the variation among the closely related taxa? If true, the markers or patterns that have been identified are unique to the species. If the answer is no, too much overlap exists with closely related groups to rely on the marker or pattern.

Molecular biologists must be aware that all taxonomic classifications are fallible. When working with closely related taxonomic groups it is always possible that the taxa will not turn out to be separate species or that they have been incorrectly identified in the taxonomic literature. In attempting to develop species diagnostic markers the species status of the taxa is being tested.

Another possibility when examining closely related taxa is that a taxonomic grade, or cline, will be discovered. Often a species is distributed along a latitudinal, longitudinal, climatic, or altitudinal gradient. If taxonomists sampled populations at ends of these environmental extremes, they might split a single species into 2 when in fact gene flow occurs freely among populations distributed throughout intermediate regions. This pattern might be revealed through extensive geographic sampling.

All of these procedures take time, thorough sampling of taxa, and careful examination of molecular characters. The danger is to assume that molecular markers developed from laboratory colonies or single field collections are representative of the entire species. These markers, especially if they originate from laboratory colonies, are a limited sample of the actual genetic variability in the field. The sequences that we have discussed are useful in separating closely related taxa because they mutate quickly. Sequences that mutate quickly vary intraspecifically. Molecular taxonomists must estimate intraspecific variation when working with closely related taxa. This dictates that a population genetics rather than a strict taxonomic approach be taken (Tabachnick and Black 1994). For example, Wesson et al. (1993) examined gene flow among populations of *Ixodes dammini* and *I. scapularis* using sequence data from the rDNA ITS1 and ITS2 regions. By comparing variability of their markers within and among taxa, they found complete overlap in sequences among these taxa. This supports recent reclassification of *I. dammini* as a junior synonym of *I. scapularis* (Oliver et al. 1993). However, if they had simply accepted the existing taxonomic status and gathered sequence information from single laboratory colonies, they might have developed primers that had no relevance to gene flow in the field.

Good molecular markers will not be developed quickly. It will require time, patience, and extensive testing in the field. Scott et al. (1993) reported that their markers have been tested in a large number of laboratories in areas in which members of the *An. gambiae* complex are present.

BIOCHEMICAL AND MOLECULAR SYSTEMATICS

Hematophagous arthropods have fascinating evolutionary histories. Ultimately, complete description of zoonotic disease cycles requires an understanding of how these systems evolved. This will require construction of phylogenies not only of the vector species but also of their hosts and the pathogens that they transmit. A number of informative books and papers on this subject have recently appeared (e.g., Kim 1985; Rai et al. 1982; Brookes and McLennan 1993; Klompen et al. 1995).

The concept of parallel evolution between hematophagous arthropods, especially more permanent ectoparasites, and their vertebrate hosts is well entrenched in the medical entomology literature. However, many hematophagous arthropods spend little time on their host (e.g., most dipteran species, some flea species, trombiculid mites), whereas others spend a large proportion of their life on the host (e.g., ticks, psoroptic, and chorioptic mange mites); still others spend almost their entire life cycle on the host (e.g., chewing and sucking lice, follicle and nasal mites). Alternative models of hematophagous ectoparasite speciation based on habitat adaptation or biogeographic distribution have received little or no attention in medical entomology or ectoparasite evolutionary biology. Analysis of the phylogenies of ectoparasites with respect to their host's phylogeny, biogeography, habitat, and life histories will indicate the relative degree to which host versus habitat have influenced arthropod ectoparasite evolution. At least 1 reason that alternative modes of speciation have not been advanced has been the absence of tools for the construction of phylogenies. Molecular and biochemical systematics promises to become a powerful tool in analyzing host and parasite evolution.

The objective of any systematic analysis of a group is to derive the true phylogenies for species in that group. This is referred to as a species tree and indicates the exact order with which species were derived in the evolution of a group. In the case of molecular characters, the derived phylogeny is referred to as a gene tree. Ideally, the species tree and the gene tree will be concordant. Problems arise when the derived phylogeny reflects the relationships among the morphological or molecular characters examined and these are independent of the true phylogeny of the species. This could occur for a variety of reasons.

The chief argument for the use of proteins and nucleic acid sequence data in systematic studies is that, in theory, sequences are largely unaffected by environmental selection pressures and therefore can stand as neutral indicators that accumulate differences at a constant rate through time. By this argument the number of accumulated differences between species should be proportional to the time elapsed since their divergence (i.e., act as a "molecular clock"). If this were strictly true, sequence data would provide a means for testing for divergence time among groups. In contrast, a shared morphological character in a group might not be controlled by the same sets of genes. Natural selection might cause convergence of function among nonhomologous genes and lead to an erroneous grouping of species using morphological data. By using a molecular systematic approach in which the same gene is examined in each taxon, it should be possible to detect molecular divergence despite morphological convergence.

The problem with this approach in practice is that there are good examples of selection acting on genes at the amino acid level (Koehn et al. 1983) as well as at the level of nucleotides (Kimura 1986), thus raising the possibility of convergence in gene sequences among species. Furthermore, analyses of amino acid sequences among taxa have shown that not all amino acid substitutions are functionally equivalent. There are selective constraints that vary among and within proteins and affect the rate with which substitutions can be tolerated. This is corroborated at the nucleotide level because the rate of synonymous substitutions is generally much higher (4.7×10^{-9} per year) than the rate of nonsynonymous substitutions (range = 0.004×10^{-9} per year [histone H4] to 2.8×10^{-9} per year [gamma interferon]) (Kimura 1986). At a still more fundamental level, tRNAs with different but synonymous anticodons are not all equally abundant in the cytoplasm. This has caused differences in codon usage among species with the result that not all synonymous substitutions can be considered selectively neutral.

These problems have resulted in the consideration of noncoding sequences for use in molecular systematic studies. Noncoding regions such as pseudogenes, introns, or internal spacers (e.g., in the rRNA cistron)

are known to have 3–5 times higher mutation rates than even synonymous sites in coding regions. Such regions are also appealing because they offer the opportunity to study sequences that are presumably devoid of function and therefore subject only to the effects of mutation and random drift. Because of high copy numbers, ease of cloning, and the ability to resolve divergence in coding as well as noncoding sequences, regions of the rDNA cistron discussed have also been considered ideal candidates for molecular systematics studies and are frequently used.

Analysis of mitochondrial DNA (mtDNA) was discussed as a tool for population genetics in Chapter 24. Analysis of mtDNA has also become a powerful tool in molecular systematics and has been used in studies of insect populations and species (Avise 1986). The mitochondrial genome is primarily maternally inherited, and there is no recombination among mitochondrial genomes. Maternal lineages can be traced to determine the phylogenies of existing populations and species independent of founders effects and selection or adaptation. This evidence cannot be directly obtained or inferred from studies of genomic systems experiencing recombination or biparental inheritance. The mitochondrial genome mutates rapidly, and for this reason intraspecific variation is frequently detectable. As expected, most of the changes in the mitochondrial genomes of closely related species involve single-base substitutions. This permits the degree of nucleotide divergence to be easily calculated and phylogenetic relationships to be derived. The disadvantages of mtDNA in invertebrate phylogenies are the high A-T content (sometimes as great as 80%) that reduces the number of character states that a nucleotide substitution can assume and the very high substitution rates observed in some genes.

Analysis of Molecular and Biochemical Data

Once a collection of isozyme mobilities, RFLP profiles, or nucleotide sequences have been recorded for a group, we are faced with the problem of analyzing these data to derive objective phylogenies. In cladistic analysis, the procedure for deriving phylogenies usually entails examining a set of homologous characters among the species to be analyzed. Homology is the correspondence of features (morphology or molecules) in different taxa caused by inheritance from a common ancestor. In the case of enzymes analyzed in biochemical systematics, homology is inferred because the enzymes from different species react with a common set of substrates in the histochemical stain. For example, all bands that appear on a gel stained from phosphoglucomutase are assumed to be homologous because they react with a common substrate and are assumed to have arisen from a common gene that coded for phosphoglucomutase and arose prior to the radiation of those species. The homology of nucleic acid sequences amplified during targeted PCR is inferred because they are amplified from the same pair of oligonucleotide primers that are specific for that gene region. The homology of patterns in hybridization assays is established because target genes that hybridize to a probe must share a high degree of sequence similarity. Assuming evolutionary homology of a set of characters, the next step involves determining the state of each character. Character states are recorded for each taxa to develop a taxa-character matrix. With biochemical data, proteins are recorded as having identical states if they have equivalent mobility during electrophoresis. With nucleic acids, each nucleotide position has 5 possible character states including an A, C, G, T, or a gap that arises from insertions and deletions.

Once a taxa-character matrix has been derived, a phylogeny can be inferred using 1 of any number of different cladistic methods. Heated debate has arisen over techniques for phylogeny reconstruction. Review of these issues is too lengthy for this chapter; recent reviews by Felsenstein (1988), Swofford and Olsen (1990), and the Li and Graur (1991) textbook provide in-depth discussions. Several excellent and low-cost software packages are available for phylogeny reconstruction. PHYLIP 3.5C is available through electronic mail from the anonymous FTP file evolution.genetics.washington.edu from Joe Felsenstein. PAUP 3.01 is available through the Illinois Natural History Survey, Champaign, Illinois. MACCLADE® is available through Sinauer Press. MEGA is available from the Institute of Molecular Evolutionary Genetics at Pennsylvania State University (e-mail address: imeg@psuvm.psu.edu).

CHOOSING TECHNIQUES FOR MOLECULAR SYSTEMATICS

Although isozymes and RFLP patterns have been used in molecular systematic investigations, it is clear that a greater number of taxonomically informative characters exist in gene sequences. A large and growing list of primers is available for molecular taxonomy of different groups, making it relatively easy to amplify a homologous gene sequence in many taxa. Simon et al. (1994) list a variety of primers that have been found to be useful in studies of mtDNA throughout the arthropods. Furthermore, recent advances in cycle sequencing have simplified the process of obtaining sequence information from amplified molecules. Black and Piesman (1994) demonstrate an approach using nested primers for PCR and sequencing that allow for rapid extraction of sequence information from taxa.

When beginning any molecular study, it is difficult to identify the appropriate sequences to examine in a particular group. There are no rules to follow at this point, and the utility of a sequence must be determined empirically. Generally, the reliance on a single sequence for phylogeny reconstruction has proved to be problematic, and most workers agree that a multiple sequence approach is optimal or even critical. To make any study feasible, sequences must be picked that can be processed quickly and reliably. There are currently no rules to follow on this either.

Current Progress

A number of molecular systematic studies on hematophagous arthropod groups have begun to appear. Xiong and Kocher (1991) examined variation in the 16s RNA mtDNA sequence among 7 species of black flies in 4 genera. Wesson et al. (1992) used ITS sequence variation among genera and subfamilies of Culicidae to reconstruct phylogenies. Black and Piesman (1994) examined the evolution of hard and soft tick taxa using sequence variation in the 16S mitochondrial rDNA gene. The higher level systematics of ticks have also been examined with the nuclear 18s rDNA gene (Klompen et al. 1995). To date only a single study has provided molecular systematic evidence for cospeciation between hosts and ectoparasites. Hafner et al. (1994) examined variation in the mitochondrial cytochrome oxidase I gene in pocket gophers and their associated chewing lice and demonstrated parallel phylogenies suggestive of cospeciation. This is, however, a host-parasite system in which there is limited opportunity for host transfer.

CONCLUSION

Molecular taxonomy is already being practiced in a number of groups of medically important arthropods and has improved the accuracy of identifications in a timely fashion during outbreaks of disease. Molecular taxonomy will be increasingly used in applications in the future, improving the quality of ecological and epidemiological studies by allowing species identification during any stage of development and permitting examination of small arthropods. Coupled with the diagnostic techniques being advanced for detection and identification of pathogens and parasites, vector molecular taxonomy will enable the analysis of vectorial capacity in local populations and even among individuals within populations. This level of resolution is unprecedented in the history of vector-borne disease.

Traditional dichotomous keys are gradually being replaced with whole organism systems based on multiple characters. This has already occurred with the development of morphological keys integrated with digitized scanning of characters or whole organisms under the DELTA programming system (Dietrich and Pooley 1994). Advances in taxonomic software have already revolutionized morphological identifications for certain medically important insects. These same computer programs will soon be applied to molecular characters. Eventually the multiplicity of phenotypes elucidated by molecular methods will be best interpreted by scanning devices connected to a dedicated microprocessor.

Medical entomologists and parasitologists have been enamored with the concept of parallel speciation between hematophagous ectoparasitic arthropods and their vertebrate hosts. Molecular systematics will allow, perhaps for the 1st time, the construction of well-resolved phylogenies to test hypotheses of parallel evolution. These phylogenies will not only increase our understanding of how these arthropod groups have evolved but will also allow us to examine the role that habitat and biogeography have played in ectoparasite evolution. In addition, analysis of the congruence between pathogen and vector phylogenies will increase our understanding of the evolutionary interface between pathogen and vectors.

ACKNOWLEDGMENTS

This chapter benefited greatly from the comments of Boris Kondratieff and Julian Crampton.

NOTES

1. The letters "s.l." and "s.s" often follow the names of members of species complexes or of species that are polytypic, meaning that they show a range of variation in taxonomic characters throughout their distribution. The abbreviations "s.l." and "s.s." stand for *sensu lato* and *sensu stricto* respectively and are Latin for "in the broad sense" and "in the strict sense." When we speak of *An. gambiae* s.l. we refer broadly to all 4 members of the species complex, but when we refer to *An. gambiae* s.s. we are referring strictly to the biological species *An. gambiae* (formerly species A). Often in polytypic species *sensu* is followed by an author designation indicating that a specimen was identified based on the characters described by that author and implying that not all descriptions of that species agree.

REFERENCES

Avise, J.C. 1986. Mitochondrial DNA and the evolutionary genetics of higher animals. *Phil. Trans. Roy. Soc.* (B)312:325–342.

Ballinger-Crabtree, M.E., W.C. Black IV, and B.R. Miller. 1992. Use of genetic polymorphisms detected by RAPD-PCR for differentiation and identification of *Aedes aegypti* populations. *Am. J. Trop. Med. Hyg.* 47:893–901.

Barker, R.H. Jr., T. Banchongaksorn, J.M. Courval, W. Suwonkerd, K. Rimwungtragoon, and D.F. Wirth. 1992. A simple method to detect *Plasmodium falciparun* directly from blood samples using the polymerase chain reaction. *Am. J. Trop. Med. Hyg.* 46:416–426.

Beckingham, K. 1981. Insect rDNA. In: H. Busch and L. Rothblum, editors, *The cell nucleus*. Vol. 10, Part A. New York: Academic Press. pp. 205–269.

Black, W.C. IV. 1993. PCR with arbitrary primers: Approach with care. *Insect Mol. Biol.* 2:1–6.

Black, W.C. IV, and J. Piesman. 1994. A phylogeny of hard and soft tick taxa based on mitochondrial 16S ribosomal DNA sequences. *Proc. Natl. Acad. Sci. USA* 91:10034–10038.

Breniere, S. F., M. F. Bosseno, S. Revollo, M. T. Rivera, Y. Carlier, and M. Tibayrenc. 1992. Direct identification of *Trypanosoma cruzi* natural clones in vectors and mammalian hosts by polymerase chain reaction amplification. *Am. J. Trop. Med. Hyg.* 46:335–341.

Brooks, D.R., and D.A. McLennan. 1993. *Parascript parasites and the language of evolution*. Smithsonian Series in Comparative Evolutionary Biology. Washington, DC: Smithsonian Institution Press.

Brust, R.A., and L.E. Munstermann. 1992. Morphological and genetic characterization of the *Aedes (Ochlerotatus) communis* complex (Diptera: Culicidae) in North America. *Ann. Entomol. Soc. Am.* 85:1–10.

Bullini, L., and M. Coluzzi. 1982. Evolutionary and taxonomic inferences of electrophoretic studies in mosquitoes. In: W.W.M. Steiner, W.J. Tabachnick, K.S. Rai, and S. Narang, editors, *Recent developments in the genetics of insect disease vectors. A symposium proceedings*. Champaign, IL: Stipes Publishing. pp. 465–482.

Clapp, J.P., R.A. McKee, L. Allen-Williams, J.G. Hopley, and R.J. Slater. 1993. Genomic subtractive hybridization to isolate species-specific DNA sequences in insects. *Insect Mol. Biol.* 2:133–138.

Coen, E.S., J.M. Thoday, and G. Dover. 1982. Rate of turnover of structural variants in the rDNA gene family of *Drosophila melanogaster*. *Nature* 295:564–568.

Crosskey, R.W. 1988. Old tools and new taxonomic problems in bloodsucking insects. In: M.W. Service, editor, *Biosystematics of hematophagous insects*. Systematics Association Special, Volume No. 37. Oxford, UK: Clarendon. pp. 133–147.

Delves, C.J., M. Goman, R.G. Ridley, H. Matile, T.H.W. Lensen, T. Ponnudurai, and J.G. Scaife. 1989. Identification of *Plasmodium falciparum* infected mosquitoes using a probe containing repetitive DNA. *Mol. Biochem. Parasit.* 32:105–112.

Dover, G.A. 1986. Molecular drive in multigene families: How biological novelties arise, spread and are assimilated. *Curr. Trends Genet.* 8:159–165.

Dietrich, C.H., and C.D. Pooley. 1994. Automated identification of leafhoppers (Homoptera: Cicadellidae). *Ann. Entomol. Soc. Am.* (in press).

Felsenstein, J. 1988. Phylogenies from molecular sequences: Inference and reliability. *Ann. Rev. Genet.* 22:521–565.

Gale, K.R., and J.M. Crampton. 1987. DNA probes for species identification of mosquitoes in the *Anopheles gambiae* complex. *Med. Vet. Entomol.* 1:127–136.

———. 1988. Use of a male specific DNA probe to distinguish female mosquitoes of the *Anopheles gambiae* complex. *Med. Vet. Entomol.* 2:77–79.

Gerbi, S.A. 1985. Evolution of ribosomal DNA. In: R.J. MacIntyre, editor, *Molecular evolutionary genetics*. New York: Plenum. pp. 419–517.

Hafner, M.S., P.D. Sudman, F.X. Villablanca, T.A. Spraling, J.W. Demastes, and S.A. Nadler. 1994. Disparate rates of molecular evolution in cospeciating hosts and parasites. *Science* 265:1087–1090.

Harris, H., and D.A. Hopkinson. 1976. *Handbook of enzyme electrophoresis in human genetics*. Amsterdam: North-Holland.

Hill, S.M., R. Urwin, and J.M. Crampton. 1991a. A comparison of non-radioactive labelling and detection systems with synthetic oligonucleotide probes for the species identification of mosquitoes in the *Anopheles gambiae* complex. *Am. J. Trop. Med. Hyg.* 44:609–622.

Hill, S.M., R. Urwin, T.F. Knapp, and J.M. Crampton. 1991b. Synthetic DNA probes for the identification of sibling species in the *Anopheles gambiae* complex. *Med. Vet. Entomol.* 5:455–463.

Hill, S. M., R. Urwin, and J.M. Crampton. 1992. A simplified, non-radioactive DNA probe protocol for the field identification of insect vector specimens. *Trans. R. Soc. Trop. Med. Hyg.* 86:213–215.

Hillis, D.M., and C. Moritz. 1990. *Molecular Systematics*. Sunderland, MA: Sinauer Associates Inc.

Hiss, R.H., D.E. Norris, C.R. Dietrich, R. F. Whitcomb, D.F. West, C.F. Bosio, S. Kambhampati, J. Piesman, M.F. Antolin, and W.C. Black IV. 1994. Molecular taxonomy using single strand conformation polymorphism (SSCP) analysis of mitochondrial ribosomal DNA Genes. *Insect Mol. Biol.* 3:171–182.

Hughes, M.A., M. Hommel, and J.M. Crampton. 1990. The use of biotin-labelled, synthetic DNA oligomers for the detection and identification of *Plasmodium falciparum*. *Parasitol.* 100:383–387.

Hunt, G.J., and R.E. Page. 1992. Patterns of inheritance with RAPD molecular markers reveal novel types of polymorphisms in the honey bee. *Theor. Appl. Genet.* 85:15–20.

Kambhampati, S., W.C. Black IV, and K.S. Rai. 1992. RAPD-PCR for identification and differentiation of mosquito species and populations: Techniques and Statistical analysis. *J. Med. Ent.* 29:939–945.

Kawasaki, E.S. 1990. Sample preparation from blood, cells and other fluids. In: M.A. Innis, D.H. Gelfand, J.J. Sninsky, and T.J. White, editors, *PCR protocols: A guide to methods and applications.* San Diego, Academic Press. pp. 146–152.

Kazmer, D.J. 1991. Isoelectric focusing procedures for the analysis of allozyme variation in minute arthropods. *Ann. Entomol. Soc. Am.* 84:332–339.

Kim, K.C. 1985. *Coevolution of parasitic arthropods and mammals.* New York: John Wiley and Sons. 800 pp.

Kimura, M. 1986. DNA and the neutral theory. *Phil. Trans. R. Soc. Lond.* (B)312:343–354.

Klompen, J.S.H., W.C. Black IV, J.E. Keirans, and J.O. Oliver Jr. 1995. Evolution of ticks. *Ann. Rev. Entom.* (in press).

Koehn, R.K., A.J. Zera, and J.G. Hall. 1983. Enzyme polymorphism and natural selection. In: M. Nei and R.K. Koehn, editors, *Evolution of genes and proteins.* Sunderland, MA: Sinauer Associates, Inc. pp. 115–136.

Li, W-H., and D. Graur. 1991. *Fundamentals of Molecular Evolution.* Sunderland, MA: Sinauer Associates, Inc.

Lopez, M.R. Inga, M. Cangalaya, J. Echevarria, A. Llanos-cuentas, C. Orrego, and J. Arevalo. 1993. Diagnosis of *Leishmania* using the polymerase chain reaction: A simplified procedure for field work. *Am. J. Trop. Med. Hyg.* 49:348–356.

Mayr, E., and P.D. Ashlock. 1991. *Principles of systematic zoology.* 2nd ed. New York: McGraw-Hill.

Miles, S.J. 1979. A biochemical key to adult members of the *Anopheles gambiae* group of species (Diptera: Culicidae). *J. Med. Entomol.* 15:297–299.

Munstermann, L.E. 1988. Biochemical systematics of nine nearctic *Aedes* mosquitoes (subgenus *Ochlerotatus*, *annulipes* group B). In: M.W. Service, editor, *Biosystematics of hematophagous insects.* Systematics Association Special Volume, No. 37. Oxford, UK: Clarendon. pp. 133–147.

Narang, S.K., P.E. Kaiser, and J.A. Seawright. 1989. Identification of species D, a new member of the *Anopheles quadrimaculatus* complex: a biochemical key. *J. Am. Mosq. Contr. Assoc.* 5:317–324.

Oliver, J.H., M.R. Owsley, H.J. Hutchinson, A.M. James, C. Chen, W.S. Irby, E.M. Dotson, and D.E. McLain. 1993. Conspecificity of the ticks *Ixodes scapularis* and *Ixodes dammini* (Acari: Ixodidae). *J. Med. Ent.* 30:54–63.

Orita, M., Y. Suzuki, T. Sekiya, and K. Hayashi. 1989. A rapid and sensitive detection of point mutations and genetic polymorphisms using polymerase chain reaction. *Genomics* 5:874–879.

Panyim, S., S. Yasothornsrikul, and V. Baimai. 1988. Species-specific DNA sequences from the *Anopheles dirus* complex—a potential for efficient identification of isomorphic species. In: M.W. Service, editor, *Biosystematics of hematophagous insects.* Systematics Association Special Volume, No. 37. Oxford, UK: Clarendon. pp. 193–202.

Paskewitz, S.M., and F.H. Collins. 1990. Use of the polymerase chain reaction to identify mosquito species of the *Anopheles gambiae* complex. *Med. Vet. Entomol.* 4:367–373.

Post, R.J., and J.M. Crampton. 1988. The taxonomic use of variation in repetitive DNA sequences in the *Simulium damnosum* complex. In: M.W. Service, editor, *Biosystematics of haematophagous insects.* Systematics Association Special Volume, No. 37. Oxford, UK: Clarendon. pp. 133–147.

Post, R.J., P.K. Flook, and M.D. Wilson. 1992. DNA analysis in relation to insect taxonomy, evolution and identification. In: J.M. Crampton and P. Eggleston, editors, *Insect molecular science.* 16th Symposium of the Royal Entomological Society of London. London: Academic Press. pp. 21–34.

Rai, K.S., D.P. Pashley, and L.E. Munstermann. 1982. Genetics of speciation in aedine mosquitoes. In: W.W.M. Steiner, W.J. Tabachnick, K.S. Rai, and S. Narang, editors, *Recent developments in the genetics of insect disease vectors.* Champaign, IL: Stipes Publishing. pp. 84–129.

Richardson, B.J., P.R. Baverstock, and M. Adams. 1986. *Allozyme electrophoresis: A handbook for animal systematics and population structure.* Sydney: Academic Press.

Saiki, R.K., S. Scharf, F. Faloona, K.B. Mullis, G.T. Horn, H.A. Erlich, and N. Arnheim. 1985. Enzymatic amplification of the β-globin genomic sequences and restriction site analysis for diagnosis of sickle cell anemia. *Science* 230:1350–1354.

Sambrook, J., E.F. Fritsch, and T. Maniatis. 1989. *Molecular cloning: A laboratory manual.* Cold Spring Harbor, NY: Cold Spring Harbor Laboratory.

Scott, J.W., W.G. Brogdon, and F.H. Collins. 1993. Identification of single specimens of the *Anopheles gambiae* complex by the polymerase chain reaction. *Am. J. Trop. Med. Hyg.* 49:520–529.

Service, M.W. 1988. *Biosystematics of haematophagous arthropods.* Oxford, UK: Clarendon Press.

Singh, R.S., and L.R. Rhomberg. 1987. A comprehensive study of genic variation in natural populations of *Drosophila melanogaster.* I. Estimates of gene flow from rare alleles. *Genetics* 115:313–322.

Sugita, Y., Y. Yamakawa, K. Takahashi, T. Nagatani, K. Okuda, and H. Nakajima. 1993. A polymerase chain reaction system for rapid diagnosis of scrub typus within six hours. *Am. J. Trop. Med. Hyg.* 49:636–640.

Swofford, D.L., and G.J. Olsen. 1990. Phylogeny reconstruction. In: D.M. Hillis and C. Moritz, editors, *Molecular systematics.* Sunderland, MA: Sinauer Associates Inc. pp. 411–515.

Simon, C., F. Frati, A. Beckenbach, B. Crespi, H. Liu, and P. Flock. 1994. Evolution, weighting, and phylogenetic utility of mitochondrial gene sequences and a compilation of conserved polymerase chain reaction primers. *Ann. Entomol. Soc. Am.* 87: 651–701.

Tabachnick, W.J. 1991. The yellow fever mosquito: Evolutionary genetics and arthropod-borne disease. *Am. Entomol.* 37:14–24.

Tabachnick, W.J., and W.C. Black IV. 1994. Making a case for molecular population genetic studies of arthropod vectors. *Parasit. Today* 11:27–30.

Welsh, J., and M. McClelland. 1990. Fingerprinting genomes using PCR with arbitrary primers. *Nucl. Acids Res.* 18:7213–7219.

Wesson, D.M., C.H. Porter, and F.H. Collins. 1992. Sequence and secondary structure comparisons of ITS rDNA in mosquitoes (Diptera: Culicidae). *Mol. Phyl. Evol.* 1:253–269.

Wesson, D.M., D.K. McLain, J.H. Oliver, J. Piesman, and F.C. Collins. 1993. Investigation of the validity of species status of *Ixodes dammini* (Acari: Ixodidae) using ribosomal DNA. *Proc. Natl. Acad. Sci. USA* 90:10221–10225

Wilkerson, R.C., T.J. Parsons, D.G. Albright, T.A. Klein, and M.J. Braun. 1992. Random amplified polymorphic DNA (RAPD) markers readily distinguish cryptic mosquito species (Diptera: Culicidae: Anopheles). *Insect. Mol. Biol.* 1:205–211.

Williams, J.G.K., A.R. Kubelik, K.J. Livak, J.A. Rafalski, and S.V. Tingey. 1990. DNA polymorphisms amplified by arbitrary primers are useful genetic markers. *Nucl. Acids Res.* 18:6531–6535.

Xiong, B., and T.D. Kocher. 1991. Comparison of mitochondrial DNA sequences of seven morphospecies of black flies (Diptera: Simuliidae). *Genome* 34:306–311.

27. COLLECTING METHODS FOR VECTOR SURVEILLANCE

Chester G. Moore and Kenneth L. Gage

INTRODUCTION

Surveillance is "an organized system of collecting data" for a subject (Bowen and Francy 1980). A vector-borne disease has at least 4 different components that are used in a surveillance program: (1) detection of disease in humans or domestic animals, (2) surveillance of vectors, (3) surveillance of pathogen activity in wild vertebrate hosts, and (4) study of weather patterns related to pathogen transmission (Bowen and Francy 1980). This chapter focuses on surveillance of vectors. A vector surveillance system is any procedure or group of procedures used to collect estimates of vector population characteristics required to predict, prevent, or control vector-borne disease.

Surveillance programs for vector-borne disease are employed to anticipate, prevent, or control disease in humans or domestic animals. The specific type of surveillance system and the methods used are determined by the objective of the overall program. Thus, it is crucial to identify the question or questions we seek to answer before designing the surveillance program. For example, if the objective is to prevent disease in humans, a surveillance program that only records the occurrence of human cases will be of little or no use. Instead, we need to measure the predictors of human cases. Depending on the type of information desired, different collection methods and equipment are required. We must know which methods and equipment best suit a given purpose.

Programs can be either intensive or extensive. In intensive studies, detailed data are collected for one or a few species in a restricted geographic area. In extensive studies, data for many species are collected over a large geographic area (Southwood 1978). Although research projects frequently are intensive, disease prevention and control programs generally involve extensive surveillance programs. In this chapter we concentrate on disease surveillance methods. However, we also point out methods that are useful in a research setting, especially those that help to answer specific questions about the ecology of vector-borne disease.

DESIGN OF SURVEILLANCE PROGRAMS

Absolute Versus Relative Density

Absolute population estimates of density per unit area (e.g., number per hectare) are essential for the proper construction of life budgets and similar studies (Southwood 1978). However, relative estimates such as catch per unit of effort (e.g., females per trap night or larvae per dip) are adequate for most surveillance systems. In a few cases, animal products (e.g., pupal skins, puparia of muscoid flies) can be sampled to provide a rough population index. If simultaneous data are collected on absolute and relative density, correction factors can be calculated that permit the computation of absolute densities (Southwood 1978).

Sampling Bias and Assumptions

Certain assumptions are implicit in all sampling and trapping procedures. The impact of different assumptions frequently becomes evident only when 2 or more sampling methods are applied simultaneously. We must recognize hidden assumptions when designing a surveillance program. For example, are all physiological stages and ages collected equally by this method? Does this trap have uniform sampling efficiency in all environments? Does the "knockdown" method really collect all the mosquitoes in a room?

More complex assumptions are reflected in decisions to sample only particular organisms. For example, we assume that house flies are not involved in transmitting any arboviral diseases of humans or domestic animals. Therefore, these insects are rarely processed for arbovirus isolation; however, when house flies were studied during an outbreak of vesicular stomatitis (VSV) in Colorado, numerous VSV (Indiana) isolates were obtained (Francy et al. 1988). The actual role of house flies in the dynamics of this disease remains speculative, however.

Sampling systems are usually biased in 1 way or another. If these biases are known and understood, they can be put to good use (intentional bias). However, when the biases in a system go unrecognized (unintentional bias), they can severely affect the interpretation of the data collected by that system. For example, entrance and exit traps can be used in malaria studies to sample only that portion of the anopheline population entering or leaving houses. Gravid traps can be used to sample only the gravid *Culex pipiens* population. This increases the likelihood of arbovirus isolation because these females have previously taken at least 1 blood meal.

However, if the objective is to estimate absolute density, but all traps have been placed along fence rows or other flight corridors, inflated estimates will be generated. Traps placed along flight corridors collect more specimens than traps located in the middle of an open field or in similar habitats, thus artificially increasing the catch. A vector surveillance program frequently involves the placement and retrieval of many traps put out and retrieved 1–5 days each week. It is tempting to place the traps in easily accessible sites for rapid servicing without considering the habits or behavior of the vector populations being sampled; the result is inaccurate data.

Placing mosquito traps near larval habitats can result in collections of larger proportions of young individuals. This is undesirable if the specimens are to be processed for arbovirus isolation because young individuals are unlikely to be infected.

The number of traps and sampling sites in a surveillance system depends on the biology and behavior of the vector being monitored and on the size of the area under surveillance. Cost is often important in surveillance. For a given cost, the most accurate estimates are obtained by taking many small samples rather than by taking fewer large ones (Southwood 1978).

Handling and Processing Specimens

For some applications, specimens need only be handled for identification purposes. For other applications (e.g., blood meal identification, ovarian dissection, pathogen isolation), specimens must be handled in special ways. It is very important that those responsible for field work clearly understand the methods by which specimens should be handled.

TICKS AND MITES

Hard Tick Collection

Ticks are actually large mites (order Parasitiformes) that have some distinctive characteristics, such as Haller's organ (Chap. 1). Many of the techniques used for collecting these ectoparasites also can be used to collect smaller mite taxa. Nonetheless, ticks are usually discussed separately. The most commonly used methods for collecting hard ticks (Ixodidae) are dragging, examination of captured hosts, and using attractants to lure ticks to a trap or collecting area (Falco and Fish 1992). Some ixodid ticks also can be collected from nest materials. No single method is likely to apply for sampling all species or life-cycle stages. Often a combination of techniques must be employed to gather the desired information.

Dragging (or flagging) involves pulling a cloth drag across vegetation where unfed ticks are questing for hosts. The questing ticks will cling to the passing drag and can be collected with forceps or by hand-picking at the end of each pass. Dragging is useful for collecting all 3 questing stages (larvae, nymphs, and adults) (Chap. 1) of many ixodid species, including *Amblyomma americanum* and members of the *Ixodes ricinus* complex (Milne 1943; Semtner and Hair 1973; and Falco and Fish 1988). Other species can be sampled by dragging only during certain life-cycle stages. For example, immature *Dermacentor andersoni* or *D. variabilis* are rarely encountered on drags, but questing adults of these species can be collected in large numbers by dragging (Philip 1937; Sonenshine et al. 1966). Conversely, larvae of the 1-host tick *Boophilus microplus* can be collected by dragging (Zimmerman and Garris 1985), but unfed nymphs and adults remain on their ungulate hosts between feedings and must be collected by other means. Off-host stages of other hard ticks, especially those species of *Ixodes* that inhabit nests, roosts, caves, or cliff habitats, are unlikely to be encountered on drags because the unfed ticks remain sequestered in these habitats until their hosts return.

Drags usually consist of a piece of cloth (about 1 m square) attached on one end to a pole. A rope is then attached to both ends of the pole, and the drag is pulled across vegetation where ticks are questing (Fig. 27.1). Weights are sometimes sewed into the side of the drag opposite from the pole to ensure that the drag stays in close contact with the vegetation (Falco and Fish 1988; Falco and Fish 1992). Dragging is typically done for a standard amount of time or distance to give a relative density estimate of the number of ticks in the area.

Another variant of the dragging technique uses a "flag" consisting of a cloth attached to one end of a long pole. The flag is then swept across vegetation where ticks are questing. Flags are most useful when ticks are questing on or near dense brush because it is difficult to pull a typical drag across this kind of vegetation.

Cylinder-shaped drags and hinged flag devices are also used. These samplers were found to be slightly less efficient than traditional tick drags for collecting larvae of *Boophilus microplus* (Zimmerman and Garris 1985). Although less efficient than traditional drags in pasture environments, the heavier weight and greater sturdiness of cylinder and hinge flag samplers might make them superior for use in areas with dense brush (Zimmerman and Garris 1985).

Ixodid ticks also can be collected by using host animals or carbon dioxide (CO_2) as attractants (Wilson et al. 1972; Koch and McNew 1981; Koch and McNew 1982; Falco and Fish 1992). Appropriate host animals are placed in cages near areas where ticks are likely to seek hosts. The animals are collected after a given period and examined for ticks. Traps baited with live animals also can be surrounded with sticky tape that

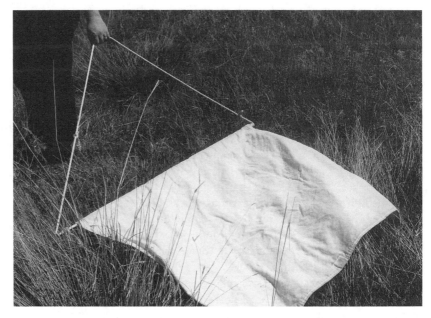

27.1   Tick drag, a standard technique in tick surveillance. Photo by L. Carter, CDC.

captures the ticks as they crawl toward the host (Koch and McNew 1981).

Many kinds of CO_2 traps have been described for collecting various ixodid ticks, including species of *Amblyomma* and *Ixodes* (Koch and McNew 1981; Kinzer et al. 1990; Falco and Fish 1992). Koch and McNew (1981) reported that a simple collecting device consisting of a 365–370-g cube of dry ice placed on a white cotton cloth (0.7 × 0.9 m) was more effective than rabbit-baited traps, foam bucket CO_2 traps baited with dry ice, or dry chemical traps. Kinzer et al. (1990) compared CO_2-baited traps with flagging and found that significantly more *A. americanum* larvae, nymphs, and adults could be collected with CO_2-baited traps than by flagging. These authors also found that traps baited with CO_2 detected adult *A. americanum* activity several weeks earlier than flagging. Falco and Fish (1992) found that drag sampling was inferior to a CO_2 sampling device for collecting *I. scapularis* larvae. However, the reverse was true for nymphal collections.

Sampling with CO_2 traps should be performed for a standard period, after which ticks can be collected from the cloth and counted. One disadvantage of CO_2 traps is that they operate over a limited range (Koch and McNew 1981; Falco and Fish 1992) compared to the area sampled by dragging or trapping and examining host animals. The effective ranges of these collecting devices and how the sampling range is influenced by meteorological factors are also difficult to determine.

Ixodid ticks also can be collected from host animals that have been trapped (Sonenshine et al. 1966; Main et al. 1982; Wilson and Spielman 1985; Falco and Fish 1992; Gage et al. 1992). The same trapping techniques described later for collecting flea hosts can be used to collect tick hosts. In some instances, trapping is the only practical means of collecting enough ticks of a certain stage. For example, immature *D. variabilis* are rarely collected by dragging but often can be found in large numbers on small mammal hosts (Soneshine et al. 1966; Gage et al. 1992).

Other techniques can be used to collect bird, lizard, or large- to medium-size mammal hosts. Avian hosts of ticks can be captured for examination by using either mist nets or ground traps (Manweiler et al. 1990). Lizard hosts, such as western fence lizards harboring *Ixodes pacificus* larvae and nymphs, can be captured by noosing (Manweiler et al. 1990). Pets or livestock can be examined for ticks without anesthesia; however, it is often necessary to restrain large livestock, such as cattle or horses, to make collecting easier and safer. Tick hosts also can be shot and then examined.

Dead hosts can be examined directly for ticks. Live wild animals should be humanely killed or anesthetized with metofane, halothane, or other suitable anesthetic, as described later for fleas, and then examined for ticks. Ticks can be removed from anesthetized or dead host animals with forceps. Collection procedures should be standardized as much as possible to minimize sampling variations related to differences between the techniques of individual collectors, the species of host or tick being sampled, the method of trapping employed, or other factors.

Another method for collecting ticks from captured live hosts is to hold hosts in the laboratory until attached ticks have completed engorgement and then detach from the host (Mather and Spielman 1986; Gage et al. 1990). Infested hosts are usually housed in wire mesh cages that are placed within a cloth bag or over a pan of water. When the ticks have completed engorgement, they fall from the host and then can be collected from the bag or pan of water.

Ticks also can be collected from dead hosts by first digesting the host's skin in trypsin and then dissolving the remaining skin and hair in potassium hydroxide (KOH). Soft tissues are destroyed, but the exoskeletons of ticks and other arthropod ectoparasites remain intact. Exoskeletons are removed from the digest solution by filtration and then collected for identification and counting (Henry and McKeever 1971). This method presumably collects all ectoparasites present on the host and is, therefore, more efficient than handpicking with forceps. Few workers, however, attempt such a labor-intensive collection procedure. Besides being very time-consuming, the method also precludes sampling the ticks or other ectoparasites for pathogenic microorganisms.

Soft Tick Collection

Sampling soft ticks (Argasidae) presents challenges that are somewhat different from those encountered while sampling hard tick populations. Some stages of certain argasid species remain on their hosts for long periods and can be collected using the techniques described above for examining hosts for ixodid ticks. Larvae and nymphs of the spinose ear tick (*Otobius megnini*) can be collected from the ear canal of the host, where they spend several weeks feeding and developing before leaving the host after the final nymphal feeding (Cooley and Kohls 1944; Oliver 1989). Larvae of most *Argas* and some *Ornithodoros* species also attach to their avian hosts for several days and can be collected directly from these animals; however, Argasids usually feed for only short periods during each stage of the life cycle. Some, such as *Otobius* adults, *Ornithodoros moubata* larvae, and probably all *Antricola* adults, do not feed at all.

Most argasids, therefore, must be collected from areas off their hosts using methods other than direct examination of host animals. Many such methods have been described; following are a few that are widely applicable. One such method is the CO_2 trap described by Miles (1968) for collecting *Ornithodoros parkeri* from ground squirrel burrows (Fig. 27.2). This CO_2 trap is fashioned from a cardboard mailing tube that has a hose connected to one end leading to a CO_2 source. The other end is fitted with a screen funnel that is open on both ends. Ticks attracted to the trap climb toward the small end of the funnel and fall into the trap, where they remain until collected. Burrows are sampled by inserting the mailing tube trap and hose into the burrow for a few hours or overnight. This allows sufficient time for ticks to be attracted to and enter the trap.

Another means of sampling argasid ticks in animal burrows has been described by Pierce (1974). *Ornithodoros moubata* were collected from warthog dens by wrapping a cloth around a spade and rubbing this "lure" on the roof of den entrances. The ticks clung to the cloth on the spade and were collected by hand-picking. Pierce also collected these ticks by sieving soil samples from the floors of warthog dens through wire mesh.

Argasid ticks often can be collected from nest material, bat guano on cave floors, undersides of tree bark, underneath loose soil or rock layers on cliff faces, or from other comparable habitats (Hopla and Loye 1983; Cooley and Kohls 1944). Small amounts of these samples can be examined for ticks by sorting the materials in a pan and using forceps or an aspirator to remove any ticks encountered. Larger amounts of nest material or other samples can be placed in a Berlese funnel or modified Tullgren apparatus (Baker and Wharton 1952; Krantz 1978). These use light and heat from a light bulb located at the top of the funnel-shaped device. Ticks and other arthropods are driven from the

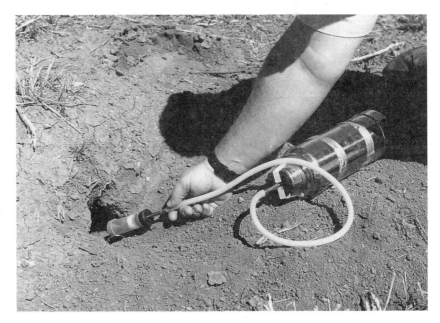

27.2   Tick trap of Miles (1968). See text for details. Photo by L. Carter, CDC.

sample material toward the bottom of the funnel, where they fall into a jar containing 70% ethanol or other collecting solution. Samples that contain small-grained material also can be sorted through soil sieves to separate ticks from debris (Hopla and Loye 1983).

Mite Collection

Mites are extremely diverse in their habits and the habitats they occupy. Thus, a wide variety of sampling techniques have been designed to sample specific species or life-cycle stages. There are, however, a few general sampling techniques, including those described for ticks, that can be adapted for most sampling situations encountered by medical entomologists.

Like ticks, mites can be collected directly from captured, shot, or restrained host animals. Some mites, such as chiggers (Trombiculidae), attach firmly to the surface of the host's body and feed for periods of many hours to a few days. These mite species can be removed from the host with fine forceps. Alternatively, the hosts can be suspended above water until the mites complete engorgement, detach, and drop from the host into water, where they can be collected. It is also possible to collect chiggers, or other fur- or feather-dwelling mites, by digesting the host's skin as was previously described for ticks (Henry and McKeever 1971).

Other mites, such as laelapids, dermanyssids, and macronyssids, which infest mammals, do not attach as firmly to their hosts as do chiggers. These mites can be collected by suspending the anesthetized or dead hosts above a white enamel pan and vigorously brushing the hosts with a pocket comb, rat-tail file, or toothbrush. The dislodged mites fall from the host's body into the pan, and they can be collected with forceps, a small brush, wetted applicator stick, or Singer aspirator (Krantz 1978). Dead mammalian or avian hosts also can be shaken vigorously in a detergent solution, which will dislodge any loosely attached mites and cause them to float free. The mites can then be recovered by pouring the detergent through a Buchner funnel that contains a filter paper for trapping the mites (Henry and McKeever 1971; Krantz 1978).

Nesting materials, soil debris, or other habitats of different off-host stages of various mite species also can be examined by collecting the material and placing it in a Berlese funnel or modified Tullgren apparatus as described for ticks (Baker and Wharton 1952; Krantz 1978). This technique is especially useful for many nest-dwelling species and for the nonparasitic nymphal and adult stages of chiggers, including those *Leptotrombidium* species whose larvae are vectors of scrub typhus. Unfed chigger larvae questing for hosts can be collected on black plates placed on the forest floor (Hubert and Baker 1963; Upham et al. 1971).

Some mites, including rhinonyssids associated with birds and some halarachnids that parasitize mammals, actually live as internal parasites of their hosts. These must be collected by postmortem examinations of various tissues. Other mites also remain on their hosts for most of their life cycles. Some of these mites, including species in the families Sarcoptidae, Psoroptidae, Demodicidae, as well as others, infest the skin of mammals and cause mange or related skin disorders. Other species, many of which are members of the superfamily Analgoidea, cause skin conditions, feather loss, or irritability in birds (Krantz 1978). Infestations of these mites are often suspected on the basis of hair loss, feather loss, or skin lesions in host animals, but definitive diagnosis requires identifying the mites themselves.

For those species infesting the skin, identification typically involves microscopic examination of skin scrapings (Meleney 1985). Scabies mites, for example, can be collected by first dipping a knife or similar tool in light mineral or machine oil and then scraping skin from the suspected infestation. These skin scrapings, still suspended in the oil, are then placed on a microscope slide, overlaid with a cover slip, and examined with a compound microscope under low power. Scrapings also can be digested in potassium or sodium hydroxide for a few hours to free the mites from the skin. The mites are then collected from the digested material by using a sugar-flotation method (Meleney 1985). Other species, such as psoroptic mites, dwell on the surface of the host's skin and can be tentatively identified with a hand lens. Definitive identification, however, requires collecting the mites by scraping and then examining the washed and stained scrapings with a microscope (Meleney 1985). Quill mites of the family Syringophilidae are internal parasites of the quill portion of feathers. They can be removed from within the quill by dissection (Krantz 1978).

Some species of astigmatid mites cause dermatitis and allergic conditions in humans (Spieksma and Spieksma-Boezeman 1967). Probably the most important of these is the house dust mite (*Dermatophagoides pteronyssus*). Although this mite is not parasitic, it is an important agent of allergic rhinitis and asthma in humans. House dust mites can be sampled by examining dust vacuumed from surfaces using a specially modified vacuum apparatus (Arlian et al. 1983). The density of mites collected can be expressed as the number of mites per gram of dust examined. Konishi and Uehara (1990) also have described a double-antibody sandwich enzyme-linked immunosorbent assay (ELISA) that can identify antigens of *D. pteronyssus* and *D. farinae* in house dust samples. The assay is very sensitive and can detect as little as 0.17 μg of antigen, approximately equivalent to one-half the amount of antigen found on a single mite.

MOSQUITOES

Eggs

Egg-sampling methods for mosquitoes (Chaps. 4 and 5) fall into 2 general categories: artificial samplers and samples from natural habitats. Artificial samplers, such as ovitraps, are placed at sampling stations to attract and sample the ovipositing female mosquito population. Artificial samplers can be used to increase the number of specimens collected or to achieve greater uniformity in a sampling system.

Methods for sampling natural habitats vary with the species of interest and the type of larval habitat. The standard 1-pt (pint) larval dipper (Fig. 27.3) is useful in assessing the oviposition activity of *Culex* and other raft-producing groups. Dipping is less effective for species that lay their eggs singly (*Anopheles*) on the water surface and is ineffective for species that oviposit on moist substrates (*Aedes*). For smaller habitats, a soup ladle can be used. Variation in results among technicians can seriously undermine the accuracy and usefulness of data collected from dipping. Several egg separators have been devised to separate *Aedes* eggs from soil and plant matter (Service 1976).

Oviposition traps (ovitraps) sample the gravid population. This can be an advantage for many epidemiologic studies when the species feeds only on humans (e.g., *Aedes aegypti*) or the proportion of blood meals from humans is known. Traps can be separated on the basis of whether they retain the ovipositing females or allow them to escape. Female-retaining traps are discussed in the following section on sampling adults. Nonfemale-retaining oviposition samplers include the Centers for Disease Control (CDC) ovitrap (Fig. 27.4) and bamboo pot for *Aedes aegypti* and other container-inhabiting *Aedes*, and oviposition pans (Fig.

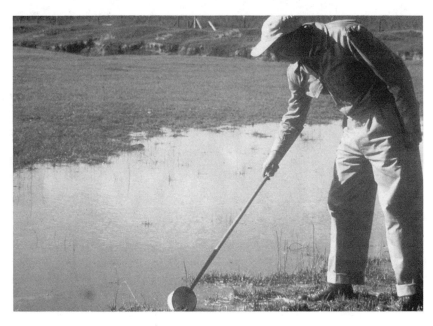

27.3 Standard 1-pt.(450 ml [ca]) larval dipper used in mosquito surveys. CDC file photo.

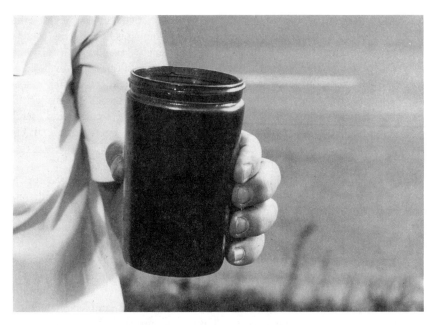

27.4   The CDC ovitrap. A hardboard paddle or paper strip is placed inside the container with about 1–1 1/2 inches (2.54–3.81 cm) of water. CDC file photo.

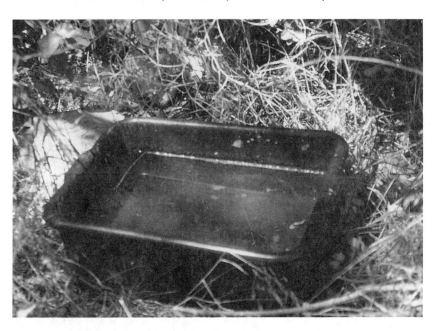

27.5   An oviposition pan consisting of a large plastic pan filled with an appropriate attractant such as a hay infusion. Photo by C.G. Moore, CDC.

27.5) (Horsfall et al. 1973; Reiter 1986) for *Culex* species. Ovitraps for *Culex* usually are larger and have an attractant or infusion. Trap placement is likely to be very important in determining response by ovipositing females. Nearby competing habitats can reduce the number of eggs collected.

Larvae and Pupae

The standard device for collecting mosquito larvae from open water is the 1-pt dipper (Fig. 27.3). Many other devices have been used, and several larval concentrators have been developed (Service 1976). Turkey basters, soup ladles, tea strainers, and similar devices are useful for sampling small larval habitats such as tree holes and scrap tires. Specialized techniques are needed for larvae of groups such as *Coquillettidia*, which attach to the roots of aquatic plants. Laird (1988) gives detailed descriptions of larval habitats and collecting methods.

Adults

A full discussion of the various traps and methods available is beyond the scope of these guidelines. Readers wishing more detailed information should consult Service (1976) or Moore et al. (1993).

Adults of many mosquito species are inactive during

the day, resting quietly in dark, cool, humid places. An index of the population density can be obtained by carefully counting or collecting the adults found in a resting station. Sampling resting adults usually provides a more representative sample of the population: teneral, postteneral unfed, blooded, and gravid females, as well as males. Population age structure also is more representative. However, different species and different gonotrophic stages sometimes prefer different types of resting sites.

Sampling resting populations is usually time-consuming, especially when looking for natural resting sites. Artificial resting stations can be constructed when suitable natural resting stations are not available. Aspirators can be used to collect resting adult mosquitoes. In addition, specimens can be collected with a sweep net, or they can be killed or immobilized by several materials (e.g., pyrethroids, chloroform, triethylamine). Knockdown collections are often used to collect mosquitoes resting inside dwellings (e.g., *Anopheles* and *Aedes aegypti*). White sheets or other materials are spread on the floor, and a pyrethroid spray is used to kill or knock down the mosquitoes resting on the walls.

Traps that do not use attractants, such as the malaise trap, give a more representative sample of the population than attractant traps, but they only sample the airborne population. A representative sample is not always desirable. For virus studies, it is better to bias collections toward collection of physiologically old females. Representative samples are highly desirable for general ecological studies and essential for estimating absolute population density. Examples of nonattractant traps include the malaise trap, ramp trap, truck trap, sticky trap, and suction trap. For details on these traps, consult Service (1976).

Animal-baited and CO_2-baited traps disproportionately attract host-seeking females. Usually, this is the population segment of greatest interest in vector-borne disease surveillance. The bait species or chemical attractant is important in trap performance. Often there is significant interhost variability in attractiveness that can affect trap performance. Other considerations are the duration of collection (especially human landing/biting collections) and time of day (especially important for species with a narrow host-seeking window). A final consideration is the need to decide whether to let mosquitoes feed (e.g., will specimens be used for blood meal identification?). CO_2-baited traps rely on the sublimation of dry ice (occasionally bottled CO_2) to provide the attractant, imitating CO_2 release by the host in animal-baited traps. Another material, 1-octen–3-ol, has recently been used either alone or with CO_2 as an attractant in bait traps (Kline et al. 1991).

Landing/biting collections, usually using humans, horses, or other domesticated vertebrates, are used to sample selected portions of the mosquito population, particularly in studies to incriminate specific vectors or in other research applications (Service 1976). When using human bait, potential health risks must be considered. During epidemics, these activities should be restricted to individuals who are naturally immune or who are receiving appropriate prophylaxis.

Many animal-baited traps have been designed (Service 1976). These are used mostly for special studies rather than for routine surveillance. One important application for these traps is to determine the probable vectors or vectors of a particular virus or other agent to a given host (for example, eastern equine encephalomyelitis [EEE] or western equine encephalomyelitis [WEE] in horses). Drop nets and tent traps (e.g., Mitchell et al. 1985) normally are left open or are suspended above the bait (human or animal). After a set period, the openings are closed or the net lowered and the trapped mosquitoes are collected (Service 1976). The Magoon trap is similar in principle to the tent trap but is sturdier in design, which provides some restraint for larger bait animals. Mosquitoes enter the trap but cannot escape, and they can be collected periodically.

Entrance/exit traps have a long history of use in malaria research. A variation with application to mosquito-borne encephalitis studies is the sentinel chicken shed (Rainey et al. 1962). The trap consists of a portable chicken shed and 1 or more removable mosquito traps. Mosquitoes attempting to enter the shed to feed are collected in the traps and can be removed the following morning.

The lard can trap (Fig. 27.6) is an economical, portable mosquito trap made from a 12-in (or larger) lard can (Bellamy and Reeves 1952). It is very effective in capturing *Culex tarsalis* and *Culex nigripalpus*. The trap has inwardly directed screenwire funnels on each end. Three pounds of dry ice (wrapped in newspaper or insulated mailer) is placed inside the can. The lard can trap also can be baited with a live chicken or other animal. An inner, double-screened enclosure can be used to prevent feeding by the trapped mosquitoes.

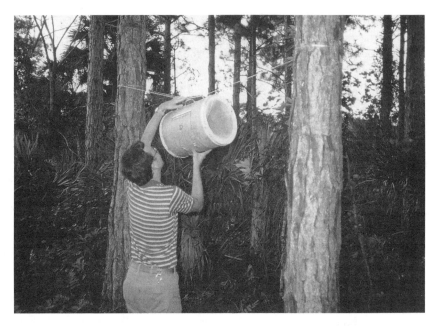

27.6   The lard can trap of Bellamy and Reeves (1952). Photo by C.G. Moore, CDC.

The Reiter gravid mosquito trap (Reiter 1983; 1987) (Fig. 27.7) samples female *Culex* mosquitoes as they come to oviposit. It therefore is selective for females that have already taken at least 1 blood meal (Reiter et al. 1986). Because they have fed at least once, they are more likely to be infected, thus reducing the work required for processing mosquito pools for virus isolation or for dissecting females for oocysts, sporozoites, or filariae. Because of the introduced bias in age and physiologic state, infection rates are, on average, higher than those obtained from light trap catches.

Many mosquito species are attracted to light, making it possible to sample adult

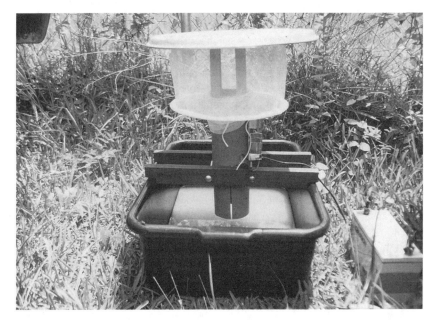

27.7   The Reiter gravid mosquito trap. Photo by R.S. Nasci, CDC.

populations between dusk and dawn. Light traps probably work by disrupting the normal behavior of flying mosquitoes. Mosquito species respond differently to these traps. Some species are not attracted to light at all and are even repelled (for example, *Cx. p. quinquefasciatus*). Light traps only sample the flying population. The catch is influenced by many factors, including light source, wavelength, and intensity. Competing light sources (including moonlight), fan size and speed, and presence or absence of screens also affect trap performance.

The placement of traps (height, location in relation to trees and other cover, proximity to breeding sites, etc.) can have a marked effect on the species and numbers of mosquitoes collected. Some trial and error placement is frequently involved in locating good trap placement sites. The light trap is usually suspended from a tree or post so the light is approximately 5–6 feet above the ground. The light traps should be placed 30 feet or more from buildings, in the tree line or near trees and shrubs. The light traps should not be near other lights, in areas subject to strong winds, or near industrial plants that emit smoke or fumes. Traps should be operated on a regular schedule from 1–7 nights per week, from just before dark until just after daylight. Dry ice, as an added attractant, increases collections of many mosquito species including *Culex tarsalis* and *Cx. nigripalpus*. A small block (3–4 lbs) of dry ice, placed in a padded shipping envelope or wrapped tightly in newspaper, is suspended beside the light trap. Because differences have been noted in the reactions of different species of mosquitoes, light trap collections should be used with other population sampling methods.

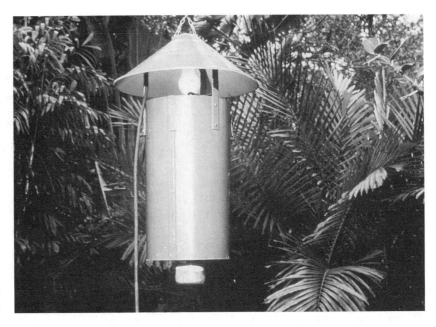

27.8 The New Jersey (or Mulhern) light trap. CDC file photo.

Light traps for mosquitoes fall into 2 general categories: large New Jersey–type light traps (Mulhern 1942) (Fig. 27.8) and small portable light traps such as the CDC light trap (Sudia and Chamberlain 1962) (Fig. 27.9). The New Jersey–type trap depends upon a 110-V source of electric power; the CDC-type trap is battery operated. Several modifications of the CDC light trap are also commercially available.

OTHER BITING NEMATOCERA

Sand Flies

Larvae of sand flies (Psychodidae) (Chap. 9) are found in decaying organic matter in animal burrows, tree holes, and other protected sites. Sampling involves digging up the burrow or extracting all material from the bottoms of tree holes.

A common method of collecting adult sand flies is the Chaniotis trap (Chaniotis 1978). This is a small, battery-operated light trap with the bulb near the bottom of the collecting chamber (Fig. 27.10). Traps are placed near animal burrows, tree buttress roots, tree holes, or other locations suspected of harboring adult flies.

Sticky plates consist of flat sheets of plexiglass or other material coated with a thin layer of castor oil or other similar medium. Sand flies are caught in the oil and can be retrieved the following day. Large-diameter disposable plastic petri dishes have also been used successfully as sticky traps (Al-Suhaibani 1990). Sticky traps are unlikely to produce specimens suitable for virus isolation because the oil interferes with the isolation system (e.g., cell culture). Landing-biting collections can be made of human-biting species.

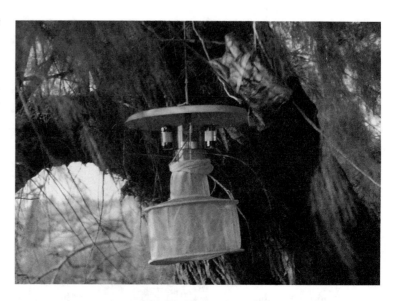

27.9   The CDC light trap of Sudia and Chamberlain (1962). Photo by C.G. Moore.

Ceratopogonid Midges

Larvae of ceratopogonids (*Culicoides* spp.) (Chap. 8) are found in habitats with high moisture; indeed, some habitats are entirely under water. Mud or other likely habitats can be sampled with a hand trowel, shovel, or other suitable device. Larvae can be collected by various salt flotation methods.

Adult ceratopogonids are collected by several types of light traps (Holbrook 1985; Weiser-Schimpf et al. 1990), including several of those described for mosquitoes.

Black flies

Larval black flies (Simuliidae) can be collected from natural habitats in streams (rocks, vegetation, or other submerged structures) or by placing strips of plastic tape in streams (Davies and Crosskey 1991).

Those species that feed on humans are generally collected by using humans as bait because few if any useful traps for these groups exist. An aluminum plaque trap for ovipositing females has been found useful in certain situations (Davies and Crosskey 1991). Light traps are not particularly attractive, and the few black flies found in these collections must be separated from all the other insects.

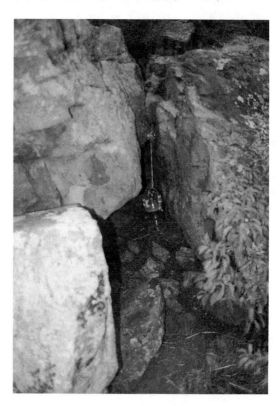

27.10   The Chaniotis trap for sand flies. Photo by C.G. Moore.

BRACHYCEROUS FLIES OF MEDICAL AND VETERINARY IMPORTANCE

Horse Flies, Deer Flies

Horse flies and other tabanids deposit their eggs on structures in or near water (emergent vegetation, sticks, rocks). These structures can be sampled to estimate oviposition. Larval tabanids can be collected from wet soil at the edges of marshes, roadside ditches, rice field borrow pits, and similar locations. Larvae of some species are found in drier habitats, usually in shady locations.

Adults can be collected in a variety of traps, such as the malaise trap, Manitoba fly trap, and the canopy trap. Trap efficiency can be increased by adding a chemical attractant such as carbon dioxide, ammonia, or octenol.

Horn Flies and Stable Flies

Horn flies (*Haematobia irritans*) and stable flies (*Stomoxys calcitrans*) are hematophagous pests of veterinary importance that belong to the family Muscidae. The stable fly is an occasional vector of equine infectious anemia virus (Foil and Issel 1991). Stable flies are an important pest of humans along Atlantic and Gulf Coast beaches of the United States. Adult stable flies and horn flies can be sampled by sweep nets or by aspirating flies coming to animal baits. The Williams, or Alsynite, trap, a type of sticky trap, is used to collect stable flies (Williams 1973).

House Flies

House fly larvae are found in manure, garbage, and various types of decomposing organic matter. Larvae can be quantitatively sampled in these habitats by a variety of methods. The "Scudder Grill" (Scudder 1947) is commonly used to estimate adult house fly densities (Fig. 27.11). It consists of a wooden frame, generally painted white, consisting of 16–24 1.9 mm wooden slats 61 cm in length. The slats are arranged on a frame with approximately 2 cm between slats. The grill is lowered over an area in which flies have congregated. As the disturbed flies begin to return to the area, the number of flies landing in a 30-second period is recorded. Several similar counts are made at each site, and an average is computed.

Estimates of fly abundance also can be obtained by counting the numbers of flies on available surfaces (e.g., walls, feeding troughs, stables, etc.). Flies can be collected in baited traps (Fig. 27.12), on sticky paper, or by sweep nets. The same techniques must be used throughout a study or control program so that data can be compared (WHO 1991). Sweep nets can be used to collect adult flies, but standardization can be a problem.

Tsetse Flies

Adult tsetse flies (*Glossina* spp.) (Chap. 10) can be collected by using a wide variety of traps. Because both males and females feed on blood, both can be collected at baits (Colvin and Gibson 1992). Electrocuting nets have been used to sample tsetse flies as well as to protect train passengers. Tsetse flies depend on both visual and olfactory cues to locate hosts, and these behaviors have been extensively exploited to

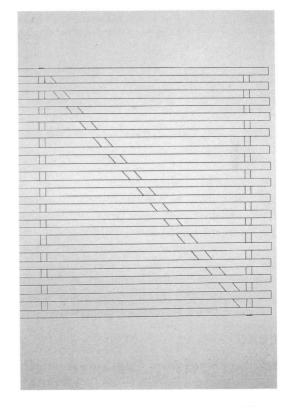

27.11   Scudder fly grid (after Pratt and Moore 1993)

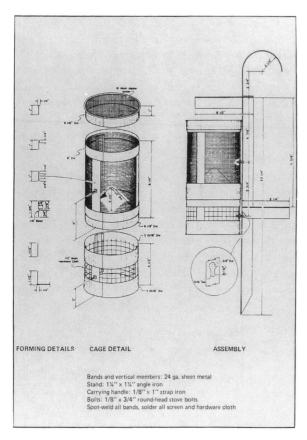

FORMING DETAILS   CAGE DETAIL   ASSEMBLY

Bands and vertical members: 24 ga. sheet metal
Stand: 1¼″ x 1¼″ angle iron
Carrying handle: 1/8″ x 1″ strap iron
Bolts: 1/8″ x 3/4″ round-head stove bolts
Spot-weld all bands, solder all screen and hardware cloth

27.12   A bait trap for house flies. From Pratt and Moore, 1993.

develop tsetse fly control programs. Tsetse flies rely on shape, orientation, brightness, contrast, movement, and color to distinguish hosts. They can thus distinguish host animals against complex visual backgrounds. Carbon dioxide is the most effective attractant, but butanone, 1-octen–3-ol, and some phenol derivatives in cattle urine are also attractive (Colvin and Gibson 1992). The latter compounds can be economically used in trapping programs.

FLEAS

Removing Fleas from Captured Animals

Probably the most common method for collecting fleas (order Siphonaptera) (Chap. 11) is to trap or shoot host animals and then examine them for fleas (Holland 1949; Stark and Kinney 1969; Haas et al. 1973; Bahmanyar and Cavanaugh 1976; Campos et al. 1985). Nonlethal traps (live traps), such as the various commercially available box or cage varieties (Fig. 27.13a), are best for collecting fleas from small rodents because fleas tend to leave dead hosts as the carcasses cool if snap traps are used.

Hosts captured in live traps should be anesthetized with metofane, halothane, or other suitable anesthetic agents before processing further (Clark and Olfert 1986). The anesthetized animal can then be placed in a white enamel pan (a depth of 20 cm or more is recommended). The animal is brushed vigorously from the tail end forward with a toothbrush, pocket comb, or other similar instrument (Fig. 27.14). The dislodged fleas fall from the host to the bottom of the pan, where they can be removed with forceps or a wetted applicator stick and placed in labeled vials for further processing. Any bedding material placed in traps to provide warmth for the host also should be examined for fleas.

Snap traps (Fig. 27.13b,c) also can be used to collect hosts for flea collection, but these traps should be checked every couple of hours or so to ensure that the hosts are collected before the fleas begin to leave the cooling carcasses. Larger rodents, such as *Rattus spp.*, often are only injured, rather than killed, in snap traps; these injured animals can drag traps a considerable distance away from the original trap site. Tethering each trap to the ground using a piece of strong but flexible wire prevents the traps from being dragged. Hosts killed in snap traps or by other means can be examined directly for fleas. However, carcasses should be treated with insecticides or anesthetic agents before examination to prevent fleas from escaping onto the investigator or into the laboratory.

Other small mammal species often must be captured using different trapping techniques. For example, the preferred means for trapping shrews is to construct pit traps. These traps consist of a smooth-sided can or jar, buried so that the top is level with the ground. Pit traps are placed in presumed runways, and animals fall into them while making their nightly rounds. Shrews do not survive well in captivity, and animals are often dead when collectors arrive. The fleas, however, usually remain in the pit trap or on the host (Holland 1949).

Collecting fleas from birds also requires special techniques. Ground-dwelling birds can be captured in traps. Other techniques, such as mist netting, are sometimes needed to live-capture adults of other bird species (Sonenshine and Stout 1970; Manweiler et al. 1990). If nests are accessible, nestling birds can be removed from their nests and examined for fleas (Hopla and Loye 1983). Fleas also can be collected from birds and large- and medium-size mammals by shooting the hosts and then inspecting the carcasses for fleas (Holland 1949).

Collecting Fleas from Burrows

Fleas can be collected from burrows by using a swabbing device. It consists of a flexible steel cable or hard rubber hose with a piece of white flannel cloth attached to the end (Vakhrousheva et al. 1989; Beard et al. 1991)(Fig. 27.15). The swab is forced down the burrow entrance; fleas mistake it for their normal hosts and cling to the cloth. The cloth is then removed from the burrow and inspected for fleas. If desired, the cloth can be placed in a plastic bag and held for later examination. Fleas within the bags can be killed by freezing, anesthetization, or insecticides. Miles (1968) also has reported capturing fleas in burrows using the CO_2 trap that was described above for collecting argasid ticks (Fig. 27.2).

Collecting Fleas from Nests and Nesting Material

Many fleas spend more time in the nests of their hosts than on the host itself. Mammalian and avian nest material can be examined for fleas by sorting the

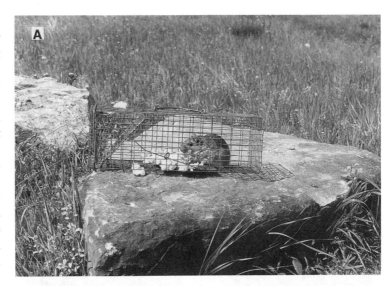

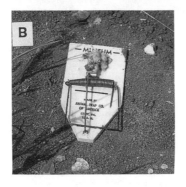

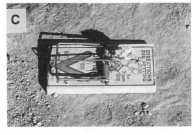

27.13 Traps for sampling mammals. (A) A wire trap for obtaining live animals, (B) and (C) Snap traps. Photos by L. Carter, CDC.

contents in an enamel pan similar to that described for brushing fleas from hosts. Although some fleas are poor jumpers, it is a good idea to treat the material with insecticides before sorting to prevent them from escaping from the pan. Nest material also can be loaded into a Berlese funnel or modified Tullgren apparatus (described later) for collecting argasid ticks and mites (Baker and Wharton 1952; Krantz 1978). Once the fleas reach the bottom of the funnel, they fall into a jar containing a saline solution or alcohol. Eggs, larvae, and pupae also can be collected from nest material, debris, or other material by sorting the samples through a series of sieves (Hopla and Loye 1983).

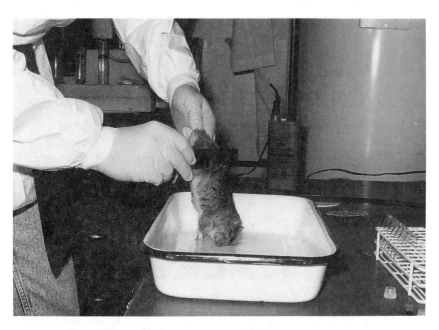

27.14   Technique for removing ectoparasites from dead or anesthetized animals. Photo by L. Carter, CDC.

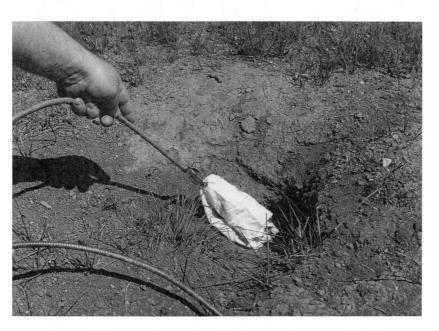

27.15   Use of the burrow swab to collect fleas. Photo by L. Carter.

Hopla and Loye (1983) also used black cardboard cards coated with honey to collect fleas (*Ceratophyllus celsus*) gathered at the entrances of cliff swallow nests (Fig. 27.16). The fleas apparently confuse the shadow created by the black squares with the approach of their swallow hosts and jump onto the cards. The honey-coated squares with the captured fleas are then covered with onion skin paper and transported to the laboratory. The fleas can be removed from the cards by soaking the samplers in a dish filled with water. The honey dissolves, and the fleas float to the surface where they can be removed easily with forceps.

Flea Indexes

The most basic data obtained from flea and rodent surveys are the number of fleas of different species found on various species of hosts. These raw data can be used to calculate various indexes, including the specific flea index (number of fleas per host of given flea and host species). Burrow, nest, or house indexes also can be similarly calculated. The percentage of hosts infested with a particular species of flea also is important. This information can be used with other rodent and vector surveillance data

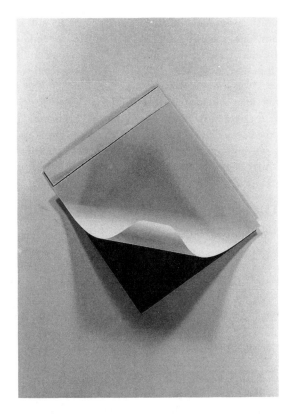

27.16 Black cardboard traps for collecting fleas. The fleas become trapped in the honey that coats the cards. Photo by C.E. Hopla.

to estimate human risks in areas with murine typhus or plague. For example, specific flea indexes of greater than 1 for *X. cheopis* infestations on rats from plague-endemic areas represent dangerously high levels of risk for the occurrence of both rat plague epizootics and human plague epidemics (Pollitzer 1954).

Many factors affect the reliability of flea indexes (Pollitzer 1954). These include host age, host species, trapping techniques, areas selected for sampling, and the fact that some hosts will be heavily infested whereas most will have few or no fleas (high variance to mean ratios for sample data). To obtain reliable indexes for comparison between different survey sites, all trapping and ectoparasite collection procedures must be standardized. Schwan (1984) has described a sequential

sampling method that can be used to determine how many host animals must be sampled before a reliable flea index is obtained for a given host/flea relationship. He reported that examining as few as 20 Nile grass rats (*Arvicanthis niloticus*) was sufficient to yield reliable specific flea indexes for infestations of either *Dinopsyllus lypusus* or *Xenopsylla cheopis bantorum*.

MISCELLANEOUS GROUPS OF MEDICAL AND VETERINARY IMPORTANCE

Triatomine Bugs

Members of the reduviid subfamily Triatominae (order Hemiptera) (Chap. 10), especially various species of *Panstrongylus*, *Rhodnius*, and *Triatoma*, transmit *Trypanosoma cruzi*, the etiologic agent of Chagas' disease, or American trypanosomiasis. Many surveillance techniques have been described for sampling these bugs in sylvatic habitats, human dwellings, and peridomiciliary structures. One common method for collecting triatomine bugs in houses or outbuildings is to use pyrethroid sprays as "excitorepellents" to flush bugs from crevices in walls, thatch roofs, or other hiding places (Piesman et al. 1985; Rabinovich et al. 1990; Garcia-Zapata and Marsden 1992; Garcia-Zapata and Marsden 1993). As bugs are flushed from their hiding places, they can be manually collected with forceps. Results of these surveys are usually expressed as the number of bugs captured per person per hour or as the number of bugs collected per house or other structure. When the latter measure is used, the searches are conducted until no more bugs can be found in each house surveyed.

The presence of triatomine bugs in houses or other artificial structures also can be determined indirectly by identifying the distinctive fecal deposits left by these insects (Schofield et al. 1986). Typically, a sheet of paper is suspended above a bed or other areas where bugs are likely to defecate after taking their nighttime blood meals (Garcia-Zapata and Marsden 1992; Garcia-Zapata and Marsden 1993). Triatomine infestations also can be detected directly or indirectly by using Gomez-Nunez boxes. These sampling devices consist of a piece of paper (approximately 20 cm × 30 cm) that is folded accordion fashion and inserted into a cardboard frame (Garcia-Zapata and Marsden 1992). Bugs are attracted to the boxes as potential resting places or refuges and defecate on the paper sampler during their visit. Although the bugs are occasionally removed from these samplers, infestations usually are identified by the presence of fecal deposits on the paper inserts. A similar device for identifying triatomine infestations in chicken coops or other peridomiciliary structures has been described by Garcia-Zapata and Marsden (1993). This simple but effective sampler consists of a section of bamboo open on one or both ends that contains strips of paper folded accordion fashion. Bugs enter these devices and defecate on the paper as described for the Gomez-Nunez box.

Triatomines also can be collected from sylvatic habitats in which they seek refuge between blood meals. Likely habitats include palm trees, hollow logs, bird or mammal nests, mammal burrows, and caves (D'Allesandro et al. 1984; Ekkens 1984). Any bugs encountered usually can be manually removed from these refuges with forceps, but considerable effort is required to excavate burrows or collect from other difficult sites. Miles et al. (1981) identified probable triatomine habitats by tracking captured mammals to their burrows, nests in hollow logs, or other refuges. Although bugs seldom existed in large numbers in any given nest, roost, or burrow, this technique was the most effective means of locating triatomines in forest ecotopes. Nest material and debris also can be placed in a pan for examination. This latter method is especially useful for collecting small nymphs (Ekkens 1984).

The winged adult triatomine bugs can be collected by using light traps or by shining a light onto a light-colored collecting area, such as a sheet, piece of canvas, or white board. The bugs can be manually gathered with forceps (Whitlaw and Chaniotis 1978; Ekkens 1981).

LICE

Two species of lice (Anoplura) (Chap. 10) are medically important: the head louse (*Pediculus capitis*) and the pubic, or "crab" louse (*Pthirus pubis*). The eggs of these insects are attached by a cement-like substance to the body hairs of the human host. Finding the eggs,

or nits, is the most practical way to check for infestations. The best estimators of louse activity are children in elementary schools, grades K–2 (Juranek 1985). Infestation rates decline with age. Suspected nits should be examined microscopically to exclude dandruff, hair spray, and other similar artifacts (Epstien and Orkin 1985). Eggs of *P. capitis* are normally found at the back of the head or around the ears. The eggs of *P. pubis* are found in the pubic hairs or, less commonly, in the eyebrows, beard, or mustache (Epstein and Orkin 1985).

SUMMARY AND CONCLUSIONS

Surveillance for the insect vectors of diseases, although complex in its own right, is only one part of an overall disease surveillance program. The particular trapping or sampling tools and schedules used depend on the disease and vectors of interest and the particular questions to be answered. Proper planning before embarking on a surveillance program will ensure that meaningful data are collected.

As our understanding of the vector-pathogen–vertebrate host relationship for a disease changes, there will likely be a need for new collection procedures. For example, individuals in only a certain physiological or behavioral state might be collected. Such specialized sampling methods are common for mosquitoes. They are less common or absent for some other groups. Just as new laboratory diagnostic methods will allow us to answer new questions (or finally answer questions that have remained unanswered for years), the availability of new collection methods might also allow us to answer previously unanswerable questions. Thus, the equipment available for surveillance defines, at least in part, what information can be collected to help us predict vector or disease activity.

REFERENCES

Al-Suhaibani, S. 1990. Field and laboratory studies of sand flies in Larimer County, Colorado. Fort Collins, CO: Colorado State University [Ph.D. thesis].

Arlian, L.G., P.J. Woodford, I.L. Bernstein, and J.S. Gallagher. 1983. Seasonal population structure of house dust mites, *Dermatophagoides* spp. Acari: Pyroglyphidae). *J. Med. Entomol.* 20:99–102.

Bahmanyar, M., and D.C. Cavanaugh. 1976. *Plague manual.* Geneva: World Health Organization. 76 p.

Baker, E.W., and G.W. Wharton. 1952. *An introduction to acarology.* New York: MacMillan Co. 465 p.

Beard, M.L., S.T. Rose, A.M. Barnes, and J.A. Montenieri. 1992. Control of *Oropsylla hirsuta,* a plague vector, by treatment of prairie dog burrows with 0.5% permethrin dust. *J. Med. Entomol.* 29:25–29.

Bellamy, R., and W. C. Reeves. 1952. A portable mosquito trap. *Mosq. News* 12(4):256–258.

Bowen, G.S. and D.B. Francy. 1980. Surveillance. In: T.P. Monath, editor, *St. Louis encephalitis.* Washington, DC: Amer. Pub. Hlth. Assoc.

Bram, R.A., editor. 1978. *Surveillance and collection of arthropods of veterinary importance.* Washington, D.C.: U.S. Dept. of Agric. Handbook No. 5.

Campos, E.G., G.O. Maupin, A.M. Barnes, and R.B. Eads. 1985. Seasonal occurrence of fleas (Siphonaptera) on rodents in a foothills habitat in Larimer County, Colorado, USA. *J. Med. Entomol.* 22:266–270.

Chaniotis, B.N. 1978. Phlebotomine sand flies (Psychodidae). In: R.A. Bram, editor, *Surveillance and collection of arthropods of veterinary importance.* Washington, D.C.: U.S. Dept. of Agric. Handbook No. 5. pp. 19–30.

Clark, J.D., and E.D. Olfert. 1986. Rodents (Rodentia): Part 4, Special Medicine: Mammals. In: M.E. Fowler, ed., *Zoo and wild animal medicine.* Philadelphia, PA: W.B. Saunders Co. pp. 727–748.

Cooley, R.A., and G.M. Kohls. 1944. *The Argasidae of North America, Central America and Cuba.* Amer. Midl. Nat. Monograph No. 1. Notre Dame, IN: Univ. Press. 152 p.

Colvin, J., and G. Gibson 1992. Host-seeking behavior and management of tsetse. *Ann. Rev. Ent.* 37:21–40.

D'Allessandro, P. Barreto, N. Saravia, and M. Barreto. 1984. Epidemiology of *Trypanosoma cruzi* in the oriental plains of Columbia. *Am. J. Trop. Med. Hyg.* 33:1084–1095.

Davies, J.B., and R.W. Crosskey. 1991. *Simulium*-Vectors of onchocerciasis. In: *Vector control series, training and information guide, advanced level* (WHO/VBC/91.992). Geneva: World Health Organization, Div. Trop. Dis.

Ekkens, D.B. 1981. Nocturnal flights of *Triatoma* (Hemiptera: Reduviidae) in Sabino Canyon, Arizona: Part 1, Light collections. *J. Med. Entomol.* 18:211–227.

Ekkens, D. 1984. Nocturnal flights of *Triatoma* (Hemiptera: Reduviidae) in Sabino Canyon, Arizona: Part 2, *Neotoma* lodge studies. *J. Med. Entomol.* 21:140–144.

Epstien, E. Sr., and M. Orkin. 1985. Pediculosis: Clinical aspects. In: M. Orkin and H.I. Maibach, editors, *Cutaneous infestations and insect bites.* New York: Marcel Dekker.

Falco, R.C., and D. Fish. 1988. Prevalence of *Ixodes dammini* near the homes of Lyme disease patients in Westchester County, New York. *Am. J. Epidemiol.* 127:826–830.

Falco, R.C., and D. Fish. 1992. A comparison of methods for sampling the deer tick, *Ixodes dammini,* in a Lyme disease endemic area. *Exper. App. Acarol.* 14:165–173.

Fay, R.W., and D.A. Eliason. 1966. A preferred oviposition site as a surveillance method for *Aedes aegypti. Mosq. News* 26:531–535.

Gage, K.L., W. Burgdorfer, and C.E. Hopla. 1990. Hispid cotton rats (*Sigmodon hispidus*) as a source for infecting immature *Dermacentor variabilis* (Acari: Ixodidae) with *Rickettsia rickettsii. J. Med. Entomol.* 27:615–619.

Gage, K.L., C.E. Hopla, and T.G. Schwan. 1992. Cotton rats and other small mammals as host for immature *Dermacentor variabilis* (Acari: Ixodidae) in central Oklahoma. *J. Med. Entomol.* 29:832–842.

Garcia-Zapata, M.T.A., and P.D. Marsden. 1992. Control of the transmission of Chagas' disease in Mambai, Goias, Brazil (1980–1988). *Am. J. Trop. Med. Hyg.* 440–443.

Garcia-Zapata, M.T.A., and P.D. Marsden. 1993. Chagas' disease: Control and surveillance through use of insecticides and community participation in Mambai, Goias, Brazil. *Bull. Pan. Amer. Health Org.* 27:265–279.

Haas, G.E., R.P. Martin, M. Swickard, and B.E. Miller. 1973. Siphonaptera-mammal relationships in northcentral New Mexico. *J. Med. Entomol.* 10:281–289.

Henry, L.G., and S. McKeever. 1971. A modification of the washing technique for quantitative evaluation of the ectoparasite load of small mammals. *J. Med. Entomol.* 8:504–505.

Holbrook, F.R. 1985. A comparison of three traps for adult *Culicoides variipennis* (Ceratopogonidae). *J. Am. Mosq. Control Assoc.* 1(3):379–381.

Holland, G.P. 1949. *The Siphonaptera of Canada.* Publication 817, Technical Bulletin 70. Ottawa, Canada: Dominion of Canada, Dept. of Agriculture. 306 p.

Hopla, C.E., and J.E. Loye. 1983. The ectoparasites and microorganisms associated with cliff swallows in west-central Oklahoma. I. Ticks and Fleas. *Bull. Soc. Vector Ecol.* 8:111–121.

Horsfall, W.R., H.W. Fowler, L.J. Moretti, and J.R. Larsen. 1973. Bionomics and Embryology of the Inland Floodwater Mosquito, *Aedes vexans.* Urbana, IL: Univ. of Illinois Press. 211 p.

Hubert, A.A., and H.J. Baker. 1963. Studies on the habitat and population of *Leptotrombidium* (*Leptotrombidium*) *akamushi* and *Leptotrombidium* (*Leptotrombidium*) *deliensis* in Malaya. *Amer. J. Hyg.* 78:131–142.

Juranek, D. 1985. *Pediculus capitis* in school children: Epidemiologic trends, risk factors, and recommendations for control. In: M. Orkin and H.I. Maibach, editors, *Cutaneous infestations and insect bites.* New York: Marcel Dekker.

Kinzer, D.R., S.M. Presley, and J.A. Hair. 1990. Comparative efficiency of flagging and carbon dioxide-baited sticky traps for collecting the lone star tick, *Amblyomma americanum* (Acarina: Ixodidae). *J. Med. Entomol.* 27:750–755.

Kline, D.L., J.R. Wood, and J.A. Comell. 1991. Interactive effects of 1-octen-3-ol and carbon dioxide on mosquito (Diptera: Culicidae) surveillance and control. *J. Med. Ent.* 28(2):254–258.

Krantz, G.W. 1978. *A manual of acarology.* 2nd ed. Corvallis, OR: Oregon State Univ. Press. 509 p.

Koch, H.G., and R.W. McNew. 1981. Comparative catches of field populations of lone star ticks by CO_2-emitting dry-ice, dry-chemical, and animal-baited devices. *Ann. Entomol. Soc. Amer.* 74:498–500.

Koch, H.G., and R.W. McNew. 1982. Sampling of lone star ticks (Acari: Ixodidae): Dry ice quantity and capture success. *Ann. Entomol. Soc. Amer.* 75:579–582.

Konishi, E., and K. Uehara. 1990. Enzyme-linked immunosorbent assay for quantifying antigens of *Dermatophagoides farinae* and *D. pteronyssus* (Acari: Pteroglyphidae) in house dust samples. *J. Med. Entomol.* 27:993–998.

Laird, M. 1988. *The natural history of larval mosquito habitats.* New York: Academic Press.

Main, A.J., A.B. Carey, M.G. Carey, and R.H. Goodwin. 1982. Immature *Ixodes dammini* (Acari: Ixodidae) on small animals in Connecticut, USA. *J. Med. Entomol.* 19:655–664.

Manweiler, S.A., R.S. Lane, W.M. Block, and M.L. Morrison. 1990. Survey of birds and lizards for ixodid ticks (Acari) and spirochetal infection in northern California. *J. Med. Entomol.* 27:1011–1015.

Mather, T.N., and A. Spielman. 1986. Diurnal detachment of immature deer ticks (*Ixodes dammini*) from nocturnal hosts. *Am. J. Trop. Med. Hyg.* 35:182–186.

Meleney, W.P. 1985. Mange mites and other parasitic mites. In: S.M. Gaafar, W.E. Howard, and R.E. Marsh, editors, *Parasites, pests, and predators.* Amsterdam: Elsevier Science. pp. 317–346.

Miles, M.A., A.A. deSouza, and M. Povoa. 1981. Chagas' disease in the Amazon Basin: Part 3. Ecotopes of ten triatomine bug species (Hemiptera: Reduviidae) from the vicinity of Belem, Para State, Brazil. *J. Med. Entomol.* 18:266–278.

Miles, V.I. 1968. A carbon dioxide bait trap for collecting ticks and fleas from animal burrows. *J. Med. Entomol.* 5:491–495.

Milne, A. 1943. The comparison of sheep-tick populations (*Ixodes ricinus* L.). *Ann. Appl. Biol.* 30:240–250.

Mitchell, C.J., R.F. Darsie, T.P. Monath, M.S. Sabattini, and J. Daffner. 1985. The use of an animal-baited net trap for collecting mosquitoes during western equine encephalitis investigations in Argentina. *J. Am. Mosq. Control Assoc.* 1(1):43–47.

Moore, C.G., R.G. McLean, C.J. Mitchell, R.S. Nasci, T.F. Tsai, C.H. Calisher, A.A. Marfin, P.S. Moore, and D.J. Gubler. 1993. Guidelines for Arbovirus Surveillance in the United States. Fort Collins, CO: U.S. Dept. of Health and Human Svcs., Centers for Disease Control. 83 p.

Mulhern, T.D. 1942. New Jersey light trap for mosquito surveys. N.J. Agric. Exp. Sta., Circ. 421 [Reprinted in *J. Am. Mosq. Control Assoc.* 1(4):411–418; 1985].

Oliver, J.H. 1989. Biology and systematics of ticks (Acari: Ixodidae). *Ann. Rev. Ecol. Syst.* 20:397–430.

Pierce, M.A. 1974. Distribution and ecology of *Ornithodoros moubata porcinus* Walton (Acarina) in animal burrows in East Africa. *Bull. Entomol. Res.* 64:605–619.

Philip, C.B. 1937. Six years' intensive observation on the seasonal prevalence of a tick population in western Montana. *Publ. Health Rep.* 52:16–22.

Piesman, J., I.A. Sherlock, E. Mota, C.W. Todd, R. Hoff, and T. Weller. 1985. Association between household triatomine density and incidence of *Trypanosoma cruzi* infection during a nine-year study in Castro Alves, Bahia, Brazil. *Am. J. Trop. Med. Hyg.* 34:866–869.

Pollitzer, R. 1954. *Plague.* Geneva: World Health Organization. 698 p.

Pratt, H.D., and C.G. Moore. 1993. Mosquitoes of public health importance and their control. Atlanta, GA: U.S. Dept. of Health and Human Services, Centers for Disease Control. 85 p.

Rabinovich, J.E., C. Wisnivesky-Colli, N.D. Solarz, and R.E. Gurtler. 1990. Probability of transmission of Chagas' disease by *Triatoma infestans* (Hemiptera: Reduviidae) in an endemic area of Santiago del Estero, Argentina. *Bull. World Health Org.* 68:737–746

Rainey, M.B., G.V. Warren, A.D. Hess, and J.S. Blackmore. 1962. A sentinel chicken shed and mosquito trap for use in encephalitis field studies. *Mosq. News* 22(4):337–342.

Reiter, P. 1983. A portable, battery-powered trap for collecting gravid *Culex* mosquitoes. *Mosq. News* 43:496–498.

Reiter, P. 1986. A standardized procedure for the quantitative surveillance of certain *Culex* mosquitoes by egg raft collection. *J. Am. Mosq. Control Assoc.* 2(2):219–221.

Reiter, P. 1987. A revised version of the CDC gravid mosquito trap. *J. Am. Mosq. Control Assoc.* 3(2):325–327.

Reiter, P., W.L. Jakob, D.B. Francy, and J.B. Mullenix. 1986. Evaluation of the CDC gravid trap for the surveillance of St. Louis encephalitis vectors in Memphis, Tennessee. *J. Am. Mosq. Control Assoc.* 2(2):209–211.

Schwan, T.G. 1984. Sequential sampling to determine the minimum number of host examinations required to provide a reliable flea (Siphonaptera) index. *J. Med. Entomol.* 21:670–674.

Schofield, C.J., N.G. Williams, M.L. Kirk, M.T.A. Garcia-Zapata, and P.D. Marsden. 1986. A key for identifying faecal smears to detect domestic infestations of triatomine bugs. *Rev. Soc. Bras. Med. Trop.* 19:5–8.

Scudder, H.I. 1947. A new technique for sampling the density of housefly populations. *Pub. Hlth. Rep.* 62:681–686.

Semtner, P.J., and J.A. Hair. 1973. The ecology and behavior of the lone star tick (Acarina: Ixodidae). Part 5, Abundance and seasonal distribution in different habitat types. *J. Med. Entomol.* 10:618–628.

Service, M.W. 1976. *Mosquito ecology: Field sampling methods.* New York: John Wiley and Sons.

Sonenshine, D.E., E.L. Atwood, and J.T. Lamb Jr. 1966. The ecology of ticks transmitting Rocky Mountain spotted fever in a study area in Virginia. *Ann. Entomol. Soc. Amer.* 59:1234–1262.

Sonenshine, D.E., and I.J. Stout. 1970. A contribution to the ecology of ticks infesting wild birds and rabbits in the Virginia-North Carolina Piedmont (Acarina: Ixodidae). *J. Med. Entomol.* 41:296–301.

Southwood, T.R.E. 1978. *Ecological methods with particular reference to the study of insect populations.* 2nd. ed. New York: Chapman and Hall.

Spieksma, F. Th.M., and M.I.A. Spieksma-Boezeman. 1967. The mite fauna of house dust with particular reference to the house-dust mite *Dermatophagoides pteronyssus* (Trouessart 1897) (Psoroptidae: Sarcoptiformes). *Acarologia* 9:226–241.

Stark, H.E., and A.R. Kinney. 1969. Abundance of rodents and fleas as related to plague in Lava Beds National Monument, California. *J. Med. Entomol.* 6:287–294.

Sudia, W.D., and R.W. Chamberlain. 1962. Battery-operated light trap, an improved model. *Mosq. News* 22:126–129.

Upham, R.W. Jr., A.A. Hubert, O.W. Phang, Y. bin Mat, and G. Rapmund. 1971. Distribution of *Leptotrombidium* (*Leptotrombidium*) *arenicola* (Acarina: Trombiculidae) on the ground in west Malaysia. *J. Med. Entomol.* 8:401–406.

Vakhrousheva, Z.P., A.D. Gorchakov, N.A. Kolupaeva, and E.G. Chernykh. 1989. The use of flannel flags for collecting fleas at the entrance of burrows of steppe rodents. *Meditsinskaya Parazitologiya i Parazitarnye Bolenzi.* 1:54–57.

Weiser-Schimpf, L., L.D. Foil, and F.R. Holbrook. 1990. Comparison of New Jersey light traps for collection of adult *Culicoides variipennis* (Diptera: Ceratopogonidae). *J. Am. Mosq. Control Assoc.* 6(3):537–538.

Whitlaw, J.T., and B.N. Chaniotis. 1978. Palm trees and Chagas' disease in Panama. *Am. J. Trop. Med. Hyg.* 27:873–881.

Williams, D.F. 1973. Sticky traps for sampling populations of *Stomoxys calcitrans*. *J. Econ. Ent.* 66(6):1279–1280.

Wilson, J.G., D.R. Kinzer, J.R. Sauer, and J.A. Hair. 1972. Chemo-attraction in the lone star tick (Acarina: Ixodidae): Part 1. Response to carbon dioxide administered via traps. *J. Med. Entomol.* 9:245–252.

Wilson, M.L., and A. Spielman. 1985. Seasonal activity of immature *Ixodes dammini* (Acari: Ixodidae). *J. Med. Entomol.* 22:408–414.

World Health Organization. 1991. *The housefly.* Vector Control Series, Training and Information Guide, Intermediate Level (WHO/VBC/90.987). Geneva, Switzerland: World Health Organization, Div. Trop. Dis.

Zimmerman, R.H., and G.I. Garris. 1985. Sampling efficiency of three dragging techniques for the collection of nonparasitic *Boophilus microplus* (Acari: Ixodidae) larvae in Puerto Rico. *J. Econ. Entomol.* 78:627–631.

28. ENVIRONMENTAL MANAGEMENT FOR VECTOR CONTROL

Carl J. Mitchell

An environment of high quality will first of all assure the biological survival of man. Gross pollution of air, land, and water is posing a global threat to survival right now. Equally threatening is the rapid depletion of nonrenewable resources that will be as critically needed by man generations hence as they are now. And, finally, the biological survival of man will demand an environment containing lesser numbers of Man himself.

One quality of the environment that should be maintained at all costs is diversity, for in the biota it promotes that biological stability without which chaos is forever imminent while in the landscape it satisfies man's innate desire for interest, beauty, and peace of mind. The biosphere is diverse beyond comprehension and it must remain so if any component of it, including man, is to survive.

—Maurice W. Provost (1973, pp. 1–2)

INTRODUCTION

The World Health Organization (WHO) Expert Committee on Vector Biology and Control defined environmental management for vector control as "the planning, organization, carrying out, and monitoring of activities for the modification and/or manipulation of environmental factors or their interaction with man with a view to preventing or minimizing vector propagation and reducing man-vector-pathogen contact"

(WHO 1980). Simply stated, environmental management for vector control includes those procedures that specifically modify the habitats of the target vector or humans to make those habitats unfavorable for the vector, or otherwise reduce human-vector-pathogen contact. Environmental management measures generally are not intended to replace other control measures but rather to complement them and contribute to the development of integrated control strategies (Fig. 28.1). Integrated vector control, thus, is "the utilization of all appropriate technological and management techniques to bring about an effective degree of vector suppression in a cost-effective manner" (WHO 1983).

Environmental management can be used in a cost-effective manner to reduce the risk of contracting a variety of vector-borne diseases (Mitchell 1987). Some environmental management practices also can adversely affect the environment (Provost 1972; 1973); therefore, careful planning during the design stage should include environmental impact assessments. Optimally, a balanced approach weighing the costs and benefits to the environment, as well as to economic and other concerns, will result in a plan compatible with the greater common good.

An extensive literature exists on environmental management for vector control. Ault (1994) and Curtis (1990) provide useful lists of recent publications. The reports by WHO (1982) and Mather and That

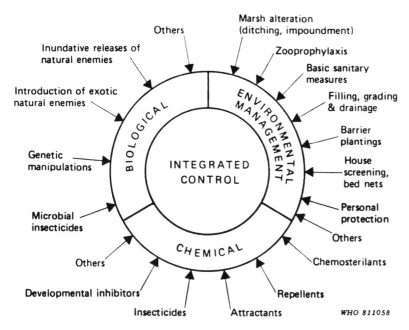

Others

Inundative releases of
natural enemies

Introduction of exotic
natural enemies

Genetic
manipulations

Microbial
insecticides

Others

Developmental inhibitors

Insecticides   Attractants

Marsh alteration
(ditching, impoundment)

Zooprophylaxis

Basic sanitary
measures

Filling, grading
& drainage

Barrier
plantings

House
screening,
bed nets

Personal
protection

Others

Chemosterilants

Repellents

BIOLOGICAL

ENVIRONMENTAL MANAGEMENT

INTEGRATED
CONTROL

CHEMICAL

WHO 811058

28.1   Diagram of the components (environmental management, chemical, biological) and their potential constituent methods to be considered in an "integrated control" approach to mosquito control. Reproduced by permission from *Manual on environmental management for mosquito control: With special emphasis on malaria vectors.* Geneva: World Health Organization, WHO Offset Publication No. 66, 1982, p. 10.

(1984) contain extensive bibliographies that include many classic references. In addition, the latter 2 publications provide instructions for implementing environmental management methods for the control of mosquito vectors of malaria, arboviral diseases, and filariasis, and the snail vectors of schistosomiasis. WHO and the United Nations Environment Programme (UNEP) have prepared a kit aimed at promoting insect and rodent control through environmental management (WHO 1991). The Panel of Experts on Environmental Management for Vector Control (PEEM), an interagency collaboration between WHO, the Food and Agricultural Organization of the United Nations, UNEP, and the United Nations Centre for Human Settlements, organizes workshops and meetings to discuss specific topics and issues periodic reports.

In this chapter, in keeping with the general theme of this book, I focus on environmental management of arthropod vectors, with examples that have proven to be successful in controlling some important vectors of arthropod-borne diseases. Mosquito control is emphasized.

HISTORICAL BACKGROUND

Some medically important insects were associated with disease in antiquity. At the end of the 1st century B.C., Vitruvius, a Roman engineer and architect, recommended that houses should not be built near marshes because mists coming from the marshes were harmful when mixed with the spirits of poisonous insects (Service 1978). Vitruvius designed a drainage system that periodically flushed the coastal marshes at high tide, a form of mosquito control widely used in modern times.

In 1901, William C. Gorgas was the first person to systematically employ antimosquito measures to control disease. Gorgas's specific objective was to control yellow fever in Havana, Cuba, but control efforts were aimed at mosquitoes in general. As a result, yellow fever was eliminated in Havana, and the incidence of malaria was reduced. Subsequently, Gorgas was placed in charge of the sanitation of the Panama Canal Zone. He proved that it was possible to control malaria as well as yellow fever by eliminating mosquito breeding habitats and by larviciding with kerosene and other petroleum oils. Because of Gorgas's successful antimosquito campaign, the United States succeeded in completing the Panama Canal whereas the French had failed to do so because of illness and death resulting from malaria and yellow fever. In 1915, the completion of the Panama Canal and Gorgas's successful control of mosquito-borne diseases were hailed as the greatest engineering and medical triumphs the world had seen.

Malcolm Watson found that of the approximately 30 species of *Anopheles* present in Malaya, only 3 species were important malaria vectors. This made malaria control practical because control efforts could be concentrated on these species. Because of similar discoveries by other pioneer malariologists working in other areas, the concept of "species sanitation" began to emerge. Species sanitation for malaria control means that attention should focus on those anopheline mosquitoes identified as the principal vectors of malaria in a specific area. For example, only about 30 of approximately 150 species of potential malaria vectors in the world have a major impact on malaria transmission (WHO 1982). Furthermore, only a few of the 30 species occur locally in a malaria focus. Consequently, the formidable task of controlling all anopheline mosquitoes in an area can be reduced to an achievable goal.

Species sanitation for malaria control led to reducing vector populations by attacking the larvae. Larviciding with petroleum oil and, especially, with paris green (copper aceto-arsenite) used as a floating dust proved effective. Larviciding was complemented by physical control methods such as destruction of the breeding habitats by drainage, filling, impounding, channeling streams into canals, and the so-called reclamation of marshes. Removing aquatic and emergent vegetation from the margins of lakes and impounding and periodically flushing breeding places by manipulating water levels also reduced populations of larvae.

Integrated control was the modus operandi of most mosquito control programs before the end of World War II, when the use of DDT and other powerful chemical insecticides became widespread. After the spectacular successes of these insecticides in controlling insect vectors of disease, especially when used as residual house sprays, other control methods fell by the wayside. More recently, public health and environmental concerns about the widespread use of pesticides and the development of insecticide resistance by vectors have stimulated renewed interest in the concept of integrated control. At the same time, heightened environmental awareness has raised concerns about the impact of all vector control activities.

EFFECTIVE VECTOR CONTROL

The elements of an effective vector control program are (1) incrimination of the vector species, (2) knowledge and understanding of vector biology and ecology, (3) surveillance, (4) public education, and (5) implementation of effective control measures.

The importance of identifying the vector species and understanding their biology and ecology is implicit in the concept of species sanitation and is basic to any successful vector control program. For example, malaria control in Trinidad resulted from the discovery that *Anopheles (Kertesia) bellator* was the major vector and the knowledge that the preferred larval habitat of this species is water collections in epiphytic bromeliads (Rozeboom and Laird 1942). Those bromeliads within a large radius of human habitations were removed and killed with sprays, thus controlling *An. bellator* and malaria. In this situation, draining swamps or eliminating other water collections would have had little impact on malaria transmission despite reducing the numbers of other mosquito species.

A surveillance system is needed to document vector densities and trends as a basis for assessing public health risks and to monitor control effectiveness (Chap. 27). A thorough public education program should be initiated prior to implementing vector control measures to assure public acceptance. Environmentally conscious vector control agencies should use an integrated approach, based on elimination of vector breeding sites through sanitation and source reduction where possible, coupled with the judicious use of chemical and biological control agents. It should be recognized that for physical, ecological, economic, or political reasons, chemical control is sometimes the only viable alternative (Provost 1977a).

MOSQUITO CONTROL

Water Impoundments

Dam construction in tropical countries has created vast artificial lakes with a cumulative capacity in excess of 15 billion cubic meters. Many of these lakes are in areas where malaria and schistosomiasis are endemic. Recently, construction of dams and irrigation projects in Sri Lanka and West Africa has led to outbreaks of

Japanese encephalitis (JE) and Rift Valley fever (RVF), respectively. Early in this century, the association of endemic malaria with artificial lakes in the southeastern United States enabled the U.S. Public Health Service and other agencies to develop strategies for control of the malaria vector, *Anopheles quadrimaculatus*, in impounded waters (USPHS and TVA 1947). These strategies proved to be highly successful in the reservoirs controlled and operated by the Tennessee Valley Authority (TVA) and have been adapted, with certain modifications, to other areas of the world with varying degrees of success. Following is a brief description of the management techniques.

Prior to impoundment, a water level management program is designed to strand drift and floatage, minimize propagation of marginal plants, and suppress aquatic plants. Proper preimpoundment preparation results in a clean water surface at all elevations between high and low levels following filling. Following impoundment, malaria mosquito control largely depends on water level management. Each reservoir has a predictable annual pattern or "rule curve" of water level changes. Such rule curves developed for the reservoirs of the TVA system serve as the bases for control of malaria vectors and of marginal vegetation necessary for their development (Fig. 28.2). During the winter period mosquito production is not a problem in temperate areas. In early spring the reservoir is filled to provide a surcharge. This surcharge strands drift and floatage as the reservoir is drawn down to a constant pool level. The constant pool level limits invasion of semiaquatic marginal vegetation into the fluctuation zone, thus providing a clean shoreline when the water is drawn down later in the season. The constant water level is maintained until anopheline mosquito production begins.

In the next phase of management, the water level is fluctuated weekly by about 0.3 m. This draw-down in the water level exposes marginal vegetation and eliminates larval habitat. Reflooding delays growth and invasion of marginal vegetation.

After a few weeks of cyclical fluctuation, a clean shoreline margin no longer occurs at the low point of the cycle, and mosquito populations begin to increase. The next phase is initiated then, which combines seasonal recession and cyclical fluctuation. Although the water level is lowered 0.3 m as before, it is subsequently raised only 0.27 m during reflooding. This seasonal recession coincides with a decrease in stream flow and an increase in the use of water downstream. The seasonal recession draws the water level sufficiently below advancing marginal vegetation to control mosquito production.

Despite successes in using water level management for mosquito control in temperate zone climates, the technique is still difficult to adapt to tropical zones in which there is no seasonal interruption in vegetation growth and mosquito production (WHO 1982). However, with good water level fluctuation and marginal drainage, mosquito production can be reduced to acceptable levels. Many important vectors of malaria do not breed in lakes. For example, members of the *An. gambiae* complex, dangerous malaria vectors in Africa, are found primarily in a wide variety of other habitats. In these situations, reducing human-mosquito contact through the use of pyrethroid-treated bed nets (Curtis et al. 1990) and other control options can be effective.

Rice Culture

The main *Culex* vectors of Japanese encephalitis probably evolved in freshwater marsh habitats. Consequently, paddy fields (irrigated rice) serve as vast artificial extensions of these habitats, and the vectors of JE breed prolifically in them (Mitchell 1977). Paddy fields also are important breeding habitats for vectors of malaria and filariasis. Overall, more than 135 pest and vector anopheline and culicine mosquito species have been found in association with riceland habitats (Lacey and Lacey 1990). To appreciate the magnitude of the problem in terms of mosquito habitat, remember that rice is the staple food of more than 50% of the world's population. Globally, more than 145 million hectares of land are used for growing rice, about 90% of which is in Asia (Mather and That 1984).

Intermittent irrigation of paddy fields for control of malaria vectors was suggested as early as 1922; this was widely used in Portugal to control *An. labranchiae* and is a well-known technique in China and Japan (Rajagopalan et al. 1990; Mogi 1993). The so-called wet

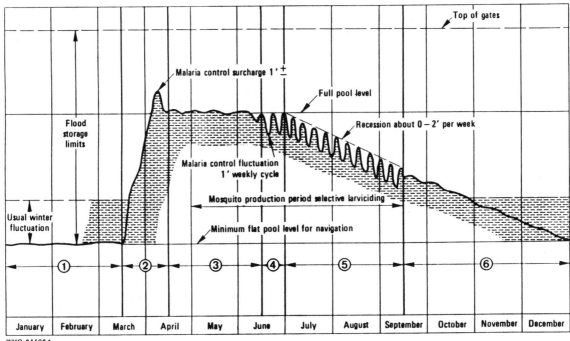

MALARIA CONTROL FEATURES OF WATER LEVEL MANAGEMENT ON T V A MAIN RIVER RESERVOIRS

WHO 811084

① **LOW WINTER FLOOD CONTROL LEVELS**
Controls growth of submerged aquatics
Permits marginal drainage and herbicidal operations

② **EARLY SPRING FILLING**
Retards plant growth
SURCHARGE
Strands drift above full pool level

③ **CONSTANT POOL LEVEL**
Provides long-range plant growth control

④ **CYCLICAL FLUCTUATION**
Destroys mosquito eggs and larvae

⑤ **FLUCTUATION AND RECESSION**
Destroys eggs and larvae
Reduces breeding area
Provides clean shoreline

⑥ **RECESSION TO WINTER LEVELS**
Permits fall shoreline maintenance and
improvement operations

28.2   Desirable phases of water level management for the control of pond-breeding anophelines on multiuse impound-ments. Reproduced by permission from *Manual on environmental management for mosquito control: With special emphasis on malaria vectors*. Geneva: World Health Organization, WHO Offset Publication No. 66, 1982, p. 10.

irrigation method of rice cultivation, a type of intermittent irrigation developed primarily to increase rice yield, also has the advantages of reducing mosquito breeding and decreasing water consumption. The method relies on supplying water according to the needs of the plants with the exception of the period of seedling transplanting (Luh 1984). During this period, which lasts about 10–15 days, the fields are filled with water to a depth of 4–6 cm. After the plants turn green, the fields are drained—contrary to conventional irrigation practice—and are intermittently flooded with a shallow layer of water that disappears by 24–48 hours through absorption, percolation, and evaporation. The interval between successive irrigations typically is 3–5 days. During the entire growing period (about 100 days), the fields are irrigated 21–26 times (Fig. 28.3).

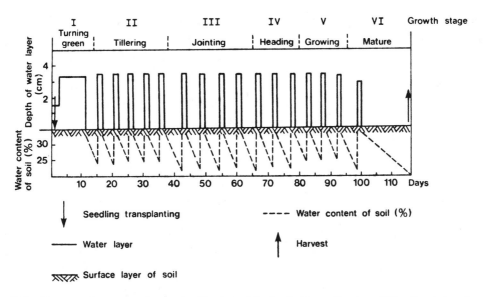

28.3 Diagram of wet irrigation method in rice cultivation in Henan Province, China. Reproduced by permission from T.H. Mather and T.T. That *Environmental management for vector control in rice fields.* Rome: Food and Agricultural Organization of the United Nations, 1984, p. 134.

The method has yielded good results in the alluvial plain of the Yellow River Basin in Henan Province, China. Larval densities of *An. sinensis* and *Cx. tritaeniorhynchus,* major vectors of malaria and Japanese encephalitis, respectively, have been dramatically reduced by the use of intermittently flooded fields compared with fields subjected to conventional irrigation (Fig. 28.4).

At present, this method can only be used successfully in areas with sandy loam soils in which the water supply is sufficient for repeated flooding. In

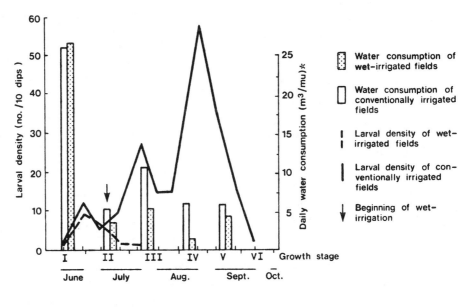

* 15 mu = 1 ha

28.4 Comparison of the larval densities of *An. sinensis* and *Cx. tritaeniorhynchus* between fields of wet and conventional irrigation. Reproduced by permission from T.H. Mather and T.T. That. *Environmental management for vector control in rice fields.* Rome: Food and Agricultural Organization of the United Nations, 1984, p. 134.

areas in which monsoon rains occur, improving drainage assists in reducing the size of risk areas.

Salt Marshes

Important vectors of malaria that breed in brackish coastal marsh habitats include *An. sundaicus* in Asia; *An. melas* and *An. merus* in Africa; *An. labranchiae, An. atroparvus,* and *An. sacharovi* in the Mediterranean; and *An. albimanus, An. aquasalis,* and *An. grabhamii* in the Americas. These species cannot develop in undiluted sea water but find suitable habitats in landlocked coastal marshes and swamps in which the water is brackish.

Excluding saline water from coastal marshes has been effective in controlling *An. sundaicus* in Malaya and *An. sacharovi* in Italy. Sluice gates exclude entry of seawater at high tides and permit the discharge of accumulated fresh water at low tides. However, some vector species such as *An. albimanus* can breed in fresh as well as brackish water. In other instances, local freshwater vectors can be more dangerous than brackish water species; therefore, saltmarsh management techniques must fit the local situation.

It is difficult to comprehend that during the early part of this century vast expanses of the United States along the West Coast (including portions of the San Francisco Bay area), the East Coast, and the Gulf Coast were practically uninhabitable during the summer months because of hordes of saltmarsh mosquitoes. The history of mosquito control in the United States is intimately related to real estate interests and saltmarsh mosquito control. Unfortunately, saltmarsh mosquito control got off to a bad start in New Jersey and neighboring states. Entire marshes were needlessly ditched, resulting in the succession of thousands of acres of saltmarsh cordgrass into solid areas of useless weeds and the concomitant loss of valuable wildlife habitat (Provost 1969a). Since then, more enlightened management has been practiced, and draining, building dikes, and excluding tidal action on salt marshes usually is not recommended. Such practices can cause entire marshes to be invaded by salt hay and other semiaquatic plants accompanied by heavy mosquito production in rain-filled depressions.

Five species of saltmarsh *Aedes* dominate the coastal zone mosquito fauna in the United States: *Ae. sollicitans, Ae. taeniorhynchus, Ae. cantator, Ae. dorsalis,* and *Ae. squamiger.* These species have similar characteristics. Eggs are laid singly on areas of the marsh subject to flooding, never directly on water. Eggs hatch when flooded by seasonal tides, storm tides, or rainfall, and adults emerge in large synchronized broods.

Salt marshes are unevenly distributed in coastal areas and are characterized by different dominant plant species in different areas of the United States. Two general types exist: a low marsh (subject to daily flooding) and a high marsh (flooded only by the year's highest tides). Mosquitoes are not produced on the low marsh because of the daily tidal action. The developmental stages of saltmarsh *Aedes* dictate that water must stand on the high marsh for a minimum of 4–10 days to produce a brood of adult mosquitoes. Production of saltmarsh *Aedes* can be prevented by altering the high marsh so that water never stands on it, by assuring that surface water on vegetated areas never lasts for more than 2–3 days, or by covering the ground completely with water and thus denying gravid saltmarsh *Aedes* suitable oviposition sites. A system of open marsh water management based on these principles has evolved that effectively controls mosquito breeding without harming the vegetation. However, the populations of other ecologically important marsh organisms often increase (Provost 1977b).

During the past decade, saltmarsh management in Florida has attempted to reconcile mosquito control and natural resource interests (Carlson et al. 1991). Rotational impoundment management is a compromise method that allows for source reduction while maintaining many of the natural functions of the high marsh. Culverts with flapgate risers through dikes are positioned throughout the marsh, thereby allowing seasonal connection with estuaries. In some situations, rotary ditching can also be used in ecologically sound source reduction programs.

Sanibel Island, off the mouth of the Caloosahatchee River in southwest Florida, represents an excellent example of mosquito control through environmental management (Provost 1969a; 1969b). During 1950, before control was begun, a single New

Jersey light trap collected 365,696 mosquitoes, mostly *Ae. taeniorhynchus*, in one night. Each winter the interior swales of Sanibel dried up, and mosquito egg deposits of up to half a billion per acre were carried over to the next rainy season. A mosquito control plan was devised based on water management. All low interior areas were connected, and a water control structure was installed that maintained a water level of about 30 inches above the average low water level. By denying adult *Ae. taeniorhynchus* places to lay eggs, and by maintaining larvivorous minnows in the pools, saltmarsh mosquito production in the interior was nearly eliminated.

Currently, wetlands are disappearing at a rapid rate in the United States and the future of those remaining is hotly debated (Alper 1992). In California, coastal wetlands now cover less than 25% of their historic area and are far from pristine (Zedler 1991). From the 1780s to the 1980s, the lower 48 states lost an estimated 53% of their original wetlands (Dahl 1990). This reduction resulted in obvious benefits to economic development and to mosquito control interests. The conquest of malaria in the southeastern United States resulted primarily from the slow but steady organization of the environment for economic and social purposes. Whereas it may have been easy for early settlers to decide to drain a mosquito-infested swamp, such decisions are no longer as clear cut. It is now understood that swamps and marshes play vital roles in the ecosystems in which they occur and thus should not always be destroyed.

Community-Based Aedes Control

Aedes aegypti is the principal vector of dengue viruses and urban yellow fever. The domestic nature of this mosquito and its container-breeding habits make it amenable to control through environmental sanitation. In the early years of the 20th century, researchers demonstrated that such control efforts could control urban yellow fever. However, when active control measures were relaxed, *Ae. aegypti* populations rapidly returned to precontrol levels. To overcome this problem, eradication techniques were developed and applied that resulted in the elimination of *Ae. aegypti* in Brazil (Soper 1963). This success was based on a vertically structured control program that could not be sustained (Gubler 1989).

Gubler (1989) has argued that a community-based approach to *Ae. aegypti* control, although slower to achieve results, is the best long-term solution. Thus, involving important community members and organizations in health education is necessary for success. Currently, several community-based programs operate in Asia and the Americas (Chan et al. 1990; Halstead and Gomez-Dantes 1992; Gubler and Clark 1993). Singapore has had a long history of successfully controlling *Ae. aegypti* and *Ae. albopictus*, mainly using environmental measures (Chan et al. 1990). Vector populations have been reduced and maintained at low levels, and there has been a dramatic reduction in the numbers of dengue and dengue hemorrhagic fever cases; however, small focal outbreaks continue to occur.

OTHER MOSQUITO AND INSECT VECTORS OF DISEASE

Space does not permit consideration of the control of other mosquitoes and insects that serve as vectors of important diseases such as filariasis (Chap. 7) and trypanosomiasis (Chap. 10); see Curtis (1990), Ault (1994), WHO (1982), and Mather and That (1984) for information on these subjects.

TICKS

Because of the distinct ecologic requirements and life histories of ticks, control strategies can be directed at the free-living stages, the feeding stages, or their vertebrate hosts. Control objectives are to make the environment inhospitable for long-term tick survival and to create an unattractive environment for tick hosts.

Jaenson et al. (1991) summarized methods for controlling members of the *Ixodes ricinus* complex, the primary vectors of Lyme borreliosis. This complex includes *I. scapularis*, which is a 3-host tick that parasitizes a wide range of hosts. Temperature and moisture are important environmental variables affecting the survival of ticks during periods when they are not attached to hosts. These variables can be manipulated through habitat modification or landscape management (Maupin et al. 1991). Landscaping with plants that are not attractive as forage for deer can reduce the population of *Ixodes scapularis* in the northeastern United States. Reduction of host availability through the use of deerproof fencing, or actually reducing the number of hosts, can be effective in some areas. Mowing and burning vegetation in some situations is a temporary solution with obvious limitations.

Physical measures to prevent tick bites include avoiding tick-infested areas, wearing light-colored, tightly woven clothing, tucking trousers into boots or high-topped shoes, regularly checking the body and pets for ticks, and being generally aware of tick-infested areas and the seasonality of tick activity.

PERSPECTIVE

The vectors of a number of important diseases can be effectively controlled by using environmental management techniques singly or in concert with other control methods. Unfortunately, the overriding theme of existing guidelines for such control is "benefit to humans," which often is narrowly construed to mean "economic" benefit. Raising the environmental consciousness of the general public to the level necessary to assure that intangibles such as overall environmental quality are taken into consideration is a challenge. The current campaign, spearheaded by the Union of Concerned Scientists and designed to alert the world to our environmental crisis, is an encouraging sign (Holden 1992).

The world's population has more than doubled in the last four decades, from 2.5 billion in 1950 to 5.3 billion in 1990. If the growth rate of the 1980s remains constant, the world's population will increase to 10.7 billion by the year 2030 (Horiuchi 1992). As a result of such population pressure, environmental concerns will become increasingly important in determining which vector control technologies are acceptable. Environmental insults associated with vector control practices are less likely to be tolerated in a climate of diminishing resources, and many current vector control practices will become unacceptable. It is therefore imperative that research efforts directed toward developing new technologies for vector control place increasing emphasis on their long-term environmental acceptability. Such attention to environmental concerns can contribute not only to the survival of man but to the survival of vector control agencies as well.

REFERENCES

Alper, J. 1992. War over the wetlands: Ecologists versus the White House. *Science* 257:1043–1044.

Ault, S.K. 1994. Environmental management: A re-emerging vector control strategy. *Am. J. Trop. Med. Hyg.* 50:35–49.

Carlson, D.B., P.D. O'Bryan, and J.R. Rey. 1991. A review of current salt marsh management issues in Florida. *J. Am. Mosq. Control Assoc.* 7:83–88.

Chan, K-L. et al. 1990. *Aedes* mosquitoes: Virus transmission and control methods. In: C.F. Curtis, editor, *Appropriate technology in vector control.* Boca Raton, FL: CRC Press. pp. 104–119.

Curtis, C.F., 1990. *Appropriate technology in vector control.* ed., Boca Raton, FL: CRC Press. 233 p.

Dahl, T.E. 1990. *Wetlands losses in the United States 1780's to 1980's.* Washington, D.C.: U.S. Department of the Interior, Fish and Wildlife Service. 21 p.

Gubler, D.J. 1989. *Aedes aegypti* and *Aedes aegypti*-borne disease control in the 1990s: Top down or bottom up. *Am. J. Trop. Med. Hyg.* 40:571–578.

Gubler, D.J., and Clark, G.G. 1994. Community-based integrated control of *Aedes aegypti*: A brief overview of current programs. *Am. J. Trop. Med. Hyg.* 50:50–60.

Halstead, S.B., and H. Gomez-Dantes, eds. 1992. Dengue, a worldwide problem, a common strategy. Proceedings of the international conference on dengue and *Aedes aegypti* community-based control. Mexico: Ministry of Health with the Rockefeller Foundation. Ediciones Copilco, S.A. de C.V. pp. 1–329.

Holden, C. 1992. Scientists' campaign to save earth. *Science* 1433:258.

Horiuchi, S. 1992. Stagnation in the decline of the world population growth rate during the 1980s. *Science* 257:761–765.

Jaenson, T.G.T., et al. 1991. Methods for control of tick vectors of Lyme borreliosis. *Scand. J. Infect. Dis. Suppl.* 77:151–157.

Lacey, L.A., and C.M. Lacey, 1990. The medical importance of riceland mosquitoes and their control using alternatives to chemical insecticides. *Am. Mosq. Control Assoc. Suppl.* 2:1–93.

Luh, P-L. 1984. Effects of rice growing on the population of disease vectors. In: T.H. Mather and T.T. That, *Environmental management for vector control in rice fields.* Rome, Italy: Food and Agriculture Organization of the United Nations. pp. 130–132.

Mather, T.H., and That, T.T. 1984. *Environmental management for vector control in rice fields*. Rome, Italy: Food and Agriculture Organization of the United Nations. 172 p.

Maupin, G.O. et al. 1991. Landscape ecology of Lyme disease in a residential area of Westchester County, New York. *Am. J. Epidemiol.* 133:1105–1113.

Mitchell, C.J. 1977. Arthropod-borne encephalitis viruses and water resource developments. Cah. ORSTOM. *Ser Ent. Med. et Parasitol.* 15:241–250.

———. 1987. The cost-effectiveness of environmental management as a vector control measure, Sixth Annual Meeting WHO/FAO/UNEP Panel of Experts on Environmental Management for Vector Control. Geneva, Switzerland: WHO 871311, VBC/87. 3:126–133.

Mogi, M. 1993. Effect of intermittent irrigation on mosquitoes (Diptera: Culicidae) and larvivorous predators in rice fields. *J. Med. Entomol.* 30:309–319.

Provost, M.W. 1969a. Man, mosquitoes, and birds. *Florida Naturalist* 42:63–67.

———. 1969b. Ecological control of salt marsh mosquitoes with side benefits to birds. Proceedings of Tall Timbers Conference on Ecological Animal Control by Habitat Management, Feb. 27–28, 1969, Tallahassee, Florida. pp. 193–206.

———. 1972. Environmental hazards in the control of disease vectors. *Environ. Entomol.* 1:333–339.

———.1973. Environmental quality and the control of biting flies. Proceedings of a symposium; Edmonton: University of Alberta Defense Research. pp. 1–7.

———. 1977a. Source reduction in salt-marsh mosquito control: Past and future. *Mosq. News* 37:689–698.

———. 1977b. Mosquito control, Coastal Ecosystem Management. In: John R. Clark, editor, *A technical manual for the conservation of coastal zone resources*. The Conservation Foundation. New York: John Wiley and Sons. pp. 666–671.

Rajagopalan, P.K. et al. 1990. Environmental and water management for mosquito control. In: C.F. Curtis, editor, *Appropriate technology in vector control*. Boca Raton, Florida: CRC Press. pp. 121–138.

Rozeboom, L.E., and Laird, R.L. 1942. *Anopheles (Kerteszia) bellator* Dyan and Knab as a vector of malaria in Trinidad, British West Indies. *Am. Jour. Trop. Med.* 22:83–91.

Service, M.W. 1978. A short history of early medical entomology. *J. Med. Entomol.* 14:603–626.

Soper, F.L. 1963. The elimination of urban yellow fever in the Americas through the eradication of *Aedes aegypti*. *Am. Jour. Public Health.* 53:7–16.

United States Public Health Service and Tennessee Valley Authority. 1947. *Malaria control on impounded water*. Washington, DC: Government Printing Office. 422 p.

World Health Organization. 1980. *Environmental management for vector control*. Geneva, Switzerland: WHO Tech. Rpt. Series, No. 649. 75 p.

World Health Organization. 1982. *Manual on environmental management for mosquito control*. Offset Publication No. 66. Geneva: World Health Organization. 282 p.

World Health Organization. 1983. *Integrated vector control*. Geneva, Switxerland: WHO Tech. Rpt. Series, No. 688. 72 p.

World Health Organization. 1991. *Insect and rodent control through environmental management: A community action programme*. Geneva: World Health Organization. 107 p.

Zedler, J.B. 1991. The challenge of protecting endangered species habitat along the Southern California coast. *Coastal Mgmt.* 19:35–53.

29. CHEMICAL CONTROL OF VECTORS

Susan Palchick

Chemicals have been used for centuries for vector control, but in recent years they have been criticized for environmental and social reasons. Nevertheless, the thoughtful use of chemical control measures can be a vital part of an integrated pest management program. Thus, it is important to know how they work, what they contain, and how they should be applied.

HISTORY

Early pesticides included botanicals such as nicotine, rotenone, and pyrethrum. Subsequently, other pesticides, such as chlorinated hydrocarbon insecticides, especially DDT (Dichlorodiphenyltrichloroethane), have become important in the control of insect-borne diseases of humans.

With the onset of World War II, a search for effective ways to control lice became important when outbreaks of typhus, trench fever, and louse-borne relapsing fever occurred. Researchers sought a chemical that could not only be safely applied to clothing and the body but also prevent reinfestation for long periods. Initially, MYL, a formulation of dinitroanisole, pyrethrins, N-isobutylundecylenamide, isopropyl crold, and pyrophyllite was used; short-lasting pyrethrum was the killing agent. But when a sample of DDT was furnished to the U.S. Department of Agriculture (USDA) in 1942, it was judged to be superior to MYL and subsequently employed. Because of the unique insecticidal properties of DDT and low manufacture cost, it was widely used for the control of disease vectors.

Residual insecticides then revolutionized vector control. When the inside surfaces of a house were sprayed with a residual insecticide, mosquitoes contacted the toxic surfaces and died before transmitting the infection. Thus, spraying with such residual insecticides as DDT (and to a lesser extent with BHC [benzene hexachloride]) became the major tool in malaria control. After a while, inhabitants opposed spraying because of socioreligious beliefs; odor and visibility of the residue; toxicity to animals, especially to chickens and ducks; and rarely, mild poisoning.

In addition to objections to residual spraying, a combination of events caused a general disillusionment with the chlorinated hydrocarbons. Increasing vector resistance to the compounds and environmental consequences of continued accumulation of the slowly degradable compounds were responsible for this disillusionment.

As the resistance of vectors and other factors began to interfere with the use of chlorinated hydrocarbon insecticides, other classes of compounds increasingly have been used. A new generation of insecticides, including synthetic pyrethroids, *Bacillus thuringiensis israelensis (Bti),* and insect growth regulators (IGRs) have become popular. These products are more expensive than DDT because they not only cost more to manufacture but must be applied more frequently. Other less-direct costs include those incurred by (1) personal safety measures, including storing and handling more hazardous compounds; (2) developing of new compounds; (3) implementing alternative methods of vector control; and (4) economic loss arising from high levels of chronic disease and from periodic outbreaks.

In addition to changes in chemicals, formulations have also changed in response to new technology and new needs of vector control. For example, wettable powders (WP) were improved technically during the 1950s. Another change in formulation has involved concentration. There has been a trend toward the application of more concentrated sprays to achieve the same or somewhat smaller dosage per unit area. This practice can reduce the amount of expensive solvent required for a given task.

CLASSIFICATION OF PESTICIDES

Insecticides are classified by chemical structure, mode of action, or formulations. These categories facilitate discussing the different pesticides and their uses.

Chemical Structure

Insecticides are inorganic or organic in origin. Today organic compounds are used more than inorganic compounds. Inorganic compounds include those of fluorine, phosphorus, and sulfur. Organic compounds are of synthetic or botanical origin. The synthetic compounds can be divided into chlorinated hydrocarbons, organophosphates, and carbamates as well as those pesticides derived from plants and other organisms (Fig. 29.1)

Chlorinated Hydrocarbon Insecticides

All chlorinated hydrocarbon (organochlorine) insecticides are aryl, carbocyclic, or heterocyclic compounds with molecular weights ranging from 291–545. In general, most of these compounds are stimulants to the nervous system. Organochlorines generally kill by contact but can also act as stomach poisons and in a few cases fumigants. The chlorinated hydrocarbons can be divided into 5 groups: DDT and its analogues, benzene hexachloride (BHC), cyclodienes and similar compounds, toxaphene and related chemicals, and the caged structures mirex and chlordecone. In spite of similarity of chemical structure and pharmacological effect, insecticides within each group can differ widely in toxicity and in their capacity for storage.

Although the organochlorine insecticides were widely and effectively used in malaria control programs from the 1940s to the 1960s, they have come into disfavor because of their persistence in the environment, wildlife, and humans. The relatively low cost of these insecticides and unavailability of complete substitutes for some uses, however, ensure their continued use in many countries. None of the cyclodienes (chlordane, heptachlor, aldrin, or dieldrin) is available in the United States. Examples of other organochlorine compounds include DDT, methoxychlor, toxaphene, and lindane.

Organic Phosphorus Pesticides

Organic phosphorus compounds (organophosphates) share a common general chemical structure, but they differ in the details of their structure, in their physical and pharmacological properties, and consequently in their uses.

The organic phosphorus compounds are generally less stable than the organochlorine compounds and can degrade in the presence of water by hydrolysis, through chemical alterations by reaction with oxygen, through heat, and through bacterial action.

Organophosphorus compounds also vaporize quickly, and thus are often rapidly lost into the atmosphere. These materials are not stored in the body fat of animals but are readily broken down and excreted through the kidneys.

These pesticides attach themselves to cholinesterase, an enzyme found in the blood of mammals that is necessary for normal nerve function. Because organic phosphorus compounds "tie up" cholinesterase, they are referred to as cholinesterase inhibitors. When the cholinesterase cannot break down acetylcholine, the nerves in the body continue to send messages to certain muscles, which make them move constantly.

Examples of organophosphorus insecticides used in vector control are chlorpyrifos, diazinon, fenthion, malathion, dichlorvos, and naled.

Carbamates

The carbamates, like the organophosphorus compounds, are cholinesterase inhibitors. They range from

CHLORINATED HYDROCARBONS

(1) DDT:
    mode of action: stomach poison and contact

(2) Methoxychlor, DMDT (Marlate, Methoxcide, Moxie, Prentox):
    mode of action: stomach poison and contact

(3) Lindane (gamma isomer of BHC (1,2,3,4,5,6-hexachlorocyclohexane)) (Agronexit,
    Ambrocide, Gamaphex, Gammalin, Gammex, Isotox, Lindacol, Lintox, Nexit, Novigam):
    mode of action: stomach, fumigant, and contact

(4) Dieldrin:
    mode of action: contact and stomach poison

(5) Chlordane:
    mode of action: contact, stomach poison and fumigant

(6) Toxaphene:
    mode of action: contact and stomach poison

(7) Mirex:
    mode of action: stomach insecticide, little contact action

ORGANIC PHOSPHATES

(8) Diazinon (Basudin, Dazzel, Diazide, Knox-out, Nipsan, Sarolex):
    mode of action: contact and stomach poison

(9) Fenthion (Baycid, Baytex, Queletox, Spotton, Tiguvon):
    mode of action: contact and stomach poison

(10) Malathion (Chemathion, Cythion, Fyfanon, Kypfos, Zithiol):
    mode of action: nonsystemic

(11) Naled (Bromex, Dibrom, Hibrom):
    mode of action: contact and stomach poison

CARBAMATES

(12) Carbaryl (Calpolin, Dicarbam, Hexavin, Murvin, Ravyon, Sevin):
    mode of action: contact and stomach poison, non-systemic

(13) Propoxur (Aprocarb, Baygon, Propion, Sendran, Suncide):
    mode of action: contact and stomach poison

BOTANICALS

(14) Rotenone (Cubor, Derris, Mexide, Noxfire, Rotacide, Nekos):
    mode of action: contact and stomach poison

(15) Nicotine:
    mode of action: stomach poison

(16) Allethrin (Bioallethrin, Evergreen, Pyrocide, Sectol):
    mode of action: contact, stomach poison and fumigant

(17) Permethrin (Ambush, Atroban, Biothrin, Evercide, Pounce, Pramex):
    mode of action: contact and stomach poison

(18) Resmethrin (Derringer, Vectrin, Scourge, Synthrin):
    mode of action: contact insecticide

INSECT GROWTH REGULATORS

(19) Methoprene (Altosid, Apex, Precor, Ovitrol):
    mode of action: insect growth regulator

CHITIN INHIBITORS

(20) Diflubenzuron (Difluron, Dimilin, Larvakil, Micromite):
    mode of action: stomach poison and contact

29.1 Names and chemical structures of common insecticides

low to high mammalian toxicity. Examples include carbaryl and propoxur.

Pesticides Derived from Plants

Insecticidal compounds derived from plant materials are referred to as botanicals. Some are used as insect repellents, others are mixed with toxicants and used as attractants in bait formulations, and still others are refined into insecticides. Botanical insecticides commonly used today come from families including nicotine sulfate (Solanaceae—tobacco), pyrethrum (Compositaceae—chrysanthemum), rotenone (Leguminosae—pea), ryania (Flacourtiaceae), and sabadilla (Liliaceae—lily).

Pyrethrum and related compounds. The insecticidally active components in pyrethrum are known collectively as pyrethrins and are the natural extracts of the plant. One of the first successful synthetic pyrethrins was the pyrethroid allethrin, first synthesized in 1949. Allethrin was followed by resmethrin, bioresmethrin, cismethrin, and other related pyrethroids. These pyrethroids are potent insecticides; all are unstable in light and air. The compounds were attractive because they lacked persistence in the environment and possessed rapid "knockdown" activity. The introduction of synergists in the 1950s reduced the cost of treatment.

In recent years a new group of pyrethroids have been synthesized that exhibit greater stability in light and air than earlier compounds. These pyrethroids are active contact insecticides, relatively involatile, stable on inert surfaces, but readily degraded by metabolizing systems, especially those of mammals and soil microorganisms.

Pesticides Derived from Other Living Organisms

Insect growth regulators (IGRs). These compounds act on the highly species-specific insect hormonal systems that control molting and metamorphosis. They have the advantage of low mammalian toxicity; some disadvantages are species specificity, time required to kill, and poor stability.

Juvenile hormones (JH) are used by insects to regulate growth and metamorphosis (Chap. 17). Only a small amount of this hormone is necessary for the larva to metamorphose into a pupae. Adding synthetic juvenile hormone (e.g., methoprene) inhibits this molting process.

Bacteria. Although usually considered biological control agents, these materials are subject to production methods similar to chemicals and are sometimes grouped with chemical control agents. *Bacillus thuringiensis israelensis* disrupts the midgut lining of mosquito and black fly larvae. *Bacillus sphaericus* is not as widely used as *Bti* but is also effective against mosquito larvae (Chap. 32).

Chitin Inhibitors

The benzoylphenylureas interfere with the formation of chitin, a major constituent of the exoskeleton of insects. As vertebrates and most plants do not form chitin, these compounds are probably safe for humans, domestic animals, wildlife, and plants. Other arthropods and some fungi, however, do form chitin and are affected by these compounds. Diflubenzuron (Dimilin®) is an example of a chitin inhibitor.

MODE OF ACTION

The way that a particular insecticide affects its target is referred to as mode of action. Various modes of action exist:

- Stomach poisons affect the vector when they are ingested and are absorbed in the digestive tract. These can be applied directly to the vector or as a systemic to the host.

- Contact insecticides enter the body wall or respiratory system and kill the vectors by contact.

- Systemics are applied to the host to combat parasites in or on the host such as fleas or botflies.

- Fumigants are volatile and enter the vector's body through the respiratory system.

- Suffocants include materials, such as oils, that clog the respiratory system via the tracheae or respiratory siphon.

- Desiccants cause the vector to dry out by disrupting the waxy layer of the cuticle.

- Repellents make the vector avoid or leave a treated surface (animal or plant). These can change the vector's behavior by preventing or reducing oviposition or feeding.

- Attractants are used to bait vectors into a trap or treated area or to confuse males of some species and prevent them from mating. Attractants include pheromones that are secreted by an insect and that influence the behavior of other individuals of the same species.

- Hormones inhibit the growth and development of the vector. They interfere with formation of the cuticle during the larval stage or they inhibit molting from the larval to pupal stage.

Formulations

The active ingredients in insecticides are rarely used in their pure form; they usually are combined with other materials in a formulation. Dry formulations include dusts, granules, wettable powders, soluble powders, and baits. Liquid formulations include emulsifiable concentrates, solutions, flowables, and aerosols. Formulations can also contain a carrier or diluent.

Adjuvants are added to change the physical or chemical characteristics of the formulation. Adjuvants can improve wetting characteristics, modify the rate of spray evaporation, improve the weatherability of the deposit, improve uniformity of the deposit, or reduce phytotoxicity. Surface active agents (surfactants) include wetting agents, emulsifiers, adhesives, and spreaders. Synergists also are added to enhance the activity of the active ingredient. Nonactive ingredients, such as diluents, are considered inert.

When choosing a formulation, certain factors should be considered: the type of pest to be controlled, application equipment required, whether the formulation will be applied indoors or outdoors, susceptibility of plants or nontarget organisms to toxicant, coverage, and drift.

Dusts

Dusts or powders contain an active ingredient and a carrier such as talc, clay, diatomaceous earth, nut hulls, or other material. Dusts penetrate dense foliage better than sprays. They also are less likely to cause plant injury because they do not contain solvents, oils, or emulsifiers. Drift onto nontarget areas can be hazardous to humans and can result in undesirable residues on plants. Drift also reduces the effectiveness of dusts

because less of the formulation actually penetrates the target area. Dusts have less residual effect than other formulations.

Granules

Granular formulations are made by applying a liquid formulation of an active ingredient to coarse particles of some type of porous material (such as clay, corn cobs, or walnut shells). Granule particles are much larger than dust particles and therefore less likely to drift.

Wettable Powders

Wettable powders resemble dusts but are formulated to mix with water. Wettable powders form a suspension rather than a true solution when added to water. Although wettable powders contain wetting agents, or "spreader-stickers," they contain no solvents; therefore, they are less likely to cause plant injury than are emulsifiable sprays containing solvents. Wettable powders do not drift as readily as dusts. Constant agitation is necessary or particles will settle out in the spray tank. The diluents in wettable powders are abrasive and can wear down pumps and nozzles.

Soluble Powders

Soluble powders (SP) are similar to wettable powders, except that they form true solutions in water. Because they dissolve completely in water they do not need constant agitation nor do they abrade equipment.

Baits

Baits are edible or attractive substances mixed with a toxicant that attract pests and subsequently poison them. These are formulated for direct application.

Emulsifiable Concentrates

Emulsifiable concentrates (EC) are solutions of active ingredient and emulsifying agent dissolved in an organic solvent that can then be mixed with water. This emulsion requires minimal agitation. After water and solvents evaporate from the treated surface, the remaining insecticide residue adheres to the sprayed surface. Because emulsifiable concentrates contain organic solvents and emulsifying agents, plants can be damaged more from them than from dusts or wettable powders.

Solutions

High concentrate solutions contain only the active ingredient or a high concentration of the active ingredient that has been diluted with oil or petroleum solvents. Ultralow volume (ULV) concentrate should be used without further dilution. Low-concentration solutions are usually in highly refined oils. They need no further dilution.

Flowables

Active ingredients that can be formulated only as a solid or semisolid are finely ground and mixed with a liquid to form a suspension. Flowables can be added to water and need only moderate agitation.

Aerosols

The active ingredient in solution in a solvent is dispersed in very small droplets. Aerosols are used in treating areas that are difficult to reach with other types of formulations and application equipment.

Slow-Release Systems

Slow-release systems blend an active ingredient with a material from which it will evaporate or be released at a controlled rate. Ingredients that are volatile or subject to environmental degradation such as sunlight remain present much longer. Microencapsulation is a form of slow-release formulation in which the active ingredient is enclosed in a material such as polyamide, neoprene, polyvinyl chloride, or polyester. The active ingredient can diffuse from the matrix. An advantage of microencapsulation is the ability to use smaller amounts of the active ingredient.

Synergists

Compounds of various kinds can increase an insecticide's toxicity to insects by promoting absorption of the insecticide or by interfering with detoxification of the insecticide. Piperonyl butoxide is an example of a methylenedioxyphenolic compound used as a synergist with pyrethroids.

VECTORS

Substantial knowledge of vector biology is necessary for a well-executed chemical control program. The location of the vector dictates the timing and type of program instituted. The following examples of chemical control of vectors illustrate the variety of tactics employed.

Hemiptera

Kissing Bugs

The primary method of reducing the incidence of Chagas' disease (Chap. 10) is chemical control of the vector *Triatoma*. Chemical control consists almost entirely of spraying dwellings and adjacent structures with chlorinated hydrocarbons and organophosphorus and pyrethroid insecticides. The pyrethroids deltamethrin, cypermethrin, and fenpropathrin and the organophosphorus fenitrothion and malathion have been widely used.

Researchers have studied penetration, metabolism, and mode of action as methods of enhancing the effectiveness of insecticides on Chagas' disease vectors. A faster penetration was obtained by varying the physicochemical properties of oily carriers and resulted in enhancement of the activity of formulated insecticides.

Modification of the vector-insecticide interaction to improve triatomicidal activity (synergism) between N-ethylmaleimide and organophosphorus insecticides as well as consecutive treatments with lindane and dichlorvos or sulfurous anhydride have been effective. These produced a mortality of *T. infestans* adults and nymphs higher than that observed in individual treatments. This synergism was used to develop an insecticide fumigant carrier that could be a promising tool for the control of Chagas' disease vectors.

Bed Bugs

Important as pests, not vectors, bed bugs warrant control because of their abundance and the effect of their bites. Bed bugs can be detected by the presence of fecal spots, eggs, and cast skins. They can be encouraged to leave their hiding places by blowing carbon dioxide or a pyrethrin aerosol into the crack or crevice. Spraying a residual insecticide on the surfaces over which the bed bugs crawl controls them. Furniture and mattresses should also be sprayed.

Anoplura

Lice

Although primarily a nuisance, lice are also vectors of typhus. Insecticidal lotions or shampoos formulated with malathion, carbaryl, temephos, or permethrin control lice on humans. In the past, lice were also controlled with lindane. Insecticide dusts can be applied to clothing and onto the body in disease-threatening situations.

A variety of methods including dips, pourons, dilute sprays, and hand applications of dusts and liquids have been used to control lice on domestic animals. Fenvalerate- or cypermethrin-impregnated ear tags have been suggested for prolonged control of lice.

Diptera

Mosquitoes

Mosquitoes are vectors for a variety of diseases. The diversity of mosquito species dictates the need for a wide variety of control approaches. Mosquito control programs target either the larval or adult stages. In larval mosquito control, the materials focus on breeding sites, where the mosquitoes naturally concentrate. Proper applications should be timed with larval development; some instars are more susceptible than others, depending on the material used. Unique breeding areas such as containers are difficult to access. Long-lasting or slow-release formulations can provide season-long control for successive broods in a breeding site.

Adult mosquito control centers around where the nuisance or vector mosquitoes are present. Applications target resting or flying mosquitoes and can include residual applications. The method of application takes advantage of resting habitats and activities.

Various materials and methods have been used to control mosquitoes, including representatives from the major groupings of insecticides. DDT is still widely used in some areas, as are several organophosphate compounds. Synthetic pyrethroids, *Bti*, and insect growth regulators are also being used.

Future mosquito control will likely consist of some new approaches, either in choice of materials or methods of application. For example, ivermectin was fed to mosquitoes and caused death, decreased egg production, and a decrease in egg production. Thus, a possible beneficial side effect of the widespread use of ivermectin in veterinary and human medicine is mosquito control. In addition, 2 new pyrethroids, ETOC™ (2 methyl–4–oxo–3–(2-propynyl) cyclopent-2–enyl chrysanthemate) and lambdacyhalothrin have been tested against organophosphorus-resistant adults of *Culex tarsalis*. Changes in application techniques include permethrin formulations with residual activity that can be used as barrier treatments around parks or daytime mosquito resting areas. When applications are made to the vegetation with a mist blower, landing counts can remain depressed for up to 10 days.

Tsetse Flies

Tsetse flies, the vectors of African sleeping sickness, can be chemically controlled with insecticides applied to screens or applied by ground or aerial spray. Attractants and hormones also can be used in conjunction with chemical methods and odor-baited targets.

In ground spraying, the insecticide is applied to the resting and refuge sites of tsetse flies, including resting sites located along the margins of roads and tracks, well-used game and cattle paths, edges of fields, and around established cattle pens. Although ground spraying is an efficient method of control, there has been concern about the continued used of persistent insecticides.

Aerial spraying involves sequential ultra–low-volume applications of a nonpersistent insecticide to the habitat using low-flying aircraft. Aerial application in tsetse control is less discriminating than ground spray procedures. In the latter, the daytime resting sites of tsetse flies can be treated selectively whereas aerial application can affect all species present.

Insecticides used include DDT, dieldrin, endosulfan, deltamethrin, and permethrin. DDT has been used since 1945; dieldrin was introduced in the early 1960s and endosulfan in the early 1970s. Endosulfan is less persistent than both DDT and dieldrin, and it is more toxic to tsetse flies. Bioaccumulation is a concern with both DDT and dieldrin. Effects on nontarget organisms are a concern with DDT, dieldrin, and endosulfan.

Deltamethrin was the first pyrethroid used successfully against tsetse flies at an operational level. After residual applications, certain crustaceans appear to be highly vulnerable. Laboratory observations indicate that administration of ivermectin to the host could adversely affect the lives and fecundity of tsetse flies. Tsetse flies are affected by ivermectin even when hosts were treated with pyrethroid several days earlier. When mosquitoes repeatedly feed on a treated animal, less ivermectin is required to produce a given effect.

Black Flies

Control of black flies lessens the incidence of onchocerciasis, or river blindness. The Onchocerciasis Control Programme in the Volta River Basin Area in West Africa included the almost weekly spraying of up to 14,000 km of rivers. Larval breeding places were sprayed with temephos by helicopter or by fixed wing aircraft beginning in 1975. Resistance to temephos has resulted in the use of the microbial insecticide *Bacillus thuringiensis israelensis* (Chap. 32).

Siphonaptera

Fleas

Use of systemic rodenticides can help to prevent the transmission of diseases such as plague, which is acquired by humans from rats and other rodents (Chap. 11). However, efforts to kill rats in the face of an epidemic of plague ironically can cause increased spread of the disease because infected fleas leave the dead rats and attack humans. Insecticides, primarily DDT, are valuable during epidemics; fleas are killed before they can leave the rats or have a chance to contact humans.

Plague control in suburban situations consists of surveillance to reveal the presence of epizootic plague and subsequent application of insecticidal dust to burrow entrances to control flea vectors. Carbaryl and permethrin dusts have been used to control rodent fleas. Carbaryl's short half-life in burrows has made repetitive applications, which are labor intensive and expensive, necessary to maintain flea control. In recent years, diazinon and bendiocarb have been used as alternatives. However, both compounds have also failed to achieve necessary levels of residual activity to control the resurgence of epizootic plague during a disease transmission season. Nesting material treated with insecticides has also been used to control fleas in burrows.

The cat flea, the most common flea in homes in the United States, also feeds on humans and dogs. Chlorinated hydrocarbon pesticides such as DDT and chlordane were once widely used to control fleas on floors and rugs; currently, the less toxic organic phosphate and carbamate pesticides as well as insect growth regulators are being used.

Arachnida

Mites

Mites are vectors for many pathogens, including the agents of rickettsial pox, scrub typhus, and Q-fever (Chap. 12). The most practical and economic way to control the vector of scrub typhus, *Leptotrombidium fletcheri*, is by using chemical compounds in the form of pesticides or repellents. Dieldrin, aldrin, chlordane, toxaphene, pyrethroids, and lindane control the scrub typhus vector. Dieldrin must be used with caution because of high mammalian toxicity. In recent years, there has been an increase in the number of new acaricides, which could result in more efficient control in the future.

Residual pesticides that last for several weeks should be used to control chiggers. Pyrethroids generally have a very short-lasting residual effect and thus are not the best way to control chiggers in grasslands over the long term. For short-term control (1–2 weeks) these pyrethroids can be suitable.

The method used to control mites depends on whether the mites are intradermal, ectoparasitic, in the dwelling place, or in the outdoor environment. Scab mites can be treated by dip treatments with materials such as lindane or by treating the bedding with insecticide granules or dust. Ivermectin also shows promise for mite control on animals.

Ticks

Because of the increased incidence of Lyme disease (Chap. 12), ticks (primarily *Ixodes*) and tick control have received considerable attention. Chemical treatments target adults or subadults and can be residual or applied directly. Acaricides are applied to vegetation, soil, houses, or animal quarters to kill resting or host-seeking ticks on domestic or wild animals. Domestic animals can be dipped, sprayed, or fitted with a collar impregnated with a volatile acaricide.

Granular acaricides such as carbaryl and diazinon can be used to control questing ticks in the fall. Control of adults continues into the spring or during the peak activity periods of nymphs and larvae, thus limiting the number of stages found on the host. Residual application of acaricides for control of *Ixodes* can be effective when applied to relatively small areas frequented by humans but are too costly when applied to large areas of forest or brush.

Permethrin can be applied directly to the burrows of white-footed mice to control subadult ticks. Permethrin-impregnated cotton can be distributed as a nesting material for the preferred host to reduce the number of immature ticks feeding on the host. Unfortunately, this treatment does not effectively kill host-seeking nymphs during the first year of application; in addition, larvae feeding on host animals other than the white-footed mouse are not controlled. The efficacy of this product depends on the diversity and abundance of the hosts.

Tick control on cattle consists of a variety of techniques, including arsenic and organophosphorous dips to eliminate *Boophilus* for cattle fever control. Topical applications of insecticides or insecticides in oil can be applied to cattle ears. Insecticide-impregnated ear tags are also used for tick control on animals. Ivermectin controls ticks in livestock.

FACTORS FOR EFFECTIVE APPLICATION OF PESTICIDES

A responsible chemical control program includes the use of a legal, registered product. The directions on the label should be followed, and the appropriate dosage administered with the proper equipment. Changes in weather and subsequent effect on application should be considered. The biology of the vector can greatly affect results; thus, knowledge about the vector and its habits is imperative. With increased resistance to many chemicals, the applicator should consider the resistance status of the target and the agricultural use of pesticides in the area.

Target Areas

Pesticides can be applied in breeding areas where immature stages are found and at the resting and feeding sites of the adult vector. Different techniques and pesticides are necessary for application of larvicides as well as for treatment of interior surfaces of buildings and exterior and/or interior spaces. The application equipment should be appropriate for the target area and species.

The extent and accessibility of the target area, the presence of vegetation or forest, and the layout of buildings determine applications and whether ground or aerial dispersing equipment is used.

Selection of Pesticides

A pesticide's biological effectiveness, possible effect on target and nontarget organisms, threat to humans and the environment posed by its proposed use, cost, transportation requirements, and the availability of suitable application equipment should be evaluated when selecting pesticides. Determination of costs should be based on the expense incurred to apply the material, not just the purchase price of the chemical.

Pesticide Formulations

Where alternative pesticide formulations are available, the least toxic to humans and the least hazardous to the environment should be given preference. Liquids can be applied in dilute or concentrated form. Dilute spray mixtures are most frequently used for high-volume applications, using large droplets to to saturate the treated surface. Extremely low volumes of more concentrated chemicals can be used, including fine sprays, mists, or aerosols—a technique known as ultra–low-volume (ULV) application.

The aim of ULV techniques is to apply the least amount of liquid, usually less than 5 liters per hectare, to achieve control of a specific organism. When such small volumes are applied, the liquid must be finely nebulized to maintain a sufficient number of droplets per unit area or per unit volume; unfortunately, such small droplets are susceptible to air disturbances. ULV application has resulted in substantial savings to vector control programs through speed of operation, reduced labor requirements, and lower handling costs. ULV cold aerosols and thermal fogs can be equally effective against a vector, but the latter use a higher volume of diluted spray per hectare. One advantage of cold aerosol application is that it does not produce a dense fog, which can constitute a traffic hazard.

Droplet Size of Sprays

The droplet size produced by spraying equipment is important from a biological point of view. Aerosols produce a "space spray" to control flying insects that persists in the air for an appreciable length of time. Alternatively, when a pesticide is employed for its residual effect on resting insects, a coarser spray can be used. Droplet size affects whether the chemical reaches its target, residual activity, effective dose available to the vector, impingement, and drift.

Dosage Rate

Dosage of pesticide is usually expressed in terms of the amount of active ingredient applied per unit area or per unit volume, depending on the type of treatment. The amount of product used is governed by the concentration of the formulation. Optimum usage of chemicals to maximize the effect requires an even and continuous dispersal of the recommended dosage over the target area in the prescribed time. The rate of emission and speed of application, therefore, must be carefully calibrated at the start of a job to ensure that the correct dosage rate is applied. Wind and temperature also can affect drift and the effectiveness of the chemical.

SUMMARY

In all regions, vector control is still largely achieved by the use of chemical pesticides. The organochlorine insecticides still play an important role, but they have been barred by many countries. Residual insecticides for indoor house spraying, the increasing numbers of cases of insecticide resistance and refractory vector behavior, the high cost and increased toxicity of many of the alternative insecticides, and opposition by environmentalists to their use are difficulties facing pesticide-based programs. A shift toward greater emphasis on environmental management and integrated methods of control with varying degrees of community participation is under way. It is likely that the use of chemicals will remain an essential component of most vector control programs for the foreseeable future; their more efficient, economic, and selective use presents a challenge.

REFERENCES AND FURTHER READING

Cavallora, R., editor. 1986. Integrated tse-tse fly control: Methods and strategies. Proceedings of the CEC International Symposium, Ispra, Italy, 1986.

Coats, J.R., ed. 1982. *Insecticide mode of action.* New York: Academic Press.

Hayes, W.J. Jr., and E.R. Laws Jr., editors. 1991. *Handbook of pesticide toxicology.* San Diego: Academic Press.

Hiller, J.A. 1987. New approaches to the chemical control of arthropod pests of livestock. *Intl. Jour. for Parasit.* 17:689–693.

Ho, T.M., and S. Ismail. 1991. Efficacy of three pyrethroids against *Leptotrombidium fletcheri* (Acari: Trombiculidae) infected and noninfected with scrub typhus. *J. Med. Entomol.* 28:776–779.

Leahey, J.P., ed. 1985. *The pyrethroid insecticides.* Philadelphia: Taylor and Francis.

Schulze, T.L., G.C. Taylor, R.A. Jordon, E.M. Bosler, and J.K. Shisler. 1991. Effectiveness of selected granular acaricide formulations in suppressing populations of *Ixodes dammini* (Acari: Ixodidae): Short-term control of nymphs and larvae. *J. Med. Entomol.* 28:624–929.

Simmons, S.W. 1959. The use of DDT insecticides in human medicine, In: P. Muller, editor, *DDT: The insecticide dichlorodiphenyl-trichloroethane and its significance*, Vol. 2. Birkhaeuser: Basel. pp. 251–502.

Thomson, W.T. 1994. *Agricultural chemicals, book I: Insecticides, acaricides and ovicides.* Fresno, CA: Thomson Publications.

Traub, R., and C.L. Wisseman. 1968. Ecological considerations in scrub typhus: Methods of control. *Bull. WHO* 39:231–237.

World Health Organization. 1992. Vector resistance to pesticides: Fifteenth report of the WHO expert committee on vector biology and control. (WHO technical report series 818.) Geneva: World Health Organization.

Zerba, E.N. 1989. Chemical control of Chagas' disease vectors. *Bio. Envir. Sci.* 2:24–29.

30. INSECTICIDE RESISTANCE

James A. Ferrari

INTRODUCTION

Insecticides have played an important role in the control of insect vectors of disease since the early 20th century. Although important advances continue to be made in the development of alternative control measures, insecticides will remain a vital part of integrated control programs for the foreseeable future. Unfortunately, the remarkable ability of insect populations to evolve resistance to every class of insecticide that has been developed (Chap. 29) often leaves control programs with few insecticide options. Even the promise of effective control by bacterial insecticides has come into question as evidence for resistance in both the field and laboratory has begun to accumulate. The study of insecticide resistance has recently undergone a renaissance of sorts with the realization that unless our understanding of the genetic, biochemical, and ecological factors that affect the evolution of resistance improves dramatically, we may lose our ability to control many important disease vectors and crop pests.

Resistance is formally defined by WHO (World Health Organization) as "the development of an ability in a strain of some organism to tolerate doses of a toxicant that would prove lethal to a majority of individuals in a normal population of the same species." This definition is adequate if we recognize that resistance has a genetic basis and is the result of a change in the genetic composition of a population as a direct result of the selective effects of a toxicant. In addition, the definition of a "normal" population is debatable.

Natural populations of most species differ genetically to varying degrees (Chap. 25). Thus, populations of a species might vary in their tolerance to a particular insecticide despite never having been subjected to insecticidal selection.

To understand the process by which resistance evolves, we must address the mechanisms that produce resistant individuals and the process that results in the proliferation of such individuals in a population. In the neo-Darwinian model of evolution by natural selection, 3 conditions are necessary to bring about the genetic change of a population. First, individuals in the population must differ genetically. Second, the genetic differences among individuals must produce an effect on some aspect of the phenotype, which is the target of selection. Third, phenotypic differences among individuals must affect their reproductive fitness; that is, some phenotypes must contribute more offspring to the next generation than others.

Genetic and phenotypic variation affecting degree of resistance ultimately arises in individuals as a result of a random mutation that leads to the modification of some normal physiological, morphological, or behavioral aspect of the phenotype. Such phenotypic changes enhance either the process of detoxification of a toxicant or the ability to avoid contact with the toxicant. When insecticide is applied, individuals possessing such mutations thus have a considerable advantage over more susceptible individuals in the population. They have a higher probability of surviving insecticide treatment and on average will contribute more off-spring than susceptible individuals to the next generation. As a result, the gene conferring resistance will increase in frequency in the population over time.

Insecticide resistance can be investigated at many levels: from the molecular characterization of genes conferring resistance and their biochemical products to the role gene products play in overcoming the toxic effects of insecticides to studies of the ecological and evolutionary forces that affect the dynamics of genes conferring resistance in populations. Indeed, the scope of the resistance problem is so broad that no single investigator has sufficient training to study resistance in a comprehensive manner. The greatest advances in understanding specific cases of resistance have resulted from the joint efforts of molecular biologists, toxicologists, physiologists, and population biologists.

TRADITIONAL APPROACHES TO THE STUDY OF INSECTICIDE RESISTANCE

The traditional approach to studying cases of resistance in species that can be colonized in the laboratory is to

1. Detect resistance in a population.

2. Collect individuals from the population and colonize them in the laboratory.

3. Subject the colony to strong insecticidal selection to increase the frequency of resistant individuals and, ideally, create a homogeneous resistant strain.

4. Characterize the genetic control of resistance.

5. Characterize the mechanism or mechanisms responsible for resistance.

Detecting Resistance

For many years, resistance was "detected" in an insect population only when it had evolved to the point where it had an obvious impact on a control program. Today the early detection and monitoring of resistance is recognized as a vital part of resistance management. Resistance management is a relatively new area of research that is directed at developing insecticide use strategies that minimize the rate of evolution of resistance. In this section some techniques for detecting resistance are discussed, but a discussion of the broader role of detection techniques in control programs is deferred until the section on resistance management.

Insecticide Bioassay Using the Diagnostic Dose

The simplest method for detecting resistance using insecticide treatment is the diagnostic dose test. The diagnostic dose is a predetermined insecticide dose that is known to be lethal to a high proportion of susceptible individuals but that a high proportion of resistant individuals can tolerate. Ideally, the choice of a diagnostic dose should be made after the genetic control of resistance has been characterized and the tolerance limits of resistant and susceptible individuals determined.

A current list of recommended diagnostic doses of many insecticides for a number of arthropod disease vectors is available from WHO, as are standardized test kits (WHO 1992). Standardized tests exist for the immature and adult stages of many vector species. For aquatic stages, insecticide is added to the water at a given concentration. For terrestrial and/or adult stages, insecticide is either applied topically or individuals are exposed to a surface treated with insecticide.

In cases where control failure is evident in the field, the diagnostic dose test can be used to confirm that resistance is the cause. There are, however, a number of problems associated with the use of diagnostic doses for detection of resistant individuals at low frequency in a population. ffrench-Constant and Roush (1990) provide a thorough discussion of the advantages and disadvantages of this method.

The Dose-Response Bioassay

A useful tool in monitoring the progress of resistance in the strain and in genetic analysis is the dose-response bioassay. In this type of assay, samples of individuals from a strain are subjected to a range of doses of insecticide chosen to produce a range of mortalities among the treated samples. This technique is described in detail by Robertson and Preisler (1992). Probit analysis (Finney 1971) can be used to characterize the response of the strain to the toxicant. If cumulative percent mortality is transformed into probit units and plotted against the logarithm of dose of

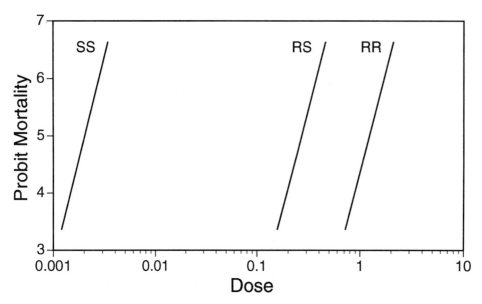

30.1   Log-dose probit mortality lines for 3 hypothetical strains. A susceptible strain (SS), a resistant strain (RR), and an F1 strain (RS) were produced by crossing the SS and RR strains. In this case, resistance exhibits incomplete dominance.

toxicant, a log-dose probit mortality (LD-P) line is obtained (Fig. 30.1). By subjecting dosage-mortality data to probit analysis, it is possible to characterize the response of a strain to a toxicant and establish the dose of insecticide necessary to kill a given percentage of treated individuals. The strain is characterized by the doses or concentrations of insecticide that kill 50%, the LD_{50}, and 95%, the LD_{95}, of treated individuals. Probit analysis provides 95% confidence intervals for these values as well as the slope of the LD-P line. Confidence intervals for LD_{50} and LD_{95} values can be used in comparisons of different strains. The slope of the LD-P line is a measure of the variability of the strain. The steeper the slope the more uniform the response of individuals to insecticide concentration. Computer programs that perform probit analysis are available in some statistical software packages (SAS Institute 1985) and for PCs (personal computers) (Raymond 1985).

Probit analysis is designed to characterize the response of a homogeneous group of organisms to a toxicant. When a genetically heterogeneous colony (recently established from a field population) is subjected to a dose-response bioassay, the resulting LD-P line should have a shallow slope, indicating that the individuals in the sample vary in their level of tolerance to the insecticide. As selection continues, the more resistant individuals increase in frequency in the colony. Thus the LD-P line will shift to the right and become steeper in slope. This will continue until the strain becomes homogeneous with respect to the tolerance of individuals (Fig. 30.2). At that point, the slope of the line reflects relatively minor variation among individuals that affects susceptibility.

When the strain stabilizes and resistance remains stable, the homogeneous resistant strain can be compared to a standard susceptible strain to determine its degree of resistance. This is most commonly done using the resistance ratio. For example, the resistance ratio at the LD_{50} is the LD_{50} of the resistant strain divided by the LD_{50} of the susceptible strain. The resistance ratio is usually calculated at the LD_{50} and LD_{95} of the strain.

Genetic Characterization of Resistance

If homogeneous resistant (RR) and susceptible (SS) strains of the species under study are available, the genetic control of resistance can be determined (Georghiou 1969; Tsukamoto 1983). First, the degree of resistance is determined in the F_1 offspring of reciprocal crosses between the resistant and susceptible strains. The relative position of the LD-P lines of the

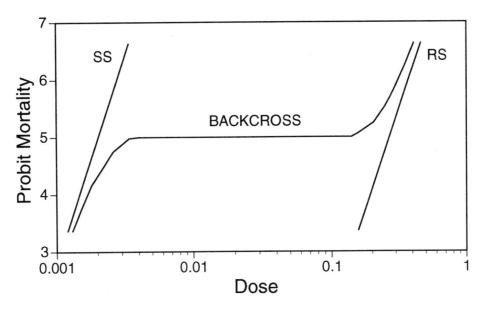

30.2 Log-dose probit mortality lines for hypothetical SS and RS strains (as described in Fig. 30.1) and the predicted response curve for individuals produced by backcrossing RS to SS individuals when resistance is caused by a single gene

reciprocal F_1's indicates whether there are so-called maternal effects on resistance. Maternal effects on resistance result from differences in cytoplasmically transmitted factors from susceptible or resistant females that affect resistance. Such effects are rare in insecticide resistance. The position of the F_1 LD-P lines relative to the susceptible and resistant parental strains indicates the degree of dominance of the resistance—if this dominance is caused by allelic differences at a single genetic locus. Evidence for polygenic resistance, in which more than one genetic locus contributes to resistance to a given insecticide, is discussed later.

The dominance of genes conferring resistance has been represented in several ways in the literature. The following system, which is based on comparison of LD-P lines, has been suggested by Georghiou (1969):

1. Completely recessive—the resistance of the F_1 is identical to that of the susceptible parental strain.

2. Incompletely recessive—the F_1 is significantly more resistant than the susceptible parental strain, but resistance is less than intermediate.

3. Intermediate—the resistance of the F_1 is the logarithmic average of the susceptible and resistant parental strains.

4. Incompletely dominant—the F_1 is significantly more resistant than intermediate but less resistant than the resistant parental strain.

5. Completely dominant—the resistance of the F_1 is identical to the resistant parental strain.

Alternatively, dominance (D) can be represented on a continuous scale using the equation:

$$D = (2F_1 - P_1 - P_2) / (P_2 - P_1)$$

where F_1 is the resistance of the F_1 and P_1 and P_2 are the resistances of the susceptible and resistant parental strains, respectively (represented as log LD_{50}). Values of D range from −1 for completely recessive resistance to +1 for completely dominant resistance. On this scale, intermediate resistance has a dominance of 0.

After the dominance of the resistance has been evaluated, the next step is to determine whether resistance is conferred by an allele of a single genetic locus (monogenic) or by multiple genetic loci (polygenic). This can be determined by either crossing F_1 individuals to produce an F_2 generation or by backcrossing F_1 individuals to either the susceptible or resistant parental strain, depending on the dominance of the resistance phenotype.

In the dose, response bioassay of the F_2 or backcross offspring, monogenic control of resistance is indicated when a clear plateau of mortality is observed across a range of doses. When resistance is intermediate, and F_1 (RS) heterozygous individuals are backcrossed to the susceptible parent, monogenic resistance will result in a dose-response curve with a clear plateau between the LD-P lines of the SS and RS individuals at the 50% mortality level, since 50% of the backcross offspring are RS heterozygotes that are unaffected over a range of insecticidal doses (Fig. 30.2). If resistance is polygenic, recombination and independent assortment of R and S alleles of different loci will occur in F_1 individuals. Backcrossing these individuals to susceptible individuals will result in offspring that include a number of genotypes that vary in their level of resistance. The shape of the LD-P line resulting from insecticide bioassay of these backcross individuals depends on a number of factors; in most cases a clear plateau will not be observed. If a number of unlinked genes contribute to resistance, the slope of the LD-P line should decrease compared to the lines for the susceptible and F_1 individuals and few backcross individuals will exhibit the level of resistance observed in the F_1.

Although in some cases backcross analysis has revealed clear-cut evidence for monogenic resistance, or at least a major gene for resistance, many complicating factors can make genetic analysis difficult. In addition, plateaus sometimes occur even for polygenic resistance (Georghiou 1969). Genetic analysis becomes considerably easier when a biochemical marker that distinguishes resistant and susceptible individuals is available, such as a difference in activity of an enzyme involved in resistance.

MECHANISMS OF RESISTANCE

In the classical approach to a comprehensive study of resistance, once a homogeneous resistant strain has been produced by laboratory selection, the next step is to determine the mechanism of resistance. Methods used to determine the mechanism of resistance vary in their sophistication. Bioassay of a resistant strain with a number of different insecticides from the same class or different classes of compounds establish the so-called cross-resistance profile of a given strain. Certain resistance mechanisms can be identified by their characteristic cross-resistance profiles. Another common technique is to carry out insecticide bioassays that incorporate synergists (substances that block certain resistance mechanisms). If resistance is eliminated when an insecticide is applied with a synergist, then the blocked mechanism is implicated in resistance. A number of relatively simple biochemical assays are available to detect increased activity of several detoxifying enzymes and reduced sensitivity of a target molecule such as acetylcholinesterase (AChE). The most sophisticated techniques involve determining the metabolism of a radiolabeled insecticide, or its rate of penetration through the insect cuticle.

In these techniques, resistance to a given insecticide in different species, or even in different populations of the same species, can be caused by different mechanisms or variants of the same mechanism. Not all of the variants will be detectable by the same techniques. For example, although organophosphate (OP) resistance in some insects is associated with elevated esterase activity against (α-naphthyl acetate substrate, not all detoxifying esterases exhibit increased activity against this substrate (Scott 1990).

Resistance Mechanisms

Resistance arises as a result of a mutation, which alters a normal physiological, morphological, or behavioral attribute of a species. Resistance mechanisms can be divided into four broad categories:

1. Reduced penetration
2. Metabolism
3. Site insensitivity
4. Behavior

Reduced Penetration

Many insecticides enter the insect through the cuticle. Cuticular changes that reduce the rate of penetration of insecticide confer resistance to a number of insecticides. Reduced penetration alone usually confers only a low level of resistance (Oppenoorth 1985). In combination with other mechanisms, however, it can potentially result in a large nonadditive increase in resistance. By slowing the rate at which an insecticide reaches its target, other mechanisms can more effectively affect the insecticide and prevent it from reaching toxic levels at the site of action. This mechanism is most readily detected through penetration studies using labeled insecticide.

Metabolic Resistance

A small group of enzymes or families of enzymes are involved in metabolic resistance. None of the enzymes involved are unique to resistant insects. Resistance is the result either of a structural change in an enzyme molecule that increases its ability to detoxify insecticide, and/or an increase in the amount of enzyme produced. The major enzyme systems involved in insecticide resistance are discussed below. For comprehensive discussions, refer to Oppenoorth (1985), Soderlund and Bloomquist (1990), and Mullen and Scott (1992).

Mixed Function Oxidases

The cytochrome P-450 dependent monooxygenases, or mixed function oxidases (MFOs), are a group of oxidative enzymes with overlapping substrate specificities. They confer resistance to a wide range of insecticides (Oppenoorth 1985). The action of these oxidases on a substrate results in products with increased water solubility that can be more readily excreted. The role of MFOs in resistance can usually be detected using the synergist piperonyl butoxide in insecticide bioassay.

Resistance by MFOs can involve structural changes or increases in the production of one or more components of this complex system (Soderlund and Bloomquist 1990).

Hydrolases

These enzymes cleave carboxylester and phosphodiester bonds. They are important in resistance to organophosphate insecticides and to a lesser extent in resistance to pyrethroids. One of the most thoroughly studied cases of resistance to insecticides in a vector species is that of organophosphate resistance caused by enhanced nonspecific esterase activity in *Culex pipiens* and *Cx. quinquefasciatus*. Resistance in these species is associated with high esterase activity in assays using (α-naphthyl acetate substrate (Dary et al. 1990). The genetic basis of high esterase activity is amplification of the esterase gene involved (Mouches et al. 1986; Soderlund and Bloomquist 1990; Devonshire and Field 1992).

Resistance caused by high nonspecific esterase activity can be most easily detected either by the synergist DEF (S,S,S-tributylphosphorotrithioate) in bioassay, or from the high esterase activity observed on electrophoretic gels or in microtiter plate–based biochemical assays. Not all hydrolases involved in resistance result in enhanced nonspecific esterase activity with (α-naphthyl acetate substrate. Malathion resistance is not associated with increased nonspecific esterase activity and is believed to caused by a specific carboxylesterase. This mechanism can be detected using the synergist TPP (O,O,O-triphenylphospate).

Gluthione-S-Transferases

This class of enzymes is important in resistance to organophosphate insecticides. Enhanced gluthione-s-transferases (GSH) transferase activity can be demonstrated with insecticide or model substrates. The synergist diethylmaleate (DEM) is sometimes useful in detecting this mechanism of resistance. Recent evidence suggests that DDT-dehydrochlorinase, a mechanism of resistance to DDT in the house fly, is a GSH-transferase (Soderlund and Bloomquist 1990).

Site Insensitivity

Resistance to several insecticide classes is conferred by alteration of the target site of the insecticide. Such alterations have been observed in neuronal enzymes and receptors, which are the targets of several classes of insecticides.

Insensitive Acetylcholinesterase

Organophosphate and carbamate insecticides are neurotoxins. These insecticides exert their effects by inhibiting the enzyme acetylcholinesterase. Many insects and other arthropods have developed resistance to these compounds through structural modification of their acetylcholinesterase. The AChE enzyme from resistant individuals is far less sensitive to inhibition than that from susceptible individuals (Hama 1983; Soderlund and Bloomquist 1990; Oppenoorth 1985). Relatively simple biochemical assays are available to detect AChE insensitivity (Brown and Brogdon 1987).

Knockdown Resistance

Knockdown resistance (kdr) received its name from the observation of insects following treatment with DDT or pyrethroids. Susceptible insects exposed to the insecticides usually results in rapid paralysis, or "knockdown." This is not observed in resistant individuals. Recent evidence indicates that these insecticides kill by acting on the voltage-sensitive sodium channel of nerve membranes. Although studies in many insects indicate that kdr-like resistance involves some form of site insensitivity associated with nerves, the exact mechanism of resistance is unknown and may involve different mechanisms in different insects (Soderlund and Bloomquist 1990). The observation of cross-resistance (a single mechanism conferring resistance to 2 unrelated classes of insecticides) to DDT and pyrethroid insecticides is a good indication of kdr resistance—at least when metabolic detoxification of these compounds is not observed. In addition, kdr-type resistance is usually genetically recessive.

Cyclodiene Resistance

Cyclodiene insecticides target neuronal gamma-aminobutyric acid (GABA) receptors. Resistance to this class of insecticides in several insects is associated with reduced sensitivity of a GABA receptor to the toxic effects of the insecticide (Soderlund and Bloomquist 1990).

Behavior

Changes in behavior that result in reduced contact with insecticide can enhance the probability of survival in a treated environment. Such changes can involve a reduced tendency to enter treated areas or the increased tendency to move away from a surface treated with insecticide when contact is made. A number of cases of behavioral resistance, alone or in combination with other resistance mechanisms, have been documented (Sparks et al. 1989).

POPULATION BIOLOGY OF RESISTANCE

Insecticide resistance has long been recognized as one of the best examples of rapid evolutionary change. Crow (1957) was the first to review population genetic aspects of insecticide resistance. Although a number of investigators have studied resistance as an evolutionary phenomenon, recently a resurgence in the application of the principles of population biology, especially population genetics, has occured in the study of resistance.

In recent years, efforts of population biologists interested in the resistance problem have been directed toward "resistance management." The goal of resistance management is to develop control strategies designed to prevent or delay the onset of resistance in populations exposed to pesticide for the first time or which cause existing resistance to decline (Croft 1990).

The first step in developing a resistance management program is to evaluate the myriad factors that can affect the rate of evolution of resistance (Georghiou and Taylor 1976; 1986), which are shown in Table 30.1. The factors are separated into 3 categories: genetic, biological/ecological, and operational. Genetic factors include properties of the genes conferring resistance, such as dominance, as well as population genetic parameters, such as the initial frequency of alleles for resistance prior to the onset of selection. Biological/ecological factors include a number of life-history parameters. These can vary widely from species to species or among populations of a single species that occur in different environments. Operational factors include properties of the insecticide used and how it is applied. Ideally, information about all of the factors listed should be available to those designing a resistance management program. Unfortunately, for most pest species and many insecticides several genetic and biological/ecological factors have not been evaluated; it is possible that the best operational factor options are still unknown.

Resistance management strategies try to take advantage of the factors that are under human control to minimize the rate of resistance evolution. Factors under human control include all of the operational factors (when there are several insecticide options available) as well as some genetic and biological/ecological

TABLE 30.1 Factors influencing the evolution of resistance

Genetic	Biological/Ecological	Operational
frequency of R alleles	generations per year	chemical nature of the insecticide
number of R alleles	number of offspring	relationship of the insecticide to those previously used
dominance of R alleles	degree of isolation, tendency and ability to migrate	persistence of residues, formulation
penetrance, expressivity, interaction of R alleles	availability of refugia	application threshold
relative fitness of R and S genotypes		selection threshold
		life stages selected
		mode of application

Adapted from Georghiou and Taylor 1986

factors. For example, when resistance exhibits incomplete dominance, applying a dose of insecticide that kills all heterozygotes makes the resistance phenotype functionally recessive. Refugia (areas in which a portion of the population remains untreated) can be artificially produced by treating some areas and leaving others untreated. If susceptible individuals predominate within the refugia, these individuals will recolonize the treated areas and mate with resistant individuals that survived treatment.

Research in resistance management, as in most areas of population biology, can be broadly divided into 2 categories, theoretical and empirical. The theoretical work depends on computer modeling to identify important factors affecting the evolution of resistance and promising control strategies. The empirical work attempts to provide information about the factors affecting the evolution of resistance and involves the experimental testing of control strategies in laboratory and field populations.

Theoretical Research in Resistance Management

Computer modeling has contributed significantly to resistance management, and several excellent reviews of this work are available (Taylor 1983; Tabashnik 1986;

1990). Computer modeling has identified key factors affecting the evolution of resistance. In addition, models have provided a simple means of investigating the efficacy of different strategies of pesticide use in resistance management schemes. An admitted shortcoming of models is that their validity depends on the assumptions made about the system being modeled. This has always been a problem in basic as well as applied population biology. Many key assumptions, such as population size, migration rates, and selection intensity, are difficult to measure in natural populations. Nevertheless, empirical population biologists and geneticists are attempting to address these problems.

Single-Locus Models

In most cases in which resistance has been analyzed genetically, resistance appears to involve a single Mendelian genetic factor (Roush and McKenzie 1987). These genetic factors can be single genes or, in cases of gene-amplification–based resistance, blocks of genes that behave as single Mendelian factors in genetic crosses. Thus, most models of the evolution of resistance have assumed that resistance is controlled by a single locus with a resistance allele, R, and a susceptibility allele, S. If p and q represent the frequencies of the S and R alleles respectively, the frequencies of genotypes SS, RS, and RR are assumed to follow Hardy-Weinberg expectations of p^2, $2pq$, and q^2 respectively (Hartl and Clark 1989 and Chap. 25). Each genotype can be assigned a "relative fitness" based on the proportion of individuals of that genotype expected to survive insecticide treatment and/or the assumed reproductive potential of each genotype.

Among the predictions of the single-locus models are that the rate of evolution of resistance will increase as reproductive potential (including generations per season) increases, as the rate of immigration of SS individuals into the treated populations decreases, and as the intensity of insecticide use increases (Taylor 1983; Tabashnik 1990). The relative fitness of resistant and susceptible genotypes in the population when selection of a particular insecticide is relaxed for one or more generations can also be important in how the frequency of the R alleles change when employing different pesticide use strategies (Taylor 1983).

Multilocus Models

Models of resistance involving more than one genetic locus can be divided into 2 broad categories: (1) Models of resistance to a single insecticide conferred by resistance alleles at 2 or more genetic loci, and (2) Models of multiple resistance (resistance to 2 or more different insecticide classes), each due to a resistance allele at a different genetic locus.

The first category of multilocus resistance models addresses the growing number of cases of resistance that do not behave in a simple Mendelian manner in genetic crosses (Tabashnik 1990). Two types of models have been used: gene models and quantitative genetic models. In gene models, allele and genotype frequencies at 2 or more discrete genetic loci are monitored over time. In quantitative genetic models individual genotypes are not followed; rather, quantitative genetic parameters such as heritability, genetic variance, and selection intensity are used to model the evolution of resistance (Via 1986).

In some cases, the results of multilocus models generally agree with those of single-locus models regarding the effects of factors such as migration and selection intensity on the evolution of resistance. In other cases, the results of multilocus models differ from those of single locus models. The disagreement may be due to different assumptions made in constructing the models and not to an inherent difference in the way these genetic systems respond to selection (Tabashnik 1986; 1990). Multilocus models of multiple resistance have been used to assess a number of resistance management strategies using mixtures of insecticides or using different insecticides in rotational schemes or mosaic patterns. These will be discussed later in the general context of resistance management strategies.

Resistance Management Strategies

Armed with the broad conclusions of computer models and common sense, modelers and control specialists have proposed a number of strategies and recommendations for effective resistance management (Georghiou 1983; Roush and Daly 1990; Tabashnik 1990). In evaluating a strategy the context in which it is to be used must be defined. Most management schemes have been developed through models that assume the initial frequency of an R allele in the population is very low, as would be expected at the start of a control program using a newly developed insecticide to which there was no cross-resistance. The bacterial insecticides are, we hope, still in this category. In many cases, however, control programs must contend with situations in which there is already a substantial frequency of individuals in the population resistant to one or more classes of insecticides and few alternative insecticides are available. Consequently, efforts have been directed at prolonging the useful life of available insecticides by using them in mixtures or rotations. Evaluation of the success of such efforts will depend on monitoring the progress of resistance in these situations. The theoretical considerations discussed below probably have little relevance to these control dilemmas.

Strategies Using Single Insecticides

Minimize Selection Pressure on Susceptible Individuals

In this strategy, insecticide is applied in a way that allows a substantial proportion of the susceptible individuals in the population to survive. This can be achieved by creating artificial refugia in which certain areas remain untreated. In models, this strategy delays the onset of resistance when the R allele is at low frequency in the population. If the number of heterozygous individuals in the population is low compared to the number of SS survivors and/or immigrants, the R allele will increase in frequency very slowly. This strategy might be feasible for some crop pests, where the goal is to keep population size below some economic threshold, but it is considered impractical in vector control programs in which target population sizes to maintain adequate disease control is lower.

Maximize Selection Against RS Individuals.

This so-called high-dose strategy calls for application of insecticide at a level designed to kill all SS and RS individuals in the population. Again, this strategy will only be effective when the frequency of the R allele is low. Using the Hardy-Weinberg equilibrium formula, it is easy to see that when the R allele frequency is low (0.001–0.0001), the overwhelming majority of R allele gene copies in a population occur in heterozygotes, with RR homozygotes occurring at low frequency. The frequency of RR survivors in a population is assumed to be so low that they would be overwhelmed by and mate with SS immigrants. Although the high-dose strategy seems to have potential, common sense argues against it in most situations. Pesticide applications never reach all individuals in a population. In addition, residual pesticides gradually decay and lose effectiveness, resulting in doses that will allow heterozygotes to survive. The economic and environmental cost of this strategy must also be considered (Georghiou 1983; Roush and Daly 1990; Tabashnik 1990).

Strategies Using More Than One Insecticide

The measure of success of strategies employing 2 or more insecticides is whether resistance to all of the insecticides when used together evolves slower than the combined time it would have taken for a population to evolve resistance to each one individually. Some models have suggested that the use of mixtures of insecticides with different modes of action, rotations in time, or spatial pattern of applications can be useful in managing resistance. The theoretical advantage of using a mixture of insecticides relies on the fact that if the frequency of R alleles at 2 genetic loci is low, the expected frequency of individuals carrying both R alleles is the product of the probability of carrying either individually. To survive exposure to both insecticides, an individual must be heterozygous for both loci, an extremely rare occurrence.

Some models have indicated that mixtures of insecticides effectively delay the onset of resistance, but their assumptions are quite restrictive and unlikely to hold in field populations (Tabashnik 1990). The use of insecticides in rotational schemes in which they are applied in some alternating sequence is also based on the low probability that an individual usually does not carry R alleles at 2 different loci. If the frequency of individuals heterozygous or homozygous for the allele conferring resistance to one insecticide increases under selection with that insecticide, they will be killed when the switch is made to a second insecticide. The switch must be made before the probability of the occurrence of double heterozygotes increased to a significant level. Some models of rotations have assumed that although genes for resistance confer a fitness advantage in the presence of insecticide, they have pleiotropic effects on other components of reproductive fitness that impose a fitness cost in the absence of insecticide. This results in a decline in the frequency of an R allele conferring resistance to one insecticide when a switch is made to another insecticide in the rotation. Various models using rotations have given mixed results in their ability to delay the evolution of resistance (Georghiou 1983; Tabashnik 1990). In addition, the assumption of a pleiotropic cost of resistance does not appear to have general validity (Roush and McKenzie 1987). Most models of the use of mosaic patterns of different insecticides have indicated that it will not be an effective resistance management strategy.

NEW AREAS OF RESEARCH

Molecular Studies

Armed with the ever-improving tools available for biochemical and molecular genetic analysis, impressive progress is being made toward understanding resistance at the molecular level. Research at the biochemical level continues to provide insight into how qualitative and quantitative changes in the enzyme systems involved in resistance and in the physiological target sites of insecticides contribute to resistance (Georghiou and Saito 1983; Soderlund and Bloomquist 1990; Mullin and Scott 1992).

Recently, molecular geneticists have made important contributions to our understanding of a number of cases of resistance. The first cases of resistance to be characterized at the molecular level were organophosphate resistance in *Culex quinquefasciatus* (Mouches et al. 1986) and the aphid *Myzus persicae* (Field et al. 1988). In both instances, resistance had previously been associated with elevated esterase activity on electrophoretic gels and in enzyme assays. It was determined that the molecular basis of the elevated activity was amplification (increase in the number of copies) of a gene coding for the esterase enzyme. In *Cx. quinquefasciatus*, individuals from an insecticide-resistant strain, Tem-R, were found to carry an estimated 250 times more copies of the esterase B1 gene (Mouches et al. 1987) and exhibit 120 times higher esterase activity (Ferrari and Georghiou 1990) than susceptible individuals. The gene has been cloned and sequenced, revealing that the amplified unit, or amplicon, is at least 30 kb (kilobase) in size, including a 2.8 kb coding sequence (Mouches et al. 1990). Hybridization studies using cDNA probes from the esterase B1 gene indicate that additional cases of esterase-associated resistance in *Culex* also involve gene amplification (Raymond et al. 1989). Gene amplification is a common mechanism of resistance to toxic substances in a number of organisms. Many cases of resistance are associated with elevated activity of detoxifying enzymes, and it is likely that a number of these cases will be found to involve gene amplification.

Recently, a number of other resistance genes have been cloned. Most of these genes have been isolated from insecticide-resistant strains of *Musca domestica* and *Drosophila melanogaster;* however, it is already apparent that the resulting DNA probes from these species will be useful for isolating homologous resistance genes in many disease vectors and crop pests.

D. melanogaster is a useful model insect for the study of resistance, because of the highly developed techniques available for genetic analysis in this species. The literature of insecticide resistance in *Drosophila* is substantial (Morton 1993). The advantages of using *D. melanogaster* for isolating resistance genes conferring target site insensitivity have been clearly illustrated in a series of studies leading to the isolation and cloning of the gene *(Rdl)* conferring resistance to dieldrin, a cyclodiene. The *Rdl* gene was found to code for a GABA receptor component. The proteins coded by the gene in resistant and susceptible strains differ in only one amino acid. A cDNA probe for the *Rdl* gene has been used to isolate a cyclodiene resistance gene from *Aedes aegypti*. The same amino acid substitution found in the resistant *Drosophila* strain was found in the resistant mosquito strain (ffrench-Constant 1993; ffrench-Constant et al. 1993; Thompson et al. 1993).

Knockdown resistance in a house fly strain has been mapped to a sodium channel gene locus, which has been partially sequenced (Williamson et al. 1993). The gene was isolated using a cDNA probe from a *Drosophila* sodium channel gene. A gene conferring resistance to the juvenile hormone (JH) analogue methoprene has been cloned in *D. melanogaster* (Wilson 1993). Several genes from the glutathion-S transferase (Wang et al. 1991; Beall et al. 1992; Cochrane et al. 1992) and cytochrome P-450 (Feyerisen et al. 1989; Carino et al. 1992; Waters et al. 1992; Koener et al. 1993) gene families have been cloned. Both structural and regulatory differences in these genes have been observed between resistant and susceptible strains (see Carino et al. 1992; Grant and Hammock 1992).

Molecular genetic studies of resistance genes will lead to a better understanding of the detoxifying proteins and altered target sites involved in resistance as well as how gene expression is regulated. This information will be useful in the design of new insecticides. Knowing the molecular genetic basis of resistance in particular cases also aids population biologists interested in the dynamics of resistance genes in populations. Knowing whether a resistance gene exhibits constitutive or inducible expression or whether resistance is due to a single gene copy or due to gene amplification can affect the methods used to study resistance in the laboratory or field. In addition, expectations of how resistance evolves will vary depending on whether resistance is conferred by a single gene or the process of gene amplification is involved.

Quantitative Genetics

A number of cases of polygenic resistance have been identified in which several genes contribute to resistance, and more than one gene is necessary to confer a high level of resistance (Chap. 25). In the case of gene amplification–based resistance, the level of resistance varies depending on the number of copies of the resistance gene an individual carries. In some populations of *Cx. quinquefasciatus* in which OP resistance is conferred by high esterase activity due to gene amplification, a wide range of esterase activities is observed among individuals, suggesting that they differ in the number of esterase genes they carry. In both polygenic resistance and gene amplification–based resistance, individuals cannot be classified into the 2 or 3 different resistance phenotypes that result when resistance is caused by a single allele at a genetic locus. Rather, individuals in a population exhibit a more or less continuous range of resistance phenotypes. These cases cannot be adequately studied using Mendelian genetic methods alone—the techniques of quantitative genetics must be employed.

A quantitative trait is any trait for which phenotypes do not fall into discrete classes. Investigators sometimes assume that a number of genes must contribute to quantitative phenotypic differences among individuals in a population, but this is not necessarily true. Even when phenotypes are the result of different combinations of 2 alleles at a single locus, the trait can be quantitative because individuals in a population differ in phenotype resulting from differences in environmental factors (e.g., nutrition) they experienced during development in addition to genetic differences. Thus, the total phenotypic variation observed among individuals (V_P) in a population is caused by genetic variation (V_G) and environmental variation (V_E). The phenotypic variation of a quantitative trait in a population is best described in statistical terms, and the methods of quantitative genetics rely on parameters generated by regression, correlation, and analysis of variance to assess the relative contribution of genetic and environmental factors to the observed variation.

Quantitative genetic techniques can provide useful information about resistance in a number of ways. When resistance results from resistance alleles at several genetic loci, it is difficult to predict changes in the frequency of resistant genotypes using simple models of selection based on the Hardy-Weinberg model for several genes. To use this model, it would be necessary to know the linkage relationships of the genes involved, the relative contribution of each resistance allele to resistance, and any gene interactions that affect the level of resistance. Rather than attempt to model the change in frequency of resistance alleles at all loci that contribute to resistance, the overall contribution of genetic differences among individuals to variation in resistance phenotypes is assessed by determining the "heritability" of resistance. Broad-sense heritability (H^2) relates to the proportion of the total phenotype variation in a population that is due to genetic differences among individuals. In response to selection, only one component of V_G, the so-called additive genetic component (V_A) of genetic variation, is important because it determines the response of a population to selection. Narrow-sense heritability (h^2) = V_A/V_P (see Firko and Hayes 1991 for a discussion of heritability in resistance and Falconer 1989 for a general discussion of quantitative genetics).

Several techniques can be used to estimate h^2 for a population. Some of these techniques measure the degree of phenotypic resemblance among relatives. These include offspring-parent regression and sib (sibling) analysis. Sib analysis involves producing a number of families of siblings and comparing the variation of resistance within families and between families. This technique has been used to assess the heritability of resistance in several agricultural pests (Firko and Hayes 1991; Tabashnik and Cushing 1989).

Another technique for estimating heritability of resistance is to monitor the change in resistance from generation to generation under controlled conditions where both the selection differential (S) and the response to selection (R) can be monitored over a number of generations (Tanaka and Noppun 1989; Tabashnik 1992). The selection differential is related to the intensity of selection (proportion of the population killed in each generation), and the response to selection is related to the change in the level of resistance from one generation to the next (Falconer 1989; Tabashnik 1992). When cumulative R is plotted versus cumulative S each generation, the regression coefficient of the line fitted to this plot is called the realized heritability, h^2 = R/S. Realized heritability can be used to predict the response to selection, R = h^2S. The information needed to calculate realized heritability is often available from laboratory selection imposed on lab colonies prior to genetic analysis, but it is rarely calculated. It can be an informative measure when the colony is representative of the field population from which it was derived. It provides a rough estimate of the resistance potential of the population but must be interpreted correctly.

It is important to understand that estimates of heritability of a population are time- and environmentally specific. The heritability of the same population can differ in various environments. Heritability of resistance in a uniform laboratory environment, for example, will probably be higher than the heritability of resistance in the field, in which environmental contributions to phenotypic variation of resistance is greater. The heritability of a trait in a population changes over time under selection. As selection proceeds, V_A (and therefore h^2) gradually decline, as the resistance genotypes increases in frequency and individuals become more uniform genetically. It can be seen then, that heritability is not only a measure of the level of resistance in a population but also a measure of the potential for change in the short term. A population consisting of mostly susceptible or mostly resistant individuals will both have low heritability for resistance. Heritability is highest when there is a range of susceptible and resistant phenotypes present close to the same frequency. Quantitative genetic techniques are also useful in characterizing resistance caused by gene amplification when some quantitative measure associated with resistance is available (Ferrari and Georghiou 1991).

STATUS OF RESISTANCE IN ARTHROPOD VECTORS

Resistance to 1 or more insecticides has been documented in more than 504 species of arthropods (Georghiou and Lagunes-Tejeda 1991). Of these, about 41% are considered of medical or veterinary importance (Table 30.2). The status of resistance in arthropod vectors has been reviewed (WHO 1992); however, information is incomplete because in many countries resistance surveys have either not been done or have included only a few insecticides. Although resistance can be documented in a species, the conclusion that resistance is widespread or that it has led to control failures does not necessarily follow. However, the presence of resistant individuals in one population of a species does indicate the potential for resistance to spread to other populations.

The impact of resistance on the control of disease vectors and on disease transmission is unknown in many cases. In some cases that have been evaluated, resistance has been implicated in control failures leading to an increase in the incidence of disease. In other cases, when resistance has been detected, little or no impact on control programs has been reported (WHO 1992). Usually, when resistance to one class of insecticide is detected, its use is discontinued and another insecticide is introduced; however, many control programs have not developed a coordinated strategy based on principles of resistance management. Such haphazard approaches to control may work in the short term but will eventually fail as resistance to all classes of insecticides becomes widespread.

An example of a highly coordinated vector control program is the WHO onchocerciasis control program (OCP) in West Africa (Le Berre et al. 1990; Curtis et al. 1993). The OCP depends on a well-planned effort to control the black fly vectors of this disease in the face of the evolution of resistance to organophosphates. Originally the organophosphate insecticide temephos provided effective black fly control, but resistance was detected in 2 species of the *Simulium damnosum* complex in 1980. Resistance spread rapidly and was found in 2 additional species in 1983. Rather than abandon temephos, the OCP developed a control

TABLE 30.2   Number of resistant species in different groups of arthropod vectors[a]

Common name	Genus	Number of species	Insecticide class[b]			
			DDT	OP	Carb.	Pyr.
Mosquitoes	*Anopheles*	56	x	x	x	x
	Aedes	19	x	x	x	x
	Culex	20	x	x	x	x
	Other	4				
Black flies	*Simulium*	9	x	x		
Sand flies	*Phlebotomus*	2	x			
Other flies		10				
Lice	*Pediculus*	2	x	x		
Bed bugs	*Cimex*	2	x	x		
Triatomines	*Triatoma*	1	x	x		
Fleas	*several*	8	x	x	x	x
Cockroaches	*Blatella*	2	x	x	x	x
	Periplaneta	2	x	x		
Ticks	*Amblyomma*	1	x	x		
	Boophilus	2	x	x	x	x
	Hyalomma	3		x	x	
	Rhipicephalus	3		x		

[a] Information from WHO (1992)
[b] OP = organophosphate; Carb. = carbamate; Pyr. = pyrethroid

strategy that involved rotating 5 different insecticidal compounds. The rotational scheme was "reactive." Decisions about which insecticide to use were based on the constant monitoring of river flow and resistance levels. It was observed that resistance to temephos declined in an area when other insecticides were used, making it possible to reintroduce it to the rotation after a time. This maintained the usefulness of temephos, which is the insecticide of choice because it causes less damage to the ecosystem than some of the other insecticides used. Now the OCP has adopted a prearranged insecticide rotation, which is less labor intensive. Computer simulations indicate that prearranged and reactive rotations will produce resistance at the same rate (Curtis et al. 1993).

Although the OCP is in many ways a model vector control program, there is no guarantee that it is the best possible program from a resistance management viewpoint. The program utilizes each of the available insecticides at the time when it will be most effective based on the prevailing conditions. Whether this is the optimal control strategy to delay resistance to all of the insecticides is unknown. The OCP is constantly reviewing its strategy and developing new tactics, and the information obtained from this "experiment in progress" will undoubtedly be useful in designing other control programs in the future.

FUTURE OUTLOOK

Theoretical work on the evolution of resistance has not yet found a pesticide use strategy that will prevent the evolution of resistance. Even if such a strategy were found to operate in computer models, the diversity of conditions that exist in actual vector populations make it unlikely that such a strategy would have general applicability. It is clear that specific control strategies will need to be devised for each species, or perhaps for each population of a species, that take advantage of the prevailing conditions. This will require detailed information on the biology of the vector under different conditions, the available insecticides and their properties, and the status of resistance (Table 30.1).

For new compounds, such as the bacterial insecticides, to which resistance is not yet widespread in the field, it is important to establish criteria for detecting resistance when it appears. Ideally, prior to use of a new insecticide, standardized bioassay methods should be developed and used to characterize a representative sample of "susceptible" populations to establish the existing natural variation in susceptibility and criteria for identifying resistance. When insecticide use begins, treated populations must be monitored periodically to detect resistance at an early stage (Keiding 1986; Brent 1986).

Once resistance has arisen in a population, its genetic control, biochemical mechanism, molecular genetic basis, and cross-resistance spectrum must be determined. In addition, the dynamics of the gene or genes involved, both when the insecticide is used and when a switch is made to an alternative insecticide, must be determined. This information will facilitate devising a control program that maximizes the useful life of the insecticide after resistance has been detected. Many existing vector control programs are now at the stage in which resistance exists to several insecticide classes and few alternative insecticides are available. In these cases, the goal is to use the available insecticides in a way that will prolong their usefulness while maintaining adequate control. Rotations can help accomplish this goal if resistance to one insecticide is found to decline when it is not used. The ability to plan effective control programs after resistance is detected will depend on how much information is available about the vector and the resistance.

Although resistance has not been discussed in the context of integrated pest management, it is obvious that the best way to prolong the useful life of safe, effective insecticides is to use them as little as possible. Whenever possible, insecticides must only be part of a comprehensive control program in which other control options play important roles.

The problem of insecticide resistance will undoubtedly continue to increase in the coming years. Scientists interested in resistance must analyze the problem at many levels, from molecular genetics through population biology. It is only through the combined efforts of individuals with varied talents and training that we will be able to address the problem and devise effective solutions.

REFERENCES AND FURTHER READING

Beall, C., C. Fyrberg, C. Song, and E. Fyrberg. 1992. Isolation of a *Drosophila* gene encoding glutathione S-transferase. *Biochem. Genet.* 30:515–527.

Brent, K.J. 1986. Detection and monitoring of resistant forms: An overview. In: National Academy of Sciences, *Pesticide resistance: Strategies and tactics for management.* Washington, D.C.: National Academy Press. pp. 298–312.

Brown, T.M., and W.G. Brogdon. 1987. Improved detection of insecticide resistance through conventional and molecular techniques. *Ann. Rev. Entomol.* 32:145–162.

Carino, F., J.F. Koener, F.W. Plapp, and R. Feyereisen. 1992. Expression of the cytochrome P-450 gene CYP6A1 in the housefly, *Musca domestica.* In: C.A. Mullen and J.G. Scott, editors, *Molecular mechanisms of insecticide resistance: Diversity among insects,* Washington D.C.: American Chemical Society. pp. 31–40.

Cochrane, B.J., M. Hargis, P. Crocquet de Belligny, F. Holtsberg, and J. Coronella. 1992. Evolution of glutathione S-transferases associated with insecticide resistance in *Drosophila.* In: C.A. Mullen and J.G. Scott, editors, *Molecular mechanisms of insecticide resistance: Diversity among insects.* Washington D.C.: American Chemical Society. pp. 53–70.

Croft, B.A. 1990. Developing a philosophy and program of pesticide resistance management. In: B.E. Tabashnik and R.T. Roush, editors, *Pesticide Resistance in Arthropods.* New York: Chapman and Hall. pp. 277–296.

Crow, J.F. 1957. Genetics of resistance to chemicals. *Ann. Rev. Entomol.* 2:227–246.

Curtis, C.F., N. Hill, and S.H. Kasim. 1993. Are there effective resistance management strategies for vectors of human disease? *Biol. J. Linn. Soc.* 48:3–18.

Dary, O., G.P. Georghiou, E. Parsons, and N. Pasteur. 1990. Microplate adaptation of Gomori's assay for quantitative determination of general esterase activity in single insects. *J. Econ. Entomol.* 83:2187–2192.

Devonshire, A.L., and L.M. Field. 1991. Gene amplification and insecticide resistance. *Ann. Rev. Entomol.* 36:1–23.

Falconer, D.S. 1989. *Introduction to quantitative genetics,* 3rd ed. New York: Longman.

Ferrari, J.A., and G.P. Georghiou. 1990. Esterase B1 activity variation within and among insecticide resistant, susceptible, and heterozygous strains of *Culex quinquefasciatus* (Diptera: Culicidae). *J. Econ. Entomol.* 83:1704–1710.

Ferrari, J.A., and G.P. Georghiou. 1991. Quantitative genetic variation of esterase activity associated with a gene amplification in *Culex quinquefasciatus. Heredity* 66:265–272.

Feyereiser, R., J.F. Koener, D.E. Farnsworth, and D.W. Herbert. 1989. Isolation and sequence of cDNA encoding a cytochrome P-450 from an insecticide resistant strain of the house fly, *Musca domestica. Proc. Nat. Acad. Sci. USA* 86:1465–1469.

ffrench-Constant, R.H. 1993. Cloning of the *Drosophila* cyclodiene insecticide resistance gene: a novel GABA receptor subtype? *Comp. Biochem. Physiol.* 104(C):9–12.

ffrench-Constant, R.H., and R.T. Roush. 1990. Resistance detection and documentation: The relative roles of pesticide and biochemical assays. In: B.E. Tabashnik and R.T. Roush, editors, *Pesticide Resistance in Arthropods.* New York: Chapman and Hall. pp. 4–38.

ffrench-Constant, R.H., J.C. Steichen, T.A. Rocheleau, K. Aronstein, and R.T. Roush. 1993. A single amino acid substitution in a gamma-aminobutyric acid subtype A receptor locus is associated with cyclodiene insecticide resistance in *Drosophila* populations. *Proc. Nat. Acad. Sci. USA.* 91:1957–1961.

Field, L.M., A.L. Devonshire, and B.G. Forde. 1988. Molecular evidence that insecticide resistance in peach potato aphids (*Myzus persicae* Sulz.) results from amplification of an esterase gene. *Biochem. J.* 251:309–312.

Finney, D.J. 1971. *Probit analysis.* Cambridge: Cambridge University Press.

Firko, M.J., and J.L. Hayes. 1990. Quantitative genetic tools for insecticide resistance risk assessment: estimating the heritability of resistance. *J. Econ. Entomol.* 83:647–654.

Georghiou, G.P. 1969. Genetics of resistance to insecticides in houseflies and mosquitoes. *Exp. Parasitol* 26:224–255.

Georghiou, G.P. 1983. Management of resistance in arthropods. In: G.P. Georghiou and T. Saito, editors. *Pest resistance to pesticides.* New York: Plenum. pp. 769–792.

Georghiou, G.P., and A. Lagunes-Tejeda. 1991. The occurrence of resistance to pesticides in arthropods. Rome: FAO.

Georghiou, G.P., and T. Saito, editors, 1983. *Pest resistance to pesticides.* New York: Plenum.

Georghiou, G.P., and C.E. Taylor. 1976. Pesticide resistance as an evolutionary phenomenon. In: Proc. 15th Int. Congr. Entomol. Washington, D.C.: Entomological Society of America. pp. 759–785,

Georghiou, G.P., and C.E. Taylor. 1986. Factors influencing the evolution of resistance. In: National Academy of Sciences, *Pesticide resistance: Strategies and tactics for management.* Washington, D.C.: National Academy Press. pp. 157–169.

Grant, D., and B.D. Hammock 1992. Genetic and molecular evidence for a *trans*-acting regulatory locus controlling glutathione S-transferase expression in *Aedes aegypti. Mol. Gen. Genet.* 234:169–176.

Hama, H. 1983. Resistance to insecticides due to reduced sensitivity of acetylcholinesterase. In: G.P. Georghiou and T. Saito, editors, *Pest resistance to pesticides.* New York: Plenum, pp. 299–231.

Hartl, D.L., and A.G. Clark. 1989. *Principles of Population Genetics,* 2nd ed. Sunderland, MA: Sinauer.

Keiding, J. 1986. Prediction or resistance risk assessment. In: National Academy of Sciences, *Pesticide resistance: Strategies and tactics for management.* Washington, D.C.: National Academy Press. pp. 279–297.

Koener, J.F., F.A. Carino, and R. Feyereiser. 1993. The cDNA and deduced protein sequence of housefly NADPH-cytochrome P450 reductase. *Insect Biochem. Mol. Biol.* 23:439–447.

Le Berre, R., J.F. Walsh, B. Philippon, P. Poudiougo, J.E.E. Henderickx, P. Guillet, A. Sékétéli, D. Quillévéré, J. Grunewald, and R.A. Cheke. 1990. The WHO onchocerciasis programme: retrospect and prospects. *Phil. Trans. Roy. Soc. Lond. B.* 328:721–729.

Morton, R.A. 1993. Evolution of *Drosophila* insecticide resistance. *Genome* 361–367.

Mouches, C., M. Magnin, J.-B. Berge, M. de Silvestri, V. Beyssat, N. Pasteur, and G.P. Georghiou. 1987. Overproduction of detoxifying esterases in organophosphate-resistant *Culex* mosquitoes and their presence in other insects. *Proc. Natl. Acad. Sci. USA* 84:2113–2116.

Mouches, C., N. Pasteur, J.-B. Berge, O. Hyrien, M. Raymond, B.R. de St. Vincent, M. de Silvestri, and G.P. Georghiou. 1986. Amplification of an esterase gene is responsible for insecticide resistance in a California *Culex* mosquito. *Science* 233:778–780.

Mouches, C., Y. Pauplin, M. Agarwal, L. Lemieux, M. Herzog, M. Abadon, V. Beyssat-Arnaouty, O. Hyrien, B.R. de Saint Vincent, G.P. Georghiou, and N. Pasteur. 1990. Characterization of amplification core and esterase B1 gene responsible for insecticide resistance in *Culex*. *Proc. Natl. Acad. Sci USA* 87:2574–2578.

Mullen, C.A., and J.G. Scott, editors. 1992. *Molecular mechanisms of insecticide resistance: Diversity among insects*. Washington D.C.: American Chemical Society.

Oppenoorth, F.J. 1985. Biochemistry and physiology of resistance. In: G.A. Kerkut and L.I. Gilbert, editors, *Comprehensive insect physiology, biochemistry and pharmacology*, Vol. 12. Oxford: Pergamon. pp. 731–773.

Raymond, M. 1985. Présentation d'un programme "Basic" d'analyse log-probit pour microordinateur. *Cah. ORSTOM sér. Entomol. Med. Parasitol.* 23:117.

Raymond, M., V. Beyssat-Arnaouty, N. Sivasubramanian, C. Mouches, G.P. Georghiou, and N. Pasteur. 1989. Amplification of various esterase B's responsible for organophosphate resistance in *Culex* mosquitoes. *Biochem. Genet.* 27:417–423.

Robertson, J.L., and H.K. Preisler. 1991. *Pesticide bioassay with arthropods*. Boca Raton: CRC Press.

Roush, R.T., and J.C. Daly. 1990. The role of populations genetics in resistance research and management. In: B.E. Tabashnik and R.T. Roush, editors, *Pesticide resistance in arthropods*. New York Chapman and Hall. pp. 97–152.

Roush, R.T., and J.A. McKenzie. 1987. Ecological genetics of insecticide and acaricide resistance. *Ann. Rev. Entomol.* 32:361–380.

SAS Institute. 1985. *SAS user's guide: Statistics*. Version 5 ed. Cary, NC: SAS.

Scott, J.G., 1990. Investigating mechanisms of insecticide resistance: Methods, strategies, and pitfalls. In: B.E. Tabashnik and R.T. Roush, editors, *Pesticide resistance in arthropods*. New York: Chapman and Hall. pp. 39–57.

Soderlund, D.M., and J.R. Bloomquist. 1990. Molecular mechanisms of insecticide resistance In: B.E. Tabashnik and R.T. Roush, editors, *Pesticide resistance in arthropods*. New York: Chapman and Hall. pp. 58–96.

Sparks, T.C., J.A. Lockwood, R.L. Byford, J.B. Graves, and B.R. Leonard. 1989. The role of behavior in insecticide resistance. *Pestic. Sci.* 26:383–399.

Tabashnik, B.E. 1986. Computer simulation as a tool for pesticide resistance management. In: National Academy of Sciences, *Pesticide resistance: Strategies and tactics for management*. Washington, D.C.: National Academy Press. pp. 194–206.

Tabashnik, B.E. 1990. Modeling and evaluation of resistance management tactics. In: B.E. Tabashnik and R.T. Roush, editors, *Pesticide resistance in arthropods*. New York: Chapman and Hall. pp. 153–182.

Tabashnik, B.E. 1992. Resistance risk assessment: realized heritability of resistance to *Bacillus thuringiensis* in diamond back moth (Lepidoptera: Plutellidae), tobacco budworm (Lepidoptera: Noctuidae), and Colorado potato beetle (Coleoptera: Chrysomelidae). *J. Econ. Entomol.* 85:1551–1559.

Tabashnik, B.E., and N.L. Cushing. 1989. Quantitative genetic analysis of insecticide resistance: variation in fenvalerate tolerance in a diamondback moth (Lepidoptera: Plutellidae) population. *J. Econ. Entomol.* 82:5–10.

Tanaka, Y., and V. Noppun. 1989. Heritability estimates of phenthoate resistance in the diamond-back moth. *Entomol. Exp. Appl.* 52:39–47.

Taylor, C.E. 1983. Evolution of resistance to insecticides: The role of mathematical models and computer simulations. In: G.P. Georghiou and T. Saito, editors, *Pest resistance to pesticides*. New York: Plenum. pp. 163–173.

Thompson, M., F. Shotkoski, and R.H. ffrench-Constant. 1993. Cloning and sequencing of the cyclodiene insecticide resistance gene from the yellow fever mosquito Aedes *aegypti*. *FEBS Letters* 325:187–190.

Tsukamoto, M. 1983. Methods of genetic analysis of insecticide. In: G.P. Georghiou and T. Saito, editors, *Pest resistance to pesticides*. New York: Plenum. pp. 71–98.

Via, S. 1986. Quantitative genetic models and the evolution of insecticide resistance. In: National Academy of Sciences, *Pesticide resistance: Strategies and tactics for management*. Washington, D.C.: National Academy Press. pp. 222–235.

Wang, J., S. McCommas, and M. Syvanen. 1991. Molecular cloning of a glutathione S-transferase overproduced in an insecticide-resistant strain of the Housefly (*Musca domestica*). *Mol. Gen. Genet.* 227:260–266.

Waters, L. C., B.J. Shaw, and L.Y. Ch'ang. 1992. Regulation of the gene for *Drosophila* P450-B1, a P450 isozyme associated with insecticide resistance. In: C.A. Mullen and J.G. Scott, editors, *Molecular mechanisms of insecticide resistance: Diversity among insects.* Washington D.C.: American Chemical Society. pp. 41–52.

WHO. 1992. *Vector resistance to pesticides.* Fifteenth report of the WHO expert committee on vector biology and control. Geneva: WHO technical report series, No. 818.

Williamson, M.S., I. Denholm, C.A. Bell, and A.L. Devonshire. 1993. Knockdown resistance (kdr) to DDT and pyrethroids insecticides maps to a sodium channel gene locus in the housefly (*Musca domestica*). *Mol. Gen. Genet.* 240:17–22.

Wilson, T.G. 1993. Transposable elements as initiators of insecticide resistance. *J. Econ. Entomol.* 86:645–651.

31. BIOLOGICAL CONTROL OF MOSQUITOES

Jennifer Woodring and Elizabeth W. Davidson

INTRODUCTION

Biological control can be broadly defined as the reduction of a target pest population by a biological control agent. The biological control agent can be a predator, pathogen, parasite, competitor, or toxin produced by a microorganism.[1] Microbial toxins are called biorational pesticides. Compared to conventional broad-spectrum insecticides, biological control has the advantage of target host specificity with correspondingly little disruption of nontarget organisms in the environment. Furthermore, it is possible that some living biological control agents can provide long-term control after a single introduction.

Modern biological control efforts began in 1889 in California when a predator was introduced to control a scale insect that was devastating the citrus industry. Since then, biological control agents have been successfully used against a variety of agricultural pests in diverse locations. For cropping systems, biological control will be an important component of several integrated pest management schemes by the year 2000. However, biological control of arthropod vectors that transmit pathogens to vertebrates has lagged behind control of agricultural pests. Most efforts have concentrated on larval mosquitoes, black flies, and manure-breeding flies (that transmit disease by contamination). This chapter focuses on mosquitoes.

Early mosquito control methods included large-scale removal or modification of breeding sites and treatment of remaining larval habitats with oils or inorganic toxins such as Paris green. Biological control became popular in the early 1900s when the mosquito fish, *Gambusia affinis*, was introduced in many countries to control larval mosquitoes. Synthetic insecticides toxic to both larvae and adults largely replaced these early control methods in the 1940s and 1950s. Interest in using biological control (and habitat modification) reemerged in the 1960s when vector populations began to develop resistance to conventional insecticides. The nematode *Romanomermis culicivorax* and the protozoan *Nosema algerae* were extensively studied because they could infect and kill mosquito larvae. Large-scale field trial results varied. Poor control was attributed to the adverse effect of environmental factors on these biological agents. Nonetheless, *Romanomermis* was first marketed in 1976. High production costs, problems with storage and transport, and the rapid development of the pathogenic bacterium *Bacillus thuringiensis* subsp. *israelensis* eventually led to its commercial demise as a biological control agent.

Bacillus thuringiensis subsp. *israelensis* (*Bti*) was discovered in 1975. Unlike the previous *thuringiensis* isolates, which had been successfully used to control several agricultural pests, *Bti* toxins killed mosquito and black fly larvae (see Chap. 32). By 1981 *Bti* was available for use as a mosquito and black fly control agent. Several firms now market *Bti*-based insecticides. Strains of *Bacillus sphaericus* that are toxic to mosquitoes have also been developed commercially.

These *Bacillus* spp. are effective when placed in a larval habitat, but control does not continue over several generations. Researchers continue to seek living agents that not only reproduce in the environment but also provide ongoing control of the target population. The fungus *Lagenidium giganteum* provides long-term control of mosquito larvae in unpolluted freshwater environments and has recently been approved by the U.S. Environmental Protection Agency (USEPA) for application as a mosquito control agent. Other biological control agents are discussed later. Transgenic organisms that produce toxins specific for vectors and reproduce in the environment are also under investigation (see Chap. 32).

Biological control requires sound ecological information about the vector population and the biological control agent(s). This chapter concentrates on fundamental principles of biological control, the ecology of

selected biological control agents for mosquitoes, and considerations for the successful implementation of biological control strategies against vector populations.

FUNDAMENTAL PRINCIPLES OF BIOLOGICAL CONTROL

Population Ecology

Considerable research has focused on parameters affecting mosquito population size (Mogi 1981, 1993; Service 1985a,b). Figure 31.1A depicts hypothetical vector population growth in the absence of exogenous mortality factors such as biological control agents (also known as natural enemies) and catastrophic mortality events. Population density increases until it reaches K, the theoretical carrying capacity that the environment can support. Once K is surpassed, intraspecific competition for food, space, or other limiting resources causes population growth to decline. When the population drops below K, competitive pressure relaxes and the population increases.

Most populations do not fluctuate around their carrying capacity because other mortality factors are present. Mortality factors are often classified as density dependent (DD) or density independent (DI). With DD factors, the percentage of mortality increases as the population becomes more dense and decreases as the population becomes less dense. DD mortality factors tend to regulate a population around an average size and to resist changes to that average size.[2] The intraspecific competition that maintains the population of Figure 31.1A around K is a DD factor. In Figure 31.1B, natural enemies function as DD mortality factors that maintain the population at a new equilibrium point below K. If a population is heavily regulated by DD factors, killing an extra percentage of larvae has no effect on the resulting adult

31.1 Population dynamics. (A) Population growth in the absence of external mortality factors. (B) Population growth with density-dependent regulation below the carrying capacity. (C) Population growth with a single density-independent mortality factor. (D) A hypothetical mosquito population subjected to a combination of density-independent and density-dependent mortality factors. See text for further details.

population because of the compensating reduction in DD mortality. In fact, overcompensation, resulting in more adults emerging, is theoretically possible.

DI mortality factors are characterized by mortality that is not proportionate to the population density. DI mortality reduces population size but does not promote population stability at a typical density. In Figure 31.1C, the hypothetical population growth curve (of Fig. 31.1A) is shown with the addition of a single DI event that kills 80% of the population. The population can return to K in the absence of further DI mortality events. DI factors can cause wide population fluctuations, depending upon their frequency and severity and the fecundity of the population subject to them. Floods, unfavorable temperature extremes, droughts, and insecticides frequently act as catastrophic DI mortality factors. Natural enemies also cause density-independent mortality. The percentage of mortality depends on the relative population sizes and on the presence of alternative hosts or prey. DI mortality can be important for mosquitoes and can partially explain their great population fluctuations.

Most populations are subject to both DD and DI mortality factors. The relative strength of each mortality factor varies with the species, season, and location. Figure 31.1D depicts a hypothetical mosquito population in a rice field (Mogi 1993) in which both DD and DI mortality factors are operating. At time zero, mosquitoes begin colonizing the rice field. The population grows rapidly, then decreases as natural enemies also colonize the field. A flood serves as a major density-independent mortality event, flushing the fields of both mosquitoes and their predators (here assumed to act in a density-dependent manner). The mosquitoes recolonize faster than the predators after a flood; thus, the mosquito population rebounds to higher than preflood levels. When the predators finally recolonize, they reduce mosquito numbers to a preflood state. Vector population resurgence is also observed after applications of pesticides that kill both the biological control agents and the vector. Pest populations usually rebound more quickly than populations of their natural enemies. Not only do pests often have life-history traits that enable them to rapidly recolonize and reproduce, but natural enemy populations often require a minimum host density to support them.

Biological control agents function as either DD or DI mortality agents. Pathogens and oligophagous predators (restricted to a few prey species) are more likely to provide DD mortality because their populations depend on the specific vector population. Unless these natural enemies can persist in the absence of the vector, they require a residual vector population to support them (at least if ongoing control is the goal). The minimum host density required by the pathogen or predator determines the size of the residual vector population. Natural enemies that provide DI mortality can maintain a vector population at low densities depending upon relative population sizes and the availability of alternate prey or hosts. Microbial toxins function as DI mortality agents that usually provide a large reduction in the vector population. In either case (DD or DI mortality), the biological control is adequate if the vectorial capacity (Chap. 3) of the vector population has been decreased to an acceptable level.

Mosquito Ecology

The ecology of different mosquito species varies considerably, but for the sake of simplification some generalizations can be made (see Mogi 1981; Service 1985b) (Chaps. 4 and 5). Mosquito populations are characterized by rapid increases and precipitous declines. The females are highly fecund. Most species also have a short generation time under warm weather conditions. Thus, mosquito populations can quickly increase when the breeding season begins or rapidly rebound after a catastrophic event. Furthermore, the adults disperse well and the females quickly colonize new habitats.

Larval habitats are quite diverse, ranging from ephemeral to permanent, from artificial to completely natural, from hoofprints to rice fields. Generally mosquitoes avoid deep or rapidly flowing water. Some species prefer sunny habitats; others are found only in shaded locations. Vectors may shift preferred habitats as the seasons change and as new habitats become available. Larvae are not evenly distributed within favored breeding sites. Within larger habitats they tend to be aggregated. For container habitats, some containers will be overutilized whereas others will be underutilized or empty.

Different mortality factors predominate in different habitats. In permanent ponds and rice fields, larvae often experience over 80% mortality, primarily from predators. In small container habitats, such as tree holes, over 80% mortality can be experienced, usually resulting from overcrowding and competition and more rarely from predators or pathogens. Mortality rates in ephemeral ponds are not well documented but probably depend upon how quickly the pond dries and whether the pond is rapidly colonized by a predator or pathogen population. DI mortality factors, such as flooding, temperature extremes, or desiccation, can be important in any of these habitats. Factors that affect mosquito population size are not completely understood, and accurate prediction of population changes requires more information.

How do these mosquito characteristics affect biological control efforts? The ideal mosquito biological control agent probably does not exist; however, analysis of existing control methods is instructive. The ideal mosquito control agent should respond to any vector population increase by rapidly colonizing new habitats and quickly producing numerous progeny. This agent should be able to efficiently find all vector individuals, survive periods of mosquito absence, and function well in any mosquito habitat.

Mosquito natural enemies usually affect the larval stages. The diversity of larval habitats, feeding behavior, and physiology probably provide an insurmountable challenge to development of any single control agent. Even within one genus, vector larvae often exhibit marked species-specific differences in susceptibility to certain microbial control agents. No single agent or formulation can be expected to provide adequate control of, for example, *Culex quinquefasciatus* in polluted wastewater, *Aedes aegypti* in human potable water containers, and *Anopheles gambiae* in hoofprints. Therefore, efficacy of biological control cannot be generalized from one agent, target, or habitat to another. A variety of potentially useful agents, formulations, and application techniques must be developed for specific target vectors and habitats.

Mosquito adults are the vectors, yet many control methods, including biological control, are directed at juvenile stages. In comprehensive control programs, both the terrestrial adults and the aquatic larvae must be monitored. The effect of decreasing larval populations on the resultant adult populations is still not well understood and deserves further study.

Types of Biological Control

Biological control can be categorized into natural and applied biological control. Natural biological control is vector reduction caused by naturally occurring biotic agents. Biological control agents are more likely to cause significant mortality in permanent habitats than in ephemeral habitats. Natural control provides greater than 80% larval reduction by DI and DD action in some habitats. Abiotic mortality factors (such as unfavorable temperatures) contribute even further to population reduction. Natural biological control alone may not reduce vector populations sufficiently to interrupt disease transmission. However, the explosion of a vector population after disruption of natural biological control (e.g., by a broad-spectrum pesticide) demonstrates the contribution of natural control.

Applied biological control is planned human intervention to add biological control agents to a site (augmentation) or to protect the agents already present (conservation). Applied biological control is a vector control option when natural biological control is insufficient. Perceived as more natural than the use of conventional insecticides, applied biological control is less likely to harm nontarget organisms. However, it is not necessarily natural because it does intervene, for example, when the timing of a pathogen outbreak is altered or artificially high numbers of a (native or exotic) natural enemy are released into the environment. The altered timing of an outbreak or the artificially high numbers of a natural enemy affect the desired control.

Augmentation is the deliberate release of natural enemies into vector habitats to reduce the pest population. Two major strategies for augmentation are inoculation and inundation. With inoculative releases, small numbers of natural enemies are introduced that are expected to reproduce in the environment and provide long-term vector suppression by means of successive generations. The inoculative approach depends on a residual vector population or on an agent that persists in the absence of the host to support the biological control agent. Inoculation is a good strategy for container habitats such as tree holes. Though the initial search for habitats is labor intensive, vector reduction results from a natural enemy that persists during periods of host absence. Inoculations also work in large, accessible habitats. Spring releases of mosquito fish into rice fields when the fields are first flooded are a good example of inoculative biological control in vector management. Both indigenous and exotic biological control agents can be introduced in augmentative biological control.

For inundative releases, overwhelming numbers of organisms are released into a vector population, which is expected to immediately decline. Inundative releases are frequently performed with microbial pathogens and are analogous to the use of chemical insecticides. Indeed, inundative control may utilize toxins produced by a microorganism in artificial culture and applied along with the pathogen. Some establishment (reproduction) of living pathogens can occur, but the progeny generations are not efficacious or numerous enough to maintain control of the pest population. The temporary decimation of the vector population leaves insufficient hosts to support establishment of this or other natural enemies. Inundative releases are most practical in large, accessible vector habitats. Inundation by biological control agents often is required to interrupt disease transmission.

Conservation manipulates the environment to optimize natural biological control by minimizing detrimental effects on natural enemies or by enhancing their efficacy. Indeed, introduced biological control agents must be conserved to be effective. To conserve natural enemies, habitats can be constructed to provide refugia during the winter or dry periods (see Chap. 32). Selective insecticides that are not toxic to the natural enemies can be used. Monitoring vector populations and applying chemical insecticides only when vector density warrants (rather than following a predetermined application schedule) can facilitate natural biological control.

Integrated pest management (IPM) is the current model for most pest control. All available methods of pest management are examined, and an optimal combination of methods is designed to provide adequate control and minimize adverse environmental side effects. More specific than most other vector control methodologies, applied biological control is a prime candidate for inclusion in IPM programs. Biological control alone is probably not sufficient for most vector control; however, it should have a place in integrated programs. Chapter 32 describes an effective IPM program for mosquitoes in the Rhine Valley of Germany.

BIOLOGICAL CONTROL AGENTS

This section surveys the pathogens and predators of mosquito larvae that have been studied as potential biological control agents.

Pathogens

Invertebrate pathogens include viruses, bacteria, protists, fungi, and nematodes. Each group or species varies in its route(s) of infection, host specificity, infectivity and virulence, prevalence in nature, dispersal and persistence mechanisms, and sensitivity to biotic and abiotic parameters. Hundreds of different pathogens and potential pathogens have been reported that infect vector insects (Roberts and Strand 1977; Roberts and Castillo 1980; Roberts et al. 1983).

Invertebrate pathogens affect their target host by 3 different, but sometimes interrelated, pathogenic strategies. The 1st strategy is patent toxicity. For example, the most successful vector control organisms to date, *Bacillus* spp., produce highly specific toxins during sporulation. The live or dead spores with accompanying toxins are applied inundatively, essentially as chemical insecticides. The 2nd strategy is invasion. The invading pathogens do not kill the host immediately upon entry into the body but rather over a period of days or weeks. These pathogens can invade vital tissues, sap host resources, or produce a lethal lesion during exit from the host. Viruses, microsporan protozoans, fungi, and nematodes usually function in this manner. Microsporans and viruses invade the larval midgut following ingestion, whereas most fungi and nematodes penetrate the cuticle to enter the target insect. A 3rd strategy involves sublethal effects. Insects surviving sublethal concentrations of toxic or invasive pathogens exhibit deformities, small size, or reduced fecundity as adults. Some viruses, protozoa, and fungi are transmitted to the next generation by sublethally infected female hosts, providing a mechanism for these pathogens to move to new habitats along with the adult insect. Transovarially transmitted pathogens of low pathogenicity can suppress a population over the course of many generations, but this is probably not a useful strategy against vectors.

Pathogens are subject to many environmental factors such as salinity, pH, oxygen availability, ultraviolet (UV) radiation, adverse temperatures, and pollution. To obtain maximal immediate and long-term success, the specific sensitivities of a pathogen must be considered when planning an application. In cases of patent toxicity, reproduction may or may not occur in target larvae, and the progeny may or may not exert further control on the target population. Establishment of these pathogens is not usually a realistic goal; thus, it is important to determine whether the toxin will remain active and whether the target insect will ingest sufficient toxin in the given habitat. In contrast, invasive pathogens often reproduce successfully and their progeny likely infect other larvae in the environment. When establishment and long-term vector population reduction are goals, the habitat and the pathogen's environmental constraints must be considered.

Natural recycling of pathogens in the environment frequently involves periods of relatively low pathogen prevalence interspersed with unpredictable epizootics (outbreaks). Favorable environmental conditions, the presence of infective pathogens, and a sufficiently dense host population (threshold density) must coincide for an epizootic to occur. The initial introduction of high densities of infective-stage pathogens often induces an epizootic in host populations that are below the characteristic threshold density. The epizootic generally cannot sustain itself for a long period because the host population is rapidly decimated. Pathogens that are able to produce new infective stages even in the absence of a host or that require a low threshold density are best suited for long-term vector suppression.

Viruses

A number of insect-pathogenic viruses have been recorded from vector insects. Although insect viruses are quite useful in microbial control of lepidopteran insect pests, no known virus pathogens appear to have good potential as microbial control agents of vectors. Viruses affect only a small percentage of most vector populations. High doses of the viruses must be ingested to infect the host, older larvae requiring even more virus than younger instars. Moreover, many can be transovarially transmitted, demonstrating that they are not effective in killing the current generation. Viruses are dispersed passively by wind, water, or an infected host. Their persistence in vector habitats is not well known. Even if a virus with good potential were to be discovered, in vivo production would be costly.

Natural mosquito populations sometimes harbor nuclear polyhedrosis viruses (NPVs), cytoplasmic polyhedrosis viruses (CPVs), and mosquito iridescent viruses (MIVs). Mosquito NPVs affect larval mosquito midguts, and the natural prevalence of the virus can occasionally reach 70%. High doses are required to cause laboratory infections. Infected adults and pupae can be found, and transovarial transmission is sometimes observed. CPVs also infect midgut cells. They stress, but do not directly kill, the affected larvae. MIVs affect aedine larvae in the snowmelt pools of northern temperate forests. Virus replicates in the fat body, muscles, and hypodermis and usually gives the larvae an iridescent blue-green or violet appearance. Most infected larvae die before pupation, but a few live to adulthood and transmit the virus transovarially. Once again, it is difficult to infect mosquitoes in the laboratory.

Bacteria

Chapter 32 provides a thorough discussion of bacteria useful in vector control.

Protista

The pathogenic protists are a diverse polyphyletic group with a wide variety of life cycles and pathogenic actions. There are perhaps more types of protists identified from mosquito larvae than any other type of pathogen. Rather than trying to generalize about their

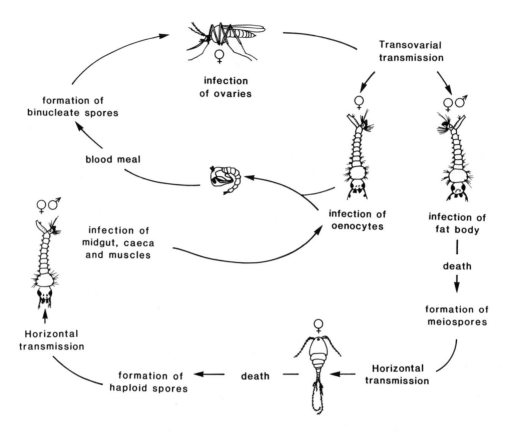

31.2 Life cycle of *Amblyospora* spp. In response to acquisition of a blood meal by the adult female mosquito, *Amblyospora* spp. undergoes sporulation, germination, and infection of the oocytes, assuring vertical transmission to the next generation. Some infected female progeny support benign infections and transmit the infection transovarially to the next generation. In male larvae and other female larvae, the microsporidian undergoes meiosis and sporulates, producing thousands of haploid spores in the fat body and killing the host. When these haploid spores are ingested by a female copepod, an asexual cycle is initiated, leading to the production and release of haploid spores. Haploid spores eaten by a mosquito larva invade the tissues and enter a sexual phase in which the parasite returns to the diploid state. Female mosquitoes thus infected can then transmit the protozoan transovarially to reinitiate the cycle. Adapted from T. Andreadis (1990) and the Society of Protozoologists.

characteristics, some of the better known mosquito pathogens are described.

Members of the phylum Microspora are the most common and extensively studied mosquito pathogens. They produce a coiled polar filament in the spore (Fig. 31.2). When spores are ingested by an appropriate host, the polar filament is forcibly ejected. If the polar filament penetrates a gut cell, the sporoplasm migrates through the filament to initiate an infection in the cell. Microspora infecting vector larvae produce single or polymorphic spore types.

Nosema and *Vavraia* spp. produce a single spore type, develop asexually, and easily infect larvae in the laboratory. Although these Microspora have a broad host range, they usually produce low mortality and do not persist in the environment. Therefore, they are not likely to be useful in vector control. *Nosema algerae* might attract more interest for use in anopheline control (*N. algerae* causes high mortality in *Anopheles* spp.) if an inexpensive in vitro production system could be devised to replace current in vivo methods, and if formulation technology could improve the ability of spores to float and survive in aquatic habitats.

Microspora that produce polymorphic spores affect a wide range of mosquito species, infect transovarially or orally, consistently produce high mortality, and persist in the environment. The discovery that a copepod serves as an intermediate host for *Amblyospora* spp. (Andreadis 1985) and recent elucidation of the complex life cycles of other polymorphic species (some of which do not require intermediate hosts) have opened the door to further development of these microorganisms. *Amblyospora* spp. provide a typical example of a complex life cycle of a microsporan pathogen (Figs. 31.2 and 31.3). Detailed laboratory and field studies of the *Amblyospora connecticus* cycle in *Aedes cantator* and the copepod *Acanthocyclops vernalis* have shown that this protozoan can produce regular epizootics in mosquito populations and can have a natural regulatory effect (Andreadis 1983; 1990). These protozoa could be introduced inoculatively. However, they do not consistently provide adequate control so they would be only one component of an integrated control program.

The ciliates *Tetrahymena pyriformis* and *Lambornella clarki* have been studied extensively. These organisms provide natural control of mosquito larvae in tree holes and are potentially useful as applied biological control agents. The infective stages encyst on and penetrate the host. They then reproduce and kill the host larva. Dead larvae can contain hundreds of mobile ciliates that forcibly exit through the cuticle. *Lambornella* has both parasitic and free-living forms. The free-living forms provide a means of persistence during periods of host absence and transform into parasitic forms in the presence of host larvae.

Fungi

Fungal pathogens generally infect a wide range of hosts; however, strain or pathotype differences in host range and virulence are

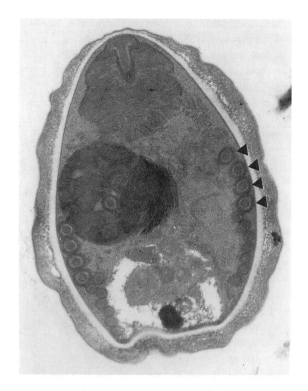

31.3A   Ultrastructure of the *Amblyopora* sp. spore, demonstrating coiled polar filament (arrow). Courtesy of T. Andreadis.

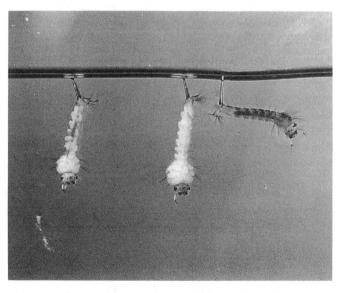

31.3B   Two mosquito larvae (left) infected with *Amblyospora* sp., with 1 healthy larva (right). Photo from the late W.R. Kellen.

well documented. To initiate an infection, viable spores must contact the host cuticle, recognize a host, and attach, germinate, and penetrate the cuticle. Vegetative growth in the hemocoel follows and leads to death of the host by starvation or invasion of vital organs. After host death, the next generation of infectious fungal forms is produced. The host can raise an immune response to fungal infection. Many pathogenic fungi of insects are characterized by a relatively slow pathology, but the mosquito pathogens that are most promising kill their hosts within 1–3 days. Fungal activity is temperature dependent and can be limited by periodic desiccation of the habitat. Most fungi have a resistant spore stage or other method for surviving periods of host absence and unfavorable abiotic conditions. Several are obligate pathogens, but many can be grown in vitro. Three fungal pathogens of mosquito larvae are recognized as having significant potential as microbial control agents: *Lagenidium giganteum*, *Coelomomyces* spp., and *Culicinomyces clavisporus*.

Lagenidium giganteum (order Lagenidiales) infects many mosquito species. This fungus can recycle among hosts every 2–3 days (Figs. 31.4 and 31.5). Its asexual zoospore survives about a day, and the sexually produced oospore can survive up to 7 years under adverse environmental conditions (Kerwin and Washino 1988).

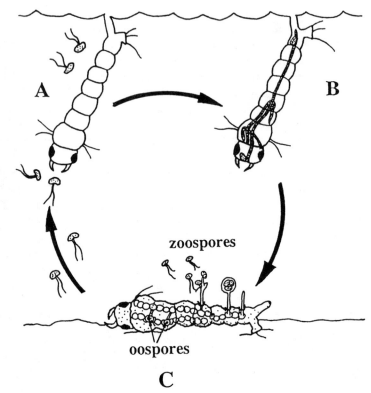

31.4 Life cycle of *Lagenidium giganteum*. (A) Motile, biflagellated zoospores locate and encyst on the cuticle (usually on the head or siphon/anal gills) of a mosquito larva. Zoospores are magnified as compared to the larva. (B) Upon penetration, mycelia extend through the hemocoel to cause (C) death of the larva, probably by starvation, within 34–72 hours. For the next few days, the hyphae forms sporangia, which develop exit tubes that release asexual zoospores to continue the cycle, or the fusion of 2 adjacent hyphal segments form sexual oospores. The oospores persist months to years, then make new zoospores to reinitiate the cycle.

Upon germination, the oospore releases zoospores similar in form and function to the asexual zoospores. Production of both zoospores and oospores in artificial culture has been accomplished (Kerwin and Washino 1986a,b). Inundation with zoospores can quickly reduce a high-density host population. Oospores can be particularly useful for control of low-density hosts because they germinate asynchronously and persist well in the environment. Endemic mycosis has been observed for several years following applications of *Lagenidium* in California rice fields. Organic pollution and high salinity rapidly inactivate zoospores, so this fungus is best used in unpolluted freshwater environments. Products based on mycelium and oospores of *Lagenidium* have been registered by the USEPA.

Coelomomyces spp. (order Blastocladiales) are obligately parasitic fungi that infect a broad range of mosquitoes and have frequently been described from natural epizootics. Attempts to infect mosquito larvae with this fungus in the laboratory were unsuccessful

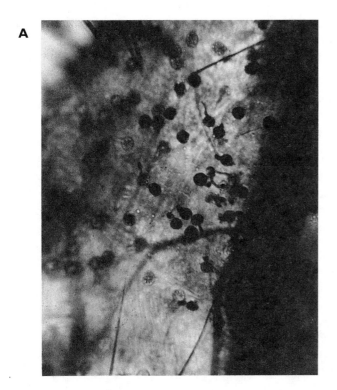

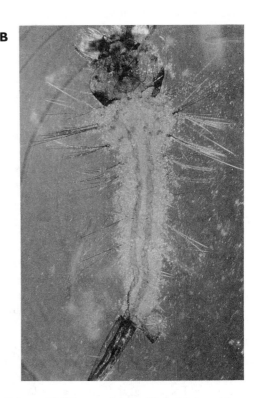

31.5 (A) Zoospores of *Lagenidium* encysted on the cuticle of a *Culex tarsalis* larva. (B) *Culex tarsalis* larva filled with *Lagenidium* hyphae. Light micrographs. Courtesy of J. Kerwin.

until the discovery of an obligate sexual generation in a copepod alternating with an asexual generation in the mosquito (Whistler et al. 1974). Each *Coelomomyces* species has an optimal copepod host. Severe infections can kill mosquito larvae; however, lightly infected mosquitoes can survive to adulthood, providing a mechanism for dispersal of the fungus. Interestingly, in adults only blood-fed females develop sporangia and are unable to reproduce. *Coelomomyces* spp. are attractive biological control agents because they persist in the same site, can kill over 90% of the vector population, and successfully establish in new locations. Because of its complex life cycle, in vitro mass production of this fungus has not yet been accomplished. More ecological information about the microcrustacean hosts will facilitate using the fungi.

Culicinomyces clavisporus (Fungi Imperfecti) infects a very broad host range among mosquitoes and readily produces infectious conidia in artificial culture.

Moreover, it tolerates fresh and brackish water. In contrast to most fungi, *Culicinomyces* spores generally must be ingested by the larvae, whereupon the spores adhere to the cuticle-lined foregut or hindgut, germinate, penetrate the cuticle, and proliferate in the larval body. The host often appears to mount an immune response to invasion by this fungus. Following death of the larva, the fungus sporulates on the surface of the dead host. Occasionally, a lightly infected larva survives to adulthood. Adult cadavers also support fungal sporulation, so this can be a means of fungal dispersal between larval habitats. Interest in development of this fungus has declined because of temperature-dependent activity, difficulties in storage (it can be dried and stored only temporarily), high dosages required for field efficacy, and lack of adequate field persistence and recycling.

Other fungi that infect vector larvae but are not considered as promising for vector control at this time include *Tolypocladium* (Fungi Imperfecti), *Leptolegnia* (Saprolegniales), and the black fly pathogen *Coelomomycidium* (Chytridiales).

Nematodes

Although insect-parasitic nematodes are not microorganisms, their small size, persistence in the environment, and utility in biological control have resulted in their inclusion in most discussions of insect pathogens. Several species of Mermithid nematodes specifically parasitize mosquito or black fly larvae, but only *Romanomermis culicivorax* has been developed for vector control. *Romanomermis* females lay eggs in the substrate of mosquito larval habitats. If the substrate desiccates, the eggs remain dormant. When the substrate is (re)covered by standing water, the eggs develop and preparasites emerge. The preparasite actively seeks a host for up to 2 days. The preparasite attaches to a host larva by means of a stylet and bores a hole through the cuticle. The nematode grows for 7–8 days in the larva (Fig. 31.6), molts to the postparasitic stage, and kills the host as it forcibly exits. The nematode then burrows into the substrate, matures to the adult stage, mates, and lays eggs. The life cycle requires at least 1 month at favorable temperatures (Petersen 1985).

Romanomermis culicivorax exhibits a relatively broad host range among mosquito species; however, it is active only in relatively warm waters and is inhibited by salinity and other environmental factors. This nematode establishes in suitable environments but often provides unpredictable control. The number of nematodes per host affects the sex ratio, with more males being produced as the parasite density in the host increases. This fact and the relatively long life cycle indicate that *Romanomermis* is best used as an inundative biological control agent (Hominick and Tingley 1984).

A large-scale production system was devised for *Romanomermis* using *Culex pipiens* larvae as hosts, and a product was marketed for a few years. Although this nematode is no longer commercially available in the United States, other parasitic nematodes of insects are produced commercially. *Romanomermis* might eventually return to large-scale production if an in vitro production method is discovered. In other countries, such as India, this nematode is reared in vivo and used on a small scale.

Predators

The most commonly studied predators of mosquitoes include many invertebrates such as predaceous insects, hydra, and flatworms and vertebrates such as fish. Predators differ from pathogens in several respects. Predators are usually polyphagous (feed on many prey species), not host-specific. Polyphagy is advantageous because predators can survive the absence of the target species; however, it can be a disadvantage for biological control when the prey sought is not the target vector. One predator can kill many animals over its lifetime whereas several microbes are generally required to kill 1 host. Predators not only seek and attack prey but also can kill more prey than they consume. Most predators are highly mobile and thus not dependent upon the

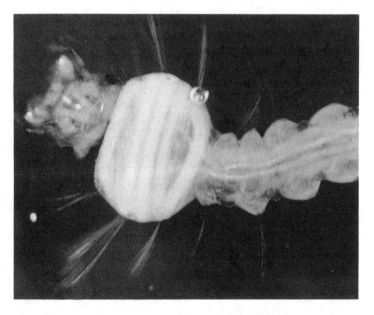

31.6 Nematode, *Romanomermis culicivorax,* coiled within the thorax of *Culex* sp. larva. Courtesy of J. Petersen.

passive dispersal utilized by many pathogens. Finally, predators are usually less sensitive than microbial pathogens to water-quality parameters.

When there is an abundance of prey, predators often display a "functional response," in which they consume more prey than usual to achieve satiation. Predators also respond to a surfeit of prey by reproducing or immigrating, which is called a numerical response. However, predators often reproduce more slowly than their prey; thus, a fecund prey population can potentially escape their influence. Immigration frequently occurs after the prey population is already significant. When the vector population overwhelms the predator population, deliberate introduction of predators can achieve the balance desirable for vector control.

Each predator species displays innate prey preferences, although quantity of prey certainly affects the actual predator diet. The presence or absence of alternate prey also affects the level of control achieved. Thus, prey species A present at low densities is sometimes ignored in favor of the more abundant species B. As the density of species A increases, the predator can switch to preferentially feeding on A over B. This switching phenomenon is possibly caused by enhanced recognition of A or simply by increased contact.

Predators vary in their ability to find prey. Those with good searching abilities are thought to be the better natural enemies. Natural enemies with good searching abilities are often found at low densities because they keep their prey/host population at a low density. Of course, the degree of polyphagy and availability of alternate hosts also affects final predator density.

The ideal predator for biological control of mosquitoes should: (1) consume large numbers of prey per predator, (2) quickly colonize new habitats, (3) prefer the vector but be able to thrive on alternate prey, (4) excel at finding prey, and (5) reproduce rapidly, producing large numbers of offspring. No predator fits this description exactly. In the following sections we will describe organisms that significantly affect mosquito populations.

Invertebrate Predators

Invertebrate predators have been introduced less often than vertebrate predators (fish). Most invertebrate introductions have been experimental rather than practical in nature. Recognition and conservation of important invertebrate predators have often been considered the appropriate methods because of high costs associated with their mass-rearing. In locations in which collecting predator eggs is fairly easy, introduction of eggs into mosquito habitats is promising. A few noninsect invertebrates have been studied for their potential as mosquito control agents. Hydra (Hydrozoa) ambush many invertebrate species in aquatic habitats. In temperate habitats they can reduce larval mosquito populations. Flatworms (Planaria and Turbellaria) can also affect larval populations. They tolerate the presence of chemical pesticides well but are very sensitive to salinity and water temperature. Many species kill more prey than they consume. Predaceous copepods have recently been studied. They provide high mortality in container habitats, and some species are easy to mass produce in the laboratory.

Several groups of insect predators feed on mosquito larvae. The Coleoptera (beetles) and Trichoptera (caddisflies) are considered the most efficient of these predators; however, at naturally occurring densities they do not yield adequate control. Dragonflies reduce both larval and adult mosquito populations but are far from specific for mosquitoes. Several Hemiptera, such as backswimmers, are aquatic predators that feed on mosquitoes.

Toxorhynchites have been reared and released as biological control agents of container-breeding mosquitoes. Larvae of *Toxorhynchites* spp. mosquitoes prey upon other mosquito larvae; the large adults feed only on nectar (Fig. 31.7). Voracious gourmands, *Toxorhynchites* larvae kill more than they can consume. When prey are absent, the larvae can withstand long periods of starvation. Because the adult female seeks containers in which to oviposit, they naturally disperse to habitats that are difficult for humans to find and treat. However, they prefer natural to artificial containers, so human intervention is needed to repeatedly treat artificial containers. Unfortunately for control efforts, this organism does not find all the natural containers harboring vectors and has a lower fecundity and a longer life cycle than most mosquitoes. Thus, the target mosquito population is reduced

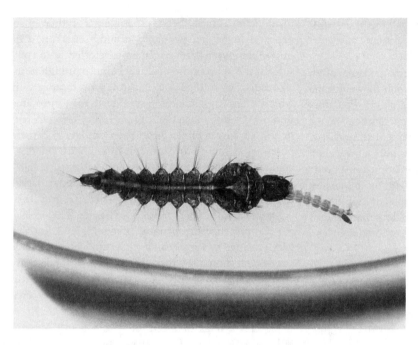

31.7 Predaceous *Toxorhynchites* larva. Courtesy of J. Lenly, Florida Medical Entomological Laboratory, Vero Beach.

which human diagenetic flukes use fish as intermediate hosts, studies to verify that a particular fish does not support fluke development are also important. The family Poeciliidae contains 2 members frequently used in mosquito control: the mosquito fish, *Gambusia affinis* (Fig. 31.8), and the guppy, *Poecilia reticulata*. Both are live-bearers about 3–6 cm long. *Poecilia* is quite similar to *Gambusia* in prey and habitat preferences; however, *Poecilia* survives better in waters with low dissolved oxygen content. *Gambusia* are the most widely disseminated predators used in biological control. Efficient predators in clear temperate waters, *Gambusia* prey on mosquitoes as well as many other invertebrates. Mosquito fish survive water temperatures as low as 13°C and overwinter in areas where ice forms only transiently on the water surface. They can gradually adapt to water temperatures above 35°C and to saltwater. In the summer, they reproduce rapidly. *Gambusia* are frequently maintained in fish farms over the winter months and released into mosquito habitats in the early spring when mosquito breeding begins.

Gambusia are surface feeders attracted to moving prey and provide the best mosquito reduction in water with little vegetation to provide larval refuges. Simultaneous release of a weed-eating species or a species with a different feeding zone can increase the levels of control. Despite the expense of rearing and transport, mosquito fish have reduced both the total cost and the number of insecticide applications required for mosquito control in Californian rice fields (Lichtenberg and Getz 1985).

Gambusia do not always reduce mosquito populations, however. Sometimes they can adversely affect populations of other predators without causing much

when *Toxorhynchites* is present but can reproduce in containers without the predator.

Copepods are microcrustaceans that are often found in the same habitats as mosquito larvae. Several species of copepods prey on mosquito larvae. *Mesocyclops aspericornis* has been shown to control *Aedes* and *Culex* spp. larvae in French Polynesia (Riviere et al. 1987; Lardeux et al. 1992), and Brazilian strains of *M. aspericornis* and *M. longisetus* were found to be effective predators of *Ae. aegypti* larvae in laboratory tests (Kay et al. 1992). A related species, *M. leukarti pilosa,* is capable of surviving in diluted sewage effluent while preying on mosquito larvae (Mian et al. 1986). In areas in which predaceous copepods can become established, they should prove to be useful control agents.

Vertebrate Predators

Fish are the predators most commonly used for mosquito control. Small fish are more likely to eat larvae than large fish. Many fish must still be tested for their efficacy and habitat requirements. In regions in

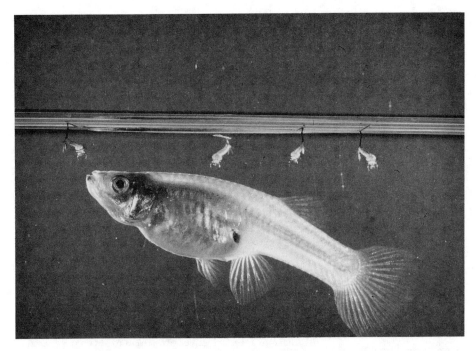

31.8 The mosquito fish, *Gambusia affinis,* shown with 4 mosquito larvae. Photo by Jack Kelly Clark, courtesy of the University of California Statewide IPM Project.

reduce vector populations. The fish are harvested when the fields are drained.

Apocheilus blochi tolerate polluted waters (and thus can be used in pit latrines) well, and *Fundulus* spp. can withstand fairly salty water. In habitats that periodically dry out, the annual fish *Cynolebias* and *Nothobranchius* can be used. These 2 species lay drought-resistant eggs. Although bats and insectivorous birds eat adult mosquitoes, the effect of flying vertebrates on adult mosquito populations is not understood.

mosquito mortality. Insufficient stocking rate is hypothesized to be a reason (Lacey and Lacey 1990). *Gambusia* have some other potential disadvantages. They eat zooplankton and allow algal blooms that are inappropriate for some habitats. Further, they can overwhelm or eat the progeny of native fish, endangered species such as the desert pupfish, or economically important fish. Because of these negative characteristics, indigenous fish should be used when possible.

Tilapia spp., *Aphyocypris chinensis,* and carp can be used for the dual purposes of vector reduction and food supply. Smaller fish are less likely to be eaten, although they are sometimes used by local people as bait. If the fish are removed before the vector season is over, their dual use will have a negative effect on biological control. Prolific fish like *Tilapia* can better tolerate reductions in population. If the fish are removed after the mosquito breeding season in the given habitat, both uses can be quite compatible. For example, in China, pisciculture practiced in rice fields helps

IMPLEMENTATION OF BIOLOGICAL CONTROL

Successful implementation of biological control requires that many ecological and economic factors be taken into consideration. Discovering a promising agent is only the first step. Its efficacy in a variety of habitats must be studied. Biosafety tests and governmental registration must be performed for microbial agents. Economic factors, including cost of production, ease of storage, transport and application, and market size, must be considered whether an organism is to be developed commercially or by a governmental organization. Governmental organizations can choose to operate at a loss if the perceived benefit to the public health is great enough; corporations cannot afford that viewpoint. This section gives an overview of important considerations for effective biological control (see Chap. 32).

Efficacy and Sustainability in Diverse Habitats

Both abiotic and biotic factors can affect the efficacy and sustainability of biological control. The suitability of a habitat should be verified at each new location; as we obtain increasingly detailed data sets for a given biological control agent, our ability to predict success or failure increases.

Abiotic aquatic conditions impact biological control. Temperature can affect a pathogen's ability to infect and the speed with which it kills the host. Pathogens from temperate locations often do poorly in warm tropical waters, and pathogens from tropical regions can be inactivated in cold waters. Predators also have optimal temperature ranges. Within natural waters, pH is not a limiting factor for most multicellular natural enemies but can sometimes be detrimental to microbial agents. The total electroconductivity and the concentration of specific ions can affect pathogen efficacy. Many freshwater species do not tolerate salt or brackish water. Organic matter or pollutants can also affect natural enemy survival and performance. Decreased oxygen availability and the sedimentation of infective spores by particulate matter have been implicated in reduced biological control. The addition of toxic agents, such as chemical pesticides, can be detrimental to a natural enemy population.

The habitat type, size, permanence, and water depth all determine which biological control agents can successfully establish in a given location. *Toxorhynchites* can be introduced to many habitats, but subsequent generations will seek out natural containers. Water impoundments that periodically dry out are not suitable for long-term establishment of many fish. Most pathogens do not provide persistent activity in deep-water habitats.

Biotic factors affecting control agent efficacy include the ecology of the agent itself, the natural history of the target species, and the presence of other interacting species. Important characteristics of the biological control agent are its host specificity and adaptation, dispersal and host-finding abilities, infectivity or capture ability, persistence mechanisms, generation time, and population age structure. Many qualities are innate; however, humans can modify the age structure and density of the population by deliberate introductions. Genetic engineering can be used to address some innate limitations of biological control agents. For the target host, the reproductive strategy, dominant type of population regulation, aggregation, diversity of breeding sites, and innate resistance to the biological control agent must be known and assessed against the characteristics of the control agent. Other interacting species can function as competitors, as alternate hosts/prey available to serve as distraction or extra food supply, or as natural enemies of the biological control agent. Vegetation can provide habitat for the control agent or serve as a refuge for the vector larvae.

Development of resistance by the vector is a possibility that cannot be ignored. Laboratory strains have been selected to be more resistant to nematode attack and bacterial toxins. Resistance to bacterial toxins has also been observed in field populations of Lepidoptera. Pathogens and predators that depend on a vector population face selective pressures to overcome escape mechanisms the vector may develop.

Commercial feasibility of biological control depends upon many factors. Biological agents capable of being produced, stored, and applied as easily as conventional insecticides but that yield long-term adequate suppression of vector populations would be ideal for control agencies. Commercial companies obtain the most profit from agents that require periodic reintroduction. The microbial toxins are quite viable commercially because they fill most of these requirements. Living agents, however, are frequently difficult to produce or store. They may provide longer ongoing control, but for disease reduction they are only effective right after application. As insecticide resistance increases among vector species and as pressures increase to minimize insecticide applications in the environment, biological control will become a more viable option.

Biosafety

Biological control agents should be evaluated in terms of their impact on nontarget organisms such as other beneficial invertebrates, detritivores, and other aquatic fauna. Most biological control agents of mosquitoes tend to be relatively innocuous to other organisms; however, fish sometimes eat the offspring of indigenous, endangered, or economically important fish.

Microbes must also be evaluated for their effect on vertebrates. Their toxic, carcinogenic, teratogenic, and allergenic properties must be determined on representative vertebrate species. To date, microbial pathogens of insects have proven to be relatively harmless to vertebrates.

Registration and Governmental Regulation

In the United States, the USEPA requires biosafety tests be performed for microbial agents to obtain registration for application and sale. Additional tests may be stipulated for genetically engineered organisms. Nematodes and predators have been exempt from these requirements. However, permission must usually be obtained to release exotic species or strains of any organism.

Mass Production of Biological Control Agents

The chief concerns of mass production of biological control agents are cost-effectiveness and retaining field performance. In vitro production methods are usually the most cost-effective. Three-dimensional systems such as fermentation tanks are generally more efficient than 2-dimensional systems (such as growing a culture on a layer of agar). In vivo systems are more complex and labor intensive than in vitro systems and are thus more expensive.

The *Bacillus* spp. and the fungi *Lagenidium* and *Culicinomyces* are facultative pathogens that can be grown in fermentors without loss of virulence. In contrast, the complex life cycle of *Coelomomyces* requires rearing both mosquito and copepod hosts to support fungal production. All viruses, most protists, and the nematode *Romanomermis* must also be grown in living hosts.

Invertebrate predators can sometimes be grown on an artificial medium or on easily reared prey. Backswimmer eggs can be collected efficiently from nature. Most studies with invertebrate predators of mosquitoes have focused on the predators' ability to reduce the target population, not on cost-effective production

techniques. The local agencies responsible for mosquito abatement usually rear larvivorous fish.

Quality control or standardization of mass-produced biological control agents is imperative to ensure field efficacy. In addition, a reliable bioassay for pathogens often uses a standard host species of a particular age, which is compared to a universally recognized international standard. Similar techniques are not generally available for predators.

Formulation

Various formulations have been developed that stabilize pathogen viability and provide long-term storage. The physical form of the final product (e.g., powder, liquid, wettable powder, or granules) can be varied to suit the habitat. Granules effectively penetrate to the water's surface and thus are used to broadcast over vegetation. The size of particles may also influence whether or not they are ingested by the target larvae. Floating particles maintain a pathogen in the larval feeding zone longer than the infective spores alone. Additives can also be included to provide sufficient aeration or moisture or to protect from UV radiation. Many microbial formulations are purposefully similar to chemical formulations to enhance acceptance with organizations that already use insecticides for vector control and to facilitate use in conventional application equipment. The specifics of formulary ingredients are usually proprietary secrets.

Formulations for multicellular pathogens and predators have not been developed yet. *Romanomermis* eggs and preparasites can be stored up to 6 months in sand. Flooding the sand cultures with water 24 hours prior to use extracts preparasites for application.

Storage and Transport

Ideally, for long-term storage, biological control agents should be maintained at room temperature (or above, in warehouses). *Bacillus* preparations and oospores of *Lagenidium* do not require special handling; however, many other pathogens must be stored at cool temperatures, properly aerated, protected from contamination, and so forth. Predators normally cannot be stored as long as some microbial pathogens. Eggs and some starvation-resistant stages can only be stored for an intermediate amount of time.

Lightweight formulations are preferred for transport because they are less expensive to ship. Pathogens or predators that must be shipped and stored in an aqueous medium are less useful than those that can be desiccated. Fish, in particular, require an aqueous medium for transport.

Application of Biological Control Agents

Organisms that can be applied with conventional insecticide application equipment are likely to be accepted by mosquito control agencies. *Bacillus* products, some protozoal and fungal spores, and *Romanomermis* preparasites can be broadcast with traditional equipment, including aircraft sprayers (though certain accommodations in the delivery pressure are sometimes necessary). In contrast, *Toxorhynchites* larvae are often spread by spoonfuls to container habitats; adult females can simply be released in an area with several containers. *Gambusia* are introduced periodically along the shore of a body of water. The ongoing use of these latter 2 organisms demonstrates that if results appear beneficial, unconventional release methods can gain acceptance. Research to define appropriate application technologies and release rates continues with many biological control agents.

SUMMARY AND FUTURE DIRECTIONS

Biological control has many perceived advantages. It is relatively natural and host specific, it can be self-perpetuating, and it does not adversely affect beneficial invertebrates. Also, biological control produces less vector resistance than single-action chemical pesticides. As attractive as biological control is in principle, in practice this technique has had limited success in vector control compared to crop pest control.

Several factors prevent biological control agents from achieving their full potential. Factors limiting microbial control agents include settling of the active agent out of the feeding zone, sensitivity of the pathogen to environmental factors, requirement for an intermediate host, limited pathogenicity or host range, and restrictions imposed by governmental agencies. Predators are often unpredictable, and in many respects their use is limited by our lack of information on their ecology, rearing, transport, and so forth. Thus, ecological expertise is more essential than for the use of insecticides. Because natural enemies are relatively specific, much effort and money can be invested to achieve control of only a few vector species. Establishing an effective natural population is challenging because of the ephemeral nature of many larval habitats and the diversity of vector habits and physiology. Even when the biological control agent establishes, the resulting control can be variable.

Research on several fronts increases the success of vector biological control. In addition to new formulation technologies, several innovative genetic approaches are being applied to microbial organisms in an attempt to extend their usefulness as vector control agents. New technologies are aimed at combining the benefits of an inundation with an introduction (see Chap. 32). Classic genetic techniques may also be appropriate for enhancing the efficacy of promising natural enemies. Although a relatively simple task, isolation of new pathogens and predators is still one of the most fruitful ways to increase the utility of biological control. As new agents are discovered and as known agents are more fully tested, studies of their ecological requirements will be critical to determining when and where they will best function. Further ecological studies of vector populations will also enhance our understanding of the best biological control strategies.

As vector control programs move toward integrated vector management, combinations of control measures will be used to provide optimal control with minimal detrimental environmental impacts. Both applied biological control and conservation of natural biological control will be components of these programs.

NOTES

1. Not all biological control practitioners include microbial toxins as agents of biological control in the strictest sense. They restrict biological control to actively reproducing organisms that provide more or less continuous control over a season or from year to year. Because microbial toxins have

been very effectively used in vector control we include them in our broad definition. Clearly, living biological control agents have different requirements for efficacy than these nonliving toxins.

2. The terms "regulation" and "control" are not used interchangeably in biological control. Population control refers to any population reduction. Regulation implies that factors are at work to maintain a population around a characteristic density.

ACKNOWLEDGMENTS

E. Davidson received support from the John D. and Catherine T. MacArthur Foundation. J. Woodring was supported by a postdoctoral fellowship from the National Institutes of Health. We are grateful to J. Kerwin, T. Andreadis, and K. Olson for manuscript review and to J. Kerwin, T. Andreadis, J. Petersen, J. Lenly, J.K. Clark, and the University of California Statewide IPM Project for illustrations. We also are indebted to S. Higgs for final preparation of Figures 31.1 and 31.4.

REFERENCES

Ahmed, S.S., A.L. Linden, and J.J. Cech Jr. 1988. A rating system and annotated bibliography for the selection of appropriate indigenous fish species for mosquito and weed control. *Bull. Soc. Vector Ecol.* 13:1–59.

Andreadis, T.G. 1983. An epizootic *Amblyospora* sp. in field populations of the mosquito, *Aedes cantator. J. Invertebr. Pathol.* 42:427–430.

Andreadis, T.G. 1985. Experimental transmission of a microsporidian pathogen from mosquitoes to an alternate copepod host. *Proc. Nat. Acad. Sci. USA* 82:5574.

Andreadis, T.G. 1990. Epizootiology of *Amblyospora connecticus* (Microsporida) in field populations of the saltmarsh mosquito, *Aedes cantator*, and the cyclopoid copepod, *Acanthocyclops vernalis. J. Protozool.* 37:174–182.

Baker, R.R., and P.E. Dunn, editors. 1990. *New directions in biological control: Alternatives for suppressing agricultural pests and diseases.* New York: A.R. Liss.

de Barjac, H., and D.J. Sutherland, editors. 1990. *Bacterial control of mosquitoes and black flies.* New Brunswick, NJ: Rutgers Univ. Press.

Hominick, W.M., and G.A.Tingley. 1984. Mermithid nematodes and the control of insect vectors of human disease. *Biocontrol News Info.* 5:7–20.

Kay, B.H., C.P. Cabral, A.C. Sleigh, M.D. Brown, Z.M. Ribeiro, and A.W. Vasconcelos. Laboratory evaluation of Brazilian *Mesocyclops* for mosquito control. *J. Med. Entomol.* 29:599–602.

Kerwin, J.L., and R.K. Washino. 1986a. Regulation of oosporogenesis by *Lagenidium giganteum*: promotion of sexual reproduction by unsaturated fatty acids and sterol availability. *Can. J. Microbiol.* 32:294–300.

———. 1986b. Oosporogenesis by *Lagenidium giganteum*: Induction and maturation are regulated by calcium and calmodulin. *Can. J. Microbiol.* 32:663–672.

———. 1988. Field evaluation of *Lagenidium giganteum* and description of a natural epizootic involving a new isolate of the fungus. *J. Med. Entomol.* 25:452–460.

Lacey, L.A., and C.M. Lacey. 1990. The medical importance of riceland mosquitoes and their control using alternatives to chemical insecticides. *J. Am. Mosq. Control Assoc.* 6(suppl. 2):1–93.

Lacey, L.A., and A.H. Undeen. 1986. Microbial control of black flies and mosquitoes. *Ann. Rev. Entomol.* 31: 265–296.

Laird, M., L.A. Lacey, and E.W. Davidson, editors. 1990. *Safety of microbial insecticides.* Boca Raton, FL: CRC Press.

Lardeux, F., F. Riviere, Y. Sechan, and B.H. Kay. 1992. Release of *Mesocyclops aspericornis* for control of larval *Aedes polynesiensis* in land crab burrows on an atoll of French Polynesia. *J. Med. Entomol.* 29:571–576.

Lichtenberg, E.R., and W. Getz. 1985. Economics of rice-field mosquito control in California. *BioScience* 35:292–297.

Mian, L.S., M.S. Mulla, and B.A. Wilson. 1986. Studies on potential biological control agents of immature mosquitoes in sewage wastewater in Southern California. *J. Amer. Mosq. Control Assn.* 2:329–335.

Mogi, M. 1981. Population dynamics and methodology for biocontrol of mosquitoes. In: M. Laird, editor, *Biocontrol of medical and veterinary pests.* New York: Praeger Publishers. pp. 140–172.

———. 1993. Effect of intermittent irrigation on mosquitoes (Diptera: Culicidae) and larvivorous predators in rice fields. *J. Med. Entomol.* 30:309–319.

Petersen, J.J. 1985. Nematode parasites. In: H.C. Chapman, editor, *Biological control of mosquitoes*. Bulletin No. 6. Amer. Mosq. Control Assoc. Lake Charles, LA. pp. 110–122.

Roberts, D.W., and J.M. Castillo, compilers. 1980. *Bibliography on pathogens of medically important arthropods: 1980. Bull. WHO* 58(Suppl.).

Roberts, D.W., and M.A. Strand, editors. 1977. *Pathogens of medically important arthropods. Bull. WHO* 55(Suppl. 1).

Roberts, D.W., R.A. Daoust, and S.P. Wraight, compilers. 1983. *Bibliography on pathogens of medically important arthropods: 1981*. Publication VBC/83.1. Geneva: World Health Organization.

Service, M.W. 1985a. Some ecological considerations basic to the biocontrol of Culicidae and other medically important insects. In: M. Laird and J.W. Miles, editors, *Integrated control of vectors*. Vol. 1. London: Academic Press. pp. 9–30.

———. 1985b. Population dynamics and mortalities of mosquito preadults. In: L.P. Lounibos, J.R. Rey, and J.H. Frank, editors, *Ecology of mosquitoes: Proceedings of a workshop*. Vero Beach, FL: Florida Medical Entomology Laboratory. pp. 185–201.

Riviere, F., B.H. Kay, J.-M. Klein, and Y. Sechan. 1987. *Mesocyclops aspericornis* and *Bacillus thuringiensis* var. *israelensis* for the biological control of *Aedes* and *Culex* vectors breeding in crab holes, tree holes, and artificial containers. *J. Med. Entomol.* 24:425–430.

Sweeney, A.W., and J.J. Becnel. 1991. Potential of microsporidia for the biological control of mosquitoes. *Parasitol. Today* 7:217–220.

Whisler, H.C., S.L. Zebold, and J.A. Shemanchuk. 1974. Alternative host for mosquito parasite *Coelomomyces*. *Nature* 251:715–716.

32. MICROBIAL CONTROL OF VECTORS

Elizabeth W. Davidson and Norbert Becker

INTRODUCTION

Microbial control can be broadly defined as the use of microorganisms (including insect parasitic nematodes) to reduce pest populations. Two types of microbial control are recognized that are similar to biological control (in which parasites or predators are used):

- Introduction or inoculation: The organisms are introduced at low population numbers, and the progeny of the released organisms are expected to establish a gradually increasing population providing long-term control. Long-term maintenance of a pathogen population generally depends on the maintenance of a minimal pest population as well.

- Inundation: Overwhelming numbers of pathogens are applied, and control is expected from the same organisms that were released. Inundative use of a microbial pathogen is similar to use of a chemical insecticide; indeed, the mechanism of control can often be a toxin that was produced by the microorganism in artificial culture and applied along with the pathogen. Some establishment of the pathogen can also occur, but the progeny generations are not generally efficacious or numerous enough to maintain control of the pest population.

As attractive as introduction is in principle, in practice this technique has had only limited success in vector control. The ephemeral nature of larval habitats, the difficulty of maintaining a pathogen population in running water, and similar factors make establishment of an effective pathogen population in vector habitats challenging. However, natural situations undoubtedly exist in which vector populations are suppressed due to an established pathogen. Inundative releases have been effective for up to a full season when natural enemies, seasonal drying, water management, or the life history of the pest itself maintain the pest population at a low level following the inundation. New technologies are aimed at combining the benefits of an inundation with an introduction.

PROPERTIES OF THE TARGET PEST

Most effective pathogens of vector insects are pathogens of the larval stages. Mosquito and black fly larvae, which are restricted to aquatic habitats, are the primary targets. The diversity of larval habitats, feeding behavior, and physiology challenge the development of microbial control agents for these insects. Vector larvae often exhibit marked differences in susceptibility to certain microbial control agents from species to species even within a single genus that can be related to feeding behavior and/or physiology. No single agent or formulation can be expected to provide adequate control of, for example, *Culex quinquefasciatus* in polluted wastewater, *Aedes aegypti* in human potable water containers, *Anopheles gambiae* in hoofprints, and black fly larvae in rapidly flowing water. Therefore, a variety of potentially useful agents, formulations, and application techniques must be developed. Efficacy of microbial control cannot be generalized from one agent or target to another.

PROPERTIES OF THE PATHOGENS

The extensive literature on the hundreds of different pathogens and potential pathogens reported from vector insects has been collected in 3 volumes published by the World Health Organization (WHO) (Roberts and Strand 1977; Roberts and Castillo 1980; Roberts et al. 1983). More recent reviews and primary publications of particular interest are cited in this chapter.

Three different, but sometimes interrelated, pathogenic strategies are utilized by insect pathogens:

- Patent toxicity: To date, the most successful vector control organisms are *Bacillus* spp., which produce highly specific toxins during sporulation. The spores, with accompanying toxins, are harvested from fermentation vessels, subjected to various formulations, and applied essentially as chemical insecticides. Target larvae die from gut poisoning within a few hours or days after ingesting a lethal dose of these toxins. The spores may or may not germinate, and the progeny of these spores may or may not exert further control on the target insect population. Examples include *Bacillus thuringiensis* and *Bacillus sphaericus*.

- Invasion: Most fungi and nematodes invade the body of the target insect through the cuticle. Microsporidian protozoa have complex intra- and extracellular life cycles that can involve more than one host, and transmission to mosquito larvae can involve ingestion of infective stages. These organisms do not kill the host immediately upon entry into the body but rather kill slowly over a period of days or weeks by invasion of vital tissues, sapping of host resources, and/or producing a lethal lesion during exit from the host. Examples include the fungus *Lagenidium giganteum*, the protozoan *Amblyospora* spp., and the nematode *Romanomermis culicivorax*.

- Sublethal effects: Insects surviving sublethal concentrations of toxic or invasive pathogens may exhibit deformities, small size, or reduced fecundity as adults. Some protozoa and fungi are transmitted to the next generation by sublethally infected female hosts, providing a mechanism for these pathogens to move to new habitats along with the adult insect (Andreadis 1990).

A BRIEF REVIEW OF PATHOGENS OF VECTOR INSECTS

Viruses

A number of insect-pathogenic viruses have been recorded from vector insects (Federici 1985). Although insect viruses are quite useful in microbial control of lepidopteran insect pests, to date none has been found that could potentially be used as a microbial control agent of vector insects (Lacey and Undeen 1986).

Bacteria

Both non–spore-forming and spore-forming bacteria have been found that are pathogenic to vector insect larvae under laboratory conditions. However, members of the genus *Bacillus* have proven most useful in microbial control of these insects. During sporulation, some *Bacillus* spp. produce one or more protein toxins that are concentrated in a parasporal inclusion, called the crystal (Fig. 32.1A). These proteins are often very toxic to susceptible larvae; but to nontarget organisms they are highly specific, exhibiting little or no activity. (Siegel and Shadduck 1990; Saik et al. 1990; Lacey and Mulla 1990).

Bacillus thuringiensis subsp. *israelensis*

A new strain of the well-known insect pathogen *B. thuringiensis* was isolated from dead mosquito larvae discovered in the Negev Desert of Israel in 1976 (Goldberg and Margalit 1977; Margalit and Dean 1985; Margalit 1990) and was named *B. thuringiensis* subsp. *israelensis (Bti)* (de Barjac 1980). *Bti* was found to exhibit a high level of insecticidal activity toward larvae of practically all mosquito species as well as black flies. *Bti* was an organism whose time was right. The efficacy and safety of lepidopteran *B. thuringiensis* strains, as well as fermentation and formulation technology, were understood by the companies producing them, the users, and the governmental regulatory agencies. Developing insect resistance to chemical insecticides and environmental concerns made microbial

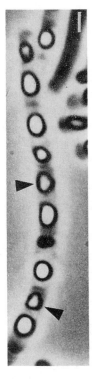

32.1A *Bacillus thuringiensis* subsp. *israelensis* sporulating cells, light micrograph. Arrows indicate parasporal crystals containing toxins.

control agents attractive, despite the cost. Thus, the remarkably rapid advance of *Bti* to registration in 1980. Currently *Bti* is commercially produced and used in many countries (Davidson 1990).

Bti produces 4 toxin proteins that bear sequence similarity to the toxins produced by lepidopteran-toxic strains of *B. thuringiensis* and are referred to as the cryIVA, B, C, and D proteins. The 5th toxin of *Bti*, called the cytA protein, shows no sequence homology to the other *B. thuringiensis* toxin proteins and is cytotoxic (Hofte and Whiteley 1989; Federici et al. 1990; Priest 1992). These toxins apparently act synergistically (Chang et al. 1993). The parasporal body is composed of several distinct particles, each of which may contain a single toxin protein (Fig. 32.1B) (Federici et al. 1990).

Specific glycoprotein receptors on the larval midgut brush border have been postulated for the *B. thuringiensis* cry toxins. The relatively nonspecific cytotoxic cytA toxin of *Bti*, however, binds to lipids. Colloidosmotic lysis is probably the common mode of action for all the *B. thuringiensis* toxins (Gill et al. 1992).

Because *Bti* is safe for most nontarget organisms, it can be readily integrated into vector control programs to provide environmentally safe control of mosquito larvae (Lacey and Undeen 1986; Davidson 1990; Mulla 1990). *Bti* has also proven to be effective against both nuisance black flies in North America and against vectors of onchocerciasis (Chap. 7) in the Onchocerciasis Control Programme in West Africa (Lacey and Undeen 1986; Molloy 1990; Guillet et al. 1990; Davidson 1990).

Bacillus sphaericus

The insecticidal strains of *B. sphaericus* also produce parasporal inclusions that contain highly potent pro-

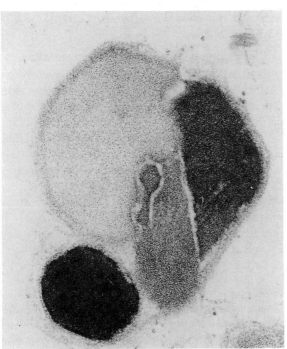

32.1B Ultrastructure of the *B. thuringiensis* subsp. *israelensis* parasporal crystal. Figs. 32.1A and 32.1B adapted from Federici et al. 1990., *Bacterial Control of Mosquitoes and Black Flies: Biochemistry, Genetics, and Applications of* Bacillus thuringiensis israelensis *and* Bacillus sphaericus, edited by Huguette de Barjac and Donald J. Sutherland. Copyright © 1990 by Rutgers, The State University. Reprinted by permission of Rutgers University Press.

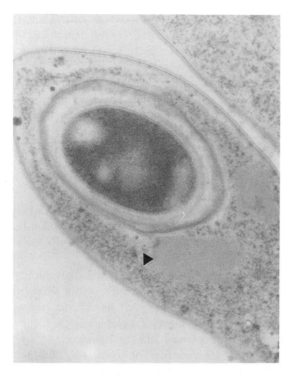

32.2 Ultrastructure of the *Bacillus sphaericus* spore and parasporal crystal. Arrow indicates paraspore. Courtesy of A.A.Yousten.

tein toxins (Fig. 32.2). However, unlike *Bti*, the toxins of *B. sphaericus* are toxic to a much narrower range of insects. Susceptibility of mosquito larvae varies from one species to another even within a genus. Certain mosquito species, such as *Cx. quinquefasciatus* and *Anopheles gambiae*, are highly susceptible to the toxins of *B. sphaericus*, whereas *Ae. aegypti* larvae are 100- to 1000-fold less susceptible (Singer 1990; Lacey and Mulla 1980; Davidson 1990; Baumann et al. 1991; Berry et al. 1991). Black fly larvae and other tested organisms are not significantly susceptible to these toxins (Lacey and Mulla 1990; Siegel and Shadduck 1990; Saik et al. 1990). Two *B. sphaericus* strains, 1593 and 2362, are the most widely used because of their high, relatively stable toxicity to *Cx. quinquefasciatus*.

The principle toxin of *B. sphaericus* is a binary toxin consisting of 2 proteins, 51.4 kDa and 41.9 kDa, respectively, both of which are required for a high level of insecticidal activity (Broadwell et al. 1990; Baumann et al. 1991; Berry et al. 1991; Priest 1992). These proteins are not homologous to the toxins of *Bti* or other *B. thuringiensis* strains. Receptor binding is apparently also important in the susceptibility of mosquito species to this toxin (Davidson 1988). The *B. sphaericus* toxins produce rapid effects on midgut cells of susceptible larvae (Charles 1987). The exact function of each of the binary toxin proteins is not yet clear; however, the 51.4 kDa protein is likely responsible for regional internalization of the 41.9 kDa protein in larval midgut cells (Oei et al. 1992). Another protein toxin of about 97 kDa, which is not homologous to either the binary toxin or to *B. thuringiensis* toxins, is also produced by *B. sphaericus* (Thanabalu et al. 1991).

Despite its more limited host range, *B. sphaericus* provides more persistent insecticidal activity than *Bti* under some conditions, and it can be readily cultured and formulated by commercial producers or local mosquito control agencies (Davidson 1990; Lacey and Undeen 1986; Lacey 1990). Local production of *B. sphaericus* has been successfully practiced in China, Brazil, Nigeria, Malaysia, and Thailand (Bhumiratana 1990; Yap 1990). *B. sphaericus* strain 2362 has been registered by the U.S. Environmental Protection Agency (USEPA).

Clostridium bifermentans serovar. *malaysia*

A mosquito larvicidal strain of *C. bifermentans* was isolated from a bacterial mixture originating from mud collected in Malaysia. It is strictly anaerobic and produces amorphous parasporal inclusions during sporulation, as well as bottle brush–like appendages. The insecticidal toxin of *C. bifermentans* serovar. *malaysia* is associated with the parasporal inclusions but declines at lysis of the sporangium, probably because of proteases present in the culture. This toxin is most active against *Anopheles* spp. larvae, a feature that makes it very attractive. The mode of action differs from that of *Bti* and *B. sphaericus* (de Barjac et al. 1990; Nicolas et al. 1990).

Fungi

Fungal pathogens of insects are characterized by relatively slow pathology, generally requiring contact between host cuticle and infectious spore, recognition of the host, spore germination, penetration of the cuticle, vegetative growth in the hemocoel, death of the host due to starvation or invasion of vital organs, and eventual emergence of the next generation of infectious fungal forms. The host sometimes raises an effective immune response to fungal infection. In general, fungi infect a wider range of hosts than bacteria; however, strain or pathotype differences in host range and virulence are well documented. Fungi are both moisture and temperature dependent, and most have a resistant spore stage or other method of survival between host infections (McCoy 1990; Carruthers and Hural 1990).

Three fungal pathogens of mosquito larvae are recognized as having significant potential as microbial control agents.

Lagenidium giganteum

This fungus undergoes both asexual and sexual cycles, infecting many mosquito species. *L. giganteum* can recycle among hosts every 2–3 days, and its sexual propagule, the oospore, is capable of survival for up to 7 years under adverse environmental conditions (Kerwin and Washino 1988). A motile, biflagellated zoospore locates and encysts on the cuticle (usually on the head or siphon/anal gills) of a mosquito larva. Upon penetration, mycelia extend through the hemocoel, resulting in death of the larva, probably by starvation, within 24–72 hours. Further asexual zoospore production follows. Alternatively, the fungus can reproduce sexually to form highly resistant oospores, which upon germination produce infectious zoospores (Lacey and Undeen 1986). Production of the oospore stage in artificial culture has been accomplished (Domnas 1981; Kerwin et al. 1986; Kerwin and Washino 1986a,b). Oospores of *L. giganteum* are particularly useful for control of low-density hosts in situations in which long-term storage, persistence, and asynchronous germination are important. Zoospores can be used to control high-density hosts. Endemic mycosis has been observed for several years following applications of *L. giganteum* in California rice fields (Lacey and Undeen 1986). Products based on mycelium and oospores of *L. giganteum* were registered by USEPA in 1991 (Kerwin 1992).

Culicinomyces clavisporus

This imperfect fungus has a very broad host range among mosquitoes and readily produces infectious conidia in artificial culture. In contrast to most fungi, *C. clavisporus* spores generally must be ingested by the larvae, whereupon the spores adhere to the cuticle-lined foregut or hindgut, germinate, penetrate the cuticle, and proliferate in the larval body. The host often mounts an immune response to invasion by this fungus. Following death of the larva, the fungus sporulates on the surface of the dead host (Sweeney 1981). Temperature-dependent activity, difficulties in storage, high dosages required for field efficacy, and lack of adequate persistence and recycling in the field have caused interest in development of this fungus to decline (Lacey and Undeen 1986).

Coelomomyces spp.

These obligately parasitic fungi infect a broad range of mosquitoes and have frequently been described from natural epizootics. Attempts to infect mosquito larvae with this fungus in the laboratory were unsuccessful until the discovery of an obligate intermediate stage in a copepod (Whistler et al. 1974). Biflagellate zygotes penetrate the mosquito larval cuticle, producing hyphal bodies and eventually mycelia in the hemocoel. Thick-walled sporangia form, which are released from the dead larva. Meiosis occurs in the sporangia, forming haploid zoospores that invade the copepod, in which another mycelium is formed. This mycelium transforms into the gametangium, which releases thousands of haploid uniflagellate gametes of either male or female mating type into the water. Fusion of 2 opposite mating-type gametes produces the biflagellated zygote, which then infects mosquito larvae (Sweeney 1981; Lacey and Undeen 1986). Heavy infections can kill mosquito larvae; however, lightly infected mosquitoes can survive to adulthood, providing a mechanism for dispersal of the fungus. Because of its complex life cycle, in vitro mass production of this fungus has not yet been accomplished.

Protozoa

There are perhaps more types of protozoa identified from mosquito and black fly larvae than any other type of pathogen. The most common and most extensively studied of these are the Microsporidia, members of the phylum Microspora. These are intracellular parasitic protozoans that produce a coiled polar filament in the spore. When spores are ingested by an appropriate host, the polar filament is forcibly ejected, penetrating and infecting the gut cells. Microsporidians infecting vector larvae include those with a single spore type and those with 2 or more spore types. *Nosema* and *Vavraia* spp. produce a single spore type, develop asexually, and are relatively easily transmitted in the laboratory. Although these Microsporidia have a broad host range, they usually produce low mortality and do not persist in the environment and are therefore not likely to be useful in vector control.

The polymorphic Microsporidia, however, are transmitted both transovarially and orally, have a wide host range, consistently produce high mortality, and persist in the environment. The simultaneous discovery in the United States and Australia of an intermediate cycle for the polymorphic microsporidian *Amblyospora* spp. in the copepod (Andreadis 1985; Sweeney et al. 1985), as well as recent elucidation of the complex life cycles of other polymorphic species (some of which do not require intermediate hosts), have opened the door to further development of these microorganisms (Sweeney and Becnel 1991).

Amblyospora spp.

In response to acquisition of a blood meal by the adult female mosquito, *Amblyospora* spp. undergoes sporulation, germination, and infection of the oocytes, assuring vertical transmission to the next generation. Some female progeny obtain a benign infection and again transmit the infection transovarially. In other infected female larvae and in male larvae, the microsporidian enters into meiosis and sporulation, producing thousands of haploid spores in the fat body, killing the larva. When these haploid spores are ingested by a female copepod, an asexual cycle is initiated, eventually leading to the production of haploid spores that are released on death of the copepod. When eaten by a mosquito larva, the haploid spores invade the tissues, in which they enter a sexual phase including cell fusion, returning to the diploid state.

Female mosquitoes thus infected can then transmit the protozoan transovarially to reinitiate the cycle (Andreadis and Hall 1979; Andreadis 1985; Sweeney et al. 1985; Andreadis 1990). Detailed laboratory and field studies of the *Amblyospora connecticus* cycle in *Ae. cantator* and the copepod *Acanthocyclops vernalis* have shown that this protozoan can produce regular epizootics in mosquito populations and has a natural regulatory effect (Andreadis 1983; 1990). These protozoa are examples of microbial control agents that can be used in inoculative releases (Sweeney and Becnel 1991).

Nematodes

Although insect-parasitic nematodes are not microorganisms, their small size, persistence in the environment, and utility in insect control have led to their being included in most discussions of insect pathogens. Eggs of mermithid nematodes are laid in the substrate of mosquito larval habitats and remain dormant unless free water is present at the proper temperature. The eggs then develop and the preparasite emerges. The preparasite actively swims until it contacts a mosquito larva, attaches to the host by means of a stylet, and bores a hole through the cuticle. The larva is not generally killed, and the nematode grows for 7–8 days in the larva, whereupon it molts to the postparasitic stage and exits, killing the host. The nematode then burrows into the substrate, matures to the adult stage, mates, and lays eggs. The life cycle can require a few weeks or a year, depending upon the temperature and nematode species (Petersen 1985). Several species of nematodes are known as specific parasites of mosquito or black fly larvae, but only *Romanomermis culicivorax* has been developed for vector control. This nematode exhibits a relatively broad host range among mosquito species; however, it is active only in relatively warm waters and is inhibited by salinity and other environmental factors. A mass production system was devised for *R. culicivorax* using *Cx. pipiens* larvae as hosts, and a product was made available for a few years (Petersen 1985). Although this nematode is no longer commercially available, other insect parasitic nematodes are produced commercially, and *R. culicivorax* could eventually return to large-scale production.

NEW DEVELOPMENTS IN MICROBIAL CONTROL OF VECTORS

Several factors stand in the way of microbial control agents achieving their full potential, including settling of the active agent out of the feeding zone, sensitivity of the pathogen to environmental factors, requirement for an intermediate host, limited pathogenicity or host range, and restrictions imposed by governmental agencies. In addition to new formulation technologies, several innovative genetic approaches are being applied to these organisms in an attempt to extend their usefulness as vector control agents.

Several *Bacillus* toxins have been cloned into organisms that normally inhabit the larval feeding zone near the water surface. *B. sphaericus* and *Bti* toxins have been inserted into the cyanobacteria *Anacystis nidulans*, *Synechococcus* spp., and *Agmenellum quadruplicatum*, producing low-to-fair toxicity (DeMarsac et al. 1987; Angsuthanasombat and Panyim 1989; Chungjatupornchai 1990; Murphy and Stephens 1992). *Bti* and *B. sphaericus* toxins have also been cloned into *Caulobacter crescentus*, which inhabits the water-air interface, again producing low-to-moderate toxicity (Thanabalu et al. 1992). Although these attempts have not yet resulted in recombinant organisms of high activity, they demonstrate the feasibility of combining the rapid activity of an inundative application with the persistence of an inoculation.

Recombination to obtain the wide host range of *Bti* and the persistence of *B. sphaericus* is an obvious goal. The *Bti* cytA and cryIVD toxin genes (Bar et al. 1991) as well as the cryIVB toxin gene (Trisrisook et al. 1990) have been cloned into *B. sphaericus* 2362, resulting in increased toxicity to *Ae. aegypti*. *B. sphaericus* binary toxin genes were cloned into both crystalliferous and acrystalliferous *Bti* without synergism or additive effects (Bourgouin et al. 1990).

Recent success in isolation of *B. thuringiensis* strains that target insects, nematodes, and even protozoa (Feitelson et al. 1992), and the discovery of mosquito larvicidal activity in *Clostridium* (de Barjac et al. 1990), confirm that many useful organisms have not yet been discovered. Although a relatively simple task, isolation of new pathogens is still one of the most fruitful ways of increasing the utility of microbial control.

A SUCCESSFUL INTEGRATED MOSQUITO CONTROL PROGRAM USING MICROBIAL CONTROL AGENTS: THE KOMMUNALE AKTIONSGEMEINSCHAFT ZUR BEKAMPFUNG DER SCHNAKENPLAGE (KABS)

History of Mosquito Control in Germany

The control of mosquitoes in Germany began in 1911 with the foundation of the first organization dealing with mosquito control in the Upper Rhine Valley, where floodwater mosquitoes constitute a tremendous nuisance nearly every summer. In the 1920s and 1930s, breeding sites were treated with petroleum oils (Bresslau and Glaser 1918; Martini 1937; Peus 1940; Eckstein 1939). During the 1950s and 1960s, chemical insecticides such as DDT were used against adult mosquitoes. However, these chemical insecticides very often produced undesirable side effects such as resistance and ecological damage.

After publication of Rachel Carson's *Silent Spring*, public awareness of environmental issues increased, and regulations controlling the application of chemicals for mosquito control were tightened. National and international organizations such as the World Health Organization supported the development of new integrated control strategies.

In the early 1970s, there were no mosquito control activities carried out in Germany. In 1975, the mosquito population in the Upper Rhine Valley was extremely high because of frequent fluctuations of the water level of the Rhine River. As a reaction to this nuisance, about 100 towns and villages on both sides of the Rhine River joined to form a voluntary mosquito control organization, the KABS. Today, the territory of the KABS covers approximately 300 river km with about 500 km^2 of inundation area (Becker and Ludwig 1983). Every member town contributes approximately 50 cents U.S. per citizen; the yearly budget of about $1.2 million serves about 2.5 million people in the KABS area. The main goal of the KABS is to reduce the abundance of mosquitoes to a tolerable level without damaging the ecologically sensitive riverbank areas. This goal has been achieved through the widespread use of *Bacillus thuringiensis* subsp. *israelensis* and the increasing use of *Bacillus sphaericus* in recent years.

The control activities of the KABS are aiming at the mosquito larvae for the following reasons:

1. Mosquito larvae are concentrated in breeding sites, whereas the adults of floodwater mosquitoes migrate out into a large area.

2. Selective biological control agents are available only for mosquito larvae.

3. It is unlikely that resistance will occur with the use of microbial control agents in the foreseeable future (McGaughey 1985; Kurtak 1986; Tabashnik et al. 1990).

The integrated mosquito control program of the KABS combines the legitimate demand of concerned inhabitants to control the mosquitoes with the requirements of environmental protection of ecologically sensitive areas.

Implementation of Microbial Control Agents in the KABS

Mapping of the Breeding Sites

The first phase of the control operations in Germany was to map the breeding sites. Each significant location was numbered for quick reference during control and for communication among the field staff. The operational area of the KABS is divided into several districts according to the morphological and topographical structure of the area. The numbering follows a system that enables a quick localization of the breeding site. For example, 01–99 indicates the district or breeding area of a community; 001–999 indicates the number of a breeding site within the specific district. The numbers follow a system from south to north. The type of breeding site is indicated by the numbers 1–9. For instance, "08–199–1" means breeding site No. 199 in District 8, which is a flooded meadow (breeding site type 1).

The ecological relationships within a region must influence the planning of the control strategy. Therefore the mapping must reflect not only the target organisms but also nontarget organisms, or rare birds or plants that can be affected by the treatment, to minimize disturbance of wildlife and the natural flora. The intervention strategy is chosen as follows:

1. Areas without restrictions have no special ecological features that could be disturbed by the intervention. Any application technique can be used.

2. Areas with rare plants or densely reeded areas are usually treated by helicopter to prevent damage to vegetation. Breeding areas of songbirds are treated by helicopters operating at high altitudes.

3. Areas in which birds of prey breed in the forest canopy are usually entered by foot and treated by hand.

4. In well-defined, limited areas of special ecological interest, no control treatments take place. These regions should contain no extensive mass breeding sites of floodwater mosquitoes.

The maps also contain information such as the elevation above sea level to indicate the sequence of floodings and the major types of vegetation. Each zone is marked with a color (e.g., dark blue = permanent water body, light blue = semipermanent water body, green = extremely temporary body, light red = thickly reeded area grown with *Phragmites communis*).

The application of microbial control agents in a mosaic-like pattern, with ecological consideration and under the supervision of biologists, allows effective as well as environmentally nonintrusive mosquito control in protected areas and nature reserves.

Entomological Evaluations

Precise knowledge of the biology and ecology of the mosquitoes is one of the most important prerequisites for successfully implementing mosquito control. In the preparation phase, baseline data are collected, including occurrence of adults and their developing stages in relation to abiotic and biotic conditions, e.g., egg-laying and hatching behavior, temperature-dependent larval and pupal development, and migration and biting behavior of the most abundant species (Becker 1989; Becker and Ludwig 1981). At regular intervals at least 10 dips are taken from each plot. Larval instars and pupae are separately recorded, and a sample of 4th instar larvae and emerged adults are identified to species.

Adult landing rate determinations and CO_2–light trap catches are conducted at regular intervals in swamps, at the outskirts of settlements, inside towns, inside houses, and at different times of the day and seasons. Different abiotic conditions, especially humidity, temperature, wind, and sunshine, are considered as well. This monitoring system provides information on the natural occurrence of mosquitoes and the success of the control intervention.

Three important mosquito populations have been distinguished in the Upper Rhine Valley:

1. Mosquitoes developing in the immediate river floodlands: In the neutral to alkaline water bodies, the polycyclic *Ae. vexans* is by far the dominant pest species during summertime; *Ae. sticticus, Ae. rossicus,* and *Ae. cinereus* are less common. Other species are insignificant.

2. Mosquito populations originating in the swampy woodlands above river level, including mostly monocyclic snowmelt mosquitoes such as *Ae. cantans, Ae. communis, Ae. punctor,* and *Ae. rusticus.*

3. *Culex pipiens,* the main pest in houses, breeds in rainwater containers and in other water bodies during summertime.

Ae. vexans is the major nuisance species during summertime, comprising more than 80% of all mosquitoes during the summer peaks of the Rhine water level. It is not unusual for several hundred to thousands of mosquito larvae per 1-L dip to be counted, which amounts to hundreds of millions of larvae per hectare water surface. *Ae. vexans* eggs diapause in the winter. Decreasing temperatures in fall, frost periods, and increasing temperatures in the spring make the larvae in the eggs respond to the hatching stimuli when the water level of the Rhine rises and the water temperature is at least 10°C. Therefore, the water peaks from April to September lead to development of

Ae. vexans and the need for mosquito control in the floodlands. During this period, the water level of the Rhine is influenced by melting snow in the Alps, which is increased by periods of continuous rainfall. There is no regularity in the time of flooding, but there is the certainty that flooding will occur one or more times during the season.

Assessment of the Efficacy of Microbial Control Agents

The basic requirement for successful use of microbial control agents is the development of effective formulations suited to the biology and habitats of the target organisms. Preparations can now be obtained as wettable powders, fluid concentrates, granules, pellets, briquettes, and tablets.

The efficacy of microbial control agents is influenced by a variety of biotic and abiotic factors: the susceptibility of the target mosquito species, the stage of development, the feeding behavior of mosquito larvae, the temperature and quality of water, the intensity of sunlight, the density of mosquito larvae populations, and the presence of filter-feeding nontarget organisms (Mulla et al. 1990; Becker et al. 1992). Characteristics of the formulation, such as potency, sedimentation rate, and shelf life, will also influence its effectiveness. Preliminary laboratory evaluation is therefore necessary to assess the potency and efficacy against the indigenous mosquito species and to assess the minimum and optimum effective dosages in small field tests.

Standardized methods have been developed to determine the LC_{50} (lethal concentration killing 50% of test larvae)/LC_{90} values using Institut Pasteur Standard (IPS) formulations for comparison purposes (e.g., IPS–82 produced by the Institut Pasteur, Paris; de Barjac 1983). The potency is expressed in international toxic units (ITUs). Bioassays are run according the World Health Organization guidelines (WHO 1981), and the results are subjected to log-probit-analysis to determine LC-values.

The optimum dosages of the most effective formulations have been determined in preliminary small-scale field tests in the Upper Rhine Valley. At least 3 replicates at each dosage (e.g., 2, 4, and 8 times the LC^{90}) were conducted, and similar untreated plots served as controls. Larval density was monitored before treatment and 1, 2, 4, and 7 days or longer following treatment.

A few hundred grams or less of powder (e.g., Bactimos®, Teknar TC®, Vectobac®) or ¹/₂–2 L of liquid concentrate (e.g., Bactimos FC®, Teknar HP-D®, or Vectobac® 12AS) per hectare are sufficient to kill all mosquito larvae. During the period of continuous high water, granule formulations are applied by helicopters. Commercially available granules based on corncobs (Bactimos® and Vectobac® granules) show excellent results when applied at rates of 8–15 kg/ha (kilogram/hectar). Locally produced sand granules can also serve as a vehicle for wettable powder formulations: 50 kg of fire-dried quartz sand (grain size 0.9–2 mm), 0.8–1.4 L litres of vegetable oil (as a binding material), and 0.9–1.8 kg *Bti* powder are mixed in a cement mixer. This mixure is sufficient for treating 2–3 ha.

Bti has a relatively brief activity after it has been applied; it thus must be frequently reapplied. In recent years pellet, briquette, and tablet formulations have provided greater residual control. For instance, larval *Cx. pipiens* in rain barrels can be effectively controlled for more than a month by *Bti* or *B. sphaericus* briquettes. Tablets containing *Bti* material sterilized by radiation to prevent contamination of drinking water can be successfully used for control of container breeding mosquitoes such *as Ae. aegypti,* the main vector of dengue fever (Becker et al. 1991). Tablets based on radiated *B. sphaericus* controlled *Cx. pipiens* breeding close to human settlements for several weeks. Fluid and powder formulations of *B. sphaericus* also provided excellent control of *Cx. pipiens* larvae up to several months under certain conditions.

When appropriately stored, most *Bti* or *B. sphaericus* preparations can be kept for a long time without losing activity; however, preparations should be retested after they have been stored for more than a year in temperate climates or after 6 months in tropical regions. Fluid concentrates can be more unstable. Powder formulations lose little of their activity even after many years of storage.

Operational Use of Microbial Control Agents in Germany

A crucial component of the German mosquito control organization is an adequately trained and efficient team as well as a smoothly functioning, tight organization. In every community with mosquito mass breeding sites, 2 persons are responsible for mosquito control, often supported by well-trained students from local universities. District leaders (experienced staff members) coordinate the control work in their districts and train the field staff. In total, about 300 persons are generally involved. The following methods are used in the KABS:

Microbial Control Agents

Today, mosquitoes in more than 90% of the KABS area are controlled exclusively with *Bti*. In routine treatments against 1st and 2nd instar larvae or in shallow breeding sites, about 125 g of *Bti* wettable powder (activity = 10,000 ITU/mg) are mixed with 10 L of screen-filtered pond water for each hectare treated and applied with a high-pressure knapsack sprayer. In deeper breeding sites or when 3rd or early 4th instar larvae are present, this dosage is doubled. Alternatively, one L of liquid *Bti* concentrate (Teknar HP-D® or Vectobac® 12AS) is mixed with 9 L of screen-filtered pond water per ha (3 x 109 ITUs per ha). When high water levels on the Rhine cause widespread inundation or when dense vegetation occurs, *Bti* sand or corncob granules are applied.

Between 1981 and 1992, about 53,000 ha of mosquito breeding sites were successfully treated with about 23 tons of *Bti* wettable powder and 20,000 L of liquid concentrate. The wettable powder was also used to produce approximately 350 tons of *Bti* sand granules.

Bacillus sphaericus preparations are increasingly being used against *Cx. pipiens molestus* in and around human settlements.

Water Management and Related Measures

The protection and encouragement of all natural predators is a very important part of the KABS integrated mosquito control program. Temporary ponds are deepened to provide permanent habitats for aquatic predators, and ditch systems are improved to facilitate fish movement. Additionally, nesting and resting habitats for swallows and bats as predators of adult mosquitoes are provided. Because predators such as fish are not affected by microbial control agents, they continue to feed upon newly hatching mosquito larvae after the breeding sites have been treated, and in some cases no further treatments are necessary.

Educational Programs

Interventions against *Cx. pipiens molestus* near houses are based on provision of information to the general public on the biology of these mosquitoes and on strategies for their control. In information sheets, tips are given on how people can control breeding sites themselves, including source reduction by environmental sanitation; protection of water containers by lids to prevent oviposition; release of larvivorous fish; observance of a "weekly dry day" (containers are totally emptied at least every 10 days); and use of *Bti* and *B. sphaericus* tablets or briquettes when other measures cannot be applied.

Success of the Intervention

Beside measuring the efficacy of the treatments 24 hours after application by dipping, the adult mosquito population is monitored by using CDC light traps twice a month from dawn to sunrise at about 40 different sites in treated and untreated areas. The comparison of the catches in treated and untreated areas permits estimation of the percentage reduction of mosquito populations. Additionally, a special bell-shaped net is used, which is fixed to a branch. When the net is open, the mosquitoes can attack the tester, who is standing under the net. After 2 minutes, the net is dropped and the mosquitoes are counted with an aspirator. In 1985, a tester received up to 350 bites in 2 minutes in untreated swamps, whereas in treated areas at the same time only 2–16 bites were counted.

These measurements have demonstrated that the program reduces the floodwater mosquito population by more than 90% each year. Mosquitoes are no longer a pest in the KABS member communities. This has been highly respected by the public, especially regarding the low cost and tremendous increase in the quality of life.

Monitoring the Environmental Impact of the Control Intervention

The direct impact of the treatments to the aquatic fauna is determined in ecotoxicological studies with the microbial control agents. Selected ponds are treated with *Bti* or *B. sphaericus,* and the development of aquatic organisms is monitored by emergence traps. All insects, especially chironomids, are sampled in treated and untreated parts of the test ponds. In laboratory and field tests during the past 10 years, none of the tested taxa (e.g., Cnidaria, Turbellaria, Rotatoria, Mollusca, Annelida, Acari, Crustacea, Ephemeroptera, Odonata, Heteroptera, Coleoptera, Trichoptera, Pisces, and Amphibia) appeared to be affected when exposed to water containing large amounts of *Bti* or *B. sphaericus* (Schnetter et al. 1981; Margalit et al. 1985; Becker and Margalit 1993). Even among the dipterans, the toxicity of *Bti* is restricted to larval mosquitoes and black flies and closely related dixids. Larval psychodids, chironomids, sciarids, and tipulids generally are far less sensitive than mosquitoes and black flies (Smits and Vlug 1990). Predatory and semiterrestrial chironomids, such as *Smitta* spp., and carnivorous larval ceratopogonids are not affected. The composition of adult insect fauna in treated and untreated regions has shown that because of the selectivity of microbial control agents no significant changes occur in the food chain. Birds, amphibians, and other organisms are not endangered by the operational use of microbial control agents.

The successful use of microbial control agents in the integrated mosquito control program in Germany requires close cooperation among authorities, scientists, industry, and the public. Although model projects cannot be identically transferred without modification from one area to another, the integrated mosquito control program in Germany can serve as a model program that demonstrates the general principles of implementation of a program using biological control agents. The cooperative program developed between the KABS and the Province of Hubei in China is an example of transfer of this technology, resulting in significant reduction in the incidence of malaria during a 3-year period (Xu et al. 1992).

REFERENCES

Andreadis, T.G. 1983. An epizootic *Amblyospora* sp. in field populations of the mosquito, *Aedes cantator. J. Invertebr. Pathol.* 42:427–430.

———. 1985. Experimental transmission of a microsporidian pathogen from mosquitoes to an alternate copepod host. *Proc. Nat. Acad. Sci. USA* 82:5574.

———. 1990. Polymorphic microsporidia of mosquitoes: Potential for biological control. In: R.R. Baker and P.E. Dunn, editors, *New directions in biological control: Alternatives for suppressing agricultural pests and diseases: Proceedings of a UCLA Colloquium.* New York: A.R. Liss. pp. 177–188.

Andreadis, T.G., and D.W. Hall. 1979. Development, ultrastructure, and mode of transmission of *Amblyospora* sp. in the mosquito. *J. Protozool.* 26:444–452.

Angsuthanasombat, C., and S. Panyim. 1989. Biosynthesis of 130-kilodalton mosquito larvicide in the cyanobacterium *Agmenellum quadruplicatum* PR–6. *Appl. Environ. Microbiol.* 55:2428–2430.

Bar, E., J. Lieman-Hurwitz, E. Rahamim, A. Keynan, and N. Sandler. 1991. Cloning and expression of *Bacillus thuringiensis* delta-endotoxin DNA in *B. sphaericus. J. Invertebr. Pathol.* 57:149–158.

Baumann, P., M.A. Clark, L. Baumann, and A.H. Broadwell. 1991. *Bacillus sphaericus* as a mosquito pathogen: Properties of the organism and its toxins. *Microbiol. Revs.* 55:425–436.

Becker, N. 1989. Life strategies of mosquitoes as an adaptation to their habitats. *Bull. Soc. Vector Ecol.* 14(1):6–25.

———. 1992. Community participation in the operational use of microbial control agents in mosquito control programs. *Bull. Soc. Vector Ecol.* 17:114–118.

Becker, N., and H.W. Ludwig. 1981. Untersuchungen zur Faunistik und oekologie der Culicinae und ihrer Pathogene im Oberrheingebiet. Mitt. dtsch. Ges. allg. angew. *Entomol.* 2:186–194.

———. 1983. Mosquito Control in West Germany. *Bull. Soc. Vector Ecol.* 8:85–93.

Becker, N., and J. Margalit. 1993. Use of *Bacillus thuringiensis* subsp. *israelensis* against mosquitoes and black flies. In: P.F. Entwistle, J.S. Cory, M.J. Bailey, and S. Higgs, editors, Bacillus thuringiensis, *an environmental pesticide: Theory and practice.* New York: J. Wiley. pp. 147–170.

Becker, N., S. Djakaria, A. Kaiser, O. Zuhasril, and H.W. Ludwig. 1991. Efficacy of a new tablet formulation of an asporogenous strain of *Bacillus thuringiensis israelensis* against larvae of *Aedes aegypti. Bull. Soc. Vector Ecol.* 16:176–182.

Becker, N., F. Rettich, M. Zgomba, D. Petric, M. Ludwig, and G. Ryba. 1992. Factors influencing the efficacy of the microbial control agent *Bacillus thuringiensis israelensis. J. Amer. Mosq. Control Assoc.* 8:285–289.

Berry, C., J. Hindley, and C. Oei, 1991. The *Bacillus sphaericus* toxins and their potential for biotechnological development. In: K. Maramorosch, editor, *Biotechnology for biological control of pests and vectors.* Boca Raton, FL: CRC Press. pp. 35–51.

Bhumiratana, A. 1990. Local production of *Bacillus sphaericus.* In: H. de Barjac and D.J. Sutherland, editors, *Bacterial control of mosquitoes and black flies.* New Brunswick, NJ: Rutgers Univ. Press. pp. 272–283.

Bourgouin, C., A. Delecluse, F. de la Torre, and J. Szulmajster. 1990. Transfer of the toxin protein genes of *Bacillus sphaericus* into *Bacillus thuringiensis* subsp. *israelensis* and their expression. *Appl. Environ. Microbiol.* 56:340–344.

Bresslau, E., and F. Glaser. 1918. Die Sommerbekampfung der Stechmucken. *Z.f.angew. Entomol.* 4:290–296.

Broadwell, A.H., L. Baumann, and P. Baumann. 1990. Larvicidal properties of the 42 and 51 kilodalton *Bacillus sphaericus* proteins expressed in different bacterial hosts: Evidence for a binary topxin. *Curr. Microbiol.* 21:361–366.

Carruthers, R.I., and K. Hural. 1990. Fungi as naturally occurring entomopathogens. In: R.R. Baker and P.E. Dunn, editors, *New directions in biological control: Alternatives for suppressing agricultural pests and diseases: Proceedings of a UCLA colloquium.* New York: A.R. Liss. pp. 115–138.

Chang, C., Y-M. Yu, S-M. Dai, S.K. Law, and S.S. Gill. 1993. High-level cryIVD and cytA gene expression in *Bacillus thuringiensis* does not require the 20-kilodalton protein, and the coexpressed gene products are synergistic in their toxicity of mosquitoes. *Appl. Environ. Microbiol.* 59:815–821.

Charles, J-F. 1987. Ultrastructural midgut events in *Culicidae* larvae fed with *Bacillus sphaericus* 2297 spore/crystal complex. *Ann. Inst. Pasteur* (Paris) 138:471–484.

Chungjatupornchai, W. 1990. Expression of the mosquitocidal-protein genes of *Bacillus thuringiensis* subsp. *israelensis* and the herbicide-resistance gene bar in *Synechocystis* PCC6803. *Curr. Microbiol.* 21:283–288.

Davidson, E.W. 1988. Binding of the *Bacillus sphaericus* toxin to midgut cells of mosquito larvae: Relationship to host range. *J. Med. Entomol.* 25:151–157.

———. 1990. Microbial control of vector insects. In: R.R. Baker and P.E. Dunn, editors, *New directions in biological control: Alternatives for suppressing agricultural pests and diseases: Proceedings of a UCLA colloquium.* New York: A.R. Liss. pp. 199–212.

de Barjac, H. 1983. Bioassay procedure for samples of *Bacillus thuringiensis israelensis* using IPS–82 standard. WHO Report TDR/VED/SWG (5)(81.3). Geneva: World Health Organization.

de Barjac, H. 1990. Characterization and prospective view of *Bacillus thuringiensis* israelensis. In: H. de Barjac and D.J. Sutherland, editors, *Bacterial control of mosquitoes and black flies.* New Brunswick, NJ: Rutgers Univ. Press. pp. 10–15.

de Barjac, H., M. Siebald, J-F. Charles, W.H. Cheong, and H.L. Lee. 1990. *Clostridium bifermentans* serovar *malaysia,* une nouvelle bacterie anaerobie pathogene des larves de moustiques et de simulies. *CR Acad. Sci. Paris* 310:383–387.

de Marsac, N.G., F. de la Torre, and J. Szulmajster. 1987. Expression of the larvicidal gene of *Bacillus sphaericus* 1593M in the cyanobacterium *Anacystis nidulans* R2. *Mol. Gen. Genet.* 209:396–398.

Domnas, A.J. 1981. Biochemistry of *Lagenidium giganteum* infection in mosquito larvae. In: E.W. Davidson, editor, *Pathogenesis of invertebrate microbial diseases.* Totowa, NJ: Allanheld, Osmun. pp. 425–450.

Eckstein, F. 1939. Die Grundlagen der Bekampfung der Stechmuckenbrut durch oberfluchenaktive Substanzen. *Zeitschr. hyg. Zool.,* 31:237–259.

Federici, B.A. 1985. Viral pathogens. In: *Biological control of mosquitoes,* AMCA Bull. No. 6. Amer. Lake Charles, LA: Mosq. Control Assn. pp. 62–74.

Federici, B.A., P. Luthy, and J.E. Ibarra. 1990. Parasporal body of *Bacillus thuringiensis israelensis:* Structure, protein composition, and toxicity. In: H. de Barjac and D.J. Sutherland, editors, *Bacterial control of mosquitoes and black flies.* New Brunswick, NJ: Rutgers Univ. Press. pp. 16–65.

Feitelson, J.S., J. Payne, and L. Kim. 1992. *Bacillus thuringiensis:* Insects and beyond. *Biotechnol.* 10:271–275.

Gill, S.S., E.A. Cowles, and P.V. Pietrantonio. 1992. The mode of action of *Bacillus thuringiensis* endotoxins. *Ann. Rev. Entomol.* 37:615–636.

Goldberg, L.H., and J. Margalit. 1977. A bacterial spore demonstrating rapid larvicidal activity against *Anopheles sergentii, Uranotaenia unguiculata, Culex univattatus, Aedes aegypti* and *Culex pipiens. Mosq. News* 37:355–358.

Guillet, P., D.C. Kurtak, B. Philippon, and R. Meyer. 1990. Use of *Bacillus thuringiensis israelensis* for Onchocerciasis control in West Africa. In: H. de Barjac and D.J. Sutherland, editors, *Bacterial control of mosquitoes and black flies.* New Brunswick, NJ: Rutgers Univ. Press. pp. 187–201.

Hofte, H., and H.R. Whiteley. 1989. Insecticidal crystal proteins of *Bacillus thuringiensis. Microbiol. Rev.* 53:242–255.

Kerwin, J.L. 1992. EPA registers *Lagenidium giganteum* for mosquito control. *Society for Invertebrate Pathology Newsletter,* 24(2):8–9.

Kerwin, J.L., and Washino, R.K. 1986a. Regulation of oosporogenesis by *Lagenidium giganteum:* Promotion of sexual reproduction by unsaturated fatty acids and sterol availability. *Can. J. Microbiol.* 32:294–300.

———. 1986b. Oosporogenesis by *Lagenidium giganteum*: Induction and maturation are regulated by calcium and calmodulin. *Can. J. Microbiol.* 32:663–672.

———. 1988. Field evaluation of *Lagenidium giganteum* and description of a natural epizootic involving a new isolate of the fungus. *J. Med. Entomol.* 25:452–460.

Kerwin, J.L., C.A. Simmons, and R.K. Washino. 1986. Oosporogenesis by *Lagenidium giganteum* in liquid culture. *J. Invertebr. Pathol.* 47:258–270.

Kurtak, D. 1986. Insecticide resistance in the Onchocerciasis Control Programme. *Parasitol. Today* 2:20–21.

Lacey, L.A. 1990. Persistence and formulation of *Bacillus sphaericus.* In: H. de Barjac and D.J. Sutherland, editors, *Bacterial control of mosquitoes and black flies.* New Brunswick, NJ: Rutgers Univ. Press. pp.284–294.

Lacey, L.A., and Mulla, M.S. 1990. Safety of *Bacillus thuringiensis* subsp. *israelensis* and *Bacillus sphaericus* to nontarget organisms in the aquatic environment. In: M. Laird, L.A. Lacey, and E.W. Davidson *Safety of microbial insecticides.* Boca Raton, FL: CRC Press. pp. 169–188.

Lacey, L.A., and A.H. Undeen. 1986. Microbial control of black flies and mosquitoes. *Ann. Rev. Entomol.* 31:265–296.

Margalit, J. 1990. Discovery of *Bacillus thuringiensis israelensis.* In: H. de Barjac and D.J. Sutherland, editors, *Bacterial control of mosquitoes and black flies.* New Brunswick, NJ: Rutgers Univ. Press. pp. 3–9.

Margalit, J., and D. Dean. 1985. The story of *Bacillus thuringiensis israelensis* (*B. thuringiensis israelensis*). *J. Am. Mosq. Control Assoc.* 1:1–7.

Margalit, J., L. Lahkim-Tsror, H. Bobroglo, C. Paskar, and Z. Barak. 1985. Biological control of mosquitoes in Israel. In: M. Laird and J. W. Miles, editors, *Integrated control of vectors.* London: Academic Press. pp. 361–374.

Martini, E. 1937. Praktische Fragen in der Stechmuckenbekampfung. *Verh. dtsch. Ges. f. angew. Ent.* 40–59.

McCoy, C.W. 1990. Entomogenous fungi as microbial pesticides. In: R.R. Baker and P.E. Dunn, editors, *New directions in biological control: Alternatives for suppressing agricultural pests and diseases: Proceedings of a UCLA Colloquium.* New York: A.R. Liss. pp. 139–160.

McGaughey, W. l985. Insect resistance to the biological insecticide *Bacillus thuringiensis. Science* 229:193–195.

Molloy, D.P. 1990. Progress in the biological control of black flies with *Bacillus thuringiensis israelensis,* with emphasis on temperate climates. In: H. de Barjac and D.J. Sutherland, editors, *Bacterial control of mosquitoes and black flies.* New Brunswick, NJ: Rutgers Univ. Press. pp. 161–186.

Mulla, M.S. 1990. Activity, field efficacy, and use of *Bacillus thuringiensis israelensis* against mosquitoes. In: H. de Barjac and D.J. Sutherland, editors, *Bacterial control of mosquitoes and black flies.* New Brunswick, NJ: Rutgers Univ. Press.

Mulla, M.S., H.A. Darwazeh, M. Zgomba. 1990. Effect of some environmental factors on the efficacy of *Bacillus sphaericus* 2362 and *Bacillus thuringiensis* (H–14) against mosquitoes. *Bull. Soc. Vector Ecol.* 15:166–175.

Murphy, R.C., and S.E Stephens. 1992. Cloning and expression of the cryIVD gene of *Bacillus thuringiensis* subsp. *israelensis* in the cyanobacterium *Agnenellum quadruplicatum* PR–6 and its resulting larvicidal activity. *Appl. Environ. Microbiol* 58:1650–1655.

Nicolas, L., S. Hamon, E. Frachon, M. Sebald, and H. de Barjac. 1990. Partial inactivation of the mosquitocidal activity of *Clostridium bifermentans* serovar. malaysia by extracellular proteases. *Appl. Microbiol. Biotechnol.* 34:36–41.

Oei, C., J. Hindley, and C. Berry. 1992. Binding of purified *Bacillus sphaericus* binary toxin and its deletion derivatives to *Culex quinquefasciatus* gut: Elucidation of functional binding domains. *J. Gen. Microbiol.* 138:1515–1526.

Petersen, J.J. 1985. Nematode parasites. In: *Biological control of mosquitoes,* AMCA Bull. No. 6. Lake Charles, LA: Amer. Mosq. Control Assn. pp. 110–122.

Peus, F. 1940. Die Stechmuckenplage und ihre Bekampfung. II. Teil: Die *Aedes* Mucken. *Zeitschr. hyg. Zool. Schadlingsbek.* 32:49–79.

Porter, A.G., E.W. Davidson, and J-W. Liu. 1993. Mosquitocidal toxins and their genetic manipulation for effective biological control of mosquitoes. *Microbiol. Rev.* 57:838–861.

Priest, F.G. 1992. Biological control of mosquitoes and other biting flies by *Bacillus sphaericus* and *Bacillus thuringiensis. J. Appl. Bacteriol.* 72:357–369.

Roberts, D.W., and J.M. Castillo, 1980. *Bibliography on pathogens of medically important arthropods: 1980.* Suppl. to Vol. 58. Geneva: Bull. World Health Organization.197 p.

Roberts, D.W., and M.A. Strand, editors. 1977. *Pathogens of medically important arthropods.* Suppl. No. 1 to Vol. 55. Geneva: Bull. World Health Organization. 419 pp.

Roberts, D.W., R.A. Daoust, and S.P. Wraight. 1983. *Bibliography on pathogens of medically important arthropods: 1981.* VBC/83.1. Geneva: Bull. World Health Organization. 324 pp.

Saik, J.E., L.A. Lacey, and C.M. Lacey. 1990. Safety of microbial insecticides to vertebrates-Domestic animals and wildlife. In: M. Laird, L.A. Lacey, and E.W. Davidson, editors, *Safety of microbial insecticides.* Boca Raton, FL: CRC Press. pp. 115–134.

Schnetter, W., S. Engler, J. Morawcsik, and N. Becker. 1981. Wirksamkeit von *Bacillus thuringiensis* var. *israelensis* gegen Stechmucken und Nontarget-Organismen. *Mittlg. dtsch. Ges. allg. angew. Entomol.* 2:195–202.

Siegel, J.P., and J.A. Shadduck. 1990. Safety of microbial insecticides to vertebrates-Humans. In: M. Laird, L.A. Lacey, and E.W. Davidson, editors, *Safety of microbial insecticides.* Boca Raton, FL: CRC Press. pp. 101–114.

Singer, S. 1990. Introduction to the study of *Bacillus sphaericus* as a mosquito control agent. In: H. de Barjac and D.J. Sutherland, editors, *Bacterial control of mosquitoes and black flies.* New Brunswick, NJ: Rutgers Univ. Press. pp. 221–227.

Smits, P.H., and H.J. Vlug, 1990. Control of Tipulid larvae with *Bacillus thuringiensis* var. *israelensis.* Proceedings of the 5th International Colloquium on Invertebrate Pathology and Microbial Control. Adelaide, Australia: Society for Invertebrate Pathology. 343 p.

Sweeney, A.W. 1981. Fungal pathogens of mosquito larvae. In: E.W. Davidson, editor, *Pathogenesis of invertebrate microbial diseases.* Totowa, NJ: Allanheld, Osmun. pp. 403–424.

Sweeney, A.W., and J.J. Becnel. 1991. Potential of microsporidia for the biological control of mosquitoes. *Parasitol. Today* 7:217–220.

Sweeney, A.W., M.F. Graham, and E.I. Hazard. 1985. Intermediate host for an *Amblyospora* sp. infecting the mosquito *Culex annulirostris. J. Invertebr. Pathol.* 46:98–102.

Tabashnik, B.E., N.L. Cushing, N. Finson, and M.W. Johnson. 1990. Development of resistance to *Bacillus thuringiensis* in field populations of *Plutella xylostella* in Hawaii. *J. Econ. Entomol.* 83:1671–1676.

Thanabalu, T., J. Hindley, S. Brenner, C. Oei, and C. Berry. 1992. Expression of the mosquitocidal toxins of *Bacillus sphaericus* and *Bacillus thuringiensis* subsp. *israelensis* by recombinant *Caulobacter crescentus*, a vehicle for biological control of aquatic insect larvae. *Appl. Environ. Microbiol.* 58:905–910.

Thanabalu, T., J. Hindley, J. Jackson-Yap, and C. Berry. 1991. Cloning, sequencing and expression of a gene encoding a 100-kilodalton mosquitocidal toxin from *Bacillus sphaericus* SSII–1. *J. Bacteriol.* 173:2776–2785.

Trisrisook, M., S. Pantuwatana, A. Bhumiratana, and W. Panbangred. 1990. Molecular cloning of the 130-kilodalton mosquitocidal delta-endotoxin gene of *Bacillus thuringiensis* subsp. *israelensis* in *Bacillus sphaericus. Appl. Environ. Microbiol.* 56:1710–1716.

Whisler, H.C., S.L. Zebold, and J.A. Shemanchuk. 1974. Alternative host for mosquito parasite *Coelomomyces. Nature* (London) 251:715–716.

WHO. 1981. Report of Informal Consultation on Standardization of *Bacillus thuringiensis* H–14. Mimeographed documents TDR/BVC/BTH–14/811; WHO/VBC/81–828. Geneva: World Health Organization. 15 p.

Xu, B.Z., N. Becker, X. Xianqu, and H.W. Ludwig. 1992. Microbial control of malaria vectors in Hubei Province, People's Republic of China. *Bull. Soc. Vector Ecol.* 17:140–149.

Yap, H.H. 1990. Field trials of *Bacillus sphaericus* for mosquito control. In: H. de Barjac and D.J. Sutherland, editors, *Bacterial control of mosquitoes and black flies.* New Brunswick, NJ: Rutgers Univ. Press. pp. 307–320.

33. GENETIC CONTROL OF VECTORS

Karamjit S. Rai

INTRODUCTION

Although the application of genetics in entomology is a relatively recent phenomenon, considerable progress has been made in genetic studies of several important disease vector species and in evaluating the use of the information thus gained for genetic control purposes. The contention that insect control is undergoing a crisis can hardly be debated. The traditional methods of control—use of synthetic organic insecticides—have in most cases proved to be ineffective and undesirable because of (a) the relatively rapid development of resistance on the part of insects treated, (b) their effects on the nontarget populations, and (c) the environmental pollution that ensues from the use of such chemicals. Consequently, several alternative types of control methods have been developed and tested in the field. These include various types of biological control methods. In simplest terms, genetic control involves any hereditary manipulation to suppress populations. Thus, genetic methods that are often termed autocidal are generally based on utilization of individuals of a particular species to control populations of *that* species. Thus, *nothing alien* is introduced into the ecological niche of a pest population. Hence, maintenance of the environment in the original untreated form can be assured.

Understandably, mechanisms for genetic control for any species can emerge only from a thorough investigation of the genetic biology of that species. Because all genetic analyses are based on controlled crosses, laboratory colonization of a candidate species becomes the first requirement for sustained genetic studies. Also, thorough knowledge of the population dynamics and ecology of the candidate vector species, under laboratory and field conditions, and the development of mass rearing techniques are necessary prerequisites for successful application of genetic control.

In this chapter the work done on genetic control of vectors with particular emphasis on various mosquito species is reviewed. The literature on the development and application of methods of genetic control in vector species is voluminous. Thus, the review is selective and field applications are emphasized over the development and laboratory and/or field evaluations of the same.

PRINCIPLES OF GENETIC MANIPULATION FOR POPULATION CONTROL

The basic principles and theoretical consideration underlying genetic control of insects have been adequately emphasized by LaChance and Knipling (1962), Craig (1963), Knipling et al. (1968), Whitten and Pal (1974), Whitten and Foster (1975), Waterhouse et al. (1976), Curtis (1985), and others. In general, because of the propagation of the sterility and/or other desirable genetic factors from one generation to the next, these methods are based on birth rather than death control. Ideally, control or replacement of a population following a single release of a desired genotype is highly desirable (Curtis 1968a), although in practice this has not yet been realized.

GENETIC CONTROL MECHANISMS

Several potentially useful mechanisms have been proposed for genetic control. Table 33.1 lists field trials that have been undertaken with vector species to evaluate the feasibility of such methods.

Sterile-Insect Technique

The sterile-insect technique (SIT) is based on the induction of sexual sterility in males through the use of radiation or chemical sterilants and on inundating natural populations with such males (Knipling 1955, 1959). To a large degree, interest in methods of genetic control of insects is a by-product of the successful application of the sterile insect release method to control the screwworm fly, *Cochliomyia hominivorax*, from the southeast and southwestern United States and the West Indian island of Curaçao in the mid-1950s (Knipling 1959).

Rai (1963, 1964a), LaChance (1967), and Curtis (1971) have provided important insights concerning the genetic basis of mutagen-induced dominant lethality in insects. Depending on the time of their application, radiation and/or chemosterilants can inhibit and completely prevent the production of gametes in insects (Rai 1964b, LaChance 1967). However, when the gametes are produced after such treatment, "sexual sterility" usually results from induction of dominant lethality in sperm and ova, caused by structural chromosomal aberrations such as loss of chromosomes or chromosome parts, particularly those that result in formation of broken ends. Mitotic anomalies such as the breakage-fusion-bridge cycles and the genetic imbalance that ensue from induction of such drastic aberrations in a developing embryo result in its death before embryogenesis is completed. Such fertilized eggs do not hatch. Although the sterile-male technique cannot be technically regarded as a type of genetic control because complete sterility cannot be inherited (NAS 1969; Rai et al. 1973), it is customary to treat it under genetic methods as described. The dominant lethal mutations that are induced in sperm of irradiated or chemically sterilized males and that result in male sterility are caused by drastic chromosomal aberrations and are hence genetic in nature.

The application of this technique for mosquito control has been reviewed by Rai (1969) and by Asman et al. (1981). In the early 1960s, this technique was tried with *Culex fatigans* (Krishnamurthy et al. 1962), *Aedes aegypti* (Morlan et al. 1962), and *Anopheles quadrimaculatus* (Weidhaas et al. 1962). All these trials were based on releases of males sterilized with radiation. The feasibility of a direct chemosterilant application to suppress an isolated desert population of *Cx. tarsalis* was investigated by Lewallen et al. (1965). Unfortunately, measured in terms of reductions of the target populations, none of these trials was successful. The reasons for these failures are fairly well understood (Rai 1969). In general, they resulted either from the use of massive doses of radiation used to sterilize males as in the case of *Ae. aegypti* (Weidhaas and Schmidt 1963) or from releases of males with reduced fitness ensuing from a long history of laboratory colonization as in *An. quadrimaculatus*. Asman et al. (1981) have listed 25 requirements that are relevant, to various degrees, for successful field application of genetic control methods.

The exploratory, small-scale pilot studies conducted in the 1960s paved the way for larger and more sustained releases using this method during the 1970s and 1980s. Patterson et al. (1970) successfully applied the sterile-male technique to control a population of *Cx. pipiens quinquefasciatus* from Sea Horse Key, a small island off the coast of Florida, following daily releases of chemosterilized males during a 10-week period. The feasibility of this method was also evaluated in the early 1970s using the same species in several villages in the vicinity of Delhi, India, under the auspices of the World Health Organization (WHO) and the Indian Council of Medical Research (WHO/ICMR) (Patterson et al. 1975; Yasuno et al. 1978), and in *Cx. tarsalis* in California (Asman et al. 1980; Reisen et al. 1981, 1982). In several of these trials, the sterile males were not fully competitive under field conditions, and immigration of fertile females from surrounding areas to experimental sites could not be effectively curtailed. Nevertheless, these studies helped to highlight the

TABLE 33.1 Field trials for genetic control of vector species

Species	Method	Location and agency	Reference
Culex fatigans	sterile male[a]	India, Govt.	Krishnamurthy et al. 1962
Culex pipiens quinquefasciatus	sterile male[b]	Florida, USDA	Patterson et al. 1970
Culex p. fatigans	sterile male[a,b]	India, WHO/ICMR	Patterson et al. 1975; Yasuno et al. 1978
Culex tarsalis	chemosterilant	California, DPH	Lewallen et al. 1965
Culex tarsalis	sterile male[a]	California, U.S. Army, USPHS	Asman et al. 1980; Reisen et al. 1981, 1982
Aedes aegypti	sterile male[a]	Florida, USPHS	Morlan et al. 1962
Anopheles quadrimaculatus	sterile male[a]	Florida, USDA	Weidhaas et al. 1962
Anopheles albimanus	sterile male[b]	El Salvador, USDA	Lofgren et al. 1974; Dame et al. 1981
Glossina palpalis gambiensis	sterile male[a]	Upper Volta, IAEA	Cuisance et al. 1978
Glossina palpalis gambiensis	sterile male[a]	Nigeria, IAEA	Lindquist 1984
Glossina morsitans morsitans	sterile male[a]	Zimbabwe and Tanzania, IAEA	Dame et al. 1981
Anopheles gambiae	hybrid male sterility	Upper Volta, WHO and ORSTOM	Davidson et al. 1970
Aedes polynesiensis	competitive exclusion	Pacific, USPHS	Rosen et al. 1976
Culex p. fatigans	cytoplasmic incompatibility	Burma, WHO	Laven 1967b
Culex pipiens	translocation heterozygote	France, EIDLM	Laven et al. 1972
Culex quinquefasciatus	cytoplasmic incompatibility/ translocation heterozygote	India, WHO/ICMR	Curtis et al. 1982
Aedes aegypti	translocation heterozygote	India, WHO/ICMR	Rai et al. 1973
Aedes aegypti	translocation heterozygote	Mombasa, E. Africa ICIPE/USAID	McDonald et al. 1977; Petersen et al. 1977
Aedes aegypti	translocation homozygote	Mombasa, ICIPE/USAID	Lorimer et al. 1976
Culex tritaeniorhynchus	translocation heterozygote	Pakistan, USPHS	Baker et al. 1979
Culex tritaeniorhynchus	translocation heterozygote	Pakistan, USPHS	Reisen et al. 1980
Culex tarsalis	translocation heterozygote	California, U.S. Army, USPHS	Asman et al. 1979

[a] Radiation-induced male sterility
[b] Chemosterilant-induced male sterility

need for additional requirements/developments to control larger target populations in future field trials.

In *An. albimanus*, a successful experimental trial resulted in the control of a relatively small isolated population at Lake Apastepeque in El Salvador (Lofgren et al. 1974). This effort was followed by a much larger experimental trial in a 20 km² area on the coastal plain of El Salvador in which approximately 1 million sterile males were released daily for a period of 4 months (Dame et al. 1981). The sterile males induced sterility in natural populations within the release zone and caused significant reductions in mosquito density. However, migration of fertile females into the study area prevented complete population control. This large-scale test was the first SIT experiment to use a genetic sexing strain (Seawright et al. 1980). Through the use of a radiation-induced translocation-inversion complex that linked propoxur resistance to the Y chromosome, females could be selectively killed by propoxur treatment in the egg stage. It was therefore possible to rear only males, which reduced the cost of production of sterile males by half (Seawright 1988).

SIT has also been applied to suppress the riverine species of tsetse flies, *Glossina palpalis gambiensis*, in Upper Volta (now Burkina Faso) (Cuisance et al. 1978) and in Nigeria (Lindquist 1984) and the savannah species *G. morsitans morsitans* in Zimbabwe and Tanzania (Dame et al. 1981). The high cost of massrearing tsetse flies and the fact that reared flies are less competitive in nature hampers the effectiveness of the technique.

Hybrid Sterility

When any 2 of the 6 sibling species in the *An. gambiae* complex are crossed, the male progeny are sterile (Davidson 1964; Coluzzi et al. 1979). Davidson et al. (1970) conducted a preliminary field trial to control a native population of *An. gambiae*, species A (see Chap. 26), near Bobo Dioulasso, Upper Volta, using such interspecific male sterility. The hybrid males released were produced by crossing females of an *An. melas* population from Liberia and males of a population of *An. gambiae*, species B, from Nigeria. They released approximately 300,000 hybrid pupae over a 2-month

period at the end of the rainy season in 1968 against a naturally declining population of species A. The results of this field trial were negative, although 75% of the males captured in the study village were sterile. Davidson et al. concluded from their results that "the sterile males were not mating on any significant scale with the natural species A females." A major flaw of this field trial can be traced to the protocol itself, whereby hybrid males produced by crossing 2 different species were utilized to compete with and control a 3rd species. Indeed, it would have been surprising if the mating and behavioral differences among the males released and females of the native population would not have come into play, particularly under field conditions. The non-Linnean designations of species A and B are synonymous with the currently used names, *Anopheles gambiae* and *An. arabiensis*, respectively (White 1975).

Cytoplasmic Incompatibility

The existence of incompatibility between certain allopatric populations of *Cx. pipiens* is well known (Laven 1967a). Such incompatibility, which can be either uni- or bidirectional and is maternally transmitted, has been ascribed to the presence of a rickettsial endosymbiont, *Wolbachia* spp., in the gonads. Thus, incompatibility ensues from the death of the sperm nucleus in an incompatible egg cytoplasm before karyogamy occurs. As a result, no progeny are produced from such incompatible crosses.

This method was field tested with successful results in a small isolated village, Okpo, near Rangoon, Burma, during an approximately 3-month period and 5–6 generations (Laven 1967b). The released incompatible male strain contained cytoplasm of a strain from Paris, France, and the genome of a Fresno, California, strain and resulted in "eradication" of the native Okpo population. Historically, this successful field trial helped generate much interest and enthusiasm in genetic methods of mosquito control. Similar cytoplasmic incompatibility exists in *Ae. albopictus* and could presumably be used for genetic control (Kambhampati et al. 1993).

Competitive Displacement

Laboratory competition between populations of *Ae. polynesiensis*, a major vector of filariasis in Polynesia, and *Ae. albopictus* resulted in elimination of *Ae. polynesiensis*. This happened both in relatively small (Gubler 1970) and in large walk-in cages in which conditions of the habitat of the 2 species were simulated (Rozeboom 1971). In small confined spaces, *Ae. albopictus* males readily inseminate *Ae. polynesiensis* females, but the eggs are infertile. Such cross-insemination sterility was considered to be an important factor in competitive displacement of *Ae. polynesiensis* in the cage populations. Rozeboom (1971) interpreted such replacement as resulting from the higher reproductive rate of *Ae. albopictus* than that of *Ae. polynesiensis*. Whatever the exact mechanism, it was hypothesized that such competitive displacement of one species by another could be used for replacing a vector or an insect pest by a nonvector or an innocuous form. A preliminary field trial was conducted on a small island in the Pacific utilizing this approach and the previously mentioned 2 species; however, the results were inconclusive (Rosen et al. 1976).

Such competitive exclusion was successfully applied to the control of a greenhouse population of race B of the Hessian fly (an agriculturally important wheat pest, *Mayetiola destructor*) by flooding it with the avirulent Great Plains race at a ratio of 9:1 with 4 releases or 19:1 with 2 releases (Foster and Gallun 1972). Competitive displacement of the native mud snail *(Ilyanassa obsoleta)* by introduced periwinkles *(Littorina littorea)* in the New England intertidal zone has been also reported (Brenchley and Carlton 1983). Thus, in theory and in practice, the concept is valid under appropriate conditions.

Chromosomal Translocations

The use of inherited sterility associated with reciprocal chromosomal translocations has been suggested for pest control (Rai 1967; Rai and Asman 1968; Rai and McDonald 1971; Curtis 1968a; Foster et al. 1972; Robinson 1976). Although the potential of this method was originally proposed by a Russian geneticist, Serebrovskii, in 1940, it was not until almost 3 decades later that its use for a number of insect species,

such as mosquitoes, tsetse flies, and house flies, was contemplated and progress made.

Because approximately 50% of the gametes formed as a result of adjacent segregation from a translocation heterozygote produce inviable zygotes, crosses involving normal individuals and translocation heterozygotes are usually semisterile. Furthermore, half the progeny surviving such crosses also inherit the same translocation and in turn pass it on to their offspring. Crosses among individuals heterozygous for the same translocation are expected to produce translocation homozygotes, translocation heterozygotes, and standard (chromosomally normal) progeny in a ratio of 1:2:1 (Fig. 33.1). Individuals homozygous for a translocation would be expected to show full fertility when mated to normal individuals with the standard chromosome arrangement because each gamete formed contains the full haploid complement. All the progeny from such matings, however, will be translocation heterozygotes and semisterile. Thus, for field releases of a single translocation, homozygotes are expected to be more efficient than heterozygotes in terms of individuals released. Twice the number of heterozygotes would be needed to introduce as many translocated chromosomes (Lorimer et al. 1972). Homozygotes are also useful in obtaining stocks of multiple translocations in which the genome is rearranged even more drastically, thereby also increasing the sterility of the progeny. This can be done by irradiating translocation homozygotes and assaying for other translocations that are then also made homozygous. Double translocation heterozygotes can also be produced by crossing individuals heterozygous for 2 different, single translocations (Hallinan et al. 1977).

In a release program in which large numbers of individuals must be reared, homozygotes are much easier to mass produce than heterozygotes because of their full fertility. Also, raising homozygotes eliminates the culling problem often associated with heterozygotes because all progeny inherit the same chromosomal rearrangement. As mentioned earlier, heterozygotes produce 50% normal progeny that have to be culled unless the translocation is very tightly linked with the male-determining locus; in that case most or all sons will be translocated and all daughters normal.

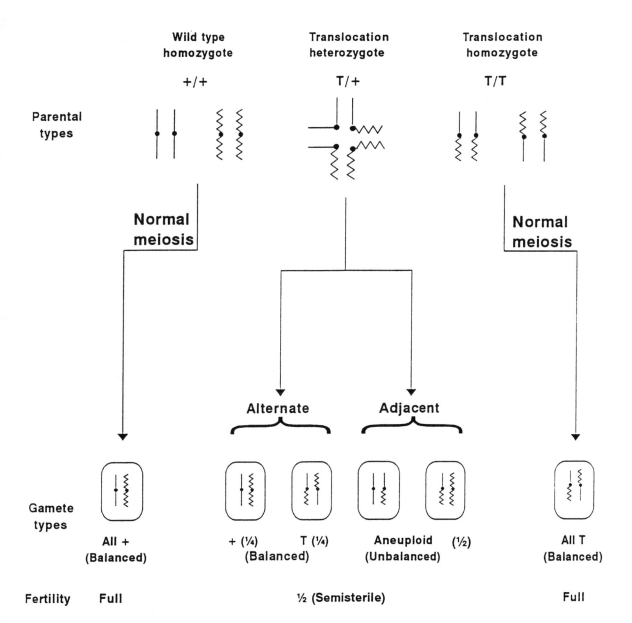

33.1   Diagrammatic representation of chromosomes in a wild-type homozygote (normal), translocation heterozygote, and translocation homozygote, illustrating the expected gamete types and the fertility of each. The centromeres are shown by a dark circle in the middle of each chromosome.

Homozygotes have also been proposed as a vehicle for driving desirable genes, such as refractoriness to parasitic diseases, conditional lethals, and so forth, into natural populations. Such genes could be located on the translocated segment and with appropriate manipulation driven to fixation in the population along with the translocation (Curtis 1968b).

Laven et al. (1972) reported the first "successful" application of a male-linked heterozygous translocation in a *Cx. pipiens* population breeding in a closed well in the village of Notre Dame near Montpellier, France, following releases over a 2-month period. The percentage of semisterile egg rafts increased to "95% or more," and the adult population in the well declined to 90% of its original level at the end of the experiment. A close scrutiny of the results indicated that other factors such as higher predator and parasite pressure in the closed well were also involved in suppressing the size of the ovipositing female population.

In *Ae. aegypti* more than 150 reciprocal translocations were induced and cytogenetically analyzed for their break points, fertility, fecundity, and transmission characteristics (Rai et al. 1974). Studies were also undertaken on the competitive mating ability of males heterozygous for the more promising of these translocations in laboratory and field population cages (Rai and McDonald 1971), and attempts were made to produce homozygotes for such translocations. Computer simulations using the available data in *Ae. aegypti* indicated the potential role of various types of sex-linked and autosomal translocations for genetic control under various release strategies (McDonald and Rai 1971).

Field work done under the sponsorship of the WHO and the ICMR at their research unit on genetic control of mosquitoes in Delhi, India, during the early 1970s described the genetic incorporation of a genetic marker and a male-linked translocation in a natural population and their maintenance for several generations following the termination of the field releases (Rai et al. 1973). This was the first demonstration of its type among any vector species. Such long-term survival of an introduced mechanism producing sterility over several generations is an essential prerequisite for successful application of the translocation method. Lorimer (1981) demonstrated the same for a population of *Ae.*

aegypti near the Kenya coast in Mombasa monitored for nearly a year after a genetic control experiment.

The use of single and double translocation heterozygotes for genetic control of *Ae. aegypti* was evaluated in villages around Mombasa, Kenya, under the sponsorship of the International Center of Insect Physiology and Ecology (ICIPE) and the U.S. Agency for International Development (USAID) by University of Notre Dame researchers (Petersen et al. 1977; McDonald et al. 1977). The targets were small village populations. Substantial (60–70%) sterility was introduced into native females during and immediately following these releases. However, no population suppression could be documented as a consequence of infiltration of *Ae. aegypti* spp. *formosus* (the jungle form) into the otherwise domestic habitat of the type form *Ae. aegypti*. The concept of population replacement through the release of translocation homozygotes was also evaluated in Mombasa. However, the results were negative because of the lack of competitiveness of the released strain under field conditions and because of behavioral differences in oviposition preference between homozygous strain released and the indigenous population (Lorimer et al. 1976).

Field releases of *Cx. tritaeniorhynchus* males heterozygous for a male-linked translocation and a pericentric inversion with 80–90% sterility at a village near Lahore, Pakistan, in 1977 (Baker et al. 1979) and 1978 (Reisen et al. 1980) showed that the released males were competitive with released laboratory colonized females and their sibling females but not with the wild females. This also suggested that prolonged laboratory colonization of the strain had selected an assortative mating behavior.

Integrated Genetic Control

An integrated strain of *Cx. quinquefasciatus* was engineered that contained cytoplasm of Paris, France, origin, and chromosomes of Delhi, India, origin including a male-linked chromosomal translocation. Males of this strain were mass-reared and released in 2 villages approximately 60 km south of New Delhi between August and November 1973 to evaluate replacement of an indigenous population through cytoplasmic incompatibility and control of residual populations through translocation sterility (Curtis et al. 1982). As a result of matings of wild females with released males, up to 68% of the egg rafts laid in the villages showed cytoplasmic incompatibility. Despite continued releases, the sterility rate in the native population plateaued and eventually declined, presumably because of a decline in emergence of virgin females in the villages and immigration of inseminated females from surrounding areas (Curtis et al. 1982). Nevertheless, compared with untreated, control villages, the releases produced partial population suppression in treated villages.

Other Mechanisms

The use of several other genetic mechanisms, e.g., meiotic drive (Hickey and Craig 1966), conditional lethal mutations (Klassen et al. 1970, Smith 1971), and deleterious recessive genes (LaChance and Knipling 1962), to suppress insect populations has also been suggested; however, the potential of not these has not yet been tested in any field trials.

SUMMARY AND CONCLUSIONS

Considerable work has been done to evaluate the feasibility of using various genetic methods to control vector populations. Except for the use of the conventional irradiated males in certain trials, the theoretically predicted long-term high levels of genetic load resulting in suppression of pest populations has not been achieved in any field releases. This often resulted from various causes, as for example, imperfect mixing and/or ethological differences in mating behavior of the released and wild males, density-dependent regulation of populations following introductions of genetic loads, lack of competitiveness of released males that can be compensated for by increasing release-native male ratios, or immigration of fertile females from regions close to release sites. Also, some of the potentially more promising field releases such as those planned by WHO/ICMR in India against relatively large urban populations of *Ae. aegypti* and *Cx. fatigans* following 5-year feasibility studies were prematurely terminated for strictly political reasons (WHO 1976). The ICIPE-sponsored releases of translocation stocks of *Ae. aegypti* in Mombasa were also terminated prematurely in mid-1970s because of the reemergence of malaria and the presumption that *Ae. aegypti* was no

longer an important vector species in Africa. Nevertheless, although the results of the field trials to date have admittedly not been startling because of the reasons discussed, they have established the validity of the scientific principle of genetic control. In no case can the lack of optimal success be ascribed to a limitation or a negative feature of the concepts involved. Furthermore, much has been learned about the field biology, ecology, and dynamics of field populations as a result of the field trials.

Recent developments in molecular genetics offer exciting possibilities for extension and possible future applications of genetic control. These are highlighted by Cockburn et al. 1984, Whitten 1986, Crampton et al. 1990, Crampton 1992, Crampton and Eggleston 1992, Eggleston 1991, Besansky et al. 1992, Curtis 1992, Kidwell and Ribeiro 1992, and others. Currently, the focus of this work is on the production of competitive transgenic strains and on the isolation of appropriate transposable elements that could be used to drive disease refractory genes into vector populations. Details of molecular manipulations of vectors are discussed by Carlson in this volume (Chap. 14).

ACKNOWLEDGMENTS

I thank Dr. A. Kumar for reading the manuscript and Tracy Frost for typesetting. The work in the author's laboratory has received support from the National Institutes of Health, Grants 2RO1 AI–21443 and 5T32 AI 07030.

REFERENCES AND FURTHER READING

Asman, S.M., P.T. McDonald, and T. Prout. 1981. Field studies of genetic control systems for mosquitoes. *Ann. Rev. Entomol.* 26:289–318.

Asman, S.M., F.B. Zaloni, and R.P. Meyer. 1980. A field release of irradiated male *Culex tarsalis*. In: C.D. Grant, Calif. Mosq. Vector Cont. Assoc., Visalia, CA. *California. Proc. Calif. Mosq. Vector Contr. Assoc.* 48:64.

Baker, R.H., W.K. Reisen, R.K. Sakai, C.G. Hayes, M. Aslamkhan, U.T. Saifuddin, F. Mahmood, A. Perveen, and S. Javed. 1979. Field assessment of mating competitiveness of male *Culex tritaeniorhynchus* carrying a complex chromosomal aberration. *Ann. Entomol. Soc. Am.* 72:751–758.

Besansky, N.J., V.J. Finnerty, and F.H. Collins. 1992. Molecular perspectives on the genetics of mosquitoes. *Adv. Genet.* 30:123–184.

Brenchley, G.A., and J.T. Carlton. 1983. Competitive displacement of native mud snails by introduced periwinkles in the New England intertidal zone. *Biol. Bull.* 165:543–558.

Cockburn, A.F., A.J. Howells, and M.J. Whitten. 1984. Recombinant DNA technology and genetic control of pest insects. *Biotech. and Genetic Engineering Rev.* 2:69–99.

Coluzzi, M., A. Sabatini, V. Petrarca, and M.A. DiDeco. 1979. Chromosomal differentiation and adaptation to human environments in the *Anopheles gambiae* complex. *Trans. Roy. Soc. Trop. Med. and Hyg.* 73:483–497.

Craig, G.B. Jr. 1963. Prospects for vector control through genetic manipulation of populations. *Bull. WHO* 29:89–97.

Crampton, J.M. 1992. Potential Application of molecular biology in entomology. In: J.M. Crampton and P. Eggleston, editors, *Insect Molecular Science*. London; San Diego: Academic Press. pp. 4–20.

Crampton, J.M., and P. Eggleston. 1992. Biotechnology and the control of mosquitoes. In: W.K. Yong, editor, *Animal parasite control utilizing biotechnology*. CRC Uniscience Volumes. Boca Raton, FL: CRC Press Inc. pp. 333–350.

Crampton, J.M., A. Morris, G. Lycett, A. Warren, and P. Eggleston. 1990. Transgenic mosquitoes: A future vector control strategy? *Parasit. Today* 6:31–36.

Cuisance, D., H. Politzar, H.M. Clair, E. Sellin, and Y. Taze. 1978. Impact des lachers des males steriles sur les niveaux de deux populations sauvages de *Glossina palpalis gambiensis* en Haute-Volta (sources de la Volta Noire). *Revue d'Élevage et de Médecine Veterinaire des Pays Tropicaux* 31:315–328.

Curtis, C.F. 1968a. A possible genetic method for the control of insect pests with special reference to tsetse flies, *Glossina* spp. *Bull. Entom. Res.* 57:509–523.

———. 1968b. Possible use of translocations to fix desirable genes in insect pest populations. *Nature* 218:368–369.

———. 1971. Induced sterility in insects. *Adv. Repro. Physiol.* 5:120–165.

———. 1985. Genetic control of insect pests: growth industry or lead balloon? *Biological J. Linnean Soc.* 26:359–374.

———. 1992. Selfish Genes in Mosquitoes. *Nature* 357:450.

Curtis, C.F., G.D. Brooks, M.A. Ansari, K.K. Grover, B.S. Krishnamurthy, P.K. Rajagopalan, L.S. Sharma, V.P. Sharma, D. Singh, K.R.P. Singh, and M. Yasuno. 1982. A field trial on control of *Culex quinquefasciatus* by release of males of a strain integrating cytoplasmic incompatibility and a translocation. *Ent. Exp. Appl.* 31:181–190.

Dame, D.A., R.E. Lowe, and D.L. Williamson. 1981. Assessment of released sterile *Anopheles albimanus* and *Glossina morsitans morsitans*. In: R. Pal, J.B. Kitzmiller, T. Kanda, editors, *Cytogenetics and Genetics of Vectors;* Proc. XVI Int. Congr. Entomol. Kyoto, 1980. Amsterdam: Elsevier. pp. 231–241.

Davidson, G. 1964. *Anopheles gambiae*, a complex of species. *Bull. WHO* 31:625–634.

Davidson, G., J.A. Odetoyinbo, B. Colussa, and J. Coz. 1970. A field attempt to assess the mating competitiveness of sterile males produced by crossing 2 member species of the *Anopheles gambiae* complex. *Bull. WHO* 42:55–67.

Eggleston, P. 1991. The control of insect-borne disease through recombinant DNA technology. *Heredity* 66:161–172.

Foster, J.E., and R.L. Gallun. 1972. Populations of the Eastern races of the Hessian fly controlled by release of dominant avirulent Great Plains race. *Ann. Entomol. Soc. Am.* 65:750–754.

Foster, G.G., M.J. Whitten, T. Prout, and R. Gill. 1972. Chromosome rearrangements for the control of insect pests. *Science* 176:875–880.

Gubler, D.J. 1970. Competitive displacement of *Aedes (Stegomyia) polynesiensis* Marks by *Aedes (Stegomyia) albopictus* Skuse in laboratory populations. *J. Med. Entomol.* 7:229–235.

Hallinan, E., N. Lorimer, and K.S. Rai. 1977. Genetic manipulation of *Aedes aegypti*. II. In: *A cytogenetic study of radiation induced translocations in DELHI strain*. Proc. XV Internat. Cong. Entomol. Washington, D.C.: Entomology Society of America. pp. 117–128.

Hickey, W.A., and G.B. Craig, Jr. 1966. Distortion of sex ratio in populations of *Aedes aegypti*. *Can. J. Genet. Cytol.* 8:260–278.

Kambhampati, S., K.S. Rai, and S.J. Burgun. 1993. Unidirectional cytoplasmic incompatibility in the mosquito *Aedes albopictus*. *Evolution* (in press).

Kidwell, M.G., and J.M.C. Ribeiro. 1992. Can transposable elements be used to drive disease refractoriness genes into vector populations? *Parasit. Today* 8:325–329.

Klassen, W., E.F. Knipling, and J.U. McGuire, Jr. 1970. The potential for insect population suppression by dominant conditional lethal traits. *Ann. Ent. Soc. Am.* 63:238–255.

Knipling, E.F. 1955. Possibilities of Insect control or eradication through the use of sexually sterile males. *J. Econ. Entomol.* 48:459–462.

———. 1959. Sterile-male method of population control. *Science* 130:902–904.

Knipling, E.F., H. Laven, G.B. Craig, Jr., R. Pal, J.B. Kitzmiller, C.N. Smith, and A.W.A. Brown. 1968. Genetic control of insects of public health importance. *Bull. WHO* 38:421–438.

Krishnamurthy, B.S., S.N. Ray, and G.C. Joshi. 1962. A note on preliminary field studies of the use of irradiated males for reduction of *C. fatigans* Wied populations. *Ind. J. Malar.* 16:365–373.

LaChance, L.E. 1967. The induction of dominant lethal mutations in insects by ionizing radiation and chemicals as related to the sterile male technique of insect control. In: J. Wright and R. Pal, editors, *Genetics of insect vectors of disease.* Amsterdam: Elsevier. pp. 617–650.

LaChance, L.E., and E.F. Knipling. 1962. Control of insect populations through genetic manipulations. *Ann. Entomol. Soc. Am.* 55:515–520.

Laven, H. 1967a. Speciation and evolution in Culex pipiens. In: J. Wright and R. Pal, editors, *Genetics of insect vectors of disease.* Amsterdam: Elsevier. pp. 251–275.

Laven, H. 1967b. Eradication of *Culex pipiens fatigans* through cytoplasmic incompatibility. *Nature* 216:383–384.

Laven, H., J. Cousserans, and G. Guille. 1972. Eradicating Mosquitoes using translocations: A first field experiment. *Nature* 236:456–457.

Lewallen, L.L., H.C. Chapman, and W.H. Wilder. 1965. Chemosterilant application to an isolated population of *Culex tarsalis. Mosq. News* 25:16–18.

Lindquist, D.A. 1984. Atoms for pest control. *Interntl. Atomic Energy Agency Bull.* 26:22–25.

Lofgren, C.S., D.A. Dame, S.B. Breeland, D.E. Weidhaas, G. Jeffery, R. Kaiser, H.R. Ford, M.D. Boston, and K.F. Baldwin. 1974. Release of chemosterilized males for the control of *Anopheles albimanus* in El Salvador. III. Field Methods and Population Control. *Am. J. Trop. Med. and Hyg.* 23:288–297.

Lorimer, L. 1981. Long-term survival of introduced genes in a natural population of *Aedes aegypti* (L.) (Diptera: Culicidae). *Bull. Ent. Res.* 71:129–132.

Lorimer, N., E. Hallinan, and K.S. Rai. 1972. Translocation homozygotes in the yellow fever mosquito, *Aedes aegypti. J. Heredity* 63:158–166.

Lorimer, N., L.P. Lounibos, and J.L. Petersen. 1976. Field trials with a translocation homozygote in *Aedes aegypti* for population replacement. *J. Econ. Entomol.* 69:405–409.

McDonald, P.T., and K.S. Rai. 1971. Population control potential of heterozygous translocations as determined by computer simulations. *Bull. WHO* 44:829–845.

McDonald, P.T., W. Hausermann, and N. Lorimer. 1977. Sterility introduced by release of genetically altered males to a domestic population of *Aedes aegypti* at the Kenya coast. *Am. J. Trop. Med. Hyg.* 26:553–561.

Morlan, H.B., E.M. McCray, Jr., and J.W. Kilpatrick. 1962. Field tests with sexually sterile males for control of *Aedes aegypti. Mosq. News* 22:295–300.

National Academy of Sciences. 1969. Insect Pest Management and Control. Vol. 3. Publication 1695. Washington, D.C.: National Academy Press. pp.196–202.

Patterson, R.S., D.E. Weidhaas, H.R. Ford, and C.S. Lofgren. 1970. Suppression and elimination of an island population of *Culex pipiens quinquefasciatus* with sterile males. *Science* 168:1368–1369.

Patterson, R.S., V.P. Sharma, K.R.P. Singh, G.C. LaBrecque, P.L. Seetheram, and K.K. Grover. 1975. Use of radiosterilized males to control indigenous populations of *Culex pipiens quinquefasciatus* Say: laboratory and field studies. *Mosq. News* 35:1–7.

Petersen, J.L., L.P. Lounibos, and N. Lorimer. 1977. Field trials of double translocation heterozygote males for genetic control of *Aedes aegypti* (L.). *Bull. Entomol. Res.* 67:313–324.

Rai, K.S. 1963. A cytogenetic study of the effects of X-irradiation on *Aedes aegypti. Caryologia* 16:595–607.

———. 1964a. Cytogenetic effects of chemosterilants in mosquitoes. I. Apholate-induced aberrations in the somatic chromosomes of *Aedes aegypti* (L.) *Cytologia* 29:346–353.

———. 1964b. Cytogenetic effects of chemosterilants in mosquitoes. II. Mechanism of apholate-induced changes in fecundity and fertility of *Aedes aegypti* (L.). *Biol. Bull.* 127:119–131.

————. 1967. Manipulation of cytogenetic mechanisms for genetic control of vectors. WHO Scientific Group on the Cytogenetics of Vectors of Disease of Man. SC/VG. 67.34. Geneva: World Health Organization. 12 p.

Rai, K.S., and S.M. Asman. 1968. Possible application of a reciprocal translocation for genetic control of the mosquito, *Aedes aegypti*. Proc. XII Internat. Cong. of Genetics, Tokyo, Japan. Tokyo: Science Council of Japan. Vol. I:164.

Rai, K.S. 1969. The status of the sterile male technique for mosquito control. In: *Sterile Male Technique for Eradication or Control of Harmful Insects*. Vienna: Internat. Atomic Energy Agency Press. pp. 107–114.

Rai, K.S., K.K. Grover, and S.G. Suguna. 1973. Genetic manipulation of *Aedes aegypti*: Incorporation and maintenance of a genetic marker and a chromosomal translocation in natural populations. *Bull. WHO* 48:49–56.

Rai, K.S., and P.T. McDonald. 1971. Chromosomal translocations and genetic control of *Aedes aegypti*. In: *The sterility principle for insect control or eradication*. Vienna: Internat. Atomic Energy Agency Press. pp. 437–452.

Rai, K.S., N. Lorimer, and E. Hallinan. 1974. The current status of genetic methods for controlling *Aedes aegypti*. In: R. Pal and M.J. Whitten, editors, *The use of genetics in insect control*. North Holland: Elsevier. pp. 119–132.

Reisen, W.K., R.K. Sakai, R.H. Baker, H.R. Rathor, K. Raana, K. Azra, and S. Niaz. 1980. Field competitiveness of *Culex tritaeniorhynchus* Giles males carrying a complex chromosomal aberration: A second experiment. *Ann. Entomol. Soc. Am.* 73:479–484.

Reisen, W.K., S.M. Asman, M.M. Milby, M.E. Bock, P.J. Stoddard, R.P. Meyer, and W.C. Reeves. 1981. Attempted suppression of a semi-isolated population of *Culex tarsalis* by release of irradiated mates. *Mosq. News* 4:736–744.

Reisen, W., M.M. Milby, S.M. Asman, M.E. Bock, R.P. Meyer, P.T. McDonald, and W.C. Reeves. 1982. Attempted suppression of a semi-isolated population by the release of irradiated males: a second experiment using males from a recently colonized strain. *Mosq. News* 42:565–575.

Robinson, A.S. 1976. Progress in the use of chromosomal translocation for the control of insect pests. *Biol. Rev.* 51:1–24.

Rosen, L., L.E. Rozeboom, W.C. Reeves, J. Saugrain, and D.J. Gubler. 1976. A field trial of competitive displacement of *Aedes polynesiensis* by *Aedes albopictus* on a Pacific atoll. *Am. J. Trop. Med. Hyg.* 25:906–913.

Rozeboom, L.E. 1971. Relative densities of freely breeding populations of *Aedes (S.) polynesiensis* Marks and *Ae. (S.) albopictus* Skuse. *Amer. J. Trop. Med. Hyg.* 20:356–362.

Seawright, J. 1988. Genetic methods for control of mosquitoes and biting flies. In: *Modern insect control: Nuclear techniques and biotechnology*. Vienna: Internat. Atomic Energy Agency, pp. 179–191.

Seawright, J.A., P.E. Kaiser, D.A. Dame, and C.S. Lofgren. 1978. Genetic method for the preferential elimination of females of *Anopheles albimanus*. *Science* 200:1303.

Serebrovskii, A.S. 1940. On the possibility of a new method for the control of insect pests. *Zool. Zh.* 19:618–630.

Smith, R.H. 1971. Induced conditional lethal mutations for the control of insect populations. In: *Sterility principle for insect control or eradication*. Vienna: Internat. Atomic Energy Agency Press. pp. 453–465.

WHO. 1976. WHO-supported collaborative research projects in India: The facts. *WHO Chronicle* 30:131–139.

Waterhouse, D.F., L.E. LaChance, and M.J. Whitten. 1976. Use of Autocidal Methods. In: C.B. Huffaker, P.S. Messenger, editors, *Theory and practice of biological control*. New York: Academic Press. pp. 637–659.

Weidhaas, D.E., and C.H. Schmidt. 1963. Mating ability of male mosquitoes, *Aedes aegypti (L.)*, sterilized chemically or by gamma radiation. *Mosq. News* 23:32–34.

Weidhaas, D.E., C.H. Schmidt, and E.L. Seabrook. 1962. Field studies of the release of sterile males for the control of *Anopheles quadrimaculatus*. *Mosq. News* 22:283–291.

White, G.B. 1975. Notes on a catalogue of Culicidae of the Ethiopian region. *Mosq. Sys.* 7:303–344.

Whitten, M.J. 1986. Molecular Biology—Its relevance to pure and applied entomology. *Ann. Entomol. Soc. Am.* 79:766–772.

Whitten, M.J., and G.G. Foster. 1975. Genetic methods of pest control. *Ann. Rev. Entomol.* 20:461–476.

Whitten, M.J., and R. Pal. 1974. Introduction. In: R. Pal and M.J. Whitten, editors, *Genetic control of insects*. Amsterdam: Elsevier/North-Holland. pp. 1–16.

Yasuno, M., W.W. MacDonald, C.F. Curtis, K.K. Grover, P.K. Rajagopalan, L.S. Sharma., V.P. Sharma, D. Singh, K.R.P. Singh, H.V. Agarwal, S.J. Kazmi, P.K.B. Menon, R. Menon, R.K. Razdan, D. Samuel, and V. Vaidyanathan. 1978. A control experiment with chemosterilized male *Culex pipiens fatigans* Wied in a village near Delhi surrounded by a breeding-free zone. *Jap. J. Sanit. Zool.* 29:325–343.

34. IMMUNOLOGIC CONTROL OF VECTORS

Stephen K. Wikel

INTRODUCTION

Blood-feeding arthropods and the pathogens they transmit are of great medical and veterinary public health importance. Annual global incidence of cases of acute malaria was estimated by the World Health Organization (WHO) to be 90–100 million, and approximately 1 million children die annually from the disease (Good et al. 1988). The primary method used to control malaria remains vector suppression (Laird 1985), despite intense efforts to develop an anti-malaria vaccine (Good et al. 1988).

Ticks are the most important vectors of disease agents in domestic and wild animal species, and they are second only to mosquitoes as transmitters of pathogens to humans (Balashov 1972). An ever-changing array of tick-borne diseases is being recognized (Hoogstraal 1981). Global incidence of Lyme borreliosis continues to increase (Steere 1989; Szczepanski and Benach 1991), and it is perceived by the population to be a significant public health concern (Barbour 1992). Importance of infection of humans and other animals with *Ehrlichia* species is gaining increasing recognition (Magnarelli 1990). A recently described rickettsial infection of immunocompetent and immunosuppressed humans, *Rochalimeaea henselae*, is thought to be transmitted by ticks (Lucy et al. 1992). Continued surveillance and the use of more sensitive methods for the detection and identification of disease causing agents

will likely result in the addition of new pathogens to the list of arthropod-borne diseases.

Microorganisms undergo complex developmental cycles within the tick (Kocan 1986). Pathogen development, vector biology, and host responses to infection and arthropod infestation are interrelated. Examination of one of these parameters without consideration of the others results in an incomplete picture of the dynamics of host-vector-pathogen interaction. Limited knowledge exists regarding activation of the pathogen and development within the arthropod vector, transmission of the disease agent, vector-induced modulation of host immunity, and the impact of the host response to the arthropod on pathogen transmission.

Host immune reactivity to vectors and the pathogens they transmit is an array of dynamic interactions. Cytokines, antibodies, and cell-mediated immune responses are critical elements concerning the establishment of infection, disease progression, and host defenses. Using induced host immunity as a control strategy for blood-feeding vectors of disease has become important. A thorough knowledge of the basic immune responses to infestation is essential if effective vaccine-based control of vectors is to be achieved. Figure 34.1 is a scanning electron micrograph of a female *Dermacentor andersoni* attached to bovine skin.

Interest in immunologically based control of arthropod vectors of disease has grown because of

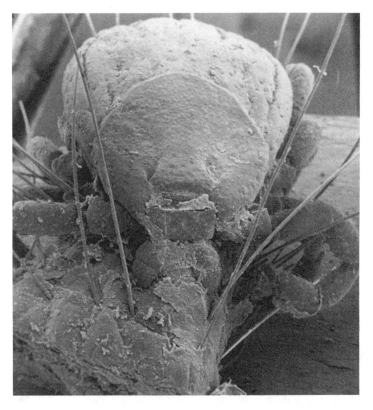

34.1 Scanning electron micrograph of female *Dermacentor andersoni* attached to bovine skin. The tick is not a "crawling hypodermic needle and syringe." Complex interactions occur at the host-vector-pathogen interface. Tick saliva contains a variety of pharmacologically and immunologically active molecules. Tick-borne pathogens undergo complex developmental cycles within the vector. Hosts acquire and express immune responses to both the vector and pathogen.

significant. New approaches for effective control must be considered.

This chapter focuses on the nature of host immune reactivity to arthropod infestation and the utilization of that information for the development of effective anti-arthropod vaccines. Research to date has been largely directed toward the control of ixodid ticks; however, vaccination-based control of rapid blood-feeders such as mosquitoes and biting flies is an attainable goal. Significant advances in biotechnology/molecular biology provide a technological basis for the successful development and delivery of anti-vector vaccines.

HOST IMMUNITY TO BLOOD-FEEDING ARTHROPODS

Arthropods stimulate a wide variety of host immune responses. A classic example is the life-threatening allergic reaction that might result from a bee or wasp sting. These are dramatic responses to arthropod-derived molecules introduced into the host. Investigation of the host-arthropod interface reveals that the full spectrum of immune responses can be stimulated. Development of immunological control strategies for blood-feeding arthropods requires a detailed understanding of the nature of host immune responses to infestation. This section examines the nature of host immune responses to blood-feeding arthropods.

Initial studies often examined the cutaneous reactions to arthropod feeding. These investigations provided useful insights into the cellular events that occurred at the bite sites of short- and long-term blood-feeding arthropods. Subsequent investigations addressed the relationships among salivary material introduced into the host, the host immune response to feeding, and the impact of those interactions upon pathogen transmission. Information gained from these

increasing vector resistance to insecticides and acaricides, which is a serious threat to animal production (Brown 1983; Solomon 1983). Anti-arthropod vaccines are target-species specific. They do not damage the environment, and meat and milk residues do not occur. These features are all significant advantages over the use of insecticides and acaricides. Economic impact of tick infestation and tick-borne diseases was estimated by the Food and Agriculture Organization of the United Nations (1984) to be approximately $7 billion per annum. The magnitude of the problem is

studies has been essential for the development of immunological control strategies for blood-feeding arthropods.

A sequential pattern of reactivity to arthropod bites was proposed by Mellanby (1946), and similar observations were subsequently made by other workers. Five stages of reactivity to arthropod feeding were described. The 1st stage was a period of sensitization with no observable skin reactivity, the 2nd phase was delayed skin responsiveness, the 3rd was immediate and then delayed skin reactions, the 4th phase consisted of only immediate skin reactivity, and the 5th pattern of the sequence was a loss of reactivity caused by possible desensitization. This general scheme for cutaneous reactivity reflects the changing pattern of immune responsiveness observed with repeated exposures to arthropod feeding.

The most extensively studied host-arthropod relationships involve ixodid ticks infesting laboratory animal species and bovines. Hosts acquire resistance to ticks, which is characterized by reduced numbers of ticks feeding, decreased size of the blood meal, reduced numbers and viability of ova, increased duration of feeding, impaired pathogen transmission, and death of ticks (Wikel 1982).

Trager (1939) examined the cutaneous responses of susceptible and resistant guinea pigs to infestation with *Dermacentor variabilis*. Ixodid ticks are pool-feeders. Histologic examination of sections prepared from tissues obtained on the 4th day of an initial tick exposure revealed only the hemorrhagic pool beneath the mouthparts. Similar sections prepared from animals expressing acquired resistance to tick feeding were very different. A mass of polymorphonuclear leukocytes had accumulated in a "pool" within the thickened and edematous epidermis at the tick attachment site. Observation of this intense reactivity caused Trager (1939) and subsequent workers to investigate the immunologic basis of host reactivity to tick bite (Wikel 1988).

The classic study by Allen (1973) of cutaneous reactivity to tick feeding reported the accumulation of large numbers of basophils at tick attachment sites on guinea pigs expressing acquired resistance. This reaction was shown to be a cutaneous basophil hypersensitivity response (CBH), which is one form of the cell-mediated immune reactivity known as delayed type hypersensitivity (DTH). Similar patterns of cutaneous reactivity were subsequently established by numerous investigators for a variety of tick-host relationships involving laboratory animals and cattle (Wikel and Whelen 1986). An intense influx of basophils to the attachment site of a *Dermacentor andersoni* larva on a tick-resistant guinea pig is shown in Figure 34.2. Note the presence of eosinophils, which act as feedback regulators of many of the biologically active molecules released by degranulating basophils. These findings provided a solid clue that host reactivity to tick feeding involved the cell-mediated immune defenses of the host.

The processing and presentation of immunogens to T-lymphocytes by macrophages or macrophage-like cells are central components in the generation of immune responses to thymic-dependent antigens. Immunogenic molecules introduced by ticks or other blood-feeding arthropods are not excluded from this process. Feeding at the skin's surface suggests that Langerhans cells are involved in processing and presentation of immunogens contained in tick saliva. Langerhans cells are found in the suprabasal position within the epidermis, and they function in a manner very similar to that of a macrophage. Nithiuthai and Allen (1984a,b,c) observed that the number of Langerhans cells surrounding tick attachment sites decreased significantly during an initial exposure to tick feeding; however, the number of Langerhans cells increased at sites of tick feeding upon hosts expressing acquired resistance. Development and expression of acquired anti-tick resistance was impaired by removal of Langerhans cells from tick-feeding sites by prior treatment with ultraviolet-B radiation. Thus, Langerhans cells function as antigen-presenting cells during tick feeding. Langerhans cells travel from the cutaneous site to the draining lymph node, where further antigen interactions with immunocompetent lymphocytes occur.

Detailed investigations of immune reactivity to hematophagous arthropods revealed complex interactions of introduced salivary immunogens with effector and regulatory pathways of the host immune system.

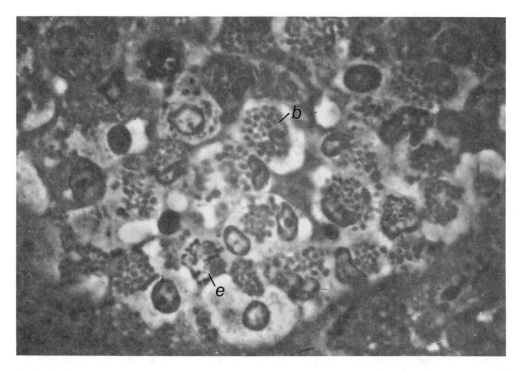

34.2 Accumulation of basophils at attachment site of *Dermacentor andersoni* larva on guinea pig expressing acquired resistance to infestation. Cutaneous basophil hypersensitivity consisting of an intense influx of basophils (b) and eosinophils (e) are present. (One micron plastic section stained with Toluidine blue O in borax, 1000x.)

Macrophages, T-lymphocytes, and their cytokines are involved in the regulation of the immune response to tick feeding (Ramachandra and Wikel 1992). Immune response effectors of acquired resistance to tick feeding include cell-mediated delayed type hypersensitivity, circulating immunoglobulins, homocytotropic antibodies, complement, and other bioreactive molecules of the immune/inflammatory response (Willadsen 1980; Wikel 1988; Brossard et al. 1991).

Primary immunoglobulin and cell-mediated immune responses are stimulated during the 1st exposure to tick feeding. The full force of an anti-tick immune response might not be effective against ticks engorging during an initial exposure of 5–10 days. Memory B and T-lymphocytes are generated as a result of this exposure to tick salivary antigens. Tick salivary gland antigens are processed by Langerhans cells, macrophages, and "macrophage-like" cells in the draining lymph nodes prior to presentation to immunocompetent B and T-lymphocytes. Antibody and cell-mediated immune responses are generated, which result in the eventual clearance of tick salivary antigens. These responses are systemic, not just limited to the tick feeding sites. Both the classical and alternative pathways of complement are likely activated, which could contribute to increased vascular permeability and slight influx of granulocytes at primary tick attachment sites. Mast cells in the vicinity of a primary feeding site are usually degranulated. Release of mast cell mediators could be caused by the action of complement-derived anaphylatoxins, C3a and C5a, and/or the direct action of saliva. Figure 34.3 is a flowchart describing the events thought to occur during a primary response to tick infestation.

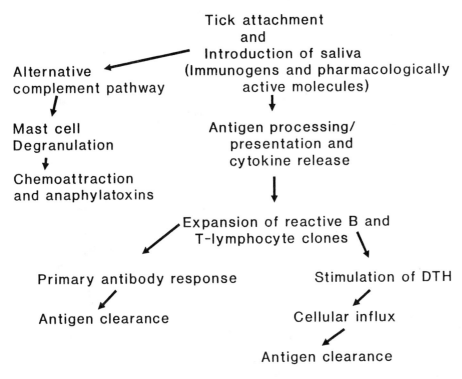

SUSCEPTIBLE HOST

Tick attachment
and
Introduction of saliva
(Immunogens and pharmacologically
active molecules)

Alternative
complement pathway

Mast cell
Degranulation

Chemoattraction
and anaphylatoxins

Antigen processing/
presentation and
cytokine release

Expansion of reactive B and
T-lymphocyte clones

Primary antibody response

Antigen clearance

Stimulation of DTH

Cellular influx

Antigen clearance

34.3   Flow diagram of the acquisition of resistance to tick infestation.

A different series of events takes place when a tick feeds upon a host resistant to infestation. The presence of preformed antibodies and effector T-lymphocytes assures an immediate response to infestation. Presence of memory B and T-lymphocytes ensures a rapid anamnestic response to introduced tick immunogens. Cytokines, activated complement components, and mediators released from various cells are likely responsible for the intense accumulation of granulocytes, particularly basophils, at the tick attachment sites. Antibodies reactive with tick saliva are present, which possibly alter the pharmacological actions of many salivary components. Cell-mediated immunity is stimulated. Basophils are "armed" with tick saliva reactive homocytotropic antibodies. Immunogens introduced during the course of feeding can then react with basophil-bound homocytotropic antibodies to cause the further release of basophil

mediators. The impact of cell-mediated immune effectors upon the tick remains to be established. Nothing is know about the possible role of cytotoxic T-lymphocytes. The cutaneous basophil hypersensitivity response is apparently a T_{H1} subset—mediated response. Figure 34.4 represents the interactions thought to occur during the expression of acquired anti-tick resistance.

Ultrastructural studies of the digestive tracts of ticks feeding upon hosts expressing acquired resistance to infestation revealed that cellular elements attracted to the attachment site damaged the engorging ixodid (Voss-McCowan 1991). The digestive tract was lined by a pseudostratified epithelium that rested on a basal lamina. Gut tissues obtained from ticks feeding upon resistant hosts were damaged. Basophils, eosinophils, and granules of both these cell types were present in the gut lumen. All elements were phagocytized by digestive tract epithelial cells. Digestive tract cell surface membranes adjacent to basophil granules were damaged. Deaths of feeding ticks were correlated with the observed ultrastructural changes. Tick antigens responsible for induction and expression of acquired resistance have yet to be clearly identified.

TICK SALIVA

Immunogens

Saliva of ticks changes in protein composition during the course of engorgement (Oaks et al. 1991). The dynamic nature of tick feeding is characterized by the

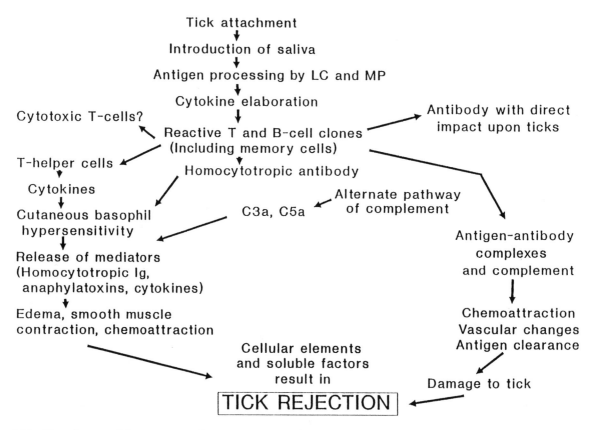

RESISTANT HOST

Tick attachment
↓
Introduction of saliva
↓
Antigen processing by LC and MP
↓
Cytokine elaboration
↓
Cytotoxic T-cells? ← Reactive T and B-cell clones → Antibody with direct impact upon ticks
(Including memory cells)
T-helper cells ← Homocytotropic antibody
↓
Cytokines
↓ Alternate pathway
Cutaneous basophil C3a, C5a ← of complement
hypersensitivity
↓ Antigen-antibody
Release of mediators complexes
(Homocytotropic Ig, and complement
anaphylatoxins, cytokines) ↓
↓ Chemoattraction
Edema, smooth muscle Vascular changes
contraction, chemoattraction Antigen clearance
↓
Cellular elements Damage to tick
and soluble factors
result in

TICK REJECTION

34.4   Flow diagram of the expression of resistance to tick infestation

introduction of a changing array of immunogens and pharmacologically active molecules into the feeding site (Ribeiro 1987a, b; Wikel 1988 Ribeiro et al. 1992). Many of these molecules have a systemic effect on the host. The alteration of host immune and inflammatory responses would facilitate tick feeding and the transmission of tick-borne pathogens.

Our understanding of the nature of tick saliva begins with an examination of the components that stimulate host antibody responses during infestation. Various molecules contained in tick saliva induce the production of host antibodies. The amounts of tick-specific immunoglobulin present during the course of infestation have been determined for several tick-host associations. Immunoblotting was used to determine

the specificities of tick-reactive immunoglobulins. The most useful information has been derived from studies involving the detection of antibodies induced by actual tick feeding. Immunization with isolated salivary gland components stimulated a very different antibody response from that elicited by exposure to saliva during engorgement.

Antibodies obtained from rabbits hypersensitized by infestation with *Hyalomma anatolicum anatolicum* were used to probe electrophoretograms by immuno-blotting fractionated saliva and a salivary gland extract derived from the sensitizing tick species (Gill et al. 1986). Antibodies reacted with 9 polypeptide bands in saliva and 17 in the extract of whole salivary glands. The salivary glands used to prepare the extract were obtained from female *H. anatolicum anatolicum* that had been allowed to engorge for 96 hours. All saliva antigens and 12 of the 17 salivary gland extract molecules reactive on immunoblotting were glycoconjugates. Immunogens appeared to be common to different stages of feeding, and their molecular weights ranged from 14.4–130.0. kDa. Three fractions isolated from sodium dodecyl sulfate polyacrylamide gels elicited skin reactions upon intradermal inoculation into rabbits previously exposed to *H. anatolicum anatolicum* infestation. Two fractions elicited immediate hypersensitivity reactions. One of those fractions, along with a 3rd extract, elicited delayed type hypersensitivity cutaneous reactions. Therefore, at least 2 of the salivary gland–derived molecules elicited both antibody and cell-mediated immune responses.

Shapiro et al. (1986) characterized the antibody responses of guinea pigs resistant to infestation with *Rhipicephalus appendiculatus*. Resistance was mediated by antibodies to several tick antigens. Immunoblot analysis revealed reactive bands in extracts of salivary glands prepared from ticks allowed to feed for different durations on nonresistant hosts. Bands recognized by immunoblotting ranged in molecular weight from 16.0–120.0 kDa. Larval and nymphal tick extracts lacked many of the adult ixodid antigens. A 90.0 kDa salivary gland–derived molecule was associated with the induction of host acquired resistance to *R. appendiculatus* infestation (Shapiro et al. 1987).

Gordon and Allen (1987) found that concentrations of tick salivary gland antigens changed during engorgement. Some of the observed concentration changes correlated with differences in skin test reactivity of tick-resistant guinea pigs to salivary gland extracts isolated at different times during feeding.

Sheep exhibiting resistance to infestation with *Amblyomma americanum* developed antibodies to salivary gland molecules of 29.0 and 35.5 kDa (Barriga et al. 1991). Several polypeptides were recognized by sera after an initial infestation but not after a 3rd exposure to tick feeding.

Amblyomma americanum, *D. variabilis,* and *Ixodes scapularis* were found to share 45.0 and 90.0 kDa salivary gland antigens (Jaworski et al. 1990). Antibodies of rabbits and rats exposed to *I. scapularis*–bound glycoproteins in salivary gland homogenates of *I. scapularis*, and *D. variabilis* (Wheeler et al. 1991). Cattle, guinea pigs, and rabbits developed cross-reactive antibodies as a consequence of infestation with either *A. americanum* or *Dermacentor andersoni* (Wikel and Whelen 1986). The possibility of cross-protective immunogens is an important area to investigate in relation to vaccine development.

The antibody responses to tick feeding are clearly complex in terms of the number of immunogenic molecules in the saliva and the changing nature of those molecules in terms of both presence and/or concentration. Development of an anti-tick vaccine directed toward salivary secretions must take into account the changing nature of the saliva and the possible requirement of multiple immunogens. Antibodies observed only in sera of resistant hosts can be effective probes for protection-inducing immunogens. Some molecules introduced during feeding might be immunodominant and totally unrelated to host protection.

Pharmacological Activity

Salivas of hematophagous arthropods contain a variety of pharmacological activities (Table 34.1) that facilitate acquisition of blood meals and transmission of disease agents (Titus and Ribeiro 1990). Arthropods benefit from the antihemostatic, vasodilatory, antiinflammatory, and immunosuppressive properties of saliva. The relationship of these activities to tick feeding has been more thoroughly investigated than other vector-host associations.

Salivary glands of engorging *D. andersoni* contain molecules that inhibit the activities of coagulation factors V and VII, thus inhibiting both the intrinsic and extrinsic coagulation pathways (Gordon and Allen 1991a). The role of these inhibitory factors in tick feeding has not been established.

Purified salivary gland antigens of *D. andersoni* generated chemotactic activity from complement component C5 (Gordon and Allen 1991b). Chemotactic reactivity resides with the anaphylatoxin C5a, which contributes to the accumulation of inflammatory cells at tick attachment sites on resistant animals. Complement component C5a is an anaphylatoxin that causes the release of mast cell and basophil mediators into the

TABLE 34.1 Pharmacological and immunological activities of hematophagous arthropod salivas

Inhibition of coagulation factors V and VII	*Dermacentor andersoni* (tick)
Chemotactic activity from complement component C5	*D. andersoni*
Apyrase activity inhibiting platelet aggregation	*Ixodes scapularis* (tick)
	Rhodinus prolixus (triatomine bug)
	Aedes aegypti (mosquito)
	Phlebotomus papatasi (sand fly)
	Glossina tachinoides (tsetse fly)
Kininase to inhibit pain that stimulates host grooming	*I. scapularis*
Anaphylatoxin inactivating activity	*I. scapularis*
Prostacyclin increases blood flow and inhibits leukocyte degranulation	*I. scapularis*

Note: Prostaglandin E2 increases blood flow to feeding site, which inhibits mast cell degranulation and neutrophil aggregation and inhibits release of host cytokines.

local tissue environment. Mast cell and basophil associated chemotactic factors most certainly are involved in cutaneous lesion formation. Histamine, leuko-trienes, prostaglandins, and other mediators affect various receptors associated with tissues at the feeding site. Increased vascular permeability, hyperemia, and sensory stimulation result from the release of these factors and the presence of acute phase molecules at the bite site. The alternative pathway of complement activation is involved in the expression of acquired resistance to tick infestation (Wikel 1979). The role of lymphocyte-derived chemotactic cytokines in generation of the tick feeding lesion remains to be established.

Ixodes scapularis saliva contains apyrase activity, which inhibits aggregation of platelets induced by platelet aggregation factor, ADP, and collagen (Ribeiro et al. 1985). Many arthropods (including the triatomine bug, *Rhodnius prolixus*; the mosquito, *Aedes aegypti*; the sand fly, *Phlebotomus papatasi*; and the tsetse fly, *Glossina tachinoides*) possess salivary apyrase activity to inhibit clotting of host blood (Ribeiro et al. 1985; Ribeiro 1987; Titus and Ribeiro 1990). Prostaglandin E2 (PGE2) in saliva of *I. scapularis* increases blood flow to the feeding site and inhibits mast cell degranulation and neutrophil aggregation (Ribeiro et al. 1985). These events facilitate tick feeding. However, the PGE2 response can enhance pain mediated by bradykinin, which stimulates increased host grooming. Saliva of *I. scapularis* contains a kininase, which inhibits bradykinin and the host pain response.

Modulation of the Host Immune Response

Ticks and their hosts live in a dynamic balance between host responses designed to inhibit tick feeding/pathogen transmission and parasite-derived strategies designed to circumvent those host defense mechanisms. Ticks and their hosts live in associations that result in prolonged exposure to the elements of the host immune system. A successful host-tick association results in the modulation of the host immune response. The ability to immunomodulate host defenses might be a factor in determining the range of host species a particular tick species can infest. The following section describes the nature of tick-induced host immunomodulation. This information is important for identifying vaccine immunogens. Host immune responses that are suppressed by the blood-feeding ectoparasite might be important in the rejection of the hematophagous arthropod. Suppression of those immune responses likely facilitates tick survival. Immunosuppressive molecules introduced by the vector should be considered as vaccine targets.

Anaphylatoxin inactivating activity was described for the saliva of *I. scapularis* by Ribeiro and Spielman (1986). Tick-mediated inhibition of anaphylatoxin blocks aspects of host-complement–dependent immune defenses directed against the feeding tick. As described earlier, host anaphylatoxin (C5a) could play a role in the cutaneous lesion induced by tick feeding upon a resistant host. The alternative complement pathway is involved in the expression of acquired resistance to ticks. *I. scapularis* saliva contains a 49.0 kDa moiety that inhibits activation of the alternative pathway of complement (Ribeiro 1987).

Prostacyclin activity has been detected in *I. scapularis* saliva, which could prevent leukocyte degranulation at the tick feeding site (Ribeiro et al. 1988). Salivary prostacyclin would also increase blood flow at the tick feeding site.

Lymphocytes obtained from guinea pigs exposed to ticks had significantly reduced in vitro proliferative responses to the T-lymphocyte mitogens concanavalin A (Con A) and phytohemagglutinin (PHA) when compared with similar cells obtained from uninfested controls (Wikel 1982b). In vitro responsiveness to the B-lymphocyte mitogen *Escherichia coli* lipopolysaccharide (LPS) was not reduced. First-infestation ConA responses were reduced by 78.7% and PHA reactivity by 60.8%. Reductions in reactivity after a 2nd infestation were 48.6% for Con A and 50.1% for PHA. Circulating antibodies induced during the 1st infestation to tick saliva probably neutralized some of the inhibitory molecules introduced during the 2nd tick feeding.

Infestation with *D. andersoni* larvae significantly reduced the ability of hosts to generate a primary antibody response against the thymic-dependent antigen, sheep red blood cells (Wikel 1985a). The immunoglobulin class (IgM) plaque-forming cell response to sheep red blood cells was reduced by 46.4% of control values by the end of a 1st tick exposure and 58.3% by the 2nd day of a subsequent infestation. Ability to produce an antibody response returned to normal within several days after termination of tick infestation. The findings of these studies indicate that host T-lymphocytes are targets of tick-induced immunosuppression.

The immune response to infectious agents is exquisitely regulated by the host cytokine network (Cannon et al. 1990). Tick salivary gland extracts from female *D. andersoni* were prepared daily during the course of engorgement. These salivary gland extracts were then tested for their ability to influence the in vitro proliferation of lymphocytes induced by B- or T-cell mitogens and to alter the elaboration of cytokines from normal macrophages and lymphocytes (Ramachandra and Wikel 1992).

Salivary gland extracts were prepared for days 0–9 of engorgement, and protein concentrations were determined. The extract was not cytotoxic to cells in the test systems. Normal T-lymphocyte responses to Con A were suppressed in the presence of salivary gland extracts by up to 68.4%, whereas proliferation induced by the B-lymphocyte mitogen *E. coli* lipopolysaccharide was enhanced. The finding of depressed in vitro T-lymphocyte reactivity to Con A was similar to the reduced responsiveness of cells derived from tick-exposed hosts (Wikel 1982b).

The same salivary gland extracts were tested for their ability to influence elaboration of cytokines by normal macrophages and lymphocytes (Ramachandra and Wikel 1992). Macrophage-derived cytokines studied were interleukin-1 (IL-1) and tumor necrosis factor (TNF). Lymphocyte-produced cytokines assayed were interleukin-2 (IL-2) and interferon-gamma (IFN-G).

Salivary gland extracts prepared on days 0–5 of engorgement suppressed IL-1 production from 89.8% on day 0 through 61.6% on day 5. Levels of TNF were reduced by extracts collected throughout the course of engorgement from 40.7–94.6%. T-lymphocyte production of IL-2 was suppressed by 14.1–31.9%, and IFN-G by 8.7–57.0%. Subsequent studies in this laboratory revealed that interleukin-4 (IL-4) levels were not altered by these salivary extracts.

Tick-induced reduction of host cytokine can impact a variety of immunoregulatory pathways essential for the development of an immune response to the blood-feeding arthropod and tick-transmitted disease agents. Reduced IL-1 levels limit host ability to activate T-lymphocytes and provide costimulatory, differentiation, and development signals for B-lymphocytes. Reduced TNF levels could result in impaired antiviral activity and decreased activation of polymorphonuclear leukocytes. Activities of IL-2 include augmentation of immunoglobulin production, promotion of natural killer-cell activities, and autocrine stimulation of T-lymphocyte growth. Interferon-gamma is an important regulator of immune function and host defenses; it promotes B-lymphocyte differentiation and immunoglobulin secretion and antiviral activity, and enhances macrophage killing.

Tick-induced modulation of host macrophage and lymphocyte cytokine responses affect many important aspects of host immune regulation and expression. Tick-induced reduction of host immunocompetence centers on the macrophage with less dramatic impact upon T-lymphocytes. Loss of appropriate macrophage-derived signals impairs the responsiveness of T-lymphocytes. The central role of macrophages in antigen processing/presentation and regulation of activities of other cells of the host defense system makes them an ideal target for parasite-induced immunosuppression. Host immune competence is only partially reduced by tick salivary gland–derived molecules. The balance between survival of the host and successful tick feeding and pathogen transmission appears to be achieved by the level of immunosuppression induced. Reduced host immunocompetence is likely a factor in the ability of the relatively small numbers of microorganisms transmitted by a feeding tick to successfully establish infection.

VACCINATION-BASED CONTROL OF VECTORS

The control of blood-feeding arthropod vectors of disease is important to medical and veterinary public health. Arthropod resistance to acaricides and insecticides is a global problem that most visibly impacts production of livestock. The rapid onset and broad-spectrum nature of acaricide resistance illustrates the major problems influencing tick control. Alternative strategies of tick suppression must be developed. One of the most promising is vaccination-induced host anti-tick immunity. Advantages of this approach over use of acaricides include target-species specificity, absence of meat/milk residues, minimal environmental consequences, ease of administration, and low cost. Slow-release vaccines can be formulated that require only one injection (under ideal circumstances); thus, less handling is necessary than when acaricides are used.

Several important points must be considered in the development of an anti-arthropod vaccine (Table 34.2).

TABLE 34.2 Factors to consider in development of anti-arthropod vaccines

Detailed knowledge of host immune response to infestation.

Utilize antibody and cell-mediated immune responses of resistant hosts to identify protection-inducing immunogens.

Characterize vector-induced modulation of host immune response. Host immune responses suppressed by the blood-feeding arthropod might damage the vector if not suppressed. Consider molecules responsible for host immunosuppression as vaccine targets.

Vaccine immunogens must have T-lymphocyte epitopes that can be "processed and presented" to immunocompetent cells of animals in a randomly bred population.

Consider the use of "novel" immunogens to which a host response would impair pathogen transmission, damage, or kill the feeding vector.

Host immune response, pathogenesis, and ectoparasite evasion strategies must be characterized for any host–blood-feeding arthropod relationship. Target immunogens must be identified that effect immune responses in a genetically heterogeneous population.

The vaccine immunogens must be effectively processed and presented to T- and B-lymphocytes of randomly bred animals. Therefore, selection of broadly reactive epitopes is essential. Several factors must be considered in the selection of vaccine immunogens. Arthropod molecules that induce host antibodies present in a susceptible host are probably not important for survival of the arthropod. Immunogen identification efforts must focus on molecules to which little or no response occurs during the susceptible phase of natural infestation. Antibodies present during the expression of acquired resistance might be important probes for protection-inducing immunogens. Molecules that induce host immunosuppression might be essential for survival of the arthropod and should be considered vaccine targets.

Do not assume that protection rests entirely with antibodies. Stimulation of an effective cell-mediated immune response might be the key to protection. Adjuvants must be selected that will stimulate the appropriate T-lymphocyte subpopulations and elicit the desired immunoglobulin isotype(s). Knowledge of the cytokine networks is very useful in directing the development of a protective immune response. Cytokine manipulation and colony-stimulating factors must be considered potential adjuvants in the development of any vaccine formulation.

The tools of biotechnology facilitate the production of immunogens for vaccine use. However, the tendency to become "sophisticated" and depend on the production of recombinant immunogens alone must be curbed. The generation of recombinant immunogens is a perfectly logical approach to vaccine development. However, to be recognized by the immune systems of the randomly bred population (in which the vaccine will be used) the molecule must have sufficient T-lymphocyte epitopes. Alternative methods for production of immunogens, such as cell culture, also must be considered. Table 34.2 provides an overview of some of the main points to consider in anti-arthropod vaccine development.

Ticks

Anti-arthropod vaccine research has focused most intensely upon the control of ixodid ticks; however, other blood- and tissue-feeding arthropods are excellent candidates for immunization-based control. Vaccine-based control of arthropods has been investigated for myiasis larvae (Sandeman 1992), stable flies (Schlein and Lewis 1976), sucking lice (Ratzlaff and Wikel 1990), and mosquitoes (Sutherland and Ewen 1974). The following examination of vaccine-based control of blood-feeding arthropods concentrates on ticks because the largest body of work has been performed with these species. Vaccines directed toward other arthropods and the future use of this approach for arthropod and vector-borne disease suppression are examined.

The vaccination against arthropods is an area of scientific endeavor that is still in its infancy. The work to date has been productive and revealing. Specific protection-inducing immunogens are being defined. Emphasis must be placed upon examination of the whole immune response to candidate immunogens to select the best approach for successful anti-tick vaccination.

A logical starting point in the quest for an anti-tick vaccine was the use of whole tick homogenates or salivary gland extracts; however, recent investigations have centered around the use of defined immunogens (Wikel et al. 1992). Trager (1939) induced resistance to infestation with *D. variabilis* by immunizing guinea pigs with an intracutaneous injection of an extract of whole larvae. Resistance was induced against a subsequent infestation with larvae of the same species. An extract of *I. holocyclus* larvae was used to induce resistance to larval challenge (Bagnall 1975). Variable levels of resistance were induced, with hosts rejecting 38–68% of infesting larvae. Examination of tick attachment sites on immunized animals revealed the presence of CBH reactions similar to those associated with the expression of acquired resistance. An extract of whole adult *Hyalomma anatolicum anatolicum* was administered to rabbits by 2 intramuscular injections and a 3rd inoculation by the subcutaneous route (Manohar and Banerjee 1992). Ticks that obtained a blood meal from immunized animals had decreased engorgement weight and egg masses and prolonged feeding times. Mean engorgement weight was reduced by 29.48%, and egg mass was reduced by 36.44%.

Characterization of acquired resistance to tick feeding demonstrated the role of tick salivary gland–derived molecules in acquisition and expression of host immunity to ticks. A logical approach to induction of anti-tick immunity was the development of a vaccine consisting of salivary gland–derived immunogens. Resistance to infestation with *B. microplus* was induced in calves by immunization with partially engorged salivary glands of the same species (Brossard 1976). Salivary glands of partially fed female *D. andersoni* were homogenized, and a 10,000 × g supernatant was used to immunize guinea pigs, which were made resistant to a subsequent infestation with larvae of the same species (Wikel 1981). Cutaneous lesions developed at tick feeding sites on vaccinated animals. Rabbits vaccinated with salivary gland extracts of *R. appendiculatus* and allowed to feed for 4 to 5 days were resistant to all 3 life-cycle stages of the tick. Engorgement weights of ticks allowed to feed on immunized animals were reduced the following amounts when compared with ixodids obtained from unimmunized controls: adults 43.4%, nymphs 44.9%, and larvae 25%.

Cattle were immunized with whole salivary gland extracts obtained from partially engorged female *H. anatolicum anatolicum* (Banerjee et al. 1990). Salivary glands were removed, homogenized, sonicated, and centrifuged at 10,000 × g at 5°C for 30 minutes. The supernatant was used as antigen I. Stored salivary glands were thawed, homogenized, and centrifuged as described and used as antigen II. Both of these antigen preparations were used to induce significant resistance to tick infestation. Both antibody and cell-mediated immune responses were induced by these immunization regimens. Determination of both immunoglobulin and cell-mediated immune responses is essential in the development of a vaccine.

The selection of partially engorged ticks as a source of protection-inducing salivary gland immunogens indicates that either the protection-inducing immunogens are only present in glands at a certain stage of engorgement or the levels of immunogen are maximal at that time.

Whole tick and salivary gland extracts are not practical for the development of a commercially acceptable vaccine because of the often low and variable levels of resistance induced. Vaccination-induced priming for development of cutaneous lesions at tick attachment sites on immunized animals is not desirable because of the potential for secondary infections and infestations. Proper selection and potentiation of a salivary gland antigen or antigens might provide a vaccine that would induce high levels of protection without sensitizing for cutaneous reactivity upon exposure to subsequent tick feeding.

Determination of vaccine efficacy is an important consideration. Extracts, fractions, and individual immunogens must be tested for their ability to induce resistance to tick feeding by actual immunization of target species. These studies are time-consuming and costly; however, they are the best measure of protection-inducing capacity of a material to be tested. An in vitro assay correlating with vaccine potency would be best because animal testing of each lot of vaccine

requires a considerable amount of time. Determination of levels of antibodies damaging a target tissue of the tick is a useful approach for in vitro testing of a vaccine. However, it is difficult to culture the desired tick cells used in such an assay.

Immunogens not associated with saliva and the development of acquired resistance have been used to induce anti-tick immunity. The use of these immunogens is appealing because they are likely not introduced into the host during feeding. However, these molecules must be accessible to immune effector elements in host blood during feeding. The most commonly used molecules are derived from tick digestive tract; however, other appropriate targets for the host immune response are hormones, elements of the nervous system, cuticle, muscle, or hemolymph proteins. In addition, tick tissue culture cells have been used successfully to induce resistance to infestation. Production of these antigens in sufficient quantities for a commercial vaccine will require recombinant protein technology or the development of novel tissue culture systems.

Primary tissue culture cells of developing *A. americanum* larvae successfully protected against a challenge infestation with adults of the same species (Wikel 1985b). Anti-tick immunity was induced by subcutaneous administration of 1 million cells, without adjuvant, on days 0, 7, and 21. Mean engorgement weight of female *A. americanum*, which fed upon immunized animals, was reduced by 74.8%, and 54.6% of challenge females died. These dramatic results were even more intriguing when it was observed that animals immunized with *A. americanum* primary tissue culture cells were also resistant to infestation with *D. andersoni* adults.

The finding of cross-protective immunity is important. A single vaccine that can protect against infestation with multiple tick species would be advantageous. *A. americanum* and *D. andersoni* are not closely related ixodid species, but the protection-inducing immunogen(s) in the primary tissue culture cells examined were not determined. Tissue culture cells are an excellent source of protection-inducing immunogens, but considerable effort is necessary to establish continuous lines of cells of the appropriate tick tissues. Achieving that goal will not be an easy task.

Guinea pigs were successfully protected against infestation by immunization with antigens consisting of midgut/reproductive tract or all internal organs of *D. andersoni* (Allen and Humphreys 1979). Host response induced by immunization with midgut/reproductive tract extract resulted in reduced engorgement by challenge females; ova produced by those ticks also were inhibited from hatching. Host antibodies might have damaged the gut of the feeding tick and altered a possibly vast array of physiological processes within the vector. A "leaky" gut allows host antibodies specific for reproductive tract to travel to the target tissues. Rats immunized with midgut tissues of *D. variabilis* developed a significant level of resistance to challenge infestation with the same tick species (Ackerman et al. 1980). The effective use of immunogens other than those of salivary gland origin was clearly established by these investigators. How long the immune effector elements of the host remain functional within the tick tissues is a question yet to be answered.

The most promising approaches to vaccine induction of anti-tick immunity center on the use of digestive tract–derived molecules. These "novel" immunogens are not introduced into the host in large quantities during the feeding process; however, they are accessible to host immune effector elements in the blood meal. Immunization with tick gut–derived epitopes is not likely to prime the host for cutaneous hypersensitivity reactions upon challenge infestation. Immunization with tick gut–derived immunogens would stimulate host immune responses, which differ from those involved in acquired resistance to tick feeding. Immunity to infestation induced by immunization with tick gut is expressed by reduced engorgement, impaired production of ova, decreased viability of ova, and death of feeding ticks. Immunization with tick digestive tract immunogens stimulates limited immune cross-reactivity with ixodid salivary gland molecules.

Tick digestive tract brushborder molecules isolated from female *A. americanum* were used to induce resistance to infestation with adults of the same species (Wikel 1988). Resistance induced with absorptive surface fragments reduced engorgement of female *A. americanum* by up to 69.8%. Females that did engorge produced fewer ova. Between 37.5 and 71.5% of challenge ticks died as a result of feeding upon hosts immunized with brushborder immunogens. Both male and female ticks were killed. Cutaneous reactions did not occur at tick attachment sites on vaccinated animals.

Biotinylated lectins were used to probe sodium dodecyl sulfate polyacrylamide gel electrophoretograms that were electroeluted to nitrocellulose (Wikel 1988). The vast majority of molecules on the lectin blot were glycosylated. Sera of animals protected against tick infestation by immunization with brushborder extract were used to identify reactive components in the extract by immunoblotting (Wikel 1988). Immunoblot and lectin blot activities were correlated. Lectin affinity chromatography has been used to isolate protection-inducing glycoconjugates.

A soluble protection-inducing immunogen has been identified in *D. andersoni* brushborder extract (D.K. Bergman, A.R. Apperson, and S.K. Wikel, unpublished observations). Preparative sodium dodecyl sulfate polyacrylamide gel electrophoresis was used to fractionate brushborder soluble extract proteins. A 74-kDa fraction induced solid immunity to challenge infestation with nymphs. Only 50% of nymphs engorged, and 90% died by the 7th day postfeeding. None of the replete nymphs molted to adults. Further purification of this soluble immunogen is in progress. Tick gut brushborder membrane-bound molecules are being fractionated and tested for their ability to induce resistance to infestation.

Opdebeeck and her colleagues (1988) immunized Hereford steers with the soluble, 100,000 × g supernatant and membrane pellet of *B. microplus* midgut. Cattle immunized with the membrane pellet blocked 91% of 3 challenge infestations, each consisting of 20,000 larvae. Vaccine-induced resistance persisted through the 7th month postimmunization. Nonionic detergent–solubilized gut membrane of larval *B. microplus* was used to vaccinate cattle (Wong and Opdebeeck 1990). Immunized cattle inhibited 78% of larvae from 2 challenge infestations, each consisting of 20,000 larvae. Immunoglobulins obtained from previously immunized and protected steers were used to purify via immunoaffinity protection-inducing immunogens. Purified antigens increased levels of induced resistance to 80% and 89% for 2 challenge trials. The protection-inducing molecules are present in adult and larval gut membranes but not in developing ova (Opdebeeck et al. 1992).

Immunization with midgut membranes induced several antigen-specific bovine immunoglobulin isotypes that were correlated with protection against infestation (Jackson and Opdebeeck 1990). Bovine IgG1 and complement fixation were correlated with resistance to tick infestation, while IgG2 and IgM isotypes were not associated with protection. Opdebeeck and Daly (1990) examined the immune responses of Hereford cattle vaccinated with *B. microplus* adult midgut membranes. In vitro lymphocyte proliferation assays prepared with cells from vaccinated animals were reactive with gut and salivary gland antigens. Antibodies produced by the same animals reacted with soluble salivary gland extracts, salivary gland membrane, soluble gut extracts, gut membrane, soluble larval extracts, and larval membranes.

Protection-inducing gut membrane immunogens were treated with 25 mM sodium metaperiodate that oxidizes carbohydrates and alters their antigenic determinants (Opdebeeck et al. 1992). Cattle vaccinated with these immunogens were not protected against tick challenge. It was concluded that carbohydrate or carbohydrate-dependent determinants maintain the specificity of the protection-inducing immunogen. A positive correlation was no longer found when antibodies from gut membrane-immunized cattle were reacted with gut membrane that had been treated with metaperiodate. Immunogold-labeled monoclonal antibodies were used to localize gut membrane antigens close to the surface of the tick digestive tract microvilli, a site likely rich in glycosylated molecules (Opdebeeck et al. 1992).

Induction of protective immunity in this system required up to 6 immunizations of an individual animal. A vaccine requiring that many inoculations to achieve potentially short-lived immunity is not practical from a commercial perspective. In response to that concern, considerable attention has been directed toward adjuvants in this system (Opdebeeck et al.

1992). A cholesterol-phospholipid implant has been devised that is not only biodegradable but also delivers the immunogen as a burst followed by a trickle over an appropriate period of time.

Important considerations in this vaccine development effort are the attention to both cell-mediated and antibody responses to immunogens, development of practical delivery systems, and the knowledge that a truly effective vaccine requires immunogens that can induce a protective anti-tick response in animals of diverse genetic backgrounds. Future progress in this system is anxiously awaited.

An elegant series of experiments designed to develop a recombinant vaccine against *B. microplus* has been recently reviewed (Tellam et al. 1992). The use of "concealed" gut-derived immunogen to induce immunity shows considerable promise. Willadsen et al. (1988) reported the successful induction of protection of bovines against *B. microplus* infestation by immunization with material isolated from semiengorged females of that species. Further purification resulted in identification of a membrane-bound glycoprotein designated Bm86 that is associated with the surface of digest cells (Tellam et al. 1992). Antibodies of vaccinated cattle to Bm86 bind to the gut digest cells and inhibit endocytosis by those cells. Tick digestion is an intracellular process, and endocytosis of blood-meal components is essential. Digest cells apparently are not lysed by the antibodies to Bm86, even though complement enhances the effect of antibody binding.

Bm86 has been well characterized (Tellam et al. 1992). This glycoprotein has a pI of 5.5. It consists of 650 amino acids and 66 cysteines, which indicates extensive intramolecular disulfide bonds. Amino acid sequence analysis revealed significant homologies with the precursor of epidermal growth factor. Apparently, Bm86 does not contain an active epidermal growth factor–like peptide. Four potential N-linked glycosylation sites have been identified. It has been speculated that Bm86 might extend some distance into the intracellular environment, making it accessible to endocytosed antibodies.

Epitope analysis has provided evidence for the existence of more than 1 protection-inducing epitope (Tellam et al. 1992). Emphasis was placed on the observation that the bacterial-expressed recombinant protein is unlikely to be correctly folded; however, it could still induce protection against infestation. This finding could indicate that at least some protection-inducing epitopes might not be conformational in nature. Recombinant Bm86 has been expressed in bacterial *Escherichia coli*, fungal *Aspergillus nidulans*, and insect cell *Spodoptera frugiperda Baculovirus* expression systems. A eukaryotic expression system was thought to be optimal because of the need for posttranslational processing and glycosylation.

Host anti-tick immunity depended on the nature of the Bm86 antigen preparation used as immunogen (Tellam et al. 1992). Immunization with native Bm86 reduced tick numbers by 61–70% and reproductive capacity by 91–93%. Vaccination with recombinant Bm86 of *E. coli* origin induced a response that reduced tick numbers by 24–27% and reproductive capacity by 77–89%. Antigen obtained from the baculovirus expression system stimulated host resistance, which reduced tick numbers by 13–34% and reproductive capacity by 63–68%. Commercial production of this vaccine dictates that recombinant Bm86 immunogen be used. It appears that levels of protection induced by recombinant-derived Bm86 would be at least as solid as those stimulated by vaccination with the native molecule. Variable levels of protection induced by recombinant Bm86, as compared with native molecules, might indicate differences in antigen processing and presentation to immunocompetent host cells. Host cell–mediated immune responses stimulated by Bm86 have not been described. It is possible that recombinant Bm86 and native Bm86 differ in their T-lymphocyte epitopes, which could explain differences in the host immune response stimulated by vaccination. A significant concern about recombinant vaccines is the potential limited number of T-lymphocyte epitopes, which could result in little or no immunogenicity when the vaccine is administered to members of a randomly bred population. This problem can possibly be corrected by incorporating into the immunogen structure a broadly recognized T-lymphocyte epitope from a different molecule.

Another interesting approach to immunological control of ticks was described by Rutti and Brossard

(1989). More than 50% of sera derived from mice infested with *I. ricinus* nymphs and rabbits infested with *I. ricinus* adults reacted with a 25 kDa antigen detected in the integument and in an extract of whole *I. ricinus*. Immunoglobulins reactive with the *I. ricinus* integument molecule bound to a 20 kDa molecule derived from the integument of female *R. appendiculatus*. Cattle immunized with the 20 kDa antigen were significantly resistant to a challenge infestation with adult *R. appendiculatus* (Rutti and Brossard 1992). Host immunoglobulins cross the tick digestive tract, and they might be capable of binding to molecules essential to the normal formation and function of the cuticle. This novel approach to tick control must be thoroughly investigated.

The main features of anti-tick vaccine research to date are summarized in Table 34.3.

TABLE 34.3   Approaches to development of anti-tick vaccine

Whole tick extracts.	Variable levels of resistance.
Salivary gland extracts.	Variable levels of resistance. Cutaneous reactions at bite sites.
Tick tissue culture cells derived from developing larvae. Effective protection achieved against sensitizing and heterologous species.	
Extract of whole tick gut. Need to identify and produce specific immunogens for commercial production.	
Isolated brush border of tick digestive tract. Need specific immunogen.	
Carbohydrate immunogen from brush border of tick gut digestive cells.	
Gut digest cell surface antigen; when blocked inhibits endocytosis.	
Integument-derived molecule used to induce resistance.	

Arthropods Other Than Ticks

Vaccination is a feasible approach for the control of both long- and short-term blood-feeding arthropods and myiasis larvae. Advances in biotechnology and the characterization of host immune responses to arthropods provide powerful tools for the development of vaccines for the control of a number of species. Examination of the literature provides useful information about potential host-arthropod relationships.

An extremely interesting series of experiments was performed in which rabbits were immunized with tissues of the mosquito *Anopheles stephensi* (Alger and Cabrera 1972). The following mosquito-derived immunogen preparations were used to vaccinate rabbits: supernatant of an extract of whole mosquitoes, pellet of whole female mosquito extract, and an extract of female mosquito midgut. Mosquitoes that obtained a blood meal from midgut-immunized rabbits had a significantly higher death rate than those *An. stephensi* that fed upon controls. Sutherland and Ewen (1974) immunized rabbits and guinea pigs with an extract of whole female *Aedes aegypti*. The fecundity of *Ae. aegypti* obtaining a blood meal from immunized hosts was reduced. These 2 studies provide evidence that immunization against mosquitoes is possible.

Mosquito gut brush border would be a likely place to look for protection-inducing immunogens; however, the role of the peritrophic membrane also must be considered. Houk et al. (1986) developed a method for isolation of mosquito gut brushborder fragments. A vaccine might be designed that consists of epitopes derived from both brush border and peritrophic membrane.

Biting flies are likely candidates for immune mediated control. The horn fly, *Haematobia irritans*, and stable fly, *Stomoxys calcitrans*, are particularly susceptible to immune effector elements in the host blood meal. Schlein and Lewis (1976) immunized rabbits with one of the following homogenates derived from *S. calcitrans*: cuticle and adhering hypodermal cells, thoracic muscles, abdominal tissues, or wing buds. Mortality of flies obtaining a blood meal from immunized animals was greater than for flies feeding on unvaccinated controls. The greatest damage occurred to flies feeding on hosts immunized with *S. calcitrans* thoracic muscles. *Glossina morsitans* that were fed on rabbits immunized with *S. calcitrans* tissues had higher rates of mortality than those engorging from unvaccinated controls (Schlein et al. 1976).

Myiasis represents an excellent opportunity for vaccine-based control of arthropods of veterinary importance.

Efforts to develop vaccines for the control of *Hypoderma* and *Lucilia* have been reviewed by Sandeman (1992).

Cattle acquire resistance to infestation with *Hypoderma bovis* and *Hypoderma lineatum*, which is directed toward the 1st instars at the cutaneous level before they migrate to the esophagus. Acquired resistance correlates with delayed hypersensitivity and not with the host immunoglobulin response. Successful vaccination against *Hypoderma* myiasis has been achieved with homogenates and metabolic products of 1st instar larvae (Sandeman 1992). The trypsinlike protease Hypodermin A helps the larva to degrade host tissue used for migration and nutrition. Hypodermin A stimulates both immediate and delayed hypersensitivity reactions, and it can degrade complement component C3. Immunization of susceptible cattle with Hypodermin A induced a response that resulted in the death of 90% of challenge larvae.

Studies to develop a vaccine against larvae of the sheep blow fly, *Lucilia cuprina*, were stimulated by the observation that afflicted sheep produced parasite-specific antibodies after infestation (Sandeman 1992). Major antigens recognized by infected sheep are derived from larval gut and salivary glands. Extracts of whole *L. cuprina* larvae are fractionated to find protection-inducing immunogens. Immunization with partially purified immunogens has resulted in up to 70% inhibition of larval development in vivo. Monoclonal antibodies have been prepared that react with internal epitopes of 1st stage larvae. Monoclonals have been identified that effect a 50% inhibition of larval growth in vitro. Those monoclonal immunoglobulins that inhibit larval growth in vitro could be used to isolate potential immunogens by immunoaffinity chromatography.

Resistance in mice to the sucking louse *Polyplax serrata* was induced by immunization with an homogenate/sonicate of whole larvae (Ratzlaff and Wikel 1990). Immunization with the "soluble" component of the extract caused a response that resulted in a reduction of 62% in the primary infestation weights of challenge lice. A cutaneous inflammatory response developed at feeding sites on immunized animals. Development of vaccines to control sucking lice is feasible, and efforts must be directed toward identification, isolation, and characterization of protection-inducing immunogens.

SUMMARY

Immunological control can be achieved for arthropods of medical and veterinary importance. Great advances have been made during the past 2 decades in the characterization of host immune responses to blood-feeding arthropods, identification of antigens involved in host reactivity to infestation, and in the development of immunological approaches to vector suppression. Only a limited number of host-arthropod associations have been examined. Extensive opportunities exist for the development of immunologically based vector suppression strategies for a number of arthropod species. Evidence exists that immunity to the arthropod impairs the transmission of vector-borne pathogens. The array of tools available to the immunologist, molecular biologist, and biotechnologist can be used to develop anti-arthropod vaccines that a few years ago were only hoped for on the "wish lists" of immunoparasitologists.

A number of fundamental elements must be considered in the development of any anti-arthropod vaccine. Those points are essential elements in the difficult quest for development of anti-arthropod vaccines.

The nature of the host immune response to infestation should be thoroughly characterized and focus on identification of immunogens that stimulate host responses. An immunogen to which a strong antibody response is induced during successful infestation is not likely to be involved in host rejection of the feeding arthropod. Those antibodies would probably be of limited value in the identification of protection-inducing immunogens for use in an anti-arthropod vaccine. Both immunoglobulin and cell-mediated immune responses must be characterized.

A very important aspect of vaccine development is a detailed analysis of any mechanisms of arthropod-mediated immunomodulation of the host. Host responses suppressed by the feeding arthropod are likely to be ones that would be potentially damaging to the survival of the ectoparasite if allowed to be fully expressed. Identification of the suppressed effector immune response(s) can provide clues to the type of protective responses that need to be stimulated and to possible target immunogens.

Selection of proper immunogens is obviously a critical factor. Emphasis should be placed on identifying new vaccine immunogens and developing reagents that can be broadly utilized in vaccine development. A parasite-derived molecule that is not highly immunogenic during the normal response to infestation might be modified to become a potent protection-inducing immunogen. An essential feature of any vaccine is the ability of the immunogens to be processed by macrophages and presented to the immunocompetent lymphocytes of a randomly bred population. Recombinant immunogens lacking broadly recognized T-lymphocyte epitopes are probably doomed to failure no matter how sophisticated the science leading to the immunogen production. Careful consideration must be given to adjuvant formulations and new delivery systems.

Anti-arthropod vaccines can become part of the tools available for vector control. They will certainly not replace acaricides and insecticides; however, their use will reduce the amount of those chemicals needed in selected settings. The technological base is in place for the development of anti-arthropod vaccines. The years ahead hold the potential for exciting research and advances. We are limited only by our perception of where we perceive the boundaries to be located.

ACKNOWLEDGMENTS

The author's research is supported by U.S. Department of Agriculture Grants 88–34116–3759 and 88–34116–4206, the Oklahoma Center for the Advancement of Science and Technology, and by an award from SmithKline Beecham Animal Health. Appreciation is expressed to Dr. Douglas K. Bergman and Dr. Rangappa N. Ramachandra for their review of the manuscript and countless helpful discussions. This manuscript is Oklahoma Agricultural Experiment Station project No. OKL 02174.

REFERENCES AND FURTHER READING

Ackerman, S., M. Floyd, and D.E. Sonenshine. 1980. Artificial immunity to *Dermacentor variabilis* (Acari: Ixodidae): Vaccination using tick antigens. *J. Med. Ent.* 17:391–397.

Alger, N.E., and E.J. Cabrera. 1972. An increase in death rate of *Anopheles stephensi* fed on rabbits immunized with mosquito antigen. *J. Econ. Entom.* 65:165–168.

Allen, J.R. 1973. Tick resistance: Basophils in skin reactions of resistant guinea pigs. *Internatl. J. Parasit.* 3:195–200.

Allen, J.R., and S.J. Humphreys. 1979. Immunisation of guinea pigs and cattle against ticks. *Nature* (London) 280:491–493.

Bagnall, B.G. 1975. Cutaneous immunity to the tick *I. holocyclus*. Ph.D. thesis. University of Sydney. 186 p.

Balashov, Y.S. 1972. Bloodsucking ticks (Ixodoidea)—vectors of disease of man and animals. *Misc. Pub. Entom. Soc. Amer.* 8:161–376.

Banerjee, D.P., R.R. Momin, and S. Samantary. 1990. Immunization of cattle (*Bos indicus* X *Bos taurus*) against *Hyalomma anatolicum anatolicum* using antigens derived from tick salivary gland extract. *Internatl. J. Parasit.* 20:969–972.

Barbour, A.G. 1992 Biological and social determinants of the Lyme disease problem. *Infect. Agents Disease* 1:50–61.

Barriga, O.O., F. Andujar, H. Sahibi, and W.J. Andrzejewski. 1991. Antigens of *Amblyomma americanum* ticks recognized by repeatedly infested sheep. *J. Parasit.* 77:710–716.

Brossard, M. 1976. Rélations immunologiques entre bovins et tiques, plus particulierement entre bovins et *Boophilus microplus*. *Acta Tropica* 33:15–36.

Brossard, M., B. Rutti, and T. Haug. 1991. Immunological relationships between host and ixodid ticks. In: C.A. Toft, A. Aeschliman, and L. Bolic, editors, *Parasite-host association: Coexistance or conflict*. Oxford: Oxford Science Publications. pp. 177–200.

Brown, A.W.A. 1983. Insecticide resistance as a factor in the integrated control of Culicidae. In: M. Laird and J.W. Miles, editors, *Integrated mosquito control methodologies*. Vol. 1. New York: Academic Press. pp. 161–235.

Cannon, J.G., R.G. Tompkins, J.A. Gelfand, H.R. Michie, G.G. Stanford, J.W.M. van der Meer, S. Endres, G. Lonneman, J. Corsetti, B. Chernow, D.W. Wilmore, S.M. Wolff, J.F. Burke, and C.A. Dinarello. 1990. Ciruculating interleukin-1 and tumor necrosis factor in septic shock and experimental endotoxin fever. *J. Infect. Diseases* 161:79–84.

Food and Agricultural Organization (of the United Nations). 1984. Ticks and tick-borne disease control. A practical field manual. Rome: Food and Agricultural Organization.

Gill, H.S., R. Boid, and C.A. Ross. 1986. Isolation and characterization of salivary gland antigens from *Hyalomma anatolicum anatolicum*. *Parasite Immun.* 8:11–25.

Good, M. F., J.A. Berzofsky, and L.H. Miller. 1988. The T-cell response to the malaria circumsporozoite protein: An immunological approach to vaccine development. *Ann. Rev. Immunol.* 6:663–688.

Gordon, J.R., and J.R. Allen. 1987. Isolation and characterization of salivary antigens from the female tick *Dermacentor andersoni*. *Parasite Immun.* 9:337–352.

———. 1991a. Factor V and VII anticoagulant activities in the salivary glands of feeding *Dermacentor andersoni* ticks. *J. Parasit.* 77:167–170.

———. 1991b. Nonspecific activation of complement factor 5 by isolated *Dermacentor andersoni* salivary antigens. *J. Parasit.* 77:296–301.

Hoogstraal, H. 1981. Changing patterns of tick-borne diseases in modern society. *Ann. Rev. Entom.* 26:75–99.

Houk, E. J., Y.M. Arcus, and J.L. Hardy. 1986. Isolation and characterization of brushborder fragments from mosquito mesenterons. *Archives Insect Biochem. Phys.* 3:135–146.

Jackson, L.A., and J.P. Opdebeeck. 1990. Humoral immune response of Hereford cattle vaccinated with midgut antigens of the cattle tick *Boophilus microplus*. *Parasite Immun.* 12:141–151.

Jaworski, D.C., M.T. Muller, F.A. Simmen, and G.R. Needham. 1990. *Amblyomma americanum*: Identification of tick salivary gland antigens from unfed and early feeding females with comparisons to *Ixodes scapularis* and *Dermacentor variabilis*. *Exper. Parasit.* 70:217–226.

Kocan, K.M. 1986. Development of *Anaplasma marginale* in ixodid ticks: Coordinated development of a rickettsial organism and its tick host. In: J.R. Sauer and J.A. Hair, editors, *Morphology, physiology, and behavioral ecology of ticks*. England: Ellis Horwood. pp. 472–505.

Laird, M. 1985. New answers to malaria problems through control? *Experientia* 41:446–456.

Lucy, D., M.J. Dolan, C.W. Moss, M. Garcia, D.G. Hollis, S. Wegner, G. Morgan, R. Almeida, D. Leong, K.S. Greisen, D.F. Welch, and L.N. Slater. 1992. Relapsing illness due to *Rochalimaea henselae* in immunocompetent hosts: implications for therapy and new epidemiological associations. *Clin. Infect. Diseases* 14:683–688.

Magnarelli, L.A. 1990. Ehrlichiosis: A veterinary problem of growing epidemiological importance. *Clin. Micro. News.* 12:145–147.

Manohar, G.S., and D.P. Banerjee. 1992. Effects of immunization of rabbits on establishment, survival and reproductive biology of the tick *Hyalomma anatolicum anatolicum. J. Parasit.* 78:77–81.

Mellanby, K. 1946. Man's reaction to mosquito bites. *Nature* 158:554.

Nithiuthai, S., and J.R. Allen. 1984a. Significant changes in epidermal Langerhans cells of guinea pigs infested with ticks (*Dermacentor andersoni*). *Immunol.* 51:133–141.

———. 1984b. Effects of ultraviolet irradiation on epidermal Langerhans cells in guinea pigs. *Immunol.* 51:143–151.

———. 1984c. Effects of ultraviolet irradiation on the acquisition and expression of tick resistance in guinea pigs. *Immunol.* 51:153–159.

Oaks, J. F., J.C. McSwain, J.A. Bantle, R.C. Essenberg, and J.R. Sauer. 1991. Putative new expression of genes in ixodid tick salivary gland development during feeding. *J. Parasit.* 77:378–383.

Opdebeeck, J.P., and K.E. Daly. 1990. Immune responses of infested and vaccinated Hereford cattle to antigens of the cattle tick, *Boophilus microplus. Vet. Immunol. Immunopath.* 25:99–108.

Opdebeeck, J. P., R.P. Lee, J.Y.M. Wong, and L.A. Jackson. 1992. Vaccination of cattle against *Boophilus microplus.* In: U.G. Munderloh and T.J. Kurtti, editors, *Proceedings of the first international conference on tick-borne pathogens at host vector Interface: An Agenda for research.* St. Paul, MN: University of Minnesota College of Agriculture. pp. 233–239.

Opdebeeck, J.P., J.Y.M. Wong, L.A. Jackson, and C. Dobson. 1988. Vaccines to protect Hereford cattle against the cattle tick *Boophilus microplus. Immunol.* 63:363–367.

Ramachandra, R.N., and S.K. Wikel. 1992. Modulation of host-immune responses by ticks (Acari: Ixodidae): Effect of salivary gland extracts on host macrophage and lymphocyte cytokine production. *J. Med. Entom.* 29:818–826.

Ratzlaff, R.E., and S.K. Wikel. 1990. Murine immune responses and immunization against *Polyplax serrata* (Anoplura: Polyplacidae). *J. Med. Entom.* 27:1002–1007.

Ribeiro, J.M.C. 1987a. *Ixodes dammini*: salivary anti-complement activity. *Exper. Parasit.* 64:347–353.

———. 1987b. Role of saliva in blood-feeding by arthropods. *Ann. Rev. Entom.* 32:463–478.

Ribeiro, J.M.C., P.M. Evans, J.C. McSwain, and J. Sauer. 1992. *Amblyomma americanum*: Characterization of salivary prostaglandins E2 and F2 alpha by RP-HPLC/bioassay and gas chromatography-mass spectrometry. *Exper. Parasit.* 74:112–116.

Ribeiro, J.M.C., G.T. Makoul, J. Levine, D.R. Robinson, and A. Spielman. 1985. Antihemostatic, antiinflammatory and immunosuppressive properties of the saliva of the tick *Ixodes dammini. J. Exper. Med.* 161:332–344.

———. 1988. *Ixodes dammini*: Evidence for salivary prostacyclin secretion. *J. Parasit.* 74:1068–1069.

Ribeiro, J.M.C., and A. Spielman. 1986. *Ixodes dammini*: Salivary anaphylatoxin inactivating activity. *Exper.Parasit.* 62:292–297.

Rutti, B., and M. Brossard. 1989. Repetitive detection by immunoblotting of an integumental 25-kDa antigen in *Ixodes ricinus* and a corresponding 20-kDa antigen in *Rhipicephalus appendiculatus* with sera from pluriinfested mice and rabbits. *Parasit. Res.* 75:325–329.

———. 1992. Vaccination of cattle against *Rhipicephalus appendiculatus* with detergent solubilized tick tissue proteins and purified 20 kDa protein. *Annals Parasitologie Humane et Comparative* 67:50–54.

Sandeman, R.M. 1992. Biotechnology and the control of myiasis diseases. In: W.K. Yong, editor, *Animal parasite control utilizing biotechnology.* Boca Raton, FL: CRC Press. pp. 275–301.

Schlein, Y., and C.T. Lewis. 1976. Lesions in hematophagous flies after feeding on rabbits immunized with fly tissues. *Phys. Entom.* 1:55–59.

Schlein, Y., D.T. Spira, and R.L. Jacobson. 1976. The passage of serum immunoglobulins through the gut of *Sarcophaga falculata. Pand. Annals Trop. Med. Parasit.* 70:227–230.

Solomon, K.R. 1983. Acaricide resistance in ticks. *Adv. Vet. Science Comp. Med.* 27:273–296.

Shapiro, S. Z., G. Buscher, and D.A.E. Dobbelaere. 1987. Acquired resistance to *Rhipicephalus appendiculatus* (Acari: Ixodidae): Identification of an antigen eliciting resistance in rabbits. *J. Med. Entom.* 24:147–154.

Shapiro, S.Z., W.P. Voigt, and K. Fujisaki. 1986. Tick antigens recognized by serum from a guinea pig resistant to infestation with the tick *Rhipicephalus appendiculatus*. *J. Parasit.* 72:454–463.

Steere, A.C. 1989. Lyme disease. *New England J. Med.* 321:586–596.

Sutherland, G.B., and A.B. Ewen. 1974. Fecundity decrease in mosquitoes ingesting blood from specifically sensitized mammals. *J. Insect Phys.* 20:655–66

Szczepanski, A., and J.L. Benach. 1991. Lyme borreliosis: Host responses to *Borrelia burgdorferi*. *Microbiol. Rev.* 55:21–34.

Tellam, R.L., D. Smith, D.H. Kemp, and P. Willadsen. 1992. Vaccination against ticks. In: W.K. Yong, editor, *Animal parasite control utilizing biotechnology*. Boca Raton, FL: CRC Press. pp. 303–331.

Titus, R.G., and J.M.C. Ribeiro. 1990. The role of vector saliva in transmission of arthropod-borne disease. *Parasit. Today*. 6:157–160.

Trager, W. 1939. Acquired immunity to ticks. *J. Parasit.* 25:57–81.

Voss-McCowan, M.E. 1991. Changes in the midgut of female *Amblyomma americanum* as a result of feeding upon hosts expressing different levels of acquired anti-tick resistance. Ph.D. dissertation. Grand Forks: University of North Dakota. 310 p.

Wheeler, C.M., J.L. Coleman, and J.L. Benach. 1991. Salivary gland antigens of *Ixodes dammini* are glycoproteins that have interspecies cross-reactivity. *J. Parasit.* 77:965–973.

Wikel, S.K. 1979. Acquired resistance to ticks. Expression of resistance by C4 deficient guinea pigs. *Amer. J. Trop. Med. Hyg.* 28:586–590.

———. 1981. The induction of host resistance to tick infestation with a salivary gland antigen. *Amer. J. Trop. Med. Hyg.* 30:284–288.

———. 1982a. Immune responses to arthropods and their products. *Ann. Rev. Entom.* 27:21–48.

———. 1982b. Influence of *Dermacentor andersoni* infestation on lymphocyte responsiveness to mitogens. *Annals Trop. Med. Parasit.* 76:627–632.

———. 1985a. Effects of tick infestation on the plaque-forming cell response to a thymic dependent antigen. *Annals Trop. Med. Parasit.* 79:195–198.

———. 1985b. Resistance to ixodid tick infestation induced by administration of tick tissue culture cells. *Annals Trop. Med. Parasit.* 79:513–518.

———. 1988. Immunological control of hematophagous arthropod vectors: Utilization of novel antigens. *Vet. Parasit.* 29:235–264.

Wikel, S.K., R.N. Ramachandra, and D.K. Bergman. 1992. Immunological strategies for suppression of vector arthropods: Novel approaches in vector control. *Bull. Soc. Vector Ecol.* 17:10–19.

Wikel, S.K., and A.C. Whelen. 1986. Ixodid-host immune interaction. Identification and characterization of relevant antigens and tick-induced host immunosuppression. *Vet. Parasit.* 20:149–174.

Willadsen, P. 1980. Immunity to ticks. *Adv. Parasit.* 18:293–313.

Willadsen, P., R.V. McKenna, and G.A. Riding. 1988. Isolation from the cattle tick, *Boophilus microplus*, of antigenic material capable of eliciting a protective immunological response in the bovine host. *Internat. J. Parasit.* 18:183–189.

Wong, J.Y.M., and J.P. Opdebeeck. 1990. Larval membrane antigens protect Hereford cattle against infestation with *Boophilus microplus*. *Parasite Immunol.* 12:75–83.

35. REARING AND CONTAINMENT OF MOSQUITO VECTORS

Stephen Higgs and Barry J. Beaty

INTRODUCTION

Many persons entering the field of vector molecular biology have little experience in the techniques, protocols, and facilities necessary to manipulate and contain arthropods that pose potential risks to humans and animals. Research involving such subjects as vector molecular biology, transgenic vectors, and vector-pathogen interactions requires containment facilities and capabilities that are rarely associated with experiments involving insects such as *Drosophila melanogaster* and *Manduca sexta* that do not transmit pathogens. There is substantial information concerning biosafety regulations and guidelines for work with human and veterinary pathogens (SALS 1980; USDHHS 1993). Guidelines for design and operation of insectaries are also available (Gerberg 1970; Gerberg et al. 1994); however, there is only limited information that describes basic requirements or guidelines for simultaneous work with vectors and pathogens (SALS 1980). In this chapter, general considerations for insectary design, operation, and biosafety protocols and practices are addressed. Mosquitoes and arboviruses are used as the principal examples of vectors and pathogens, respectively, although many of the practices and protocols are applicable to other groups. For those interested in other types of vectors, selected references describing the laboratory maintenance of some groups are provided. The insectary at the Arthropod-borne and Infectious Diseases Laboratory (AIDL) is described and used as an example of how biosafety concerns and issues can be addressed effectively and economically.

THE INSECTARY: GENERAL CONCEPTS OF CONTAINMENT

For our purposes, a secure insectary must address issues of both vector and pathogen containment and prevention of human infections. The biosafety requirements for work with pathogens and vectors are difficult to reconcile. For example, the maintenance of minimum air exchanges required for work with pathogens can preclude attainment of relative humidity levels necessary for mosquito survival. It might not be possible to satisfy all of the ideal conditions; however, there can be no compromise regarding vector and pathogen containment.

Specific containment requirements depend upon the types of vectors and/or infectious agents to be studied. In terms of the latter (including arboviruses and protozoa), defined biosafety practices and facilities have been promulgated. For example, work with some arboviruses, such as certain indigenous strains of arboviruses that do not cause disease in vertebrate hosts, may require biosafety level (BL)-1 facilities and practices (USDHHS 1993). Work with more dangerous pathogens, for example, yellow fever virus, can require BL-3 facilities and practices. BL designation can vary for a particular pathogen depending upon the nature of the work. Propagating the pathogen in an arthropod vector can require a higher BL of containment than if cell culture is used. Certain exotic and especially dangerous viruses are categorized as BL-4 pathogens, which can only be studied in high-level containment facilities, such as the Centers for Disease Control and Prevention (CDC) Special Pathogens Branch laboratory, Atlanta, Georgia. For some pathogens, personnel can be protected from infection by vaccination; indeed it is sometimes compulsory. It is recommended that before personnel commence work with pathogens, a serum sample be drawn and deposited in an appropriate cryobank. Regular (e.g., annual) screening of sera for antibodies reactive with the epitopes of the pathogens under study is suggested. In the event of an unexplained human illness, these sera can be referred to in order to ensure that it is not laboratory-related. It is vitally important that proposed work with vector-borne pathogens adhere to the appropriate regulations and that all investigators receive authorization to conduct experiments through their respective Institutional Biosafety Committees. Appropriate government authorities, such as the U.S. Department of Agriculture (USDA), must be consulted and permission received before importation of pathogens or the transfer of these between laboratories. Similar procedures must be followed for movement of arthropod vector species to another location.

Biosafety requirements for work with vectors are less well defined than for pathogen work and depend upon the pathogen and the vector species, whether or not vectors will be infected or transformed, etc. It is important to realize, however, that secure containment of vectors is imperative regardless of their experimental status. Frequently the vector species is not indigenous to the area in which the laboratory is located; escape and establishment of the vector in the area could result in new disease transmission cycles or in new pest problems. Researchers must always consider this potential and realize that reservoir hosts can exist in close proximity to the facility. Pathogens of both humans and other vertebrates such as domestic livestock must be treated with equal regard. The presence of an insectary invariably sensitizes coworkers to

issues involving vectors, and escaped arthropods can become a public relations disaster. Multiple escapes of uninfected vectors will not be viewed sympathetically by colleagues and coworkers. Escape of an infected vector will lead to closure of the facility by Institutional Biosafety officers even if no one is bitten. The potential risks of pathogen egress from the facility outweigh all other concerns.

Insectary design should prevent escape of an arthropod. At the very least, an insectary consists of limited-access, sealed room(s), preferably without windows, and with multiple-door access to the vector colonies and manipulation areas. Under normal circumstances, this minimal insectary design will prevent vector escape, especially if the insectary staff are well trained and vigilant. All who work in the insectary must be instilled with the idea that all vectors are infected and dangerous, that any vector that escapes is to be considered infected and must be located and destroyed immediately, and that safety and security always take precedence over expediency. For certain vectors (e.g., *Culicoides* spp.,) it might be impossible to locate an escapee. In such cases, procedures must be adopted to take this into account (Hunt and Tabachnick 1995). Experiments to determine the probability of an individual vector passing from one area of the insectary to another are recommended (Hunt and Tabachnick 1995). These data will indicate if additional precautions need to be implemented in order to ensure that no vector can escape from the facility.

INSECTARY DESIGN AND OPERATION: RECOMMENDATIONS

Ingress and Egress

As stated earlier, insectary design should include a restricted entrance; access should be strictly limited to scientists and support personnel who are trained in vector containment and manipulation procedures. Appropriate biohazard information notices should be prominently placed upon the entrance door. The entrance door should lock automatically. For large insectaries with many users, coded push-button locks are an efficient mechanism for restricting access. The entrance into the insectary should preferably be via a series of doors that constitute sequential barriers to vector escape. The doors should provide sufficient space in the adjacent vestibules for personnel to close the door behind them before opening the next one. All doors within the insectary should open inward and close automatically. By opening inward, an escaped arthropod will be pushed back into the insectary. Two contiguous doors must never be opened simultaneously. Interconnected electromagnetic locking systems can be installed to ensure that one of a pair of contiguous doors is always locked. Cloth sheets or zippered screens can be fixed across doorways as an additional barrier to prevent arthropod escape by dislodging them from clothing while exiting. Dehumidifiers and fans blowing air into the insectary can be positioned within vestibules to create an environment that will prevent a vector from exiting the insectary.

Colony Rooms

Within the insectary, all surfaces, including walls, ceilings, shelves, and counter tops, should be painted white so that an escapee can be easily located and killed. Gloss finishes that are easily wiped clean are preferable because the insectary atmosphere is frequently humid. Finishes should ideally be resistant to disinfectants and other chemicals, for example formaldehyde, to facilitate periodic fumigation. The relatively high humidity generally precludes the use of untreated absorbant material such as wood; indeed, the use of such organic materials is actually prohibited for BL-3 facility construction. Air ducts, lighting fixtures, and all other openings must be sealed or screened with mesh of a size that precludes egress by arthropods. Rooms should be windowless. Low ceilings with recessed lights that are flush with the ceiling are preferred. Floors should be light colored, smooth, and easily disinfected. No floor coverings should be used that could create pools of water suitable for breeding of vectors. Minimal equipment and supplies should be kept in the insectary. This reduces potential hiding places for a loose arthropod. Furniture and racks, etc., should be movable to allow easy cleaning.

Where it is essential to maintain different arthropod species or strains, it is preferable to keep each in separate rooms or designated areas. Infected arthropods should be double-caged (in cages within a cage)

and be housed in rooms separate from uninfected colony mosquitoes. When insectary space is limited, rooms can be modified to contain multiple rooms. Solid-walled or screened sections with self-closing doors within rooms are acceptable. If the pathogen under study can infect immature stages of arthropods (e.g., transtadially and transovarially), then progeny of potentially infected adults should be in rooms/sections separated from uninfected colonies as described.

Because excellent references are available that provide details on rearing different species (Gerberg 1970; Gerberg et al. 1994; e.g., Munstermann et al., in Singh and Moore 1985), routine procedures are not detailed in this chapter. Briefly, larvae should be reared in closed containers and inspected daily. Pupae should be removed within 24 hours and transferred to suitable emergence containers. All equipment, material, and solutions (including water) used to rear mosquitoes must be sterilized before disposal. An autoclave is a useful, if not essential, item of insectary equipment. Arthropod eggs can be resistant to chemicals and must not be allowed to enter drains in which larvae can eventually hatch. Waste water "traps" can be plumbed into the drainage system or below each sink. When a designated volume of water accumulates in these, disinfectant can be added or a heating element can be used to boil the water. Following treatment, a valve can be opened to release the sterilized water into the drain.

When rearing very large numbers of uninfected mosquitoes, it is almost inevitable that some will get loose. Any mosquito escapee must be destroyed immediately. It should be emphasized to insectary personnel that if they see a loose mosquito, they must remain in the room until it is destroyed. Mosquitoes should be destroyed with a swatter or mechanically aspirated (not operated by mouth suction) and then destroyed. They should not be destroyed with the naked hand because pathogens from a squashed vector can enter open wounds or abrasions. Insect traps can be used to kill a loose insect, but the type of trap and attractant must be suitable for the type of arthropod and insectary conditions. Traps releasing CO_2, although suitable for field use, may not operate efficiently under laboratory conditions with constant directional ventilation. Electrocutor-type traps with ultraviolet (UV) light as an attractant may not be suitable for some species because of specific sensitivities to light of certain wavelengths. Surveillance oviposition traps may be strategically placed in the insectary. These should be inspected weekly to ensure that loose mosquitoes are not breeding. No unmonitored open water sources (for example, waste water in sinks, beakers, etc.) should exist in the insectary because these provide potential breeding sites for mosquitoes. Similarly, no food sources should be available.

Different containment procedures must be followed when working with nonmosquito vectors, including other Dipterans such as species of *Culicoides* (Fahrner and Barthelmess 1988; Jones 1960; Hunt 1994; Hunt and Tabachnick 1995). For example, when rearing ticks (Jellison and Philip 1933; Jones et al. 1988; Waladde et al. 1991), cages can be placed on a platform standing in an oil bath. Racks of cages can be placed on a platform with an integral moat filled with oil. Dislodged ticks will sink in the oil and die. Details for rearing fleas under laboratory conditions are also available (Hudson and Prince 1958; Wade and Georgi 1988).

Vector Manipulation

Manipulation is defined here as any experimental procedure of a vector or modification of normal vector state prior to experimentation. Experimental procedures with vectors, for example, infection with viruses or genetic manipulation, should not be conducted in main rearing rooms where an escapee might infiltrate the colonies. Manipulation rooms can be cooler than rearing rooms, and this lower temperature confers the advantage that an escapee can be relatively slow and therefore easily located and destroyed. However, a suitable relative humidity must be maintained throughout the manipulation period to ensure vector survival. This is particularly important for small vectors and if procedures have involved prior water deprivation. Control of humidity within a specific microenvironment is sometimes necessary. For example, newly laid eggs destined for microinjection must be slightly desiccated at a stage particularly sensitive to water loss. When a suitable degree of drying has been achieved, fatal water loss is prevented by covering the eggs with water-saturated oil (McGrane et al. 1988).

Any manipulation procedure should be designed to cause minimal handling stress to the vector and yet satisfy the appropriate BL requirements. When working with BL-3 pathogens, all procedures, including mosquito inoculations and oral infections, must be performed in a suitable biosafety cabinet, and infected mosquitoes must from then on be housed under BL-3 containment conditions. As described earlier, vectors should be collected using mechanical aspirators (Fig. 35.1) and manipulated using forceps, or other instruments that can be sterilized if necessary. Throughout any manipulation procedure, a constant tally of the numbers being used must be maintained. Only small numbers (10–15) of arthropods should be out of their container at a given time. Accurate records must be kept to determine that all manipulated vectors are accounted for throughout the experimental period. Vector manipulation frequently requires that the arthropods be anesthetized, which can be achieved most simply by chilling vectors in a refrigerator. Differences in susceptibility to cold must be determined to avoid killing them. For example, *Ae. aegypti* is relatively susceptible to cold whereas *Ae. triseriatus* and most temperate zone species of *Culex* are not. Carbon dioxide gas is a useful alternative method of immobilization but must also be used with caution. Once anesthetized, vectors can be maintained in a torpid state by performing manipulations on a chill table (Fig. 35.1). A glass plate placed on ice can be used, but melting ice and condensation can be a problem. Larvae can be anesthetized by immersion in ice-cold water but only for short periods because low temperatures will stop respiration and larvae can drown. When vectors must perform a particular activity (e.g., in forced salivation and forced mating), they can be chilled briefly and then immobilized by removing the legs and wings (Fig. 35.2) and sometimes even the head. Additional preparation to maximize success of the procedure may be necessary, e.g., mosquitoes may have to be starved for 24–48 hours to promote feeding. If adult mosquitoes of a particular age are required, pupae can be held in mosquito breeder containers (Fig. 35.2) that automatically separate emerged adults from immature stages and permit easy collection of adults without the need for chilling and aspiration. Behavioral manipulation, for example,

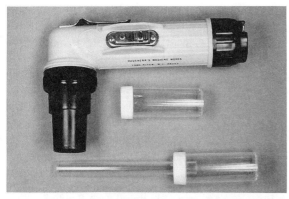 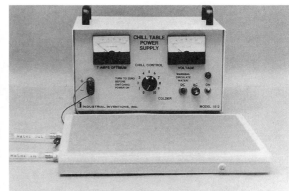

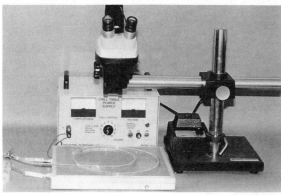 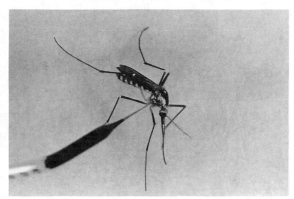

35.1   *Top left:* Mechanical aspirator (Hausherr's Machine Works). *Top right:* Chill table (Industrial Inventions Inc). *Bottom left:* Apparatus for intrathoracic inoculation. *Bottom right:* Intrathoracically inoculated mosquito.

induction of egg laying at a particular time, can be achieved through environmental control. Vectors must be shielded from ambient cues, e.g., natural temperature fluctuations and daylight entering through windows. By blood-feeding at a particular time, depriving females of a suitable oviposition medium, and carefully controlling light regimens, mosquitoes can be induced to lay eggs within well-defined periods. To eliminate problems associated with using vertebrates as a source of blood meals, artificial feeders (Rutledge et al. 1964) can be used to present precise numbers of pathogens in a blood meal to the arthropod. Various designs, membranes, and protocols are available for different vector-pathogen types (Cosgrove et al. 1994; Hastriter et al. 1980, 1981; Hunt and McKinnon 1990; Kogan 1990; Rutledge et al. 1964; Waladde et al. 1991) (Fig. 35.3).

For some species of mosquitoes it is possible to maintain colonies by using artificial feeders and blood substitutes (Kogan 1990; Dr R.J. Wood, personal communication). Nonhematophagous species, for example *Toxorhynchites amboinensis*, or male mosquitoes, can be used to propagate some pathogens (Rosen 1981). The midgut infection barrier (Chap. 4) can be circumvented by intrathoracic inoculation of these individuals that then become infected but pose no threat of transmitting the pathogen by bite because neither ingests blood.

Once manipulation is completed, vectors can be transferred to suitable containers for recovery. Because mosquitoes can be uncoordinated during this recovery period, it is generally wise to house them in containers that do not contain open water sources in which they

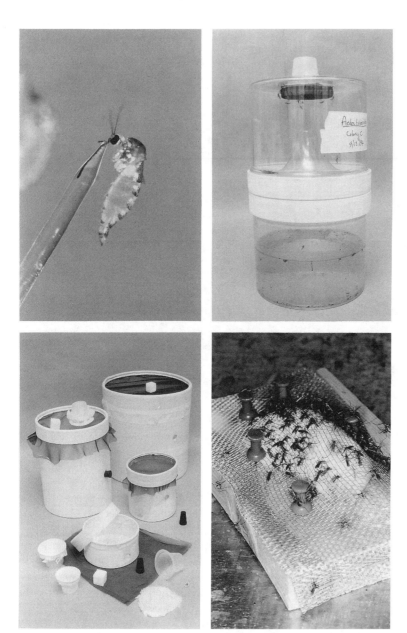

35.2 *Top right:* Immobilized mosquito salivating into capillary. *Top left:* Mosquito breeder (BioQuip Products). Mosquitoes emerge from pupae held in the lower chamber and fly upward for easy isolation in the upper chamber. *Bottom left:* Cardboard cartons and accessories used to house small groups of mosquitoes. *Bottom right:* Mosquitoes feeding on a restrained mouse, as used for general colony maintenance.

can drown. Where facilities are limited, experimental vectors can be contained in cages within environmental cabinets with controlled temperature, lighting, and humidity. These can even be used to maintain small colonies; however, these cabinets should be kept in secure screened rooms or other suitably restricted access areas.

Vertebrate Containment

Rooms housing vertebrates, even if uninfected, must be physically separated from rooms containing mosquitoes by at least a solid wall and multiple-screened or solid doors. This prevents any loose anautogenous arthropods from obtaining blood meals required for egg production. Vertebrates that have been used to feed infected arthropods should be euthanized in the area or removed to secure designated rooms. Transfers of vertebrates or arthropods between areas should be in secure and unbreakable containers. Housing, care, and experimental procedures for vertebrates must be preapproved and satisfy the requirements of appropriate institutional and government bodies.

General Housekeeping

A strict insectary maintenance and cleaning regime should be implemented. The insectary should be kept clean and all rooms regularly inspected to ensure that containment measures do not deteriorate. Screens and cages should be checked routinely for holes. All equipment such as humidifiers and lights should be examined to ensure that they are functioning correctly.

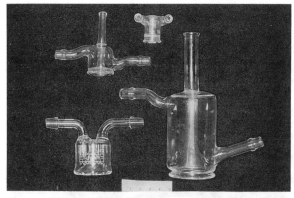
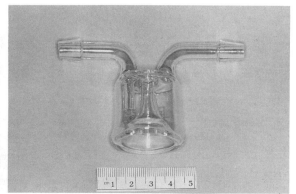
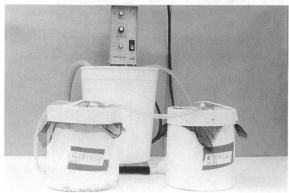
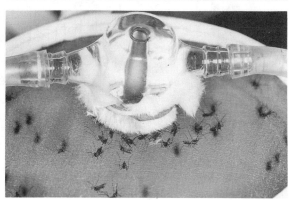

35.3 *Top left:* Various designs of glass feeders used to present blood meals to mosquitoes. *Top right:* Detail of glass feeder. Water is pumped into the feeder's water jacket via the left inlet tube and exits via the right outlet tube. *Bottom left:* Apparatus used for orally infecting mosquitoes. Water at 37°C is circulated through the feeder, which is held on top of cartons of mosquitoes. *Bottom right:* Detail of glass feeder with mosquitoes probing through a mouse-skin membrane to reach the blood meal.

THE INSECTARY OF THE ARTHROPOD-BORNE AND INFECTIOUS DISEASES LABORATORY (AIDL)

AIDL was established at Colorado State University in 1987. A windowless area of the basement was modified to provide a 2,000 sq ft containment insectary facility in compliance with safety requirements promulgated by the American Mosquito Control Association and SALS (1980) (Fig. 35.4). This facility, and equipment and practices used here, are maintained at the level required for BL-2 containment, with specified areas approved for BL-3 containment. The AIDL

insectary is used here as a model to demonstrate how mosquito vectors can be safely maintained.

Many AIDL features have been implemented at relatively low cost. Most of the practices are simply common sense. These are briefly described so that those who work with infected or genetically manipulated vectors can incorporate these features into their insectary design. In most circumstances it should be feasible to modify existing insectaries to satisfy the necessary requirements.

To access AIDL areas in which mosquitoes are housed, 4 separate doors with automatic closers must be entered. Doors fit tightly against foam on the doorjambs

A.   Autoclave
A.a.c.   *Aedes aegypti*, colony
A.a.e.   *Aedes aegypti*, experimental
A.t.c.   *Aedes triseriatus*, colony
A.t.e.   *Aedes triseriatus*, experimental
BL-3.a.   BL-3 containment area
BL-3.b.   BL-3 tissue culture/vector manipulation.
C.p.c.   *Culex pipiens*, colony
C.p.e.   *Culex pipiens*, experimental
Ent.   Entrance
Em.e.   Emergency exit
M.c.   Main corridor
V.c.   Vertebrate containment (BL-3)
V1.   Vestibule 1 (with shower)
V2.   Vestibule 2
V3.   Vestibule 3
W.C.   Toilet

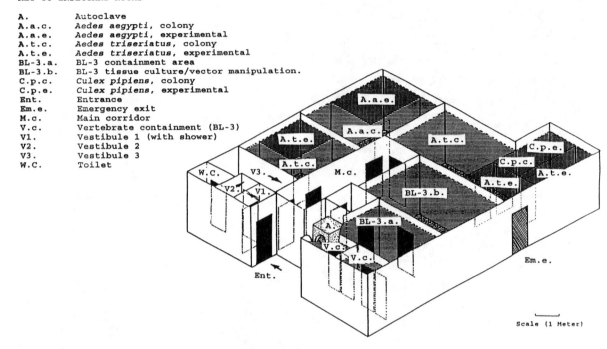

35.4 Plan of the insectary at the Arthropod-borne and Infectious Diseases Laboratory (AIDL), Colorado State University.

and have brushes fitted at the base. The first door has a combination lock, the code of which is restricted to authorized persons. Large signs are posted to indicate that entrance is restricted to suitably vaccinated persons (Fig. 35.5). Windows in the first 2 doors allow researchers to ensure that neither of these doors are ever opened simultaneously. All other internal doors have overlapping white cloth sheets stapled to the door frames to dislodge mosquitoes and inhibit fly-through (Fig. 35.5). Internal doors can be opened only once the preceding door is closed.

Separate rooms are designated for colonies of each mosquito species. This simplifies the maintenance of the different environmental conditions necessary to rear the different species. The AIDL insectary also has rooms designated for tissue-culture with a biosafety cabinet suitable for working with BL-3 category pathogens, including recombinant viruses (Fig. 35.4), for manipulating mosquitoes (e.g., virus inoculation), and for housing infected vertebrates. The latter are

housed in high efficiency particulate air (HEPA) filtered cubicles in a room where an escaped mosquito cannot enter and so cannot feed on the infected animals. Refrigerators and closed cupboards used to store supplies are all placed in a central corridor, not in rearing rooms.

Air in the insectary is maintained at pressure negative to the connecting part of the building and each room within the insectary is at negative pressure to the adjoining corridor. When doors are opened, air therefore enters each insectary room to prevent mosquitoes from flying out into the corridor. All exhaust air is passed through ceiling vents fitted with filters. In rooms designated for BL-3 pathogen research, the air is HEPA filtered. The insectary has an independent air handling system with generator backup to run ventilation and emergency lighting in the event of power failure. Safety lights are distributed throughout the insectary to guide personnel to exits in the event of an emergency evacuation.

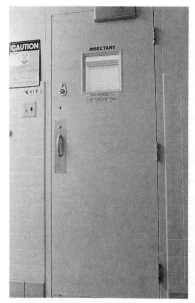

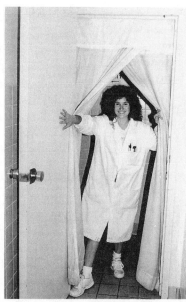

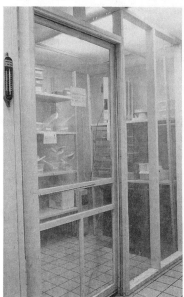

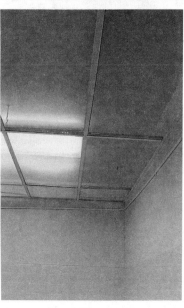

All AIDL insectary walls, ceilings, counter tops, and shelves are white. To facilitate cleaning and fumigation of rooms, surfaces have been painted with a glossy epoxy paint that can withstand exposure to formaldehyde; equipment and floors are also light-colored. A suspended ceiling constructed of panels of wire mesh is positioned below the room ceiling. This constitutes the first barrier to prevent a mosquito from entering the ventilation system. The panels are designed so that sections can be easily removed to replace lights and air filters (Fig. 35.5).

Insectary illumination is provided by fluorescent tubes, located to provide even lighting. These are operated by timers to control light to dark regimes suitable to maintain continual mosquito breeding. A sunset-sunrise simulation control system connected to incandescent bulbs allows gradual changes in the illumination to closely mimic dawn to dusk conditions as required by some species to induce oviposition. Temperature and humidity are controlled using simple household radiators and humidifiers. These are permanently plumbed into the water system. A backup humidifier and radiator is available in each room. Screening is fitted to humidifiers to prevent mosquito entrance. Environmental conditions are monitored using thermohygrographs. Using this relatively "low technology" system, we have never lost valuable mosquito stocks through failure of suitable environmental conditions.

35.5 The AIDL Insectary. *Top left:* Main entrance door with appropriate signs. *Top right:* Overlapping cloth sheets stapled across internal door to dislodge mosquito escapees from clothing. *Bottom left:* Partitioned area containing cages of manipulated mosquitoes. *Bottom right:* Suspended ceiling panels.

Large cages housing colony mosquitoes are kept in the main rearing room area, but within each room screened, partitioned areas contain experimental vectors (Fig. 35.5). This is not an ideal situation, but is necessary to conserve space. It would be better to have separate rooms to contain infected mosquitoes of each species, but this would require duplication of the appropriate temperature, humidity, and photoperiod regimens for each species. The experimental vectors are kept in cardboard ice cream cartons with black mesh fabric fixed to the top to facilitate visual inspection (Fig. 35.2). Experimental details are provided on color-coded tape. A stoppered hole in the side, sealed with tape, allows easy sampling using a vacuum pump or battery-operated aspirator (Fig. 35.1). Sugar cubes and inverted cups of water with muslin covers are placed on top of the mesh (Fig. 35.2). These are autoclaved before disposal because mosquitoes may salivate and release pathogens when feeding. Restrained mice are used for blood-feeding (Fig. 35.2). Before removal, restrainers are carefully inspected for hidden mosquitoes. Mice used to feed infected mosquitoes are sacrificed immediately upon removal.

A pass-through autoclave is used to sterilize all potentially infectious material prior to removal from the insectary (Fig. 35.4). This includes the water in which larvae have been reared, containers used to house mosquitoes, all mosquitoes, all material potentially contaminated with virus/recombinant DNA, all garbage, mouse cages/bottles, and mouse bodies. Some plastic containers cannot withstand autoclaving. Water is decanted from these into large cooking pots and autoclaved. The plastic pans are placed in the autoclave (without pressurized steam injection) and left to heat to 60°C for 30 minutes to kill eggs, etc.

The AIDL insectary is an example of how an existing facility can be modified to provide secure containment for potentially dangerous vectors. Engineered and commercially available facilities (e.g., room-sized environmental chambers) might be more sophisticated and allow more precise control of environmental conditions, and so forth; however, the successful operation of the AIDL insectary for almost 10 years demonstrates that it is possible to satisfy all of the conditions required for secure containment of vectors and pathogens at relatively little cost.

SUMMARY

In conclusion, when working with arthropods capable of pathogen transmission, it is imperative that no arthropod escapes and no accidental infection occur. The arthropods must be reared in secure insectary facilities, and strict practices are essential. This chapter describes how necessary measures can be implemented and uses a working high-containment insectary to illustrate how these can be implemented in practical terms.

ACKNOWLEDGMENTS

The authors gratefully thank Mr. L.H. Thopson (Microbiologist/Biosafety Officer, Arthropod-borne Animal Diseases Laboratory, USDA-ARS, Laramie, WY 82071) for critically reviewing the manuscript and Dr. R.B. Craven (Biosafety Officer, Division of Vector-borne Infectious Diseases, Centers for Disease Control and Prevention, Fort Collins, CO 80521) for his comments on the chapter and for supplying a prepublication copy of a DVBID safety manual. Dr. W.J. Tabachnick and Dr. G.J. Hunt (Arthropod-borne Animal Diseases Laboratory, USDA-ARS, Laramie, WY 82071) and Dr. R.J. Wood (School of Biological Sciences, University of Manchester, UK) kindly supplied preprints of manuscripts. This research was supported in part by the John D. and Catherine T. MacArthur Foundation and by Grants AI25629, AI32543, and AI34014 from the National Institutes of Health.

SOME SPECIALIST INSECTARY SUPPLIERS

There are numerous suppliers of equipment that is suitable for use in insectaries and for rearing various species of arthropods. Below are some suppliers of specialist equipment. Mention of a trade name, proprietary product, or specific equipment does not constitute a guarantee or warranty by the authors and does not imply its approval to the exclusion of other products that can be suitable.

BioQuip Products. 17803 LaSalle Ave., Gardena, CA 90248-3602. Tel. (310) 324-0620; fax (310) 324-7931.

Hausherr's Machine Works. 1186 Old Freehold Road, Toms River, NJ 08753. Tel. (908) 349-1319; fax (908) 286-4919.

Industrial Inventions Inc., 694 Village Road West, Lawrenceville, NJ 08648. Tel. 609.275.1500

REFERENCES AND FURTHER READING

Clements, A.N. 1992. *The biology of mosquitoes, Volume 1: Development, nutrition and reproduction.* London: Chapman and Hall.

Cosgrove, J.B., R.J. Wood, D. Petric, D.T. Evans, and H.R. Abbott. 1994. A convenient mosquito membrane feeding system. *J. Am. Mosq. Control Assoc.* 10:434–436.

Fahrner, J., and C. Barthelmess. 1988. Rearing of *Culicoides nubeculosus* (Diptera: Ceratopogonidae) by natural and artificial feeding in the laboratory. *Vet. Parasitol.* 28:307–313.

Gerberg, E.J. 1970. *Manual for mosquito rearing and experimental techniques.* American Mosquito Control Association Inc. Bulletin 5. Selma, CA.: American Mosquito Control Association. 109 p.

Gerberg, E.J., D.R. Barnard, and R.A. Ward. 1994. *Manual for mosquito rearing and experimental techniques.* American Mosquito Control Association Inc. Bulletin 5 (revised). Lake Charles, LA: American Mosquito Control Association. 98p.

Hastriter, M.W., and D.C. Cavanaugh. 1981. An apparatus for colonizing fleas (Siphonaptera) and collecting pupal cocoons. *J. Med. Entomol.* 18:251–52.

Hastriter, W.M., D.M. Robinson, and D.C. Cavanaugh. 1980. An improved apparatus for safely feeding fleas (Siphonaptera) in plague studies. *J. Med. Entomol.* 17:387–88.

Hudson, B.W., and F.M. Prince. 1958. A method for large-scale rearing of the cat flea *Ctenocephalides felis felis* (Bouche'). *Bull. WHO* 19:1126–1129.

Hunt, G.J. 1994. A procedural manual for the large-scale rearing of the biting midge *Culicoides variipennis* (Diptera: Ceratopogonidae). Springfield, VA: National Technical Information Service. USDA Research Service, ARS-121. 68 p.

Hunt, G.J., and C.N. McKinnon. 1990. Evaluation of membranes for feeding *Culicoides variipennis* (Diptera: Ceratopogonidae) with an improved artificial blood-feeding apparatus. *J. Med. Entomol.* 27:934–937.

Hunt, G.J., and W.J. Tabachnick. 1995. Handling small arbovirus vectors during biosafety level 3 agricultural containment: *Culicoides variipennis sonorensis* (Diptera: Ceratopogonidae) and exotic bluetongue viruses. *J. Med. Entomol.* (in press).

Jellison, W.L., and C.B. Philip. 1933. Technique for routine and experimental feeding of certain ixodid ticks on guinea pigs and rabbits. *Public Health Report* 48(33):1081–1082.

Jones, L.D., C.R. Davies, G.M. Steele, and P.A. Nuttall. 1988. The rearing and maintenance of ixodid and argasid ticks in the laboratory. *Anim. Technol.* 39:99–106

Jones, R.H. 1960. Mass-production methods in rearing *Culicoides variipennis sonorensis. J. Econ. Entomol.* 53:731–35.

Kogan, P.H. 1990 Substitute blood meal for investigating and maintaining *Aedes aegypti* (Diptera: Culicidae). *J. Med. Entomol.* 27:709–712.

McGrane, V., J.O. Carlson, B.R. Miller, and B.J. Beaty. 1988. Microinjection of DNA into *Aedes triseriatus* ova and detection of integration. *Am. J. Trop. Med. Hyg.* 39:502–510.

Rosen, L. 1981. The use of *Toxorhynchites* mosquitoes to detect and propagate dengue and other arboviruses. *Am. J. Trop. Med. Hyg.* 30:177–183.

Rutledge, L.C., R.A. Ward, and D.J. Gould. 1964. Studies on the feeding reponse of mosquitoes to nutritive solutions in a new membrane feeder. *Mosq. News* 24:407–419.

SALS 1980. Laboratory safety for arboviruses and certain other viruses of vertebrates. *Am. J. Trop. Med. Hyg.* 29:1359–1381.

Singh, P. and R.F. Moore, editors. 1985. *Handbook of insect rearing.* 2 vol. New York: Elsevier.

USDHHS. 1993. *Biosafety in microbiological and biomedical laboratories.* 3rd ed. Washington, D.C.: U.S. Government Printing Office.

Wade, S.E., and J.R. Georgi. 1988. Survival and reproduction of artificially fed cat fleas, *Ctenocephalides felis* Bouche' (Siphonaptera: Pulicidae). *J. Med. Entomol.* 25:186–190.

Waladde, S.M., S.A. Ochieng', and P.M. Gichuhi. 1991. Artificial-membrane feeding of the ixodid tick *Rhipicephalus appendiculatus* to repletion. *Exper. and Appl. Acarol.* 11:297–306.

INDEX

Attractant traps, 479
Auchmeromyia spp., 303
Augmentation, as biological control, 533
Austrosimulium sp*p.*, *99*, 100
Austrosimulium pestilens, 104
Autogeny
    in biting midges, 113
    in culicine mosquitoes, 88
    hormones and, 293
    in sand flies, 121
Autonomously replicating sequence (ARS), 223
Avian malarias, 82, 176
Avoidance of high-risk areas, as disease control method, 22

Babesia spp., 170
Babesia bigemina, 3, 17, 170, 171
Babesia bovis, 171
Babesia divergens, 171
Babesia major, 171
Babesia microti, 171, 329
Babesiosis, 170–71
Bacillary angiomatosis, 156
Bacillus sphaericus, 505, 531, 551–52, 558, 559
Bacillus subtilis, 175
Bacillus thuringiensis complex, 389, 505, 509, 530–31, 550–51, 558, 559
Bacteria. *See also Bacillus thuringiensis*
    binding proteins for cell wall components of, 388
    as chemical control agents, 505
    as microbial control agents, 550–52
    as symbionts, 357
Bacteria-inducible proteins, 377–78
Baits, insecticides as, 506
Bait traps, 479, *484*
Balancer chromosomes, 270–71
Barriers, to infection with Lacrosse virus, 68–70. *See also* Midgut barrier; Peritrophic matrix
Bartonella bacilliformis, 124
Bartonellosis, 117, 124
Basophils, 579
Bed bugs. *See also Cimex lectularius*
    control of, 134, 507
    disease agents transmitted by, 134
    as hemimetabolic vectors, 133
    hepatitis B virus and, 55
    insecticide resistance in, *525*
    life cycle of, 133
    morphology of, 133

Behavior, of vectors. *See also* Feeding behavior
    activity patterns, 36–37
    evolution of hematophagy, 35–36
    fixed-action programs, 34–35
    host location, 37–40
    host preference and receptor specificity, 37
    insecticide resistance and, 518
    mechanisms inhibiting host-seeking, 40–42
    metamorphosis and, 44
    overwintering, 43
    preoviposition, 44–45
    receptor physiology and, 36
    resting, 42–43
    sugar-feeding, 43
    swarming, 43
Bendiocarb, 509
Benzene hexachloride (BHC), 503
Benzoylphenylureas, 505
Bertram, D. S., 411
Beta-oxidation, 359
Bicoid gene, 267–68
Binding proteins, for bacterial cell wall components, 388
Biochemical markers, in genetic mapping, 191
Biochemical systematics, 464–66
Biochemical taxonomy, 446
Biological control. *See also* Microbial control
    agents of, 534–43
    definition of, 22, 530
    fundamental principles of, 531–34
    future directions in, 546–47
    history of, 530–31
    implementation of, 543–46
Biological transmission, 54–55, 57–61
Bionomics. *See also* Habitats
    of biting midges, 113
    of black fly, 104–106
    of kissing bugs, 130–31
    of lice, 135
    of sand flies, 119–22
    of tsete fly, 140
Biosafety
    of biological control agents, 544–45
    insectary practices and facilities, 595–96
BIOSYS–1 (computer program), 431
Bironella spp., 73
Biting midges. *See also Culicoides* spp.
    bionomics of, 113
    characteristics of, 110–11

Cell-to-cell communication, 390
Cellia subgenus, 74, 79
Cellular immunity, in insects, 378–85
Cellulose acetate gel electrophoresis (CAGE), 443
Centers for Disease Control and Prevention (CDC), Special
        Pathogens Branch laboratory, 596
Central European encephalitis (CEE), 170
Central nervous system (CNS)
        control of mosquito behaviors and, *45*
        sensory receptors and, 36
Ceratitis capitata, 187
Ceratophyllus celsus, 148
Ceratopogonidae, *304*
Ceratopogonid midges, 482
Chagas, Carlos, 132
Chagas' disease, 129, *130,* 131–33, 314, 377, 507. *See also*
        Trypanosoma cruzi
Chandlerella spp., *115*
Chaniotis trap, 481–82
Chaoborus americanus, 180
Charybdotoxins, 376
Chelicerata, 10, 12–20. *See also* Mites; Ticks
Chemical control, of vectors. *See also* Insecticides; Resistance
        classification of pesticides, 503–505
        factors for effective application of, 510–11
        history of, 502–503
        modes of action in, 505–507
        vector biology and, 507–10
Cheng, M. L., 418
Chiggers, 16–17, *18,* 476
Chikungunya fever, *93*
China, biological control program in, 559
Chitin, 326, 360, 505
Chloramphenicol acetyl transferase (*CAT*), 244
Chlorinated hydrocarbon insecticides, 502, 503
Cholera, 377
Chromosomal translocations, as genetic control method,
        568–70
Chromosomes
        balancer chromosomes, 270–71
        chromosome specific libraries, 200–201
        evolution and, 183–84
        organization of in mosquitoes and nematocerous flies,
        181–82
Chronic sleeping sickness, *142*
Chronological age, 412–13
Chymotrypsins, 184, 231
Cimex hemipterus, 133
Cimex lectularius, 133, 309. *See also* Bed bugs
Cimicidae, 129, *304*

Circadian cycle, of bloodsucking insects, 26
Circulatory system, of insects, 351–54
Cis-Acting DNA elements, 243–45
Citric acid cycle, *358*
Cloning, of mosquito genes, 235. *See also* Molecular genetics
Clostridium bifermentans serovar. *malayi,* 552
Cnephia pecuarum, 98
Coagulocytes, 373
Cochliomyia hominovorax, 22, 137, 565
Cockburn, A., 418
Cockroaches, insecticide resistance in, *525*
Coelomomyces spp., 538–39, 553
Coelomomyces stegomyiae, 294
Coelmomycidium spp., 540
Coen procedure, for species identification, *450*
Coevolution, of vectors and parasites, 347
Coleoptera, 541
Coleoptericin, 375
Collection and collecting methods. *See also* Traps and trapping
        for black flies, 482
        for brachycerous flies, 483–84
        for fleas, 484–87
        for lice, 488
        for midges, 482
        for mites, 476–77
        for mosquitoes, 477–81
        for sand flies, *120,* 481–82
        for ticks, 472–76
        for triatomine bugs, 487–88
Colony rooms, in insectary, 597–98
Colorado potato beetle, 360, 364, 367
Colorado State University, Arthropod-Borne and Infectious
        Diseases Laboratory (AIDL), 601–604
Colorado tick fever (CTF), 66, 170
Coluzzi, M., 418
Commensalism, definition of, 20
Community-based control programs, for *Aedes* spp., 499
Competitive displacement, as genetic control method, 568
Conditional lethal mutations, 571
Congo virus, *115,* 116
Contact insecticides, 505
Contig mapping, 200–201
Control, of vector populations
        of anopheline mosquitoes, 77–78
        of bed bugs, 134
        biological methods of for mosquitoes, 530–47
        of biting midges, 114
        of black flies, 107
        chemical methods of, 502–11
        of culicine mosquitoes, 89–90

Ticks (*Continued*)
  insecticide resistance in, *525*
  life cycle of, 17, *18,* 160–61
  morphology of, 160
  public health and, 575, 576
  salivary glands of, *338, 339, 340*
  species complexes of, 441
  vaccines against, 27–28, 585–89
  water balance of, 29–30
Tilapia spp., 543
T lymphocyte, 578–80
Tolypocladium spp., 540
T1 family, of retrotransposons, 187
Toxicants, definition of, 21
Toxins, of *Bacillus* spp., 550–52, 555
Toxorhynchites spp., 73, 75, 87, 88, *96,* 541–42, 544
Toxorhynchites splendens, 178, *180*
Tracheal system
  and alimentary canal, 300
  of generalized insect, *8,* 10
Trans-Acting DNA elements, 245
Transcription, gene expression and analysis of, 241–42
Transfection, of cultured cells, 243–45
Transformation systems, in genetic mapping, 203–204. *See also* Molecular genetics
Transgenic strains, in molecular genetics, 216–17, 571
Transovarial transmission, 163
Transport, of biological control agents, 545–46
Transposable DNA elements, 186–87, 222, 571
Transposons, 186, 216, 222
Transseasonality, of arboviruses, 64, 66
Transtadial transmission, 70, 163
Traps and trapping. *See also* Collection and collecting methods; specific types of traps
  placement of, 481
  of tsete flies, 141
Trench fever, 136
Triatoma spp., 389, 507. *See also* Kissing bugs; Triatomine bugs
Triatoma infestans, 38, 130, 309, 363, 507. *See also* Kissing bugs
Triatoma megista, 132
Triatoma sanguisuga, 132
Triatominae, 129, *304, 338, 339, 340*
Triatomine bugs
  collection of, 487–88
  insecticide resistance in, *525*
Trichodectes canis, 134
Trichoptera, 541
Tris-borate-EDTA (TBE) buffer, *445*
Tris-citrate (TC) buffer, *445*

Trombiculidae. *See* Chiggers
Trophocytes, 349
Trypanosoma spp., 129, 141–44
Trypanosoma brucei complex, 142–44, 329. *See also* Sleeping sickness
Trypanosoma congolense, 142
Trypanosoma cruzi, 29, 129, 131–33, 343, 388, 389, 463. *See also* Chagas' disease
Trypanosoma equiperdum, 142
Trypanosoma evansi, 29, *142*
Trypanosoma minasense, 132
Trypanosoma rangeli, 132
Trypanosoma simiae, 142
Trypanosoma uniforme, 142
Trypanosoma vivax, 142
Trypanosomiasis, 141–44
Trypsins and trypsin-like proteins, 30, 184, 231, 236–37, 239, 330
Tsete fly. *See also Glossina* spp.
  alimentary structure of, *306, 308*
  bionomics of, 140
  collecting methods for, 483–84
  control of, 141, 508
  disease agents vectored by, 141–44
  energy metabolism in, 360, 366, 367
  host-parasite interactions in, 140–41
  life cycle of, *139,* 140
  life table of, *406*
  molecular taxonomy of, 441
  morphology of, 139–40
  peritrophic matrix of, 319
  salivary glands of, *338, 340*
Tsutsugamushi fever, 16
Tularemia, 156, 167–68
Tumor necrosis factor (TNF), 336, 342, 583
20-hydroxyecdysone, 282, 283
Ty elements, 222
Typhoid, 377
Typhus, 134–35, 136, 155

Ultralow volume (ULV) concentrate, in insecticides, 507, 510
Ultrastructure
  of digestive tracts of ticks, 579
  of fat body, 349–50
  mosquito physiology and, 277–81
  of peritrophic matrix and PM-secreting cells, 322–24
Union of Concerned Scientists, 500
United Nations Environment Programme (UNEP), 493
U. S. Agency for International Development (USAID), 570